Expeditionary Surgery at Sea

Matthew D. Tadlock • Amy A. Hernandez
Editors

Expeditionary Surgery at Sea

A Practical Approach

Springer

Editors
Matthew D. Tadlock
Department of Surgery
Naval Medical Center San Diego
San Diego, CA, USA

Amy A. Hernandez
Department of Surgery
Naval Medical Center San Diego
San Diego, CA, USA

Declaration of Interest: The views expressed in this book are those of the authors and do not necessarily reflect the official policy or position of the Department of the Navy, Department of Defense, nor the US Government.

Funding: This research did not receive any specific grant from funding agencies in the public, commercial, or not-for-profit sectors.

Conflict of Interest Statement: The authors declare no conflict of interest

ISBN 978-3-031-21892-7 ISBN 978-3-031-21893-4 (eBook)
https://doi.org/10.1007/978-3-031-21893-4

This Springer imprint is published by the registered company Springer Nature Switzerland AG
The registered company address is: Gewerbestrasse 11, 6330 Cham, Switzerland

First, we dedicate this book to the military service members who stand at the ready to protect their nation and the ideals it represents and especially to those who have made the ultimate sacrifice defending their families, friends, and homeland. Second, we dedicate this book to our spouses. Ricky and Jackie, thank you for your patience and support when we have been deployed and missed countless days and nights at home. Caring for our nation's Sailors, Marines, Soldiers, Airmen, and the men and women of our partner nations is a privilege; therefore we lastly dedicate this book to all the physicians, nurses, corpsman, medics, and members of the military medical team who have and will care for those who go into harm's way.

Disclaimer

This work is not an official publication or statement of policy from the U.S. Army, U.S. Navy, U.S. Air Force, the Department of Defense, or any other governmental or military agency. The opinions expressed herein are those of the editors and authors, and do not represent the views of the Department of Defense, any military or civilian medical facility or group, or any other governmental or military agency.

No editor or author of this book received or will receive any royalties, reimbursement, or payments in any form. All proceeds from the sale of this work that would normally go to the editors will be donated to the Navy-Marine Corps Relief Society and to provide this book to deploying maritime surgical teams.

Foreword

The role of a General Surgeon in our Naval Service is unique, challenging, and extremely rewarding. Our operational assignments, which span the globe and include both land and sea, make us unique when compared to both our military and civilian counterparts. Our sea-based deployments, whether aircraft carrier based (CVN), amphibious based (Fleet Surgical Team (FST)), or on a modified platform (Expeditionary Resuscitative Surgical System (ERSS)), require that we both function without a "safety net" and at the full scope of our training. Our land-based deployments, either with the United States Marine Corps (USMC) or supporting our sister Services, often have many of the same challenges and typically add the dimension of directly supporting ground combat. Even many of our shore-based assignments include small critical access facilities overseas in which we are the sole surgeon and interact with host nation medical facilities. Additionally, we are often called upon to serve as medical advisors to our line leadership, extending our role. While challenging for obvious reasons—managing everything from the mundane to complex injuries such as Dismounted Complex Blast Injuries (DCBI)—these roles are all opportunities for which the rewards include the ability to directly care for those who go in harm's way as well as to self-develop as both clinicians and leaders.

This book, *Expeditionary Surgery at Sea: A Practical Approach*, has been designed to serve as companion to *Front Line Surgery*, now in its second edition, with a focus on the aforementioned sea-based environment. As highlighted in the first chapter, the mission of our Navy is to win wars, deter aggression, and maintain freedom of the seas as a key component of the National Defense Strategy. Our role in Navy Medicine is to ensure medical readiness for that mission and enhance survivability of our servicemembers during conflict. The book is organized into five parts covering key topics and authored by military health care providers from our military and our partners in the United Kingdom that incorporate the lessons learned from almost two decades of conflict applied to that maritime domain.

Part I is an overview of the maritime environment which covers the history of surgery at sea, current sea-based platforms, relevant mechanisms of injury, and includes some extremely practical information on preparing for a ship-based deployment and effectively communicating as a leader. The second part is focused on topics related to the evaluation and care of patients outside of the operating room (OR) or maritime intensive care unit (ICU). It covers triage and mass casualty incidents (MCIs), effective utilization of diagnostic resources, and practical pearls of wisdom from experienced members of the maritime health care team such as nurses and independent duty corpsmen (IDCs) who are integral to the care of the surgical patient throughout the continuum of care. This part also introduces the maritime surgical team to the roles and responsibilities of these providers and limitations of Role 1 shipboard medical departments. The next two parts focus on surgical and critical care at sea—reflecting the challenges mentioned above. Part III covers all aspects of elective and emergent surgical care, including the operative environment, role of anesthesia, and sections on our extended scope of practice including urologic, gynecologic, and hand injuries. It also covers some of the critical questions in surgery—when do I operate and what do I do in the OR during a challenging case? Both questions are extremely relevant in this environment as those "safety nets" are oftentimes literally out of reach. The next section (Part IV) is largest as it gives an overview of critical care, trauma, and burn management. In Chaps. 20 through 31, the reader will find reviews of critical care capabilities and management at sea, how to manage damage control resuscitation (DCR) with limited resources, a logical approach to orthopedic injury stabilization and neurosurgical emergencies, and treatment of unique ship-based mechanisms of injury such as closed space burns and drowning. There are also two key chapters on prolonged casualty care (PCC) and patient transport—critical when the operational environment needs to be considered while making medical decisions. The final part covers humanitarian and disaster relief (HADR), which is another core mission set in which maritime surgical teams play a key role. In this part you will find chapters on bioethics, pediatric patients, and unique populations such as detainees and treatment of pirates, all derived from real-world experience.

Overall, this is a great book and one which I wish I had during my deployment fresh out of surgical training to the USS Kitty Hawk (CV-63) during OIF 1 (and subsequent one). This book is unique in that it is not only written for the naval surgeon, but for all members of the maritime surgical team. While I was prepared from my training what was then Naval Medical Center Bethesda (now Walter Reed National Military Medical Center) for what was a very busy (clinically and operationally) deployment, many of these lessons I had to learn myself. With this guide you will be even better prepared to "care for those who go in harm's way."

Fair winds and following seas

Eric Elster

School of Medicine
Uniformed Services University of the Health Sciences
Bethesda, MD, USA

Preface

Since the navies of the world have been going to sea, they have had embarked provider(s) who manage all injuries and illnesses that can occur on a naval warship. Written by the English barber-surgeon John Woodall, *The Surgions Mate* (1617) was the first comprehensive textbook on naval medicine, surgery, and drug therapy. It covers everything from the management of seasickness, constipation, and fracture management to surgical procedures such as trephination and amputation. Similarly, *Expeditionary Surgery at Sea* is broad in its scope because modern maritime surgical teams, like the seagoing barber-surgeons during the age of sail, may be called on to care for a wide variety of surgical and nonsurgical conditions.

Combat trauma and expeditionary maritime surgery are team sports. Therefore, this book is not just for surgeons but all members of the team. It is written for and by all members of the maritime surgical team, including those nonsurgical providers (e.g., Independent Duty Corpsmen) who will be sending patients to seagoing surgical teams.

While inevitably there will be some overlap (e.g., damage control surgery and resuscitation), this book is meant to complement *Front Line Surgery*. Martin and Beekley's original comprehensive handbook, now in its second edition, is filled with lessons learned, techniques, and practical information for the combat surgeon and their team. It has served as an outstanding resource for me and countless surgeons on combat deployments. Similarly, *Expeditionary Surgery at Sea* provides lessons learned and practical information from those with deployed maritime experience and is structured similarly in terms of the overall book organization and practical straightforward tone. Like *Front Line* Surgery, each chapter starts with a BLUF box (Bottom Line Up Front).

With U.S. National Defense Strategy shifting to the vast Indo-Pacific region, non-naval surgical teams from the Air Force and Army have and will be called on to embark on naval warships. This book is for them too. Admittedly, the topic of *Expeditionary Surgery at Sea* is very niche, but I hope this book will have a broad appeal. This edition has one chapter describing surgical care at sea from the perspective of the United Kingdom. If we are lucky enough to have a second edition, my hope is to solicit contributions from other international navies to share unique lessons learned and best practices.

This book would not be here if not for two people. First is Matt Martin. Matt was a mentor to myself and Amy at the beginning of this process in getting this book started. Thank you for your encouragement and guidance! Second is Amy Hernandez. Thank you for your desire to pay it forward to the next maritime surgical team(s)! I remember Amy asking me over 5 years ago for any guidance I could give from my experiences as a carrier surgeon to help her prepare for her first deployment as a Ship's Surgeon. This book is the result of those initial conversations. Finally, to all of those surgical teams at home and those I have had the privilege to deploy with (on sea or land), thank you for your partnership, professionalism, and mentorship in caring for Sailors, Soldiers, Airmen, and Marines.

San Diego, CA, USA Matthew D. Tadlock

Preface

After completing general surgery residency in 2017, I had 1 week to prepare before flying out to meet my ship—the aircraft carrier USS Carl Vinson (CVN 70). My husband was on a pre-deployment field exercise. My childcare provider and young child had never been alone for long periods of time. In the weeks leading up to my graduation not only was I overwhelmed trying to get my household and loved ones ready to function without me on shore, but I had the additional stress of having no idea what to expect or how I was going to function at sea. I was at a loss from the basic knowledge of "what should I pack?" to the complex decision-making of "how do I decide what to operate on?" I was exasperated because I was not the first Navy surgeon going to a ship for the first time … yet I had NO IDEA what to expect.

Over the course of deployment, issues presented themselves regularly, many not unexpected nor out of the ordinary. Had I known about them ahead of time, I could have worked with my team to make a plan. Talking with other surgeons, listening to other members of the team, even reading posts on online forums demonstrate that my experience as Ship's Surgeon was far from uncommon. These types of experiences are even more frustrating for members of the team with limited to no military experience, like surgeons who trained at civilian institutions.

I resolved to stop perpetuating the problem and be part of the solution, so I created a lengthy turnover document and packing list not only for my replacement but also for all my colleagues who would be deployed on ships after they graduated. I started getting requests to send them to surgeons I had never met. In talking about this situation with my co-editor, he suggested we think "bigger" to help on a global level. So here is my "turnover document" to all members of future maritime surgical teams. It will not solve all problems, but it should help, guide, prepare, and prevent many of them. Best of luck!

San Diego, CA, USA — Amy A. Hernandez

Expeditionary Surgery at Sea: Top 10 Lessons Learned

1. **There is no true maritime surgical capability without blood**. This includes stored whole blood (best), a Walking Blood Bank (WBB) capability (better), and component therapy (minimum). Practice all aspects of your ship's WBB capability BEFORE YOU NEED IT!
2. **Expeditionary Surgery as Sea is a TEAM SPORT**! In the resource-constrained maritime environment, each member of the team plays a critical role to bring vital experience, insight, and knowledge.
3. Understand the capabilities and limitations of the shipboard medical departments referring patients to you; if they are asking you a clinical question, they need your help. **You have the ability, so always be AVAILABLE and AFFABLE!**
4. The same is true for interactions with line leadership. Many of them have no medical knowledge, so it is up to the maritime surgical team to bridge the gap by understanding the operational environment to **communicate efficiently and effectively.**
5. No matter the platform, expeditionary surgery at sea **is austere surgery.** You must know more than one way to perform common diagnostics and operations.
6. You have three imaging modalities you must be proficient with:

    (a) X-ray
    (b) Point of Care Ultrasound (POCUS)
    (c) Diagnostic laparoscopy—**the surgical team is the abdominal CT scan**

7. Prepare for the following as they will happen and **you WILL manage them!**

    (a) Hand and finger orthopedic injuries requiring surgical management
    (b) Gynecologic and urologic surgical emergencies
    (c) Advanced endoscopic emergencies

8. Mass casualty incidents (MCIs) occur when the number of patients or the severity of injuries exceeds the capabilities or resources of the surgical team. **One or two severely injured patients can result in an MCI for any shipboard medical department**! Prepare your team ahead of time.

9. Distributed Maritime Operations (DMO) and Expeditionary Advanced Base Operations (EABO) are happening now; consequently, **all shipboard medical departments must prepare for Prolonged Casualty Care (PCC) now!**
10. Remember the principles of the maritime surgical Authorized Medical Allowance List (AMAL):

    (a) **Review EVERYTHING in your spaces (equipment, instruments, and consumables) before deployment** (if you can).
    (b) "You get what you get, and don't throw a fit." BUT …
    (c) … MacGyver or tactically acquire critical equipment and consumables when needed.
    (d) PAY IT FORWARD! If the AMAL needs to be changed, work through the system to change it! Don't only change it for your ship/team.

Contents

Part I
Maritime Surgery Overview

Chapter 1
Overview of Current Maritime Surgical Platforms and Operational Environments: Part 1—United States Navy and Marine Corps

Debra M. Lowry, Michael G. Johnston, Jan-Michael Van Gent, Matthew D. Tadlock, and Theodore D. Edson

How inappropriate to call this planet Earth when it is quite clearly Ocean.

Arthur C. Clarke

Author deployment experience	
Debra M. Lowry	Flight Surgeon, 31st Marine Expeditionary Unit, embarked on the USS Essex (LHD-2), WESTPAC, INDOPACOM Area of Responsibility, 2010
	Ship's Surgeon, USS Ronald Reagan (CVN-76), WESTPAC, INDOPACOM Area of Responsibility, 2016–2017
	Force Surgeon, Special Purpose Marine Air-Ground Task Force–Crisis Response–Central Command, Operation Inherent Resolve, CENTCOM Area of Responsibility, 2018–2019

D. M. Lowry (✉)
Navy Medicine Readiness and Training Command Camp Pendleton, Camp Pendleton, CA, USA
e-mail: debra.m.lowry.mil@health.mil

M. G. Johnston
USS Gerald R. Ford (CVN-78), Norfolk, VA, USA
e-mail: michael.g.johnston2.mil@health.mil

J.-M. Van Gent
The Red Duke Trauma Institute, Memorial Hermann Hospital, Houston, TX, USA

M. D. Tadlock
Department of Surgery, Naval Medical Center San Diego, San Diego, CA, USA
e-mail: matthewtadlockmd@gmail.com

T. D. Edson
1st Medical Battalion, Camp Pendleton, CA, USA
e-mail: theodore.d.edson.mil@health.mil

M. D. Tadlock, A. A. Hernandez (eds.), *Expeditionary Surgery at Sea*,
https://doi.org/10.1007/978-3-031-21893-4_1

Author deployment experience	
Michael G. Johnston	Staff Surgeon, Fleet Surgical Team-4, embarked on the USS Iwo Jima (LHD-7), Operation Enduring Freedom, Fifth Fleet Area of Responsibility, 2011–2012
	Medical Director and Staff Surgeon, Forward Resuscitative Surgical System, Alpha Surgical Company, Combat Logistics Battalion-7, Marine Expeditionary Brigade, Operation Enduring Freedom, Camp Leatherneck, Afghanistan, 2014
	Officer in Charge, Role 2 Light Maneuver team, embarked on French ship Tonnerre (L9014), Exercise Vois Belleau 100, Fifth Fleet Area of Responsibility, 2017–2018.
	Staff Surgeon, Role 2 Light Maneuver Team NE 6160, embarked on the USS Hershel "Woody" Williams (ESB-4); Provided embarked Role 2 Surgical Support, AFRICOM Area of Responsibility, 2020 and 2021
Jan-Michael Van Gent	Assistant Officer in Charge, Forward Reconnaissance Surgical Team 1, VPOTUS PNG, Papua New Guinea, 2018
	Staff Surgeon, Forward Resuscitative Surgical System, Alpha Surgical Company, Cobra Gold, INDOPACOM Area of Responsibility, 2019
	Staff Surgeon, Forward Resuscitative Surgical System, Alpha Surgical Company, Northern Viper, INDOPACOM Area of Responsibility, 2020
Matthew D. Tadlock	Flight Surgeon, Carrier Air Wing Three (CVW-3), embarked on the USS Harry S. Truman (CVN-75) in support of Operation Iraqi Freedom, Fifth Fleet Area of Responsibility, 2004–2005; supporting Humanitarian Aid Disaster Relief (HADR) operations following Hurricane Katrina, 2005
	Resident Surgeon, USNS Mercy (T-AH-19), Pacific Partnership, Micronesia and Papua New Guinea, 2008
	Ship's Surgeon, USS Carl Vinson (CVN-70), WESTPAC, INDOPACOM Area of Responsibility, 2011–2012
	Officer in Charge, Forward Resuscitative Surgical System/Shock Trauma Platoon, Charlie Surgical Company, Native Fury, CENTCOM Area of Responsibility, 2016
	Chief of Trauma, NATO Role 3 Multinational Medical Unit, NATO Resolute Support and Operation Freedom's Sentinel, Kandahar Airfield, Afghanistan, 2017–2018
	Staff Surgeon, Expeditionary Resuscitative Surgical System Pacific, 2019–2020; Provided embarked Role 2 Surgical Support, INDOPACOM Area of Responsibility, 2020
Theodore D. Edson	Ship's Surgeon, USS Kitty Hawk (CV-63), Northern Pacific Cruise, INDOPACOM Area of Responsibility, 2003–2004
	Assistant Officer in Charge, Forward Resuscitative Surgical System/Shock Trauma Platoon, Operation Iraqi Freedom, Al Qaim, Iraq, 2005–2006
	Director Surgical Services, Surgical Shock Trauma Platoon, Operation Iraqi Freedom, Taqaddum, Iraq, 2006–2007
	Officer in Charge, Forward Surgical Team, Operation Enduring Freedom, Lagman, Qalat, Afghanistan, 2010–2011
	Staff Surgeon, Expeditionary Resuscitative Surgical System 11, 2013–2014; Provided embarked Role 2 Surgical Support, CENTCOM Area of Responsibility, 2013–2014
	Officer in Charge, Forward Resuscitative Surgical Trauma team, Operation Freedom Banner, INDOPACOM Area of Responsibility, 2021

BLUF (Bottom Line Up Front)

1. Understanding the capabilities and limitations of the varied and diverse platforms of the United States (U.S.) Navy and United States Marine Corps (USMC) is critical to successful patient outcomes when providing U.S. Navy Health Service Support (HSS).
2. There is a phased health care system (levels of care, Roles, or echelons) and continuum of care that extends from actions taken at the point of injury (POI) with Role 1 unit-level medical care to Role 2 forward resuscitative damage control resuscitation (DCR) and damage control surgery (DCS) capabilities to Role 3 platforms and finally Role 4 definitive care.
3. En route care (ERC) and patient transport in the U.S. Armed Forces can take three forms: casualty evacuation (CASEVAC), medical evacuation (MEDEVAC), or aeromedical evacuation (AE).
4. Amphibious assault ships such as a Landing Helicopter Dock (LHD) or Landing Helicopter Assault (LHA) are Causualty Receiving and Treatment Ships (CRTS) for the Amphibious Ready Group/Expeditionary Strike Group (ARG/ESG). When a surgical team is embarked, they provide Role 2 capability with the ability to be augmented in order to receive surge casualties.
5. Aircraft carriers (CVN) are not CRTS, but maintain Role 2 capability for force protection of the Carrier Strike Group (CSG).
6. Expeditionary Resuscitative Surgical System (ERSS) teams are adaptive force packages with DCR and DCS subunits that can be deployed to a variety of austere environments and commonly have to set up Operating Rooms (ORs) in atypical spaces when augmenting shipboard Role 1 medical departments.
7. Despite scalable and robust ability, Role 2 CVN surgical teams, Fleet Surgical Teams (FSTs), and austere (i.e., ERSS) surgical teams are essentially single-surgeon teams limited by availability of skilled triage and first responder care, resuscitation capability (i.e., blood products), anesthesia support, supplies, and skilled critical care capability.
8. Designed to be functional in 1 h, the Forward Resuscitative Surgical System (FRSS) is outfitted to perform up to 18 major surgical procedures over 48 h without resupply. In combination with the Shock Trauma Platoon (STP), the Surgical Platoon is capable of providing the full spectrum of DCR.
9. Hospital Ships provide a robust 1000-bed capacity Role 3 capability with specialized medical and surgical care, critical care, and advanced diagnostic capabilities for both support of military and non-military missions. They can deploy at various strengths, depending on the mission requirements.

10. In the modern operational setting, the patient evacuation process is not always linear. Roles/echelons can be bypassed based on urgency, efficiency, expediency, or due to operational considerations.
11. Distributed Maritime Operations (DMO) and Expeditionary Advanced Base Operations (EABO) require the U.S. Navy and USMC to operate in and their medical forces to provide prolonged casualty care in more disaggregated and resource-limited environments. They are happening now, so be prepared!

Introduction

The mission of the United States (U.S.) Navy is to maintain, train, and equip combat-ready naval forces capable of winning wars, deterring aggression, and maintaining freedom of the seas as part of the National Defense Strategy. Navy Medicine's purpose is to provide health services to support this mission and enhance survivability throughout the maritime domain. Maritime domain is defined as all areas and things of, on, under, relating to, adjacent to, or bordering on a sea, ocean, or other navigable waterways, including all maritime-related activities, infrastructure, people, cargo, vessels, and other conveyances. Naval surgical teams can be assigned or placed in any of these areas in order to provide a surgical capability. This chapter introduces the different Roles of care along the continuum of evacuation and examples of each Role of care that may be encountered within the maritime domain, including common U.S. Navy and United States Marine Corps (USMC) surgical platforms, and discusses the implementation of Distributed Maritime Operations (DMO) and Expeditionary Advanced Base Operations (EABO).

Continuum of Care

Joint Publication 4-02 defines the Health Service Support (HSS) mission as mitigating the effects of wounds, injuries, and disease on a unit's effectiveness, readiness, and morale. This is accomplished by disease prevention and a phased health care system (levels of care, Roles, or echelons) that extends from actions taken at the point of injury (POI) or illness to evacuation from a theater for definitive treatment at a hospital in the continental United States (CONUS) [1].

The primary objective of the HSS is to conserve the commander's fighting strength. This is accomplished by providing health promotion and disease prevention in the area of operations, preservation of life, limb, and function, and the restoration and stabilization of the patient's physiological condition to allow for strategic medical evacuation (MEDEVAC). These objectives are met through the implementation of best medical practices and ensuring the delivery of highest possible standard of care.

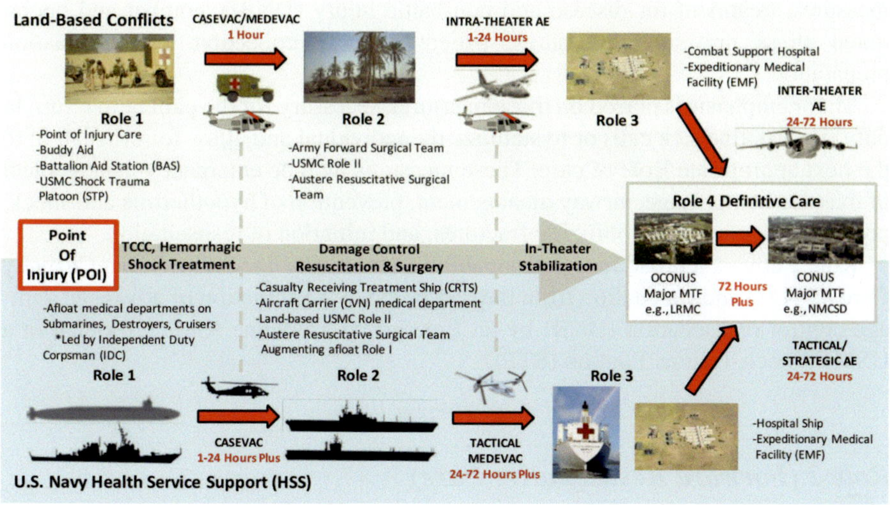

Fig. 1.1 Current Paradigm of Combat Casualty Care: Maritime- compared to Land-based continuum of care [2, 3]. *USMC* United States Marine Corps, *CASEVAC* Casualty evacuation, *MEDEVAC* Medical evacuation, *AE* Aeromedical evacuation, *OCONUS* Outside the Continental United States, *CONUS* Continental United States, *MTF* Medical Treatment Facility, *LRMC* Landstuhl Regional Medical Center, *NMCSD* Naval Medical Center San Diego (Source: Matthew D. Tadlock, MD. Adapted from Bailey et al. [2, 3])

Figure 1.1 compares the continuum of care between the paradigm instituted during the last 20 years of land-based conflict in Iraq, Afghanistan, and Syria and current U.S. Navy HSS [2, 3]. In the deployed setting, continuum of care typically follows a progressive manner from POI self-aid or buddy care to definitive treatment and return to duty. U.S. military and North Atlantic Treaty Organization (NATO) doctrine utilizes Roles of care to describe battlefield medical capabilities, also described for the United Kingdom in Chap. 2. Over the last 20 years, in well-established theaters of operation involving a defined battle space, these evacuation chains were fairly set. Each higher Role/echelon represents an expanded capability. An injured patient was expected to be evacuated along with increasing echelons of care. However, in the modern operational setting, this evacuation process is not always linear. Roles/Echelons can be bypassed based on urgency, efficiency, expediency, or due to operational considerations.

Role 1 (First Responder Care)

Role 1 refers to unit-level medical care centered on self-aid, buddy aid, combat lifesaver, and/or medic care. Typically, this is performed in a Battalion Aid Station (BAS) in the field or medical department on a ship. The focus is immediate lifesaving measures, treatment for disease and non-battle injury (DNBI), combat and operational stress preventive measures, patient casualty collection, and evacuation preparation.

Major emphasis is placed on those measures necessary for the patient to return to duty (i.e., routine sick call) or to stabilize the individual and allow for evacuation to the next appropriate Role of care. These measures include emergency management of massive hemorrhage, airway management, prevention of hypothermia and shock, protecting wounds, immobilizing fractures, and initiation of resuscitation.

Role 1 covers a broad range of capabilities, including Tactical Combat Casualty Care (TCCC) and evacuation from the battlefield to the initiation of advanced damage control resuscitation (DCR) by an Emergency Medicine (EM) physician in a USMC Shock Trauma Platoon (STP).

Role 2 (Forward Resuscitative Care)

Role 2, possessing a greater DCR capability through the ability to address non-compressible hemorrhage, is a continuation of Role 1 care. It also provides damage control surgery (DCS). Depending on the platform, Role 2 resuscitation capabilities include whole blood (cold stored or from a Walking Blood Bank (WBB)) and/or component therapy with packed red blood cells (PRBCs) and fresh frozen plasma (FFP). Role 2 capabilities also may include radiograph and ultrasound imaging, limited laboratory services, dental support, combat and operational stress control (COSC), and preventive medicine (PVNTMED). Role 2 platforms typically have a limited holding capability and finite resources, and interventions are focused on the preservation of life, limb, and eyesight with expedient evacuation.

U.S. Navy and USMC HSS utilize multiple Role 2 platforms that vary in terms of resources, overall footprint, and holding capability. Those platforms with increased capability are often referred to as Role 2 Enhanced (R2E) and provide basic secondary health care built around a primary surgical capability, including intensive care unit (ICU) and ward beds along with the other Role 2 ancillary capabilities. Role 2E has higher holding capability, allowing for further stabilization and deferred evacuation. These patients can be evacuated to a Role 4 without evacuation to a Role 3, depending on availability and stability. U.S. Navy examples include aircraft carrier (CVN) medical departments, Fleet Surgical Teams (FSTs), and Expeditionary Medical Units (EMUs). The USMC Role 2 is also scalable and can boast prolonged holding capability, depending on the configuration.

Role 3 (Theater Hospitalization Capability)

Role 3 care expands the support initiated at the Role 2 and typically has a prolonged, but often limited (i.e., 72 h) holding capability, depending on the theater of operations, operational conditions, and availability of MEDEVAC assets to facilitate transfer to a Role 4 facility.

Role 3 capabilities include initial and ongoing DCR, DCS, initial and secondary wound care, surgical subspecialty care (e.g., ophthalmology, oral maxillofacial surgery, neurosurgery), and prolonged postoperative treatment. Depending on the personnel and configuration, these robust capabilities may also include advanced burn management, advanced radiology (i.e., Computed Tomography (CT) scan), obstetrics, gynecology, pediatrics, internal medicine, medical sub-specialty care like cardiology, optometry, behavioral health, occupational health, physical therapy, medical logistics, and blood banking services. This allows for essential care to either return the patient to duty or stabilize the patient to ensure they can tolerate evacuation to a Role 4.

In the maritime environment, only hospital ships (i.e., the USNS Mercy (T-AH-19) or USNS Comfort (T-AH-20)), shore-based forward hospitals (e.g., Naval Hospital Guam), or a shore-based forward deployed Expeditionary Medical Facilities (EMFs) are Role 3 platforms (Fig. 1.1). EMFs are primarily designed to provide Role 3 care supporting ground-based operations, but can also support concurrent air and maritime operations. These scalable tents or container-based platforms have a fairly large footprint and are capable of providing a 50-bed or 150-bed expeditionary hospital that doctrinally is capable of initial operational capability at 72 h, but take up to 10 days before it is fully operational [4].

Role 4 (Definitive Care)

Role 4 represents the most definitive medical care available within the military health care system. Role 4 facilities are staffed to provide the full spectrum of surgical, medical, and post-injury rehabilitative care. The major CONUS military medical treatment facilities (MTFs) serve as Role 4 facilities. The only Role 4 facility outside the OCONUS is Landstuhl Regional Medical Center (LRMC).

Patient Movement and En Route Care (ERC) Capability

Patient movement along the continuum of care can be accomplished by regulated or unregulated conveyance via ground, sea, or air. Currently, patient transport in the U.S. Armed Forces can take three forms: casualty evacuation (CASEVAC), MEDEVAC, or aeromedical evacuation (AE). CASEVAC is the movement of casualties using a lift of opportunity. These aircrafts do not have embedded medical equipment or medical staff. MEDEVAC is patient movement with pre-designated aircraft equipped and staffed with medical attendants providing en route care (ERC). They are properly marked with a Red Cross and employed in accordance with the Geneva Conventions. AE refers to the movement of patients under medical supervision between higher echelons of care, typically Role 3 to Role 4. The U.S. Air Force has the only AE capability; their Critical Care Air Transport Teams (CCATTs) have an intensivist physician typically overseeing the care.

The U.S. Navy currently does not have designated doctrinal MEDEVAC or AE capabilities. The U.S. Navy's ERC only recently became a program of record with defined manning, training, and equipping requirements and projected operational employment. Current U.S. Navy doctrine dictates that the ERC system will provide for the uninterrupted continuation of patient care during movement. ERC is typically provided by nurses and/or corpsmen in two-person teams and encompasses ongoing ventilation support and resuscitation, physiologic monitoring, and administration of intravenous medication for analgesia, amnesia, and blood pressure support for up to two critically ill casualties for no more than 8 h [5].

Maritime Surgical Platforms

U.S. Navy surgical support can be provided on a variety of maritime platforms. With the introduction of smaller teams capable of providing austere surgical care (e.g., Expeditionary Resuscitative Surgical System (ERSS)), a damage control surgical resuscitation capability can be deployed to even smaller surface or subsurface vessels.

Understanding how medical assets are distributed requires a familiarization with U.S. Navy ship taxonomy and organization. United States Ship (USS) is a combatant vessel carried on the naval register and crewed by military personnel. A United States Naval Ship (USNS) is a non-commissioned ship owned by the U.S. Navy but operated by the Military Sealift Command (MSC) and crewed primarily by MSC civilians. All U.S. Navy ships have an associated class or model and number and are named according to naming conventions and policies that must be approved by the Secretary of the Navy, under the direction of the President, and in accordance with the rules of Congress on naming Navy Ships. As each new ship is commissioned it is assigned a subsequent number within that class. For example, CVN denotes Aircraft Carrier—nuclear propulsion. Currently, there are 11 active aircraft carriers including ten Nimitz class carriers (lead ship USS Nimitz (CVN-68)) and one Ford class carrier (lead ship USS Gerald R. Ford (CVN-78)).

The U.S. Navy is divided into two Fleet forces, the Pacific Fleet and the Atlantic Fleet (previously known as the Fleet Forces Command). These two Fleets are further divided into subordinate Fleets numbered according to geographic Area of Responsibility (AOR). Fleet assets are commonly deployed in aggregate operations as either a Carrier Strike Group (CSG) or the Amphibious Ready Group/ Expeditionary Strike Group (ARG/ESG). Both of these groups are capable of performing multiple mission sets.

The CSG mission is to control sea lanes and project naval power. The CSG core is an aircraft carrier supported by cruisers, destroyers, submarines, and auxiliary ships. A CSG typically embarks a Navy Air Wing when deployed.

The ARG/ESG is responsible for projection of maritime forces from sea to shore. To accomplish this mission they embark Marines, aircraft, and amphibious craft. The Marines are organized into a Marine Expeditionary Unit (MEU) of about 2200 that are embarked on the ships of the ARG/ESG. The ARG/ESG is composed of a "big deck" amphibious assault ship such as a Landing Helicopter Dock (LHD) or Landing Helicopter Assault (LHA) as well as additional smaller amphibious ships. Currently, there are seven active Wasp class LHDs and two active America class LHAs. The main difference between current active LHDs and LHAs is that the LHAs do not have a well deck to receive small amphibious craft. However, they do have an enlarged hangar deck and enhanced aviation capabilities compared to an LHD. Future LHAs will re-incorporate the well deck [6]. In addition to an LHD or LHA, the ARG/ESG will also deploy with smaller amphibious ships including landing platform dock (LPD), landing ship dock (LSD), and amphibious command ships (LCC). Only the 11 CVNs and nine LHD/LHAs routinely deploy with a surgical team and are configured with operating room (OR) and ICU spaces. The LPDs also possess smaller OR and ICU spaces and can embark a surgical team to support disaggregate operations outside of the ARG/ESG construct.

Aircraft Carrier (CVN)

While underway, the CVN serves as the flagship for the CSG. The primary role of the carrier and its air wing is to provide primary offensive firepower, while the other ships that are part of the CSG provide defense and support. Typically, the CSG will include at least one cruiser, a destroyer squadron, submarines, and logistic ships supplying fuel, ammunition, and food.

Table 1.1 shows the basic complement and medical complement/spaces of an aircraft carrier. With the ship's company (~3500), the embarked Air Wing (~2000), and the additional personnel in the surrounding vessels of the CSG (~2000), the CVN medical department provides Role 2 U.S. Navy HSS for approximately 7500 personnel. The CVN medical department is manned by a single general surgeon, a critical care nurse (CCRN), and either a certified registered nurse anesthetist (CRNA) or anesthesiologist along with several other officers enlisted. Table 33.1 lists a full complement for the medical and dental staff on board a CVN. The oral maxillofacial surgeon assigned to the dental department can also provide advanced airway management, experienced surgical assistance, and limited anesthesia support. There is no stored blood or blood products, but CVNs have an active WBB program, usually run by the surgeon. Facilities include a central medical space (one deck below the hangar bay) and six peripheral medical aid stations called battle dressing stations (BDS) distributed throughout the ship.

Unlike the LHD/LHA of an ARG/ESG, the carrier is not intended to be a Casualty Receiving and Treatment Ship (CRTS); rather its role is to force health protection of the strike group. However, in the past CVNs have received multiple casualties

Table 1.1 Aircraft Carrier (CVN) and Amphibious Readiness Group/Expeditionary Strike Group (ARG/ESG) Ship Class complements, organic medical personnel, and medical spaces

	CVN	LHD	LHA	LPD	LCC	LSD
Ship's Company	3500	1070	1204	386	842	330
Marines[a] or Air Wing Embarked	2000	1800[a]	1900[a]	800[a]	0	500[a]
Medical Corps	5	2	2	1	1	1
Dental Corps	5	1	1	1	0	1
Hospital Corpsmen	30	24	19	11	12	9
Operating Rooms (ORs)	1	2 (6)[b]	2	2	1 Minor	0
Intensive Care Unit (ICU) Beds	3	14	3	0	0	0
Ward Beds	52	45	23	24	20	8
Battle Dressing Stations (BDSs)	6	6	4	4	1	1

CVN nuclear-powered aircraft carrier, *LHD* landing helicopter dock, *LHA* landing helicopter assault, *LPD* landing platform dock, *LCC* landing craft control, *LSD* landing ship dock

[a] Indicates the number of Marines that can embark onto an amphibious ship in addition to Ship's Company

[b] Typically, two formal ORs but with appropriate personnel could have a maximum of six formal ORs

during spontaneous disaster relief missions (see Chap. 33) and have had additional surgical teams embarked to support specific missions.

Fleet Surgical Team (FST)

FSTs are medical assets assigned to the Pacific and Atlantic Fleets. FSTs are used to augment an established medical department aboard Casualty Receiving and Treatment Ships (CRTS). The composition of the FST allows for Role 2 support through an expanded surgical and resuscitative capability, laboratory and blood bank services, ICU and ward care, and limited ERC capability. These units are not part of ship's company; rather they are an embarked amphibious group asset.

The typical composition of an FST includes a single general surgeon, a CCRN, either a CRNA or anesthesiologist, and a Certified Perioperative Nurse (CNOR), along with a Family Medicine (FM) or Internal Medicine (IM) physician, a psychologist, and ten corpsmen. The FST is led by the CATF (Commander, Amphibious Task Force) Surgeon. The CATF Surgeon can be any medical specialty and is typically a Commander or Captain.

After troops debark for ship-to-shore movement, specific ships of the ARG/ESG are designated as CRTS to provide forward resuscitative surgical capability (Role 2) to the Landing Force (LF) during amphibious operations. Most commonly the LHD/LHA is utilized as the CRTS since it is the largest ship of the ARG/ESG. LHD/LHAs have laboratory (including blood bank) and radiology capabilities to support surgical suites. During amphibious operations, CRTS are staffed as necessary to provide DCR, DCS, and prolonged patient care. The CATF Surgeon may designate other amphibious ships as secondary CRTS. These may include any class ship with the capability to receive and treat casualties if appropriate medical materiel and personnel are available to provide resuscitative care. Ships normally designated as secondary CRTS include LPD, LSD, and LCC class ships. As seen in Table 1.1, all of these ships have varying bed capacities and do not have intrinsic medical staff to support Role 2 care without augmentation by an FST or another surgical team.

Expeditionary Resuscitative Surgical System (ERSS)

Small, austere, single-surgeon resuscitative teams have gone by multiple names in Navy Medicine over the past 18 years: ERSS (primarily maritime-based), Damage Control Surgery Team (DCST, primarily land-based), and Role 2 Light Maneuver (R2LM). However, none have truly been a program of record until recently. Although historically an ERSS/DCST/R2LM team had seven to nine personnel, the current and official term for these austere U.S. Navy multipurpose single-surgeon teams is ERSS and they are composed of seven personnel [7].

ERSS is an *adaptive force package* of seven personnel that consists of two functional subunits:

1. DCR team to include an EM physician, CCRN, another advanced provider, and a corpsman
2. DCS team to include a general surgeon, anesthesia provider (either a CRNA or anesthesiologist), and a Surgical Technologist (ST) (Navy Enlisted Classification (NEC) L23A).

While divided into two functional subunits, the DCS team rarely functions independently unless providing augmentation to a Submarine (Table 1.2), where typically only the DCS team is deployed. The other advanced provider on the DCR team has been sourced from a variety of backgrounds for a given team, including Physician Assistants (PAs), Independent Duty Corpsmen (IDCs), or EM Registered Nurses (RNs). The corpsman has also been sourced from multiple communities to include Respiratory Therapy (NEC L32A) or Field Medical Services (NEC L03A). In addition to the Officer In Charge (OIC), typical collateral duties on ERSS include Blood Officer, Supply Officer, Training Officer, and Controlled Substances Officer [7]. The current doctrine states that the 7-person ERSS does not have an organic ERC capability; this will be provided by a separate two-person ERC team made up of a nurse and a corpsman [7].

The ERSS operates in the designated battle space through available shipboard platforms (to include subsurface), buildings of opportunity, pre-designated host nation facilities, and other resource-limited maritime environments. ERSS teams can be deployed in a number of variants based on mission-specific requirements and supported platform or unit space constraints. The official anticipated variant configurations and their manning, capacity, and footprint are noted in Table 1.2. ERSS should be able to achieve operational capability within 1 h of arrival at the

Table 1.2 Anticipated mission-specific Expeditionary Resuscitative Surgical System (ERSS) configurations and capabilities, adapted from OPNAVINST 3501.408 [4]

Configuration	Functions	Proposed capacity	Manning/footprint
Surface Ship or Ashore	DCS and DCR	4 major surgeries	7 people
(Complete set of personnel, equipment, and supplies[a])		6 other procedures	26 watertight cases
			2300 lb
			274 cubic feet (cu ft)
Surface Ship or Ashore	DCS and DCR	2 major surgeries	7 people
(Optimized for employment aboard surface combatants [DDG, LCS])		3 other procedures	14 watertight cases
			1200–1500 lb
			157 cu ft
Submarine	DCS only	1 major surgery	3 people
(Optimized for employment aboard submarines)		2 other procedures	7 watertight cases
			650 lb
			120 cu ft

DCS damage control surgery, *DCR* damage control resuscitation, *DDG* destroyer, *LCS* littoral combat ship

[a]Variant 1 consumables can be fully resupplied by a Push Package contained in 15 watertight cases totaling 1500 lb and 178 cu ft

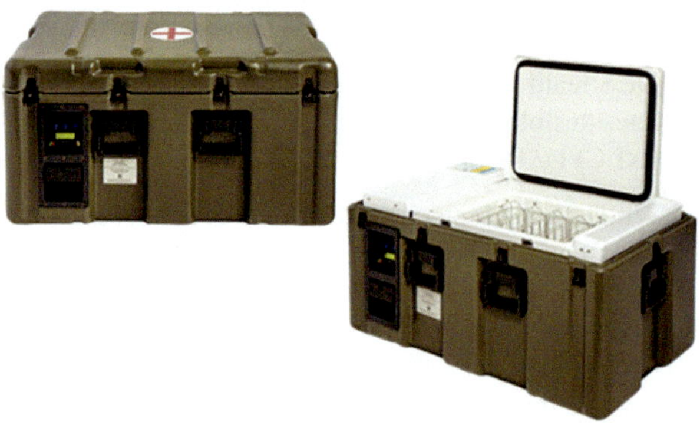

Fig. 1.2 Pelican case blood refrigerator typically used by Expeditionary Resuscitative Surgical System (ERSS) teams. (Source: AX567 technical specifications. Available at: https://csafeglobal.com/wp-content/uploads/2020/05/CSafe_AX56L_DataSheet_USLetter_screen.pdf)

designated location and, following initial intervention, be prepared to hold up to ten patients for up to 96 h. In the maritime environment, ERSS teams can augment nearly any Role 1 or Role 2 shipboard medical department, including those without formal OR spaces such as Destroyers (DDG) or Expeditionary Sea Base (ESB) ships and those with formal OR spaces (i.e., LHD, LHA, LPD). Suggested work spaces outside the formal OR include the hangar bay, mess deck, or forward sonar room of a DDG class vessel, the starboard flight deck storage locker on an ESB class vessel, and the most forward treatment room of the medical department on an LSD class vessel [7]. See Chap. 12 for more discussion with Fig. 12.3 showing an ERSS setup on a DDG.

ERSS teams must rely on the host organization to provide all Base Operating Support (BOS), external communication infrastructure, and force protection. It does not have any organic medical regulating or ERC capabilities. Therefore, in any environment and particularly the maritime environment, the ERSS capability is partially dependent on the resources of the shipboard medical department being augmented and the acuity and severity of the casualties being managed. **While the subsurface ERSS variant doctrinally only performs DCS, a blood resuscitation capability is implied; without proper resuscitation (i.e., blood products), life-saving DCS is not possible** [7].

If there is no WBB capability or stored blood on the ship being augmented, ERSS teams are limited to carrying what fits in their pelican case blood refrigerator (Fig. 1.2), which is approximately 40 total units of a mixture of low-titer O whole blood, PRBCs, and thawed FFP. ERSS also has tranexamic acid (TXA) in its formulary, but no platelets or cryoprecipitate. Its ability to obtain fresh whole blood from a WBB is completely dependent on the supported unit's manning, resources, and pre-screening prior to deployment.

ERSS does not have a sterilizer, but does carry Cidex© and must otherwise rely on external standard (i.e., larger unit's equipment) and non-standard (i.e., ship's oven) methods as described in Appendix B of the Joint Trauma System Clinical Practice Guideline "Acute Traumatic Wound Management in the Prolonged Field Care Setting (CPG ID: 62) [8]." ERSS teams also have the capability to do an i-STAT whole-blood analysis and perform hand-held bedside ultrasound.

While ERSS teams have successfully augmented and integrated with deployed shipboard Role 1 medical departments, there are no ERSS-specific outcomes data to suggest there is a benefit. However, there is some low level of evidence (i.e., case series) showing the potential benefit and favorable outcomes of care provided in the non-maritime deployed environment of single-surgeon austere resuscitative surgical teams [9].

Hospital Ship (T-AH)

The U.S. Navy has two hospital ships (T-AH): the USNS Mercy (T-AH-19) whose home port is San Diego, CA and the USNS Comfort (T-AH-20) whose home port is Norfolk, VA. Commissioned in the 1970s as commercial oil tankers, they were converted to hospital ships in the mid-1980s. Originally built for a short life span, this has been extended through maintenance and extensive refits. They are operated by a crew of civilian mariners, and when deployed embark a mission-shaped medical department relying on other ships for defense against external threats.

The primary T-AH mission is to provide a rapidly responsive, flexible, mobile medical capability for Role 3 combat casualty care in support of U.S. Navy battle forces, amphibious task forces, and forward deployed Army, Navy, Air Force, and Marine forces. The secondary T-AH mission is to provide a mobile hospital service for peacetime military operations, limited humanitarian missions, and use by appropriate U.S. Government agencies involved in disaster or humanitarian relief. Only the President or Secretary of Defense can deploy hospital ships in support of non-military missions.

A Role 3 capability, the T-AH has a 1000-bed capacity including 100 ICU beds, 400 intermediate care beds, 500 minimal care beds, and 12 ORs. Additionally, they have advanced capabilities to include a CT scanner, ICU, and an interventional radiology (IR) suite. Full staffing for the ship includes 1214 members in order to support 1000 beds; however, staffing is varied and scalable depending on the mission. The last times a hospital ship was deployed in support of combat casualty care were during Operation Desert Shield/Desert Storm (1990–1991) when both the USNS Mercy (T-AH-19) and the USNS Comfort (T-AH-20) were activated and during Operation Iraqi Freedom (2002–2003) when only the USNS Comfort (T-AH-20) was activated. However, hospital ships deploy frequently in support of both elective humanitarian missions and spontaneous disaster relief (see Chaps. 32 and 33) [10].

United States Marine Corps (USMC) Surgical Platoon

The USMC has organic medical assets consisting of Navy Medicine personnel that can be attached to an amphibious-based MEU or a Marine Air-Ground Task Force (MAGTF). The USMC's mission is to be a dynamic and mobile naval expeditionary force-in-readiness, prepared to operate in response to a number of contingencies [11]. To be able to meet this mission, the USMC must maintain a capability for rapid movement over long distances and in close proximity to kinetic operations. To meet this mandate, medical assets supporting USMC operations need to maintain the capability to provide resuscitation to trauma patients while being light and mobile enough for transportation by available U.S. Navy and USMC air, land, and sea assets.

Currently, full spectrum trauma resuscitation for the USMC is centered on the combining of a STP and a Forward Resuscitative Surgical System (FRSS) into a Surgical Platoon. The STP can be thought of as an Emergency Room with blood resuscitation and procedural capabilities (e.g., chest tubes, central venous access) that can deploy with USMC assets embarked with an ARG/ESG at sea or with the FRSS within a Surgical Platoon. The Table of Organization and Equipment (TO&E) for the FRSS was designed to be able to be transported by a single MV-22. Table 1.3

Table 1.3 Personnel that make up both the United States Marine Corps (USMC) Shock Trauma Platoon (STP) and Forward Resuscitative Surgical System (FRSS) [12–15]

	Total personnel	Surgeon	Anesthesia provider	EM physician	PA/ IDC	CCRN	EM RN	Corpsman	ST
STP	18	0	0	2	2	0	2	12	0
FRSS	8	2	1	0	1	1	0	1	2

EM emergency medicine, *PA* physician assistant, *IDC* independent duty corpsman, *CCRN* critical care registered nurse, *RN* registered nurse, *ST* surgical technologist

describes the number and type of personnel that staff both the STP and FRSS. Of note, the two FRSS surgeons could be two general surgeons or one general and one orthopedic surgeon. Designed to be functional in 1 h, the FRSS is outfitted to perform up to 18 major surgical procedures over 48 h without resupply. The Surgical Platoon is capable of providing the full spectrum of DCR, particularly the ability to address non-compressible hemorrhage. It also provides ERC personnel to allow for continued resuscitative support during the transport of critically injured patients to theater Role 3 assets [12, 13].

Following the initial maneuver warfare phases of Operation Iraqi Freedom (OIF) and Operation Enduring Freedom (OEF), a major lesson learned was that the FRSS could not operate optimally without the STP in situations involving multiple casualties. USMC missions in CENTCOM have evolved into counter-terrorism operations within a defined battle space. That, combined with a desire to increase organic capability to manage increasingly complex traumatic injuries, has resulted in a steady increase in equipment, personnel, and overall footprint which has significantly impacted STP/FRSS transportability and maneuverability. Between 2005 and 2012, there was an incremental increase in the weight of the FRSS Authorized Medical Allowance List (AMAL) from 2985 to 7310 lb with a concurrent increase in the cube size from 425 cubic feet (cu ft) to 1266 cu ft [14, 15].

The 2018 National Defense Strategy, Force Design 2030, and General Berger's Commandant's Planning Guidance have placed a renewed emphasis on the mission of the USMC to return to its maritime roots as a naval expeditionary force-in-readiness. These three governing philosophies require the USMC to shift its emphasis from the Middle East to resume its partnership with the U.S. Navy, prepared to "operate in actively contested maritime spaces in support of fleet operations" in order to meet national objectives of force projection and control of the sea lines, particularly in the Indo-Pacific areas of operation. To respond to this renewed emphasis, each of the three active Medical Battalions has begun to experiment with the development of various configurations of a Forward Resuscitation Surgical Team, similar to U.S. Navy ERSS teams. In the early process of development, these second-generation USMC teams share a common goal of maintaining a robust forward resuscitative surgical capability while allowing for scalability to adapt to the operational setting and objectives through improved mobility and deployability; in other words, they seek to gain flexibility through changing capacity while not sacrificing capability [11, 16].

The Future Is Now: Distributed Maritime Operations (DMO) and Expeditionary Advanced Base Operations (EABO)

In 2018, largely in response to the potential for peer or near-peer conflict in the Western Pacific, the Chief of Naval Operations (CNO) released *A Design for Maintaining Maritime Superiority, 2.0* with the following mission statement: "The

United States Navy will be ready to conduct prompt and sustained combat incident to operations at sea. Our Navy will protect America from attack, promote American prosperity, and preserve America's strategic influence. U.S. naval operations—from the seafloor to space, from the blue water to the littorals, and in the information domain—will deter aggression and enable resolution of crises on terms acceptable to the U.S. and our allies and partners. If deterrence fails, the Navy will conduct decisive combat operations to defeat any enemy." In addition to increasing fleet size, to meet this mission, the U.S. Navy will "continue to mature the Distributed Maritime Operations (DMO) concept." *A Design for Maintaining Maritime Superiority, 2.0* complements the 2018 National Defense Strategy and the Commandant of the Marine Corps Planning Guidance. DMO will follow three basic tenants: disruptive, modular, and reconfigurable. The U.S. Navy and USMC have been tasked to learn how to conduct DMO, Littoral Operations in Contested Environment (LOCE), and USMC EABO operations. During EABO, the USMC envisions reinforced platoon size units with the ability to maneuver around the theater of operations including island hopping and the ability to fire anti-ship cruise missiles while fighting alongside U.S. Navy forces. For HSS, U.S. Navy and USMC medical assets must possess greater agility and flexibility to provide operational commanders with a range of operations that enable more responsive support for DMO and EABO. The continuum of care for DMO requires a more decentralized and non-linear continuum of care that is optimized across all Roles of care than currently exists [11, 16, 17].

While the DMO and EABO concepts are still being developed, from a practical standpoint those providing U.S. Navy HSS must have the mindset that DMO/EABO operations are happening now as these operational concepts mature. DMO/EABO operations will require individual components of the naval force to be more geographically dispersed and operating in a disaggregate status, connected by a "comprehensive operational architecture" of new and developing technology to provide sea control over a larger geographic area. What does this mean for surgical teams supporting these operations? U.S. Navy Role 1 and Role 2 maritime- and land-based medical assets will have to provide prolonged care in austere maritime and littoral environments compared to previous operational paradigms (Fig. 1.1).

Maximizing survivability for increasing numbers of casualties over longer distances will also require improved patient evacuation and ERC capabilities. The inherent challenges of distance and movement will require extended patient-holding capabilities in more disaggregated and resource-limited environments. This will challenge medical capabilities to become more adaptive, agile, and modular. These new capabilities will need to be integrated across Fleet platforms to provide the Fleet and Marine Corps with responsive and task-organized capabilities aligned to meet the mission requirements of DMO/EABO operations. To support these operations, the U.S. Navy is currently developing a new class of hospital ship utilizing the catamaran hulled Expeditionary Fast Transport (EPF) platform. The new medical variant EPF ships will provide a Role 2 Enhanced (R2E) care capability to include DCR, DCS, and limited ICU and ward holding capability while transferring injured patients to a higher level of care [18]. These new hospital ships, formal ERC and

ERSS programs, and the developing USMC second-generation surgical teams will all be integral to successful current and future DMO/EABO operations.

Maritime Single-Surgeon Team Limitations

While each is a scalable capability, regardless of the overall team size, at their core each CVN, FST, and ERSS are single-surgeon teams. The document defining the ERSS capabilities states "One or two severely injured or critically ill patients can very quickly task-saturate the most-experienced, austere surgical team. The ERSS operates most efficiently and effectively with immediate (as soon as safely possible) medical evacuation … Depending on patient injury pattern and stability, holding multiple patients for more than 12 or 24 h may significantly degrade the ERSS capability and the team's ability to take on more patients [7]." Similarly, while CVN and FST maritime surgical teams and their medical departments may have more personnel, space, and holding capacity, these principles still apply. While highly capable of successfully performing DCR and surgery during any mass casualty situation, each maritime single-surgeon team is limited by the availability of skilled triage and first responder care (e.g., TCCC), resuscitation capability (i.e., blood products), anesthesia support, supplies (i.e., sterilization of instruments and consumables), and skilled critical care capability.

Another limitation is that none of these shipboard medical departments or maritime single-surgeon teams have organic fellowship-trained intensivists to care for critically ill or injured patients in the perioperative period while awaiting evacuation. During the operational paradigm of the last 20 years of land-based conflicts (Fig. 1.1), Role 2 expeditionary surgical teams were typically within 30–60 min from POI. Following DCR and DCS, patients were rapidly transferred to in-theater Role 3 hospitals staffed with critical care teams led by surgeon and non-surgeon fellowship-trained intensivists [18–21]. After additional surgical intervention (if needed), further intensivist-led stabilization was required for many casualties. This included advanced airway and respiratory support, extracorporeal membrane oxygenation (ECMO), and continuous renal replacement therapy (CRRT). The most critically ill of these patients were transported out of the theater to a Role 4 within 72–96 h of injury via CCATT [19–22]. This type of critical care capability (particularly ECMO and CRRT) may not be immediately available during DMO/EABO operations depending on the mission, in-theater assets, and the time/distance from a robust Role 3 capability. Therefore, maritime surgical teams *and* shipboard medical departments must be prepared to provide Prolonged Casualty Care during DMO/EABO operations [3]. Because of the global coronavirus disease 2019 (COVID-19) pandemic, Navy Medicine has started flexing its maritime critical care muscle by deploying intensivist-led COVID-19 response teams (see Chaps. 20 and 21) to augment Role 2 shipboard medical departments with a spectrum of critical care capabilities. In a contested DMO/EABO environment, these types of intensivist-led critical care teams will be crucial to optimal patient outcomes [3].

Conclusion

U.S. Navy surgical teams will deploy to support maritime and littoral operations. Understanding the capabilities and limitations of these varied and diverse platforms will be critical to successful patient outcomes when providing U.S. Navy HSS. While the U.S. Navy and USMC are developing the DMO and EABO concepts, these types of operations are happening now. Therefore, no matter the platform, maritime surgical teams must be prepared to provide prolonged care in diverse expeditionary and resource-constrained environments during this time of transition.

Declaration of Interest The views expressed in this chapter are those of the authors and do not necessarily reflect the official policy or position of the Department of the Navy, Department of Defense, nor the US Government.

Funding This research did not receive any specific grant from funding agencies in the public, commercial, or not-for-profit sectors.

Conflict of Interest Statement The authors declare no conflict of interest.

References

1. Joint Health Services. Joint Publication 4-02. 2018. https://www.jcs.mil/Portals/36/Documents/Doctrine/pubs/jp4_02ch1.pdf.
2. Bailey J, Spott MA, Costanzo GP, Dunne JR, Dorlac W, Eastridge BJ. Joint trauma system: development, conceptual framework, and optimal elements. San Antonio, TX: Fort Sam Houston, U.S. Department of Defense, U.S. Army Institute for Surgical Research; 2012. https://jts.amedd.army.mil/assets/docs/publications/Joint_Trauma_System_final_clean2.pdf.
3. Tadlock MD, Gurney J, Tripp MS, et al. Between the devil and the deep blue sea: a review of 25 modern naval mass casualty incidents with implications for future Distributed Maritime Operations. J Trauma Acute Care Surg. 2021;91(2S Suppl 2):S46–55.
4. Secretary of the Navy. OPNAVINST 3501.176D. Required operational capabilities and projected operational environment for the role 3 navy expeditionary medical facility. 2016. https://www.secnav.navy.mil/doni/Directives/03000%20Naval%20Operations%20and%20Readiness/03-500%20Training%20and%20Readiness%20Services/3501.176D.pdf.
5. Secretary of the Navy. OPNAVINST 3501.409. Required operational capabilities and projected operational environment for the en route care system. 2021. https://www.secnav.navy.mil/doni/Directives/03000%20Naval%20Operations%20and%20Readiness/03-500%20Training%20and%20Readiness%20Services/3501.409.pdf#search=3501%2E409.
6. Navy.mil. Amphibious Assault Ships - LHD/LHA. https://www.navy.mil/Resources/Fact-Files/Display-FactFiles/Article/2169814/amphibious-assault-ships-lhdlhar/.
7. Secretary of the Navy. OPNAVINST 3501.408. Required operational capabilities and projected operational environment for the role 2 light maneuver expeditionary resuscitative surgical system. 2021. https://www.secnav.navy.mil/doni/Directives/03000%20Naval%20Operations%20and%20Readiness/03-500%20Training%20and%20Readiness%20Services/3501.408.pdf.
8. Rapp J, Plackett TP, Crane J, Lu J, Hardin D, Loos P, Kelly R, Hall A, Murray C, Keenan S, Shackelford S. Acute traumatic wound management in the prolonged field care setting

(CPG ID: 62). https://jts.amedd.army.mil/assets/docs/cpgs/Wound_Management_PFC_24_Jul_2017_ID62.pdf.
9. Bingham J, Satterly S, Eckert M. Austere resuscitative and surgical care in modern combat operations. Curr Trauma Rep. 2021;7:53–9. https://doi.org/10.1007/s40719-021-00214-0.
10. Sobocinski, ABB. Answering the call: stateside deployments of U.S. Navy Hospital Ships. 2020. https://www.navy.mil/Resources/Blogs/Detail/Article/2268234/answering-the-call-stateside-deployments-of-us-navy-hospital-ships/.
11. Headquarters Marine Corps. D B. Commandant's planning guidance. 38th Commandant of the Marine Corps. 2019. https://www.hqmc.marines.mil/Portals/142/Docs/%2038th%20Commandant%27s%20Planning%20Guidance_2019.pdf?ver=2019-07-16-200152-700.
12. Marines.mil. Health Service Support Operations. USMC. MCWP 4-11.1. 2012. https://www.marines.mil/Portals/1/MCWP%204-11_1.pdf.
13. Chambers LW, Rhee P, Baker BC, et al. Initial experience of US Marine Corps forward resuscitative surgical system during Operation Iraqi Freedom. Arch Surg. 2005;140(1):26–32.
14. Lowe D HM, Wing V. Marine corps expeditionary medicine: determining clinical requirements for the Forward Resuscitative Surgery System AMALs. Naval Research Center (Report No. 13-12L). 2013.
15. Hill M GM, Konoske P, Pang G. Marine corps operational medicine: determining medical supply needs of the forward resuscitative surgery system and the shock trauma platoon. Naval Health Research Center (Report No. 05-30). 2005.
16. Mattis J. Summary of the National Defense Strategy of the United States of America. https://dod.defense.gov/Portals/1/Documents/pubs/2018-National-Defense-Strategy-Summary.pdf.
17. Department of Defense. A design for maintaining maritime superiority, Version 2.0. 2018. https://media.defense.gov/2020/May/18/2002301999/-1/-1/1/DESIGN_2.0.PDF.
18. USNI News. M S. new details of Austal's EPF hospital ship emerge. 2021. https://news.usni.org/2021/03/05/new-details-of-austals-epf-hospital-ship-emerge.
19. Ingalls N, Zonies D, Bailey JA, et al. A review of the first 10 years of critical care aeromedical transport during operation Iraqi freedom and operation enduring freedom: the importance of evacuation timing. JAMA Surg. 2014;149(8):807–13.
20. Grathwohl KW, Venticinque SG. Organizational characteristics of the austere intensive care unit: the evolution of military trauma and critical care medicine; applications for civilian medical care systems. Crit Care Med. 2008;36(7 Suppl):S275–83.
21. Zonies D, DuBose J, Elterman J, et al. Early implementation of continuous renal replacement therapy optimizes casualty evacuation for combat-related acute kidney injury. J Trauma Acute Care Surg. 2013;75(2 Suppl 2):S210–4.
22. Cannon J, Pamplin J, Zonies D, et al. Acute respiratory failure. Mil Med. 2018;183(Suppl 2):123–9.

Chapter 2
Overview of Current Maritime Surgical Platforms and Operational Environments Part 2: United Kingdom and The Royal Navy

Jonathan J. Matthews and Rex Kinnear-Mellor

England expects that every man will do his duty.

Horatio Nelson

Author deployment experience	
Jonathan J. Matthews	Resident Surgeon, Primary Casualty Receiving Facility, RFA Argus, Operation Telic 1, Northern Arabian Gulf, 2003 Staff Trauma & Orthopaedic Surgeon, Joint Force Medical Group, Operation Herrick 11, Camp Bastion, Afghanistan, 2010
	Staff Trauma and Orthopaedic Surgeon, Joint Force Medical Group, Operation Herrick 14, Camp Bastion, Afghanistan, 2011
	Clinical Director, Role 2 Afloat, RFA Cardigan Bay, International Mine Countermeasures Exercise, Northern Arabian Gulf, 2013
	Staff Trauma and Orthopaedic Surgeon, Primary Casualty Receiving Facility, RFA Argus, Exercise Sabre Dawn, English Channel, 2013
	Staff Trauma and Orthopaedic Surgeon, ANSF Medical Mentoring Team, Operation Herrick 19b/20, Camp Bastion, Shorabak, Afghanistan, 2014
	Clinical Director, Role 2 Afloat, HMS Ocean, Exercise Joint Warrior, Western Approaches, Scotland, 2015
	Clinical Director, Role 2 Afloat, RFA Mounts Bay, Operation Mounts Bay 16, Establishment and Validation/Assurance Phase, 2015; Operational Phase, supporting contingency operations in southern Mediterranean, 2016
	Clinical Director, Role 2 Afloat, RFA Mounts Bay, Operation Ruman, supporting Humanitarian Assistance and Disaster Relief (HADR) operations following Hurricanes Irma and Maria, Caribbean, 2017
	Clinical Director, Combined Role 2 Afloat Exercise with U.S. Navy Expeditionary Resuscitative Surgical System team embarked on the RFA Cardigan Bay, Exercise Azraq Serpent, Bahrain, 2018
	Staff Trauma & Orthopaedic Surgeon, Role 2 Afloat, HMS Queen Elizabeth, Westlant 18, Fixed Wing Fast Jet Trials, Eastern Seaboard, USA, 2018

J. J. Matthews (✉)
HMS Vivid, Plymouth, Devon, UK
e-mail: jonathanmatthews@nhs.net

R. Kinnear-Mellor
Maritime Deployed Hospital Group, HMS Excellent, Portsmouth, UK
e-mail: rex.kinnear-mellor793@mod.gov.uk

M. D. Tadlock, A. A. Hernandez (eds.), *Expeditionary Surgery at Sea*,
https://doi.org/10.1007/978-3-031-21893-4_2

Author deployment experience	
Rex Kinnear-Mellor	Resident Anaesthetist, Joint Force Medical Group, Operation Herrick 11, Camp Bastion, Afghanistan, 2014
	Staff Anaesthetist, Role 2 Afloat, HMS Queen Elizabeth, Westlant 18, Fixed Wing Fast Jet Trials, Eastern Seaboard, USA, 2018
	Clinical Director, Role 2 Afloat, RFA Mounts Bay, Operation Barytone, supporting Humanitarian Assistance and Disaster Relief (HADR) operations following Hurricane Dorian, Caribbean, 2019
	Clinical Director, Role 2 Afloat, HMS Queen Elizabeth, Operation Fortis, UK Carrier Strike Group, 2020
	Clinical Director, Role 2 Afloat, HMS Queen Elizabeth, Operation Fortis, UK Carrier Strike Group deployment to the Indo-Pacific, 2021
	Clinical Director, Role 2 Afloat Capability, Maritime Deployed Hospital Group, 2019–Present

BLUF (Bottom Line Up Front)

1. Deployed Hospital Care within the maritime environment is delivered in North Atlantic Treaty Organization (NATO) defined Medical Treatment Facilities (MTFs).
2. The Operational Patient Care Pathway (OPCP) is initiated at the point of wounding with pre-hospital care delivered by pre-hospital practitioners and Role 1 MTFs supported by Role 2 Afloat (R2A) MTFs (deployed hospital care forward) and maritime Role 3 (MR3) MTFs (deployed hospital care rear) before final transfer to Role 4 definitive care.
3. An R2A MTF delivers damage control resuscitation (DCR) including damage control surgery (DCS) across a number of different maritime platforms to a standard capability of 2-1-2–two resuscitation beds, one operating table, and two critical care beds.
4. R2A teams are staffed to deliver "limb and life-saving" DCS with only general surgeons and orthopaedic surgeons.
5. The Bay Class Landing Ship Dock (LSD) and Queen Elizabeth Class (QEC) aircraft carriers have MTFs on board equipped to host R2A teams with fixed operating tables and surgical lights as well as blood storage fridges, resuscitation, and critical care beds.
6. Bespoke smaller 1-1-1 R2A teams can be deployed onto smaller platforms such as Type 45 destroyers as operational requirements demand. The Commando Forces Surgical Group (CFSG) has the capability to deploy a forward surgical team in the maritime environment if required to support the littoral activities of the Royal Marines.
7. The MR3 MTF is delivered by the primary casualty receiving facility (PCRF) on board the RFA Argus.
8. MR3 can deliver specialised "in-theatre" surgical care as the PCRF is staffed with plastic, ear-nose-throat, neurosurgical, maxillary-facial, ophthalmic, and urologic surgeons as well as general and orthopaedic surgeons.

9. The full capability of MR3 delivers a maximum 100-bed capacity with four resuscitation bays, four operating tables, 10 intensive care beds, 20 high-dependency beds, and 70 low-dependency beds. It can also deploy at various strengths, including a "PCRF lite" option with a 25-bed capacity with two resuscitation bays, two operating tables, five intensive care beds, 10 high-dependency beds, and 10 low-dependency beds.
10. Due to the prolonged timelines frequently encountered in the Maritime environment, the R2A MTF is equipped to hold patients for up to 48 h if required prior to further evacuation down the OPCP. The MR3 MTF can hold patients for 2–4 days if required.

Introduction

North Atlantic Treaty Organization (NATO) Medical Treatment Facility (MTF) Role definitions [1, 2] *are summary definitions for capability of military medical facilities in order to facilitate interoperability between NATO nations.* These include:

1. **Role 1 MTF–medical response capability**. A Role 1 MTF is a national responsibility focusing on provision of primary health care, specialised first aid, triage, resuscitation, and stabilisation.
2. **Role 2 MTF–initial surgery response capability**. A Role 2 MTF provides an initial surgical response capability and is characterised by its ability to perform *surgical interventions* in addition to performing reception and triage of casualties and resuscitation and treatment of shock to a higher level than Role 1 facilities. There are two main types of Role 2 MTFs:

   (a) A **Role 2 basic MTF** must provide a surgical capability, including *damage control surgery (DCS)* and surgical procedures for emergency surgical cases, to deliver life, limb, and function-saving medical treatment. The surgical capability should be provided within medical timelines.
   (b) A **Role 2 enhanced MTF** must provide all the capabilities of the Role 2 basic, but has *enhanced capabilities* as a result of additional facilities and greater resources, including the capability of stabilising and preparing casualties for strategic aeromedical evacuation.

3. **Role 3 MTF–hospital response capability**. A Role 3 MTF provides secondary health care at theatre level. This facility must provide all the capabilities of the Role 2 Enhanced MTF and be able to conduct *specialised surgery, care, and additional services* as dictated by mission and theatre requirements.

4. **Role 4 MTF–definitive hospital response capability**. A Role 4 MTF offers the full spectrum of definitive medical care that cannot be deployed to theatre or will be too time-consuming to be conducted in theatre. Role 4 MTFs normally provide definitive care, surgical and medical specialist procedures, reconstructive surgery, and rehabilitation.

Operational Patient Care Pathway (OPCP)

In the maritime environment, the operational patient care pathway (OPCP) [2] demonstrated in Fig. 2.1 is facilitated by Role 2 afloat (R2A) MTFs (Deployed Hospital Care Forward) and the maritime Role 3 (MR3) MTFs (deployed hospital care rear) supporting Role 1 units on board surface platforms and submarines which treat patients from the point of injury.

The maritime medical scheme of manoeuvre (SoM) seen in Fig. 2.2 provides a template for medical planning for operations and can be adjusted around individual tasking's requirements. Limitations of individual platforms, availability of air assets, and transfer times between echelons of care also influence which team formats are deployed for particular operations.

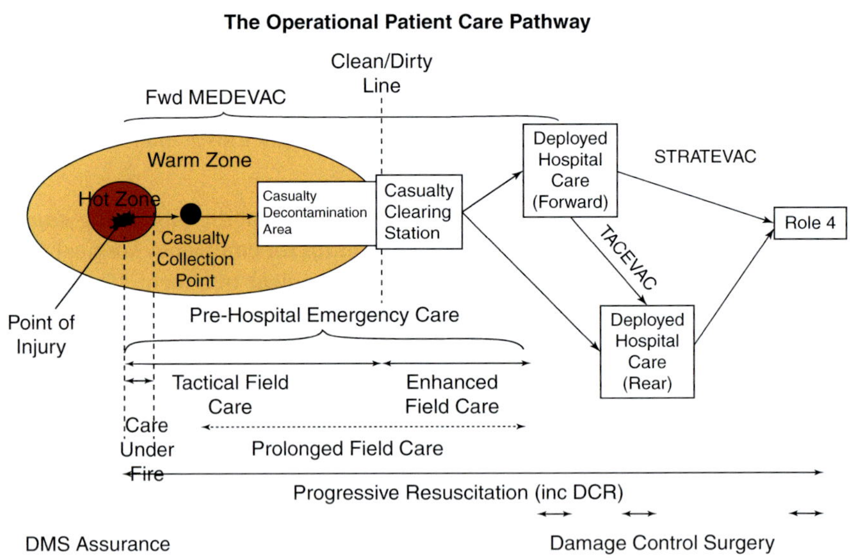

Fig. 2.1 The operational patient care pathway (OPCP) [2] (Source: Royal Naval Medical Service, used with permission)

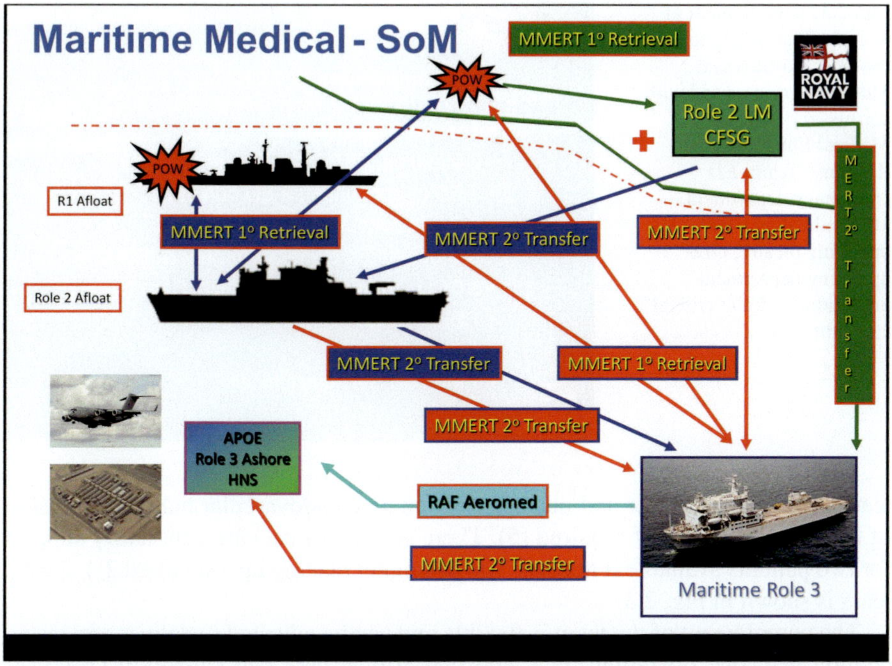

Fig. 2.2 Maritime medical scheme of Manoeuvre (SoM) (Source: Royal Naval Medical Service, used with permission). *R1* role 1, *MMERT* Maritime Medical Emergency Response Teams, *Role 2 LM* role 2 light manoeuvre, *CFSG* Commando Forces Surgical Group, *RAF* royal air force, *APOE* aerial port of embarkation, *HNS* host nation support

Role 2 Afloat (R2A)

The R2A capability is essentially a Deployed Hospital Care Forward team able to deliver damage control resuscitation (DCR) on board a suitable vessel at sea. There are two teams held at readiness within the Royal Navy with one team at 48 h to move (readiness state 1) and the second team at 5 days to move (readiness state 2). The standard R2A capability has two resuscitation beds, one operating table, and two critical care beds (2-1-2 capability). Due to the prolonged patient transfer times in the maritime environment, the R2A team is equipped to hold patients for up to 48 h. An R2A MTF is the first echelon of care in the operational patient care pathway able to deliver a surgical capability [3]. R2A-deployed hospital care should be delivered within 2 h from the point of wounding according to NATO timelines [4].

The R2A MTF is a flexible capability. The standard team will deliver a 2-1-2 capability. The trained resuscitation team is complemented with digital plain radiography and ultrasound imaging. There is a blood bank available able to store blood products and a capacity to deliver an emergency donor panel (EDP) if required. The

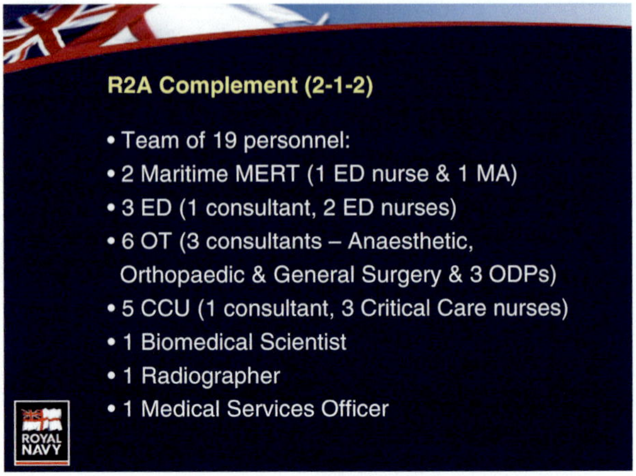
R2A Complement (2-1-2)
• Team of 19 personnel:
• 2 Maritime MERT (1 ED nurse & 1 MA)
• 3 ED (1 consultant, 2 ED nurses)
• 6 OT (3 consultants – Anaesthetic, Orthopaedic & General Surgery & 3 ODPs)
• 5 CCU (1 consultant, 3 Critical Care nurses)
• 1 Biomedical Scientist
• 1 Radiographer
• 1 Medical Services Officer
ROYAL NAVY

Fig. 2.3 Complement of Role 2 afloat (R2A) team (Source: Royal Naval Medical Service, used with permission). *MERT* Medical Emergency Response Team, *ED* emergency department, *MA* medical assistant, *OT* operating theatre, *ODP* operating department practitioners, *CCU* critical care unit

team is trained to deliver and manage resuscitative endovascular balloon occlusion of the aorta (REBOA) if required [5]. There is also critical care ventilatory support for two patients available if needed. The personnel making up a standard 2-1-2 R2A team is shown in Fig. 2.3.

The complement of the team is flexible and can be adjusted to deliver one resuscitation bed, one operating table, and one critical care bed capability (1-1-1) if required due to individual tasking's requirements and platform constraints with space, etc. A medical proof of concept exercise (Azraq Serpent 2018) allowed the opportunity for a United States (U.S.) Navy Expeditionary Resuscitative Surgical System (ERSS) team to deploy onto one of the Bay Class platforms–the RFA Cardigan Bay [6]. This team was utilised in a serial (training scenario) during the exercise to establish a secondary operating position within the medical complex. This showed that the standard R2A team deployed to Bay Class platforms could be supplemented by an additional small surgical team to increase the capability offered and allow a third patient to be treated concurrently. As such, the increased capability offered by the additional 1-1-1 team would flux between:

3-1-2 (allowing three triage category 1/2 casualties to be treated concurrently)
OR
2-2-2 (allowing two casualties to have DCS as required concurrently)
OR
2-1-3 (allowing three casualties to receive critical care prior to rearward evacuation to Role 3/4).

The Maritime Medical Evacuation Response Teams (MMERT) can be deployed separately to the main 2-1-2 team. On the Queen Elizabeth Class (QEC) aircraft carriers, the Primary Care team can provide the pre-hospital team; however, this can be supplemented as dictated by medical estimate planning. The Biomedical Scientist (BMS) is able to run the blood bank and EDP if required and can also deliver basic blood tests to guide the delivery of DCR by the R2A team. The standard 2-1-2 R2A capability is supplied to be able to deal with 10 triage Category 1 patients, 10 triage category 2 patients, and 40 triage category 3 patients over a 72-h period before first-line resupply.

Maritime Role 3 (MR3)

The MR3 MTF is delivered by the primary casualty receiving facility (PCRF) in the form of a 100-bed facility on board the RFA Argus. The RFA Argus is not a designated hospital ship as it carries weapons systems and has other military Roles, and therefore it cannot be protected by the Geneva Convention of 1949. This allows increased versatility of the PCRF, enabling it to position itself within a battle group much closer to the point of wounding to facilitate accelerated casualty evacuation times which would not be possible with a designated hospital ship operating under the protection of the Red Cross. Therefore, during its operational medical deployment in the Iraq conflict in 2003, it went to the Northern Arabian Gulf as a grey vessel [7] and was able to position itself within the maritime battle group and receive casualties directly from the point of wounding as well as from Role 2 MTFs ashore.

The PCRF is arranged over three decks beneath the flight deck. The four resuscitation bays have access to diagnostics including portable X-ray, ultrasound, 64-slice Computed Tomography (CT), and laboratory facilities including haematology, biochemistry, blood transfusion, and microbiology. The full capability delivers 4/4/10/20/70 with a maximum 100-bed capacity, four resuscitation bays, four operating tables, 10 intensive care beds, 20 high-dependency beds, and 70 low-dependency beds. It can also deploy at various strengths including a "PCRF lite" option of 2/2/5/10/10 with a 25-bed capacity, two resuscitation bays, two operating tables, five intensive care beds, 10 high-dependency beds, and 10 low-dependency beds.

Unlike R2A MTFs, which are staffed only by general and orthopaedic surgeons, the MR3 MTF has a multidisciplinary surgical team including the addition of plastic, ear-nose-throat, neurosurgical, maxillary-facial, ophthalmic, and urologic surgeons. This surgical team is able to deliver "in-theatre" surgery as well as DCS. The PCRF is also equipped to hold patients for 2–4 days prior to the evacuation to definitive care at Role 4 MTFs.

Commando Forces Surgical Group (CFSG)

The Commando Forces Surgical Group (CFSG) can support the littoral activities of the Royal Marines both ashore and with smaller Forward Surgical Teams afloat if required. The CFSG delivers a Role 2 Capability ashore. However, it does have the capability to deliver a 1-1-1 MTF in the form of a Forward Surgical Team onboard an appropriate maritime platform if needed.

Platforms

R2A MTFs are primarily deployed on the Bay Class Landing Ship Dock (LSD) and QEC aircraft carriers. Both have permanent infrastructure on board to support the R2A team. This includes an operating theatre with fixed standing operating tables and surgical lights as well as designated resuscitation bays and critical care beds. In addition, blood fridges allow the provision of blood products and the activation of an EDP if required. The three Bay Class amphibious landing ships (one pictured in Fig. 2.4) are highly versatile and well-proven platforms for the delivery of R2A-deployed hospital care. R2A MTFs based on Bay Class platforms have been used across a number of recent operations ranging from the delivery of Humanitarian Assistance and Disaster Relief (HADR) following a hurricane in the Caribbean [8] to supporting contingency operations in the Gulf [9] and Mediterranean. Both QEC aircraft carriers (one pictured in Fig. 2.5) within the Royal Navy can accommodate a 2-1-2 R2A capability.

The MR3 MTF is on board the RFA Argus, pictured in Fig. 2.6. This is a 28,000 tons Royal Fleet Auxiliary (RFA) vessel, whose primary purpose is as a PCRF. Its

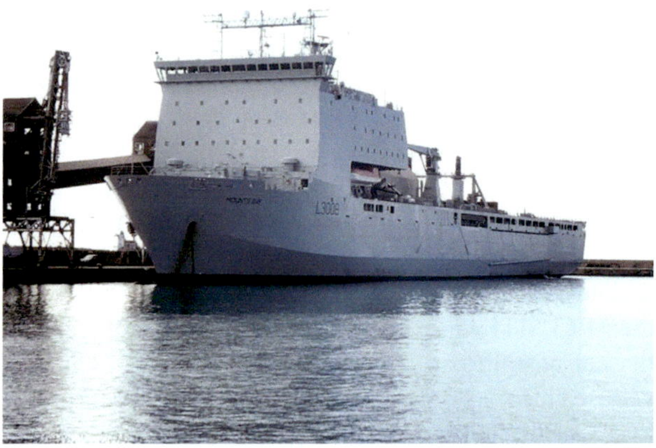

Fig. 2.4 The RFA Mounts Bay (bay class) (Source: Photo courtesy of Jon J. Matthews, MD)

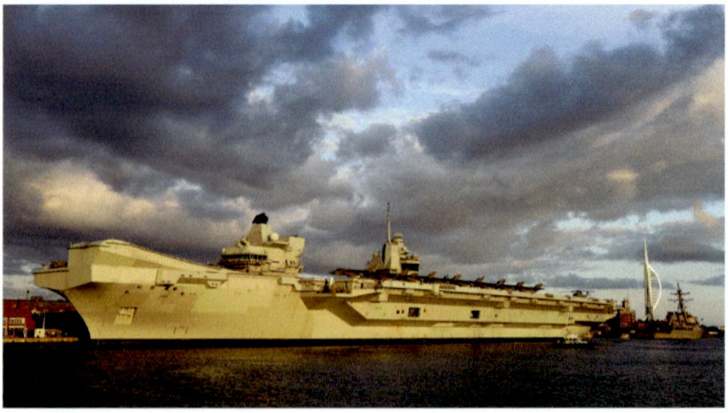

Fig. 2.5 The HMS Queen Elizabeth (QEC) (Source: Photo courtesy of Jon J. Matthews, MD)

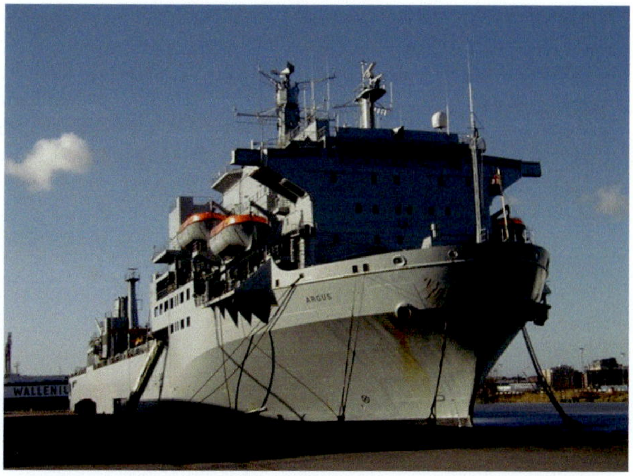

Fig. 2.6 The RFA Argus (Source: Photo courtesy of Jon J. Matthews, MD)

secondary function is as a helicopter platform, and much of its 175-meter length is taken up with a flight deck. It is well proven as a PCRF, having delivered MR3-deployed hospital care on a number of operations ranging from supporting kinetic activities in the Iraq conflict in 2003 [7] to HADR support during the Ebola outbreak in Sierra Leone in 2014–2015 [10].

Conclusion

The Royal Navy operates within NATO doctrinal timelines and delivers Deployed Hospital Care across a number of maritime platforms. DCR is delivered at defined echelons of medical care in a progressive manner with capabilities being able to deliver DCS at R2A MTFs and more specialised "in-theatre" surgery by a multidisciplinary surgical team at MR3 before further evacuation to Role 4. MMERT can be deployed within R2A or MR3 MTFs, or alternatively can deploy separately as required within the OPCP. The R2A team can be adjusted and tailored to match the requirements of the tasking and available platform. Standard R2A teams deliver a 2-1-2 capability primarily on the QEC aircraft carriers and Bay Class platforms but 1-1-1 teams can and have been deployed onto smaller platforms such as Type 45 Destroyers as operational requirements demand [11].

References

1. Allied Joint Doctrine for Medical Support, Allied Joint Publication – 4.10 (AJP-4.10), Edition C, Version 1, dated September 2019.
2. The operational patient care pathway, JSP 950 Leaflet 1-4-1.
3. Tye S, et al. The surgical aspects of role 2 afloat. J R Nav Med Serv. 2013;99(3):146–8.

4. The Ministry of Defence. Allied Joint Publication, Allied Joint Doctrine for Medical Support 2015; AJP 4-10(B), Ch1, Para 1.1.6, sub-Para 3.
5. Rees P, Waller B, Buckley AM, Doran C, Bland S, Scott T, Matthews J. REBOA at role 2 afloat: resuscitative endovascular balloon occlusion of the aorta as a bridge to damage control surgery in the military maritime setting. J R Army Med Corps. 2018;164(2):72–6. https://doi.org/10.1136/jramc-2017-000874. Epub 2017 Dec 20. PMID: 29269480.
6. Matthews JJ. Increasing role 2 afloat capability on the bay class – lessons identified from Azarq serpent. J R Nav Med Serv. 2018;104:165–8.
7. Matthews JJ, Mercer SJ. 'War Surgery at Sea': maritime trauma experience in the gulf war. J R Nav Med Serv. 2003;89(3):123–32.
8. Matthews JJ. Operation RUMAN: role 2 afloat delivering humanitarian aid and disaster relief operations in the Caribbean. J R Nav Med Serv. 2018;104:159–64.
9. Matthews JJ, Heames RM. International mine countermeasures exercise 2013: role 2 afloat. J R Nav Med Serv. 2013;99(3):133–4.
10. Gibson S, Gay D. Maritime radiology on operation GRITROCK. J R Nav Med Serv. 2016;102:12–3.
11. Mellor A, et al. Role 2 afloat in a type 45 destroyer: return to contingency. J R Nav Med Serv. 2017;103:103–10.

Chapter 3
The Ship's Surgeon and Surgery at Sea: A Brief History

Matthew D. Tadlock, Amy A. Hernandez, and Benjamin T. Miller

If you be constrained to use your saw, let first your patient be well informed of eminent danger of death by the use thereof; prescribe him no certainie of life, and let the work be done with his owne free will, and request, and not otherwise.

The Surgion's Mate, 1617, John Woodall, on amputation

Author deployment experience	
Matthew D. Tadlock	Flight Surgeon, Carrier Air Wing Three (CVW-3), embarked on the USS Harry S. Truman (CVN-75) in support of Operation Iraqi Freedom, Fifth Fleet Area of Responsibility, 2004–2005; supporting Humanitarian Aid Disaster Relief (HADR) operations following Hurricane Katrina, 2005
	Resident Surgeon, USNS Mercy (T-AH-19), Pacific Partnership, Micronesia and Papua New Guinea, 2008
	Ship's Surgeon, USS Carl Vinson (CVN-70), WESTPAC, INDOPACOM Area of Responsibility, 2011–2012
	Officer in Charge, Forward Resuscitative Surgical System/Shock Trauma Platoon, Charlie Surgical Company, Native Fury, CENTCOM Area of Responsibility, 2016
	Chief of Trauma, NATO Role 3 Multinational Medical Unit, NATO Resolute Support and Operation Freedom's Sentinel, Kandahar Airfield, Afghanistan, 2017–2018
	Staff Surgeon, Expeditionary Resuscitative Surgical System Pacific, 2019–2020; Provided embarked Role 2 Surgical Support, INDOPACOM Area of Responsibility, 2020

M. D. Tadlock (✉) · A. A. Hernandez
Department of Surgery, Naval Medical Center San Diego, San Diego, CA, USA
e-mail: matthewtadlockmd@gmail.com; amyhern7@gmail.com

B. T. Miller
Cleveland Clinic, Cleveland, OH, USA

M. D. Tadlock, A. A. Hernandez (eds.), *Expeditionary Surgery at Sea*,
https://doi.org/10.1007/978-3-031-21893-4_3

Author deployment experience	
Amy A. Hernandez	Battalion Surgeon, 7th Engineer Support Battalion, Operation Enduring Freedom, Camp Leatherneck, Afghanistan, 2011
	Ship's Surgeon, USS Carl Vinson (CVN-70), WESTPAC, INDOPACOM Area of Responsibility, 2017
	Department Head, Federal Emergency Management Agency (FEMA) and Defense Support of Civilian Authorities (DSCA), COVID-19 Community Vaccination Center mission, St. Louis, MO, USA, 2021
Benjamin Miller	Staff Surgeon, Fleet Surgical Team-6, embarked on the USS Bataan (LHD-5), Operation Inherent Resolve, Fifth Fleet Area of Responsibility, 2017
	Staff Surgeon, forward deployed Naval Hospital Guam, 2018–2020

BLUF (Bottom Line Up Front)

1. The first ship's surgeon in Western literature is Machaon as described in Homer's eighth century BC epic poem, *The Iliad.*
2. In Ancient Greece in the Age of Manpower, the Athenian Navy had the trireme *Therapeia* (431 BC), which may have served as an early hospital or casualty receiving ship.
3. M. Satrius Longinus (AD 138) was **medicus** of the trireme *Cupid.* **Medici** were early Roman military medical practitioners.
4. In the early 1300s, the first known sea-going provider described specifically as a surgeon is Venetian barber-surgeon Master Gualtieri.
5. By 1512 at the end of the Age of Discovery, naval barber-surgeons were common in the British Royal Navy, and the terms "surgeon" and "surgeon's mate" were first introduced into naval service.
6. In 1617, barber-surgeon Thomas Woodall, Surgeon General of the British East India Company, published *The Surgion's Mate*, an early textbook on surgical care at sea.
7. Throughout the Age of Sail (1600–1850), embarked surgeons were common on merchant and naval vessels throughout Europe and the United States (U.S.).
8. Two advances in U.S. naval surgery occurred during the American Civil War. The first U.S. Navy hospital ship, the USS Red Rover, was utilized in 1862. Chloroform was administered by the Ship's Surgeon on the USS Kearsarge during an upper extremity amputation in 1864; the first documented surgical procedure using anesthesia on board a U.S. naval warship.
9. In 1910, on the battleship USS South Carolina (BB-26), the first known blood transfusion was performed on board a U.S. naval warship. By World War I, blood transfusions were commonly performed for a hematocrit less than 25. During World War II, both damage control surgery and whole-blood resuscitation were commonly performed on U.S. naval warships and hospital ships.

10. Women had to overcome not only the barriers of a male-dominated surgical profession but also those of the male-dominated seafaring world. In 1997, Dr. Beth Jacklic was the first woman Ship's Surgeon in the U.S. Navy, serving on the USS George Washington (CVN-73).

Introduction

Sea travel, integral to the evolution of civilization, has enabled global migration, exploration, commerce, and war. As humans traveled further and further from land for increasingly longer periods of time, they developed medical and surgical conditions requiring treatment at sea. Infectious diseases, nutritional deficiencies like scurvy, and injuries sapped the crew's effectiveness. From Antiquity through the Middle Ages a wide variety of practitioners have embarked on warships and merchant vessels to treat illness and injury underway. By the Renaissance and the Age of Discovery, all European warships and some merchant vessels had at least two crew members providing both medical and surgical care at sea: the ship's surgeon and surgeon's mate. As medicine and surgery have matured, naval surgeons have pioneered surgery and resuscitation at sea. While the history of the Ship's Surgeon is intimately linked to all aspects of maritime medicine, this chapter focuses on surgical care at sea.

The Age of Manpower (~800 BC to AD 1450)

Ancient Greece (~800–322 BC)

The history of the ship's surgeon begins with the first known naval amphibious assault in military history, the Trojan war (twelfth or thirteenth century), when nearly 1200 Greek ships landed in what is now modern-day Turkey [1]. Homer's epic poem, *The Iliad*, written in eighth Century BC, describes the last weeks of the war, including vivid descriptions of up to 184 war wounds and their management [2]. Five warrior-physicians are also depicted, including Achilles and the brothers Machaon and Podalirius, sons of Aesculapius, the Greco-Roman god of medicine. While Podalirius was a physician, he did not perform surgical procedures. Mentioned 11 times in *The Iliad,* only Machaon was described as a surgeon [3, 4]. In an early description of combat casualty care under fire, he treats Spartan King Menelaus after he was injured by a Trojan arrow; Machaon "…ran…and approached the injured King…Then he saw the wound, where the arrow was embedded, he extracted it, sucked out the blood and he applied herbal salves …" [3]. Some authors have labeled Machaon the "father of surgery [4]" or even the first western trauma surgeon [3]. He is also the first ship's surgeon described in Western literature. As art often

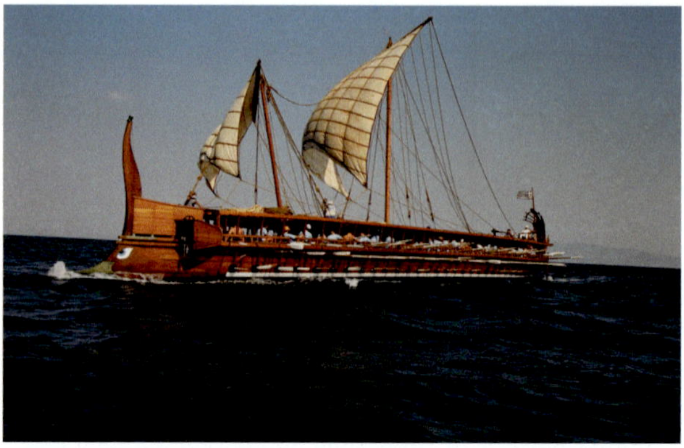

Fig. 3.1 An HS Olympias trireme replica. It was built in 1987, funded by the Hellenic Navy, and is now purely on exhibit. During the original sea trials, each oarsman required at least 1 L of water per hour or 8 L per person during a full day of rowing [5]. (Source: Hellenic Navy. Available at: https://www.hellenicnavy.gr/en/history-tradition/ships-museum-exhibits/trireme-olympias.html)

imitates or depicts real life, perhaps *The Iliad* indicates that physicians and/or surgeons routinely embarked on sea voyages in Ancient Greece as early as 800 BC.

During the era of Athenian sea power and Classical Greece (~480–322 BC), the primary warship was the light and maneuverable trireme, named after the staggered three tiers of oars that propelled it (Fig. 3.1) [1, 5, 6]. There are no known descriptions of specific Athenian naval surgeons, but as early as 431 BC. its fleet included the trireme *Therapeia* (Greek for "cure" or "heal"), which was perhaps a hospital ship as the Greeks named vessels for their purpose [7, 8]. The *Therapeia* may have been used during naval battles as a casualty-receiving ship to ferry the wounded to shore for definitive treatment.

As naval tactics included ramming and/or boarding enemy triremes [6], surgeons likely managed injuries from both blunt and penetrating trauma. Hippocrates (~460–377 BC) and his followers established Western medical tradition during this era of Athenian sea power. Hippocratic case studies and other writings give contemporary descriptions of medical conditions as well as wound care, traumatic injury, and surgical disease. Fistula-in-ano related to naval service is even described. The countless hours Athenian rowers spent seated on the wooden thwarts of triremes was listed as the cause [6, 9] and treatment included linen fistula plugs, powdered horn suppositories, myrrh applications, and the use of cutting setons to open the fistula [9, 10].

The Imperial Roman Navy (~27 BC to AD 180)

The Republic of Rome did not become an empire until it achieved maritime mastery of the Mediterranean [1, 11]. Established in 27 BC, the Roman navy peaked during the reign of Hadrian (AD 117–138). Hadrian's navy also left the first direct evidence of medical men at sea [12]. A tombstone in Naples, the home port of the Fleet of Misenum, bears the name of the Roman "M. Satrius Longinus, Medicus Duplicarius" of the trireme *Cupid* (c. 138) [12, 13]. **Medicus** or **medici** was the Roman term used for practitioners of military medical and surgical care [14–17]. Other tombstones suggest that the triremes *Faith* and *Tiger* had Greek **medici** as well. "Duplicarius" indicates that the medici received double pay for their naval service. However, for their Roman army counterparts, there is no evidence of double pay for these land lubbers! Perhaps this extra compensation existed to entice surgeons to sea, as it was less popular and more dangerous than army service [8, 12, 13, 16].

Aesculapius, part of the Misenum fleet, was also likely a hospital ship, as the Romans also named things based on their purpose [7, 8, 16]. Each Roman trireme was assigned a ship's surgeon for every 200 men [8, 12, 16]. There are no known details of specific operations performed by the Roman army and naval surgeons; however, archeologists have found contemporary surgical instruments, including scalpels, sounds (dilators), hooks, probes, retractors, speculums, bone forceps, bone saws, and the novel spoon of Diocels, designed to remove arrows [8, 17–19].

The Middle Ages (AD ~476–1453)

In the seventh century, Greek physician and surgeon Paul of Aegina (AD 625–690) gives written evidence of physicians going to sea [7]. His writings cover many aspects of surgery, including tracheotomy, hernia repair, drainage of hepatic abscesses, and subcutaneous mastectomy for gynecomastia [20]. He also urged physicians to bring textbooks with them when they travel to the desert, fields, and "… at sea on board of ships, where such diseases suddenly break out on us." Treatments for sea sickness, drowning after shipwrecks, and treating lice while embarked are also described [21]. Further evidence of embarked surgeons or physicians during the Middle Ages is the mention of **metge**, the Catalan word for physician or surgeon in the *Consolato Del Mare,* a medieval compendium of maritime Mediterranean law [12]. During the Crusades, particularly the Fifth Crusade, there is evidence of both physicians and surgeons going to sea and the vessels carrying them serving as hospital ships (1217–1221) [22]. Even in the Middle Ages, art reflected the realities of life and the dangers of sea travel. Francesco De Barberino's (1264–1348) Italian poem, "The Dangers of the Sea and How in part to Avoid them," recommends one should not embark on a sea voyage without a priest, barber, or doctor, but of these, it is the physician that would have "all things needful" [7, 8, 12].

During the Middle Ages, priests, monks, and other clergy members routinely practiced both medicine and surgery. However, because of gradual changes in Catholic papal policy between 1131 and 1237, this became forbidden, leading to the rise of barber-surgeons throughout Europe [23, 24]. Skilled in the use of sharp instruments–razors, scissors, and knives–they learned to perform surgical procedures, likely from experienced priests and monks [25, 26].

The first known ship's surgeon, though not a physician, was Master Gualtieri. Venetian archives from 1300 indicate that he treated many wounded on Venetian galleys and had a long career paid by the state [7, 27]. By the early 1300s sea-going barber-surgeons were common in the Republic of Venice. The Italian city-state required chaplains, physicians, and university-trained, licensed barber-surgeons to embark on galleys during war and trading expeditions. In 1322, the High Council of Venice decreed, "that one practitioner of medicine shall accompany those galleys for rendering service to the merchants and crews receiving the same salary as is customary for a surgeon" [16]. Assisted by "barbierotti," a precursor to the surgeon's mate, these Italian ship's surgeons were part of the captain's mess, well paid, and even participated in trading activities to make extra money with permission. Apparently serving as a sea-going barber-surgeon was a lucrative endeavor! Venetian vessels trading throughout Europe likely disseminated the idea of embarked barber-surgeons, and by 1512 barber-surgeons were common on English warships [8, 12, 25, 27, 28].

The Age of Discovery (~1450–1600)

Early European pan-global exploration of the seas caused catastrophic loss of life, largely from scurvy. Columbus' flotilla of exploration (1492–1497) carried embarked physicians. Vasco da Gama sailing around the Cape of Good Hope in 1497 had no personnel with medical training. Upon his return to Portugal, only 95 of the original 150 flagship personnel survived the voyage [2, 9]. However, Ferdinand Magellan's decision to bring surgeons on his 1519 circumnavigation of the globe did not improve his crew's chances of survival. He began the expedition with five ships and 265 men, including a surgeon and three barber-surgeon assistants. Unfortunately, only his flagship returned, with only 18 survivors; of the four medical providers in the expedition, only one barber-surgeon survived [8, 27]. Even a physician or surgeon aboard in this era did not prevent deaths from scurvy.

British Sea Power

Developments during the reign of King Henry VIII (1491–1547) not only impacted English naval dominance, but also naval medicine and surgery. Adopting the practices of Venetian warships, British surgeons had to be licensed after 1511. By 1512 the Royal Navy had a nascent medical service, and the terms "surgeon" and "surgeon's mate" were first introduced into naval service. In 1540 Henry VIII began refitting warships with two tiers of heavy guns, revolutionizing naval warfare and forever changing the types and severity of injuries seen by naval surgeons. This year also saw the Guild of Surgeons formally incorporated with the Company of Barbers.

The Royal Company of Barber-Surgeons would last over 200 years, finally splitting in 1745. This guild of professional surgeons would develop into today's Royal College of Surgeons [25, 28, 29].

The Father of Sea Surgery

Barber-surgeon John Woodall (1569–1643), though not a member of the Royal Navy, is known as the "Father of Sea Surgery." A contemporary of William Harvey, he was appointed the first Surgeon General of the British East India company in 1613. Like many barber-surgeons of the era, he started as an apothecary apprentice in the early 1600s. His textbook, *The Surgion's Mate*, published in 1617, aimed to standardize medical and surgical care at sea. Woodall described the instruments (Fig. 3.2) and medicines to include in the surgeon's chest and indications for their use. He also described scurvy and urged the use of citrus fruits to prevent and treat it, pre-dating both Captain James Cook and Royal Naval Surgeon James Lind by nearly 150 years! In 1633, Woodall, appointed Master of the Barber-Surgeons guild, inspected naval medical chests before warship deployments. Later, he trained and certified Royal Naval Surgeons. While Surgeon General, he also routinely cut hair [30–33]! By the early seventeenth century, Dutch, Spanish, Portuguese, French, and British navies had ship's surgeons in regular service. And, given the dangers of whaling, Dutch and German whaling ships also required embarked surgeons by 1610 [26, 27].

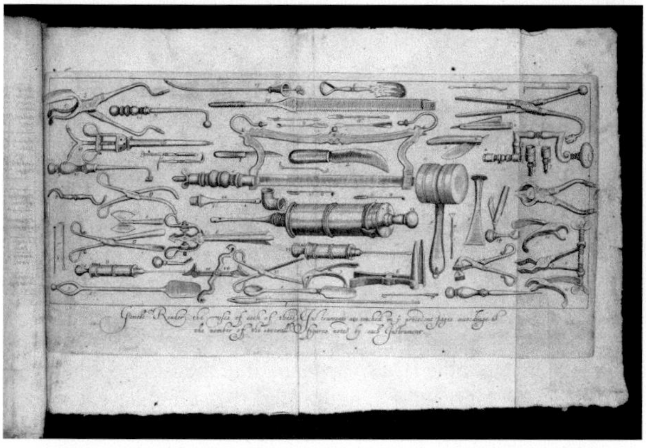

Fig. 3.2 Inventory of instruments required of naval and merchant ship surgeons. From the 1639 second edition of Woodall's *The Surgion's Mate* or "Military & Domestique Surgery: Discovering … ye method and order of ye Surgeons chest, ye uses of the Instruments, the vertues and Operations of ye medicines, with ye exact Cures of wounds…". (Source: Public domain image, not in copyright. Available at: https://wellcomecollection.org/works/scgbe675)

The Age of Sail (~1600–1850)

Naval tactics in the Age of Sail consisted of firing a "broadside" of cannon loaded with different types of shots, including cannon balls, chain shot, and grape shot (multiple small balls). Exploding bulwarks sent showers of splinters into the air, tearing into soft tissues. Round shot cut sailors in half, eviscerated abdomens, and shattered extremities. Hand-to-hand combat with cutlasses severed nerves, tendons, or arteries. Tomahawks sliced off cheeks and fractured skulls. Pikes and pistol shots caused penetrating torso injuries [29]. Even merchant or whaling ship work was dangerous. Sailors toppled from masts, tumbled through hatchways, or fell overboard. Diseases like dysentery, malaria, yellow fever, typhus, beriberi, and scurvy scuttled many crew members down to the often unsanitary and cramped sick bay [34]. "The tenure of a sailor's existence," observed one naval surgeon, "is certainly more precarious than any other man's" [35].

Surgical operations were usually performed in the cockpit (Fig. 3.3) or in the junior officers' quarters on the orlop deck below the waterline. In the ship's depths, the wounded were protected from enemy fire and surgeons lurched less in heavy seas, but right above the ship's hold, the cockpit reeked of bilge. Surgeons worked by the glow of lanterns swaying from beams overhead, further cramping a small

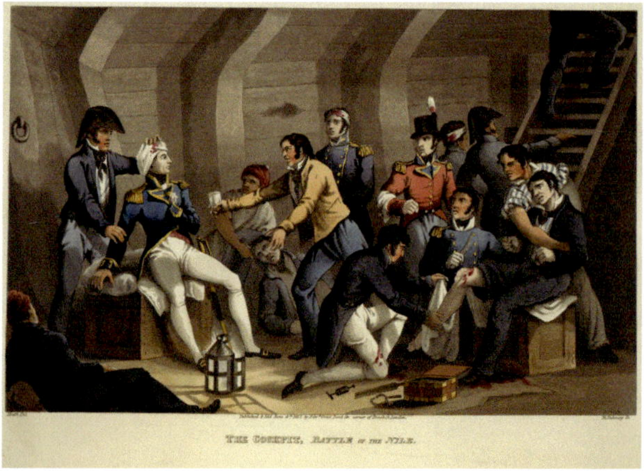

Fig. 3.3 Depiction of the cockpit of the HMS Vanguard after the 1798 Battle of the Nile. On the left is British hero Vice-Admiral Horatio Nelson. In the battle he suffered a full-thickness scalp laceration down to bone over his right eye. Also depicted is his prior left arm amputation that occurred after he was shot with a musket ball during another naval battle in 1797. On the right, the ship's surgeon is about to perform a right leg amputation with the patient seated, instead of supine. Performing surgery while the patient was seated was common during the Age of Sail. (Source: Public domain image, not in copyright. Source: Illustrated by M. Heath. Image taken from *Historic, military, and naval anecdotes of particular incidents which occurred to the armies of Great Britain and her allies in the Long-contested War, Terminating in the Battle of Waterloo* by Edward Orme. Available at: https://commons.wikimedia.org/wiki/File:The_Cockpit,_battle_of_the_Nile_-_Orme%27s_Historic,_military,_and_naval_anecdotes_(1819),_opposite_67_-_BL.jpg)

space [36]. As the ship went to quarters, surgeons prepared an operating platform by lashing a mess table to the deck. Injured sailors were tied to the operating table and gagged to muffle their screams [37]. Author, physician, and surgeon's mate on the HMS Cumberland, Tobias Smollet, describes shipboard patient care in his fictional 1748 novel, *Roderick Random*, "…I was much less surprised that people should die on board, than that any sick person should recover" [38].

Robert Young, serving on the HMS Ardent, described the care of patients after the Battle of Camperdown in 1797, "I was employed in operating and dressing till near four in the morning, the action beginning about one in the afternoon. So great was my fatigue that I began several amputations under a dread of sinking before I should have secured the blood vessels. Ninety wounded were brought down during the action, the whole cockpit, deck cabins, wing berths…were covered with them…. Melancholy cries for assistance were addressed to me from every side by wounded and dying and piteous moans and bewailing from pain and despair" [39]. There was no notion of triage [40] in this description of the cockpit at war during the Age of Sail; it appears the injured were treated on a first come, first served basis.

Without anesthesia, surgery under the Age of Sail was limited. Major abdominal or thoracic operations were unknown. Injured patients were often operated on in the sitting position (Fig. 3.3). Occasionally head injuries were trepanned [41]. Extremity amputation was the most common operation, done for a shattered, hemorrhaging limb [42]. After a tourniquet was applied, the amputation was performed in a "circular" fashion: the skin, subcutaneous tissues, and muscles were sliced in sweeping, concentric circles with a knife and the bone divided with a saw [7, 29, 43]. Even if patients survived an operation, without antisepsis, half of them later succumbed to postoperative sepsis [42]. Despite these less-than-ideal and by modern standards, beyond austere working conditions, skilled ship's surgeons saved lives at sea and have always been valued shipmates.

Notwithstanding these early descriptions of harrowing surgery at sea, the majority of personnel losses were not from injury. During the Napoleonic Wars with the French Republic (1792–1804) and the French Empire (1804–1805), Royal Navy losses at sea were estimated at approximately 100,000 fatalities, with only 6% from enemy action [44]. The majority of injuries from enemy action were from cannon shot or resultant debris (~60%). Other causes of injury included small arms fire (~20%) and burns and boarding injuries (~20%) [40].

The American Revolutionary War

In the weeks before the Second Continental Congress founded the United States (U.S.) Navy by voting to fund two warships on October 13, 1775, surgeons sailed around Boston on the armed schooners of General Washington's "ad-hoc" navy. However, skilled American surgeons and the sharp tools of their trade were in short supply. At the start of the war, wanted ads in New England area newspapers sought out "properly qualified" surgeons to embark on privateer vessels. In the months leading up to the October 1776 Battle of Valcour Island on Lake Champlain, General Benedict Arnold had difficulty finding surgical support for the 15-ship fleet he commanded. In a letter to General Horatio Gates, he is desperate for a surgeon **and** supplies: "I don't think it prudent to go without a Surgeon…the Surgeons Mate of Colonel Arthur St. Clair's Regiment has a good Box Medicines & will Incline to go with the Fleet, I wish he could be sent here, or someone who will answer to kill a man Secundum Artem. I Can procure a Case of Capital Instruments here,-nothing but the Surgeon & some few articles…prevents our proceeding…." While Arnold is in want of a surgeon, he wryly alludes to the limitations of contemporary surgical care, seeking a surgeon to kill a man "with skill" or "according to the art" (Secundum Artem). A few days later General Gates was able to deliver Stephen McCrea, "appointed First Surgeon to this Fleet under your Command. he has Instruments & Medicines, two things much in request with you" [45].

Much of American maritime and naval tradition was adopted from the British. Published and distributed to the fleet in early December 1775, the first printed document of U.S. Navy regulations, "Rules for the Regulation of the Navy of the United Colonies of North America," mostly the work of John Adams, was adapted or copied verbatim from similar Royal Navy documents. Adams listed the monthly pay for the ship's surgeon and the surgeon's mate, $21 1/3 and $13 1/3 per month, respectively. By comparison, the ship's captain was paid $32, lieutenants $20, and the carpenter $15 [46].

The Age of Steam and Iron (~1850–1915)

The American Civil War

By the beginning of the American Civil War in 1861, the Age of Sail in naval warfare was coming to an end. Union naval warships were hybrid steam and sail ships, with each successive class of warship having a diminished sailing profile. Ether and chloroform, anesthetics discovered back-to-back in the 1840s, had revolutionized surgery in the years before the Civil War. A staggering 80,000 operations are thought to have been performed under anesthesia between 1861 and 1865 [47]. Surgeons, of course, brought these anesthetics to the war at sea.

Three miles offshore from Cherbourg, France, after the battle between the USS Kearsarge and the CSS Alabama in 1864, USS Kearsarge surgeon John M. Browne performed an upper extremity amputation on an injured quarter gunner. "Chloroform was administered, with happy results" [48] Browne observed drily, performing perhaps the first surgical operation under anesthesia on an American warship at sea. Despite Browne's success, he had resorted to operating in the ship's fore-hold because the USS Kearsarge lacked adequate medical space for procedures. Converting non-medical spaces into operating rooms (ORs) was common, as the cockpit had been transformed for surgery in line-of-battle ships during the Age of

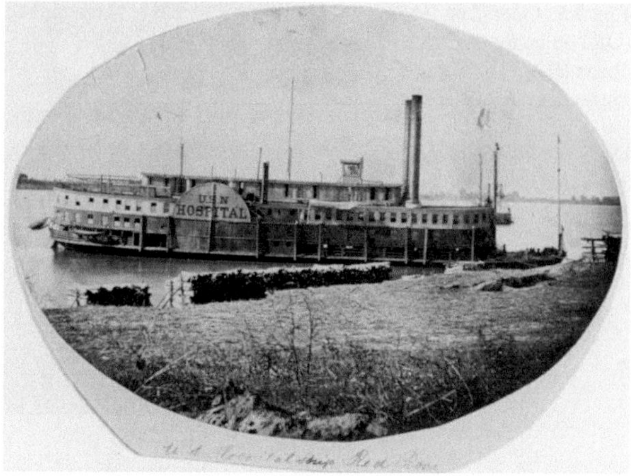

Fig. 3.4 The USS Red Rover (1862–1865) tied up on the Western Rivers during the Civil War. (Source: U.S. Naval History and Heritage Command Photograph. Government publication, not in copyright. Available at: https://www.history.navy.mil/content/history/nhhc/our-collections/photography/numerical-list-of-images/nhhc-series/nh-series/NH-59000/NH-59653.html)

Sail. However, designated space for surgical operations afloat had already been built on at least one ship in the U.S. Navy.

The USS Red Rover (Fig. 3.4), a captured Confederate barracks ship, was refitted as the U.S. Navy's first hospital ship in 1862. "Bathrooms, laundry, [an] elevator for the sick from the lower to the upper deck, [and an] amputating room" were installed [49]. Surgery of the era evidently included little more than extremity amputations. Serving in the western flotilla on the Mississippi River and its tributaries, the USS Red Rover was staffed by medical officers and "a regular corps of nurses," comprised entirely of men. But a few months after her launch, the Sisters of the Holy Cross offered to care for the USS Red Rover's wounded, becoming the first women to serve aboard a U.S. Navy ship. By the war's end, the USS Red Rover had evacuated and treated 2947 injured Soldiers and Sailors [50].

Battleships and Blood Transfusions

As steam replaced sails and the cockpit became the engine room, naval surgeons were often left to treat casualties in the wardroom, usually above the waterline and exposed to enemy fire. But after battleship broadsides had obliterated wardrooms, killing or wounding everyone inside, navies worldwide recognized the need for protected medical spaces. By 1906, following Russia's lead, the U.S. Navy installed its first Battle Dressing Station (BDS) behind armor. In the BDS, medical officers and enlisted personnel triaged and applied first-aid to wounded Sailors [22].

Additional protected medical spaces were soon added to the fleet. Battleships boasted a sick bay, isolation ward, pharmacy, radiography, and an OR. The OR housed all the recent advances in surgery: electric lighting, adjustable operating table, surgical scrub area, ventilation, and autoclave to sterilize surgical instruments (Fig. 3.5) [51]. At the same time, advances in antisepsis and pathology had expanded

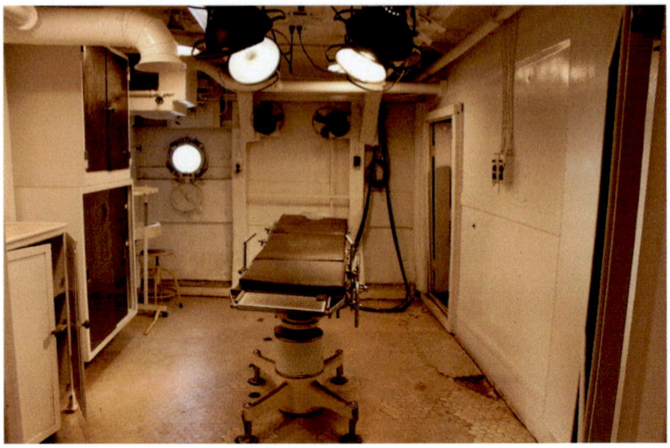

Fig. 3.5 Operating Room (OR) on board the USS Texas (BB-35). (Source: Photo courtesy of Texas Parks and Wildlife Department—Battleship Texas Archives)

surgery. Procedures once thought unnecessary or impossible (like abdominal operations) were pioneered, paving the way for advances in surgery at sea.

As early as 1909, Ship's Surgeon W. S. Pugh performed a nephrectomy on board the cruiser USS Tacoma (CL-20) in Port Limon, Costa Rica, on a Sailor who had been stabbed in the flank. Months later, while the USS Tacoma (CL-20) was off the coast of Nicaragua, another Sailor developed appendicitis. Using ether anesthesia, Pugh performed a 10 minute appendectomy through a 1 ¼-inch incision [52].

Pugh's practice of administering his own anesthesia at sea was common. In fact, anesthesia at sea had changed little since the Civil War. Few ships carried trained anesthetists, thus leaving the management of anesthesia up to the surgeon. Drop ether, spinal anesthesia, or intravenous sodium thiopental were anesthetic options underway. For amputations, some surgeons preferred a tourniquet and limb cooling with refrigeration anesthesia. A petty officer often assisted the surgeon by evaluating the color, breathing, and pulse of the patient under anesthesia [22]. Assessing vital signs this way was also useful for treating patients in hemorrhagic shock.

During exercises off New England in 1910 on the battleship USS South Carolina (BB-26), a Sailor's arm was caught in an ammunition car and severed at the shoulder. Surgeon R. B. Williams ligated the bleeding axillary vessels and upon feeling the wan Sailor's pulse race to 140 beats per minute, decided to attempt a blood transfusion. A shipmate's radial artery was cannulated and whole blood transfused through a rubber catheter into the injured Sailor's antecubital vein. After 42 min of transfusion, "all symptoms of shock had disappeared." The patient and donor went on to make a full recovery [53]. By World War I, injuries at sea with hematocrit less than 25% were routinely treated with whole-blood transfusion [22].

However, advances in resuscitation and surgery, could not fully prepare medical personnel for the devastating naval warfare of World War I. At the Battle of Jutland in 1916, German shells ignited improperly stowed cordite in British gun turrets, spreading fire through the ships. Over 6000 British sailors perished in a single engagement, more than 10% of the entire fleet's force. Many drowned. Most who survived suffered severe burns. In caring for these sailors, naval surgeons left some of the earliest descriptions of inhalation injuries, resuscitated burn victims with intravenous fluids, and pioneered skin grafting for burn injuries, a rare instance of naval medicine advancing surgery [22, 54, 55].

World War II (1939–1945)

The years preceding World War II had propelled surgery closer to the modern era. Surgical training was standardized, specialized, and included curricula on trauma surgery and wound care. U.S. Navy surgeons, nurses, and enlisted medical personnel on board hospitals and warships in European and Pacific theaters brought advances in surgery to the battle's front lines [56, 57]. The current U.S. Navy concept of a forward Expeditionary Resuscitative Surgical System (ERSS) described in Chap. 1 is nothing new. During World War II, surgeons were routinely deployed on destroyers without formal ORs. After assembling an operating table, they performed procedures and administered their own anesthesia in the wardroom or sick bay. In rough seas, surgeons sometimes strapped themselves to the operating table using a specially made belt (Fig. 3.6) [58–60]!

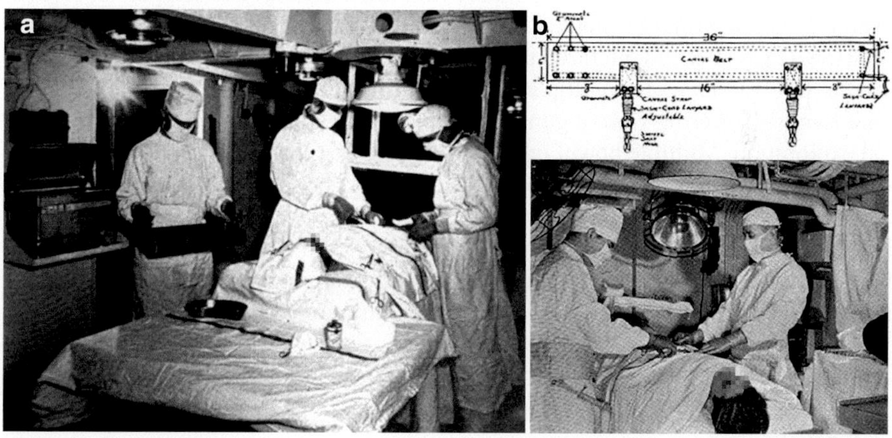

Fig. 3.6 (**a**) Major surgery is being performed on board the USS Boyle (DD-600) in the wardroom using a custom-made table designed specifically for use in the wardrooms of destroyers during World War II [58]. (**b**) Operative setup of the sickbay on board a destroyer. Note the surgeon is secured to the operating table using a specially designed canvas belt (top of figure) [59]. (Source: Government publication, not in copyright)

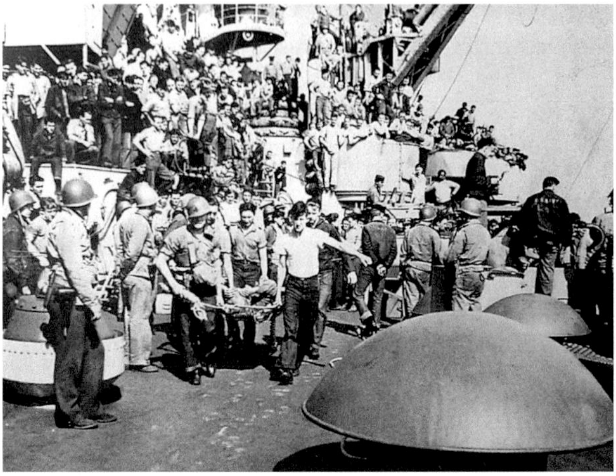

Fig. 3.7 Wounded Rangers brought aboard the USS Texas (BB-35). (Source: Photo courtesy of Texas Parks and Wildlife Department—Battleship Texas Archives)

Normandy

In the gray predawn of June 6, 1944, 14-inch guns on the battleship USS Texas (BB-35) opened up on German artillery positions atop the cliffs of Pointe du Hoc on Normandy's coast. Two hours later, the second U.S. Army Ranger Battalion staggered ashore at the foot of Pointe du Hoc on a ribbon of beach at low tide and scaled its 100-foot cliffs under withering enemy fire. The next day, two Higgins boats sent ashore returned with 34 wounded Rangers and 28 Prisoners of War to be triaged on the USS Texas (BB-35), pictured in Fig. 3.7 [61]. Many were critically injured, so a second OR was set up for multiple operations to be performed simultaneously [62]. One Ranger, suffering from a gunshot wound to the abdomen, underwent abdominal exploration. Multiple bowel injuries were found and he could not be saved, succumbing later to peritonitis and shock. Other Rangers underwent wound debridement and shell fragment extraction and were later transferred to a hospital ship bound for England [63]. The second Ranger Battalion found and destroyed the German battery on Pointe du Hoc, but at a terrible cost–after 2 days of combat, nearly two-thirds of the battalion were killed, wounded, or missing in action [64].

Iwo Jima

The U.S. Navy's "scoop-and-sail" tactic, used during early amphibious invasions in the Pacific, aimed to provide surgical care to wounded Marines within 12 h [65]. Casualties at the beachhead were triaged and loaded into empty Landing Ships, Tank (LSTs) that had dumped their materiel and troops ashore. Once aboard the LSTs (Fig. 3.8), casualties were re-triaged and moved to ships with surgical

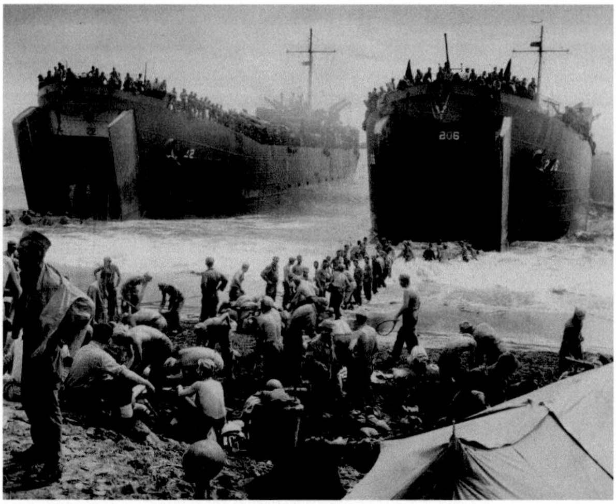

Fig. 3.8 Landing Ship, Tank (LST) unloading cargo onto the beach. They were built during World War II to support amphibious operations–able to land vehicles, cargo, and troops directly onto the shore. During the amphibious assault at Iwo Jima in 1945, four LSTs were augmented with surgical teams. (Source: Government publication, not in copyright. Available at: https://www.archives.gov/files/research/military/ww2/photos/images/ww2-151.jpg)

capabilities if needed. This cumbersome process led to delays in care, so some of the LSTs were augmented with surgical teams or four surgeons and 27 pharmacist mates (modern-day rate equivalent to hospital corpsmen), providing surgical care nearer to the point of injury [57, 60]. Four of these Hospital Landing Ships, Tank, or LST(H)s, floated offshore from Iwo Jima in February 1945, ready to receive casualties from ambulance boats leaving the invasion beachhead [57, 65].

27 min after the first Marines landed on Iwo Jima, casualties began arriving alongside the USS LST(H)-931 (many ships in this class were not formally named) [66]. During a 6½-h period on D-Day, from 9:00 AM to 3:30 PM, 2230 casualties were evacuated to the LST(H)s, the equivalent of six casualties per minute [67]. On board the LST(H)s, BDS resuscitation teams administered tetanus shots, sulfa antibiotics, and whole blood from the ship's "walking blood bank"[57]. The LST(H) surgeons operated around the clock, performing extremity amputations and exploratory laparotomies for penetrating abdominal injuries. By the time mobile surgical units were established ashore on D-Day plus nine, over 2000 casualties had been treated on board the USS LST(H)-931 [66].

The hospital ship USS Solace (AH-5), standing further out to sea, received casualties just 45 min after the initial assault. Next day, she was at full capacity and en route to Saipan. The USS Solace (AH-5) made two more trips back to Iwo Jima, eventually evacuating 2000 casualties. After Iwo Jima, hospital ships were brought even closer to the invasion beachhead to provide earlier definitive surgical care, a practice that would continue during the Korean War, Vietnam War, and the first Gulf War in 1991 [65].

Korean (1950–1953) and Vietnam (1955–1975) Wars

Four World War II–era hospital ships, taken out of mothballs, modernized, and equipped with contemporary medical equipment, provided support during the Korean War. Afloat off Korea, the USS Consolation (AH-15) was the first hospital ship ever to receive casualties via rotary wing aircraft, a routine practice during the Vietnam War. Faster evacuation times made possible by helicopters resulted in improved casualty survival in Korea and Vietnam. Even casualties with devastating vascular injuries, if quickly evacuated from the battlefield, were candidates for surgical repair.

Before the Korean War, vascular injuries were nearly always ligated, though this often resulted in extremity amputation or death. But surgeons operating in mobile hospitals in Korea pioneered successful vascular repair techniques in combat zones. By the Vietnam War, surgeons downrange were performing autogenous vein grafting, end-to-end anastomosis, and thrombectomy [68].

While on patrol in Quang Ngãi, Vietnam, in August 1969, a Marine private first-class was injured by a mine, suffering multiple penetrating extremity wounds. He was immediately evacuated by helicopter to the USS Valley Forge (CV-45), an amphibious assault ship. On board the ship, C.E. Cassidy, surgeon of Surgical Team Bravo, noted several fragment wounds to the Marine's arms and legs, including a "large… through and through" penetrating wound of the left thigh and no distal pulses. Immediately whisked to the OR, the Marine was found to have a "contusion and obstruction" of the left superficial femoral artery. Cassidy quickly ligated and resected the injured artery, and then bypassed the injury with a 10 cm ipsilateral saphenous vein graft, the first and only description of successful vein grafting or vascular anastomosis performed at sea. The Marine made a complete recovery and was later fit for full duty [69].

Women Surgeons at Sea

Much of maritime and medical history omits women by nature because they were excluded from participating in the military and medicine. In the 1700s while some "doctoresses" had unofficial shore-based practices, there were too many barriers for women to not only get a formal medical education but to purchase tools and secure a job on a ship all while hiding her sex. Additionally, society viewed the few female nurses formally employed by hospital ships negatively. Therefore, women at sea had their start in maritime medicine as unpaid volunteer "incorporated wives." Often these women would assist male surgeons in managing patients after traumatic injury or in a nursing capacity performing dressing changes. During the Napoleonic Wars at the 1798 Battle of the Nile, Nelly Giles assisted the ship's surgeon of the HMS Bellerophon in caring for 201 casualties, all while in her third trimester [70]!

In the Crimean Wars of 1853–1856, the professionalization of nursing led to the demise of the negative views of female nurses. In 1901–1902, Queen Alexandra's Royal Naval Nursing Service began, and in 1908 the U.S. Navy formed the Navy Nurse Corps [70].

In the 1800s, it was not uncommon for naval officers or the captains of merchant vessels to bring their wives and sometimes daughters to sea. American Captain Almon Stickney of the *Cicero* brought his wife, Mary, during the whaler's 1880–1881 cruise. With a parrot perched atop her shoulder, it was Mary Stickney who managed all patients with traumatic injuries and documented their care in her diary, including an ax to the foot and a gaff hook to the leg [26, 71].

Dr. Elizabeth Ross was the first woman to officially serve as a civilian ship surgeon on the voyage of the *Glenlogan* to Yokohama and Hong Kong in 1913. Dr. A. Nancy Miller was the first woman to officially serve as a civilian physician in a military capacity on the merchant ship *Britannia.* During World War II, serving as an armed troopship, the *Britannia* was fatally shelled en route to Karachi in 1941. Luckily, Dr. Miller survived and cared for many of the wounded. Despite having equal credentials to their fellow Glasgow University graduates, both of these women only had the opportunity to serve in these roles because of a lack of available male providers [70].

In 1993, U.S. Congress repealed Title 10 USC 6015 allowing women to serve on combatant vessels [72]. However, it was not until 1997, shortly after completing her general surgery residency that Dr. Beth Jaklic checked onto the USS George Washington (CVN-73) as the first female Ship's Surgeon in U.S Navy history.

These women overcame not only the barriers of a male-dominated surgical profession but also held the vital leadership role of Ship's Surgeon in the male-dominated seafaring world, opening the doors for women to follow. Less than three decades since Dr. Jaklic's tour, a woman leading the surgical team aboard a U.S. Navy ship has become routine. Since 2006, greater than 20% of the billets for surgeons on U.S. aircraft carriers and Fleet Surgical Teams (FSTs) have been filled by women.

Conclusion

Surgery at sea has come a long way since Homer's warrior surgeon Machaon provided basic traumatic wound care during the amphibious assault at Troy and the gruesome cockpit surgery performed during the Age of Sail. Today's surgical teams embarked on U.S. Navy warships can provide rapid, mobile, expeditionary damage control resuscitation and surgery anywhere in the world. Surgery and combat casualty care will surely evolve, and as they do, intrepid maritime surgical teams and Ship's Surgeons will persist in pioneering surgical and resuscitative advances at sea.

Declaration of Interest The views expressed in this chapter are those of the authors and do not necessarily reflect the official policy or position of the Department of the Navy, Department of Defense, nor the US Government.

Funding This research did not receive any specific grant from funding agencies in the public, commercial, or not-for-profit sectors.

Conflict of Interest Statement The authors declare no conflict of interest.

References

1. Paine LP. The sea and civilization: a maritime history of the world. 1st ed. New York: Alfred A. Knopf; 2013.
2. Galanakos SP, Bot AG, Macheras GA. Pelvic and lower extremity injuries in Homer's Iliad: a review of the literature. J Trauma Acute Care Surg. 2015;78(1):204–8.
3. Koutserimpas C, Samonis G. Machaon: the first trauma surgeon in Western history? J Wound Care. 2018;27(10):659–61.
4. Filippou D, Tsoucalas G, Panagouli E, Thomaidis V, Fiska A. Machaon, son of Asclepius, the father of surgery. Cureus. 2020;12(2):e7038.
5. Pryor JH, Jeffreys E. The age of the dromōn: the Byzantine navy ca. 500–1204. Leiden: Brill; 2011.
6. Hale JR. Lords of the sea: the epic story of the Athenian navy and the birth of democracy. New York: Viking; 2009.
7. Taylor JS. Military and naval medical men in Roman and medieval times. Mil Surg. 1917;40:589–94.
8. Roddis LH. A short history of nautical medicine. New York: P. B. Hoeber; 1941.
9. Hippocrates AF. The genuine works of Hippocrates. London: Printed for the Sydenham Society; 1849.
10. Soliman F, Sturgeon G, Hargest R. Revisiting an ancient treatment for transphincteric fistula-in-ano 'There is nothing new under the sun' Ecclesiastes 1v9. J R Soc Med. 2015;108(12):482–9.
11. Stavridis J. Sea power: the history and geopolitics of the world's oceans. New York: Penguin Press; 2017.
12. Mann WL. The origin and early development of naval medicine. US Nav Inst Proc. 1929;55(9):772–82.
13. Simpson JY. Was the Roman army provided with medical officers? Edinburg: Sutherland and Knox; 1856.
14. Milne J. Surgical instruments in Greek and Roman times. Oxford: Clarendon Press; 1907.
15. Bliquez LJ. The tools of Asclepius: surgical instruments in Greek and Roman times. Leiden: Brill; 2015.
16. Taylor JS. A retrospect of naval and military medicine. US Nav Med Bull. 1921;15(15):561–626.
17. Brocke T, Barr J. The history of wound healing. Surg Clin North Am. 2020;100(4):787–806.
18. Brill JB, Harrison EK, Sise MJ, Ignacio RC. The history of the scalpel: from flint to zirconium-coated steel. Bull Am Coll Surg. 2018;103(2):34–8.
19. Kosmidis IA, Katonis P, Bisbinas I, Trompoukis C. Orthopedic medical instruments: from antiquity to modern times--a historical essay. J Trauma Acute Care Surg. 2013;74(2):692–8.
20. Gurunluoglu R, Gurunluoglu A. Paul of Aegina: landmark in surgical progress. World J Surg. 2003;27(1):18–25.
21. Adams F. The seven books of Paulus Aegineta. Translated from Greek. With a commentary embracing a complete view of the knowledge possessed by the Greeks, Romans, and Arabians

on all subjects connected with medicine and surgery, in three volumes. London: Sydenham Society; 1844-1847.
22. Mann WL. Medical tactics in naval warfare. US Nav Med Bull. 1926;24(2):1–94.
23. Amundsen DW. Medieval Cannon law on medical and surgical practice by the clergy. Bull Hist Med. 1978;52(1):22–44.
24. Mitchell PD. Medicine in the crusades: warfare, wounds, and the medieval surgeon. New York: Cambridge University Press; 2004.
25. Robinson JO. The barber-surgeons of London. Arch Surg. 1984;119(10):1171–5.
26. Druett J. Rough medicine: surgeons at sea in the age of sail. New York: Routledge; 2000.
27. Goethe H, Watson EN, Jones DT. Handbook of nautical medicine. Berlin: Springer; 1984.
28. Dobson J. Barber into surgeon. Ann R Coll Surg Engl. 1974;54(2):84–91.
29. Watt J. The injuries of four centuries of naval warfare. Ann R Coll Surg Engl. 1975;57(1):3–24.
30. Woodall J, Müller I. The surgions mate: the first compendium on naval medicine, surgery and drug therapy (London 1617). In: Edited and Annotated by Irmgard Müller. Classic texts in the sciences. 1st edn. Cham: Springer: Imprint: Birkhäuser; 2016. p. 1. (online resource (VI, 343 pages 152 illustrations, 48 illustrations in color).
31. Watt J. The surgery of sea warfare from the galley to the nuclear age. Trans Med Soc Lond. 1980;97:1–15.
32. Longfield-Jones GM. John Woodall, surgeon general of the East India company. Part I: events leading to Woodall's appointment. J Med Biogr. 1995;3(1):11–9.
33. Longfield-Jones GM, Woodall J. Surgeon general of the East India company. Part II: a consideration of the provision made for treating injuries and diseases at sea. J Med Biogr. 1995;3(2):71–8.
34. Brown K. Poxed and scurvied: the story of sickness and health at sea. Annapolis: Naval Institute Press; 2011.
35. Evans A. Journal kept on board the United States frigate constitution, 1812. Penn Mag Hist Biogr. 1895;19(2):152–69.
36. Sobocinski A. Under the lantern light: navy medicine in the war of 1812. Grog. 2012;7(3):4–7.
37. Estes JW. Naval surgeon: life and death at sea in the age of sail. Canton: Science History Publications; 1998.
38. Smollett T, Blewett D. Roderick random. London: Penguin Books; 1995.
39. Watt J. The burns of seafarers under oars, sail and steam. Injury. 1980;12(1):69–81.
40. Crumplin MK. The death of an admiral--surgery and medicine in Nelson's Navy. J R Nav Med Serv. 2012;98(1):48–53.
41. Fredriksen JC. Surgeon of the lakes: the diary of Dr. Usher Parsons, 1812–1814. Erie: Erie County Historical Society; 2000.
42. Langley HD. A history of medicine in the early U.S. Navy. Baltimore: Johns Hopkins University Press; 1995.
43. Plain JJ. Concise, practical remarks on the treatment of wounds and fractures. New York: John Holt; 1775.
44. Haycock DB, Archer S. Health and medicine at sea, 1700–1900. Woodbridge: Boydell Press; 2009.
45. Gordon MB. Naval and maritime medicine during the American revolution. Ventnor: Ventnor Publishers; 1978.
46. United States. Continental congress. Rules for the regulation of the navy of the united colonies of North America. Washington, DC: Naval Historical Foundation, Inc.; 1944.
47. Cutter L, Clarke T Jr. Anesthesia advances during the civil war. Mil Med. 2014;179(12):1503.
48. Browne J. Report of Surgeon Browne, U.S. Navy, U.S.S. Kearsarge, regarding the treatment of those wounded in the engagement between that vessel and the C.S.S. Alabama, July 23, 1864. Official Records of the Union and Confederate Navies in the war of the rebellion (ORN), vol. 1, no. 3; 1864. p. 69–71.
49. Wise G. Letter from Quartermaster Wise, U.S. Army, to Flag-Officer Foote, U.S. Navy describing the new hospital boat Red Rover. ORN. 1862;1(23):153–4.

50. Adams W. Red Rover: first hospital ship of the U.S. Navy. Proc US Nav Inst. 1968;94(11):789.
51. Power HI. Battleship Texas. College Station: Texas A&M University Press; 1993.
52. Pugh WS Jr. Report of surgical cases from the USS Tacoma. US Nav Med Bull. 1910;4(2):171–80.
53. Williams RB. Direct transfusion of blood in a case of shock and hemorrhage. US Nav Med Bull. 1910;4(3):372–5.
54. Watt J. Some forgotten contributions of naval surgeons. J R Soc Med. 1985;78(9):753–62.
55. Wallace AF. The influence of the Battle of Jutland on plastic surgery. Clin Plast Surg. 1983;10(4):657–63.
56. Nahrwold DL, Kernahan PJ. A century of surgeons and surgery: the American College of Surgeons 1913–2012. Chicago: American College of Surgeons; 2012.
57. Falciola V, Waisel DB. Surgical and anesthetic challenges aboard non-hospital ships in the Pacific during world war II. J Anesth Hist. 2018;4(4):214–21.
58. Mrazek C. Wardroom operating table for destroyers. US Nav Med Bull. 1944;43(5):1044–6.
59. Tomlinson WL. Problems in surgery on a destroyer. US Nav Med Bull. 1945;45(5):977–81.
60. Tadlock MD, Gurney J, Tripp MS, et al. Between the devil and the deep blue sea: a review of 25 modern naval mass casualty incidents with implications for future distributed maritime operations. J Trauma Acute Care Surg. 2021;91(2S Suppl 2):S46–55.
61. USS Texas: War Diary, June 1-30, 1944. Office of Naval Records and Library (RG 38). College Park: National Archives and Records Administration; 1994.
62. Interview with CAPT (ret.) James A Naismith. Conducted by Tom Holland, October 8, 2000. 2000 battleship Texas crew Reunion. Texas Parks and Wildlife Department - Battleship Texas Archives; 2000.
63. USS Texas: Historical Account of Medical Department Activities during World War II. December 1, 1945. Washington, DC: Bureau of Medicine and Surgery, Department of the Navy; 1945.
64. Lane RL, Mäkelä R. Rudder's rangers. 1st ed. Manassas: Ranger Associates; 1979.
65. Lane DA. Hospital ship doctrine in the United States navy: the Halsey effect on scoop- and-sail tactics. Mil Med. 1997;162(6):388–95.
66. USS LST-931: General Action Report, Iwo Jima, Nanpo Shoto, 22 March 1945, and War Diary, February 1945. College Park: Office of Naval Records and Library (RG 38), NARA; 1945.
67. Schwartz JL. Experiences in battle of the Medical Department of the Navy. In: The history of the Medical Department of the United States Navy in world war II, vol. I. Washington, DC: United States Government Printing Office; 1953. p. 63–132.
68. Rich NM, Baugh JH, Hughes CW. Acute arterial injuries in Vietnam: 1,000 cases. J Trauma. 1970;10(5):359–69.
69. Vietnam Vascular Registry. Records, privacy and declassification Division of the Office of the Secretary of Defense, Washington, DC; 2 Aug 1969.
70. Stanley J. From cabin 'Boys' to captains: 250 years of women at sea. Stroud: The History Press; 2016.
71. New Bedford whaling museum research library Mss 95. Sub-group 2: Mary J. Stickney Papers, 1858-1880 [1 volume].
72. Marra J, O'Sullivan S, Burger S. Women in the Navy Medical Corps. https://mccareer.org/2021/01/28/throwback-thursday-classic-post-women-in-the-navy-medical-corps/. Accessed 15 Oct 2020.

Chapter 4
Mechanisms of Injury During Modern Naval Operations

Matthew C. Vasquez, Diego A. Vicente, and Matthew D. Tadlock

Naval combat offered nowhere to run, no foxholes to dive into.

The Last Stand of the Tin Can Sailors, 2004, James D. Hornfischer

Author deployment experience	
Matthew C. Vasquez	Staff Surgeon, Fleet Surgical Team-3, embarked on the USS Essex (LHD-2) with Amphibious Ready Group/13th Marine Expeditionary Unit, WESTPAC, Fifth Fleet Area of Responsibility, 2018–2019
Diego A. Vicente	Ship's Surgeon, USS Harry S. Truman (CVN-75), Operation Inherent Resolve, AFRICOM Area of Responsibility, 2015–2016
	Officer in Charge, Role 2 Light Maneuver team, embarked on the USS Hershel "Woody" Williams (ESB-4), 2020; Provided embarked Role 2 Surgical Support, AFRICOM Area of Responsibility, 2020
Matthew D. Tadlock	Flight Surgeon, Carrier Air Wing Three (CVW-3), embarked on the USS Harry S. Truman (CVN-75) in support of Operation Iraqi Freedom, Fifth Fleet Area of Responsibility, 2004–2005; supporting Humanitarian Aid Disaster Relief (HADR) operations following Hurricane Katrina, 2005
	Resident Surgeon, USNS Mercy (T-AH-19), Pacific Partnership, Micronesia and Papua New Guinea, 2008
	Ship's Surgeon, USS Carl Vinson (CVN-70), WESTPAC, INDOPACOM Area of Responsibility, 2011–2012
	Officer in Charge, Forward Resuscitative Surgical System/Shock Trauma Platoon, Charlie Surgical Company, Native Fury, CENTCOM Area of Responsibility, 2016
	Chief of Trauma, NATO Role 3 Multinational Medical Unit, NATO Resolute Support and Operation Freedom's Sentinel, Kandahar Airfield, Afghanistan, 2017–2018
	Staff Surgeon, Expeditionary Resuscitative Surgical System Pacific, 2019–2020; Provided embarked Role 2 Surgical Support, INDOPACOM Area of Responsibility, 2020

M. C. Vasquez (✉) · D. A. Vicente · M. D. Tadlock
Department of Surgery, Naval Medical Center San Diego, San Diego, CA, USA
e-mail: matthew.c.vasquez.mil@health.mil; diego.a.vicente.mil@health.mil; matthewtadlockmd@gmail.com

M. D. Tadlock, A. A. Hernandez (eds.), *Expeditionary Surgery at Sea*,
https://doi.org/10.1007/978-3-031-21893-4_4

BLUF (Bottom Line Up Front)

1. The shipboard and flight deck environments are potentially dangerous. Be prepared for a wide variety of injury patterns.
2. The most common non-fatal injuries during routine operations are extremity injuries, particularly to the hands and fingers.
3. The most common fatal mishaps are "man overboard" and drowning events.
4. Though they are not common, collisions and combat-related mishaps can significantly damage hull integrity and cause mass casualty incidents (MCIs).
5. Flight deck mishaps are uncommon, but a wide variety of injuries can occur from both flight deck equipment and aircraft during mishaps and MCIs.
6. Independent Duty Corpsmen (IDC) are a critical link in the maritime trauma system and should be trained and mentored appropriately.
7. While rare, electrocution injuries are almost universally fatal.
8. Aircraft ejection, though designed to save aircrew lives, can cause significant internal and external injuries.
9. In modern naval warfare and during routine operations, common injury patterns include burn and inhalation injuries, traumatic brain injury (TBI), long bone fractures, hypothermia, drowning, and aspiration injuries.

Introduction

Over the past 50 years, there have only been six combat-related shipboard trauma events causing injury or death (77 injuries, 57 fatalities) (Table 4.1). The most recent of these, occurred in October 2000 when the USS Cole (DDG-67) was attacked by

Table 4.1 Known attacks on United States (U.S.) Navy Vessels, 1970–2020

Year	Ship	Mechanism	Estimated complement	Injured (%)	Fatal (%)
1972	USS Goldsborough (DDG-20)	Coastal Artillery Fire	354	2 (0.56)	3 (0.8)
1987	USS Stark (FFG-31)	Air Missile Attack	220	21 (9.5)	37 (16.8)
1988	USS Samuel B. Roberts (FFG-58)	Naval Mine	205	10 (4.9)	0
1991	USS Princeton (CG-59)	Naval Mine	330	3 (0.9)	0
1991	USS Tripoli (LPH-10)	Naval Mine	2358	4 (0.17)	0
2000	USS Cole (DDG-67)	Bomb/explosion	338	37 (10.9)	17 (5)
		Totals	3805	77 (2)	57 (1.5)

DDG destroyer, *FFG* frigate, guided missile, *CG* cruiser, *LPH* landing platform helicopter

a suicide bomber resulting in 47 injuries and 17 fatalities. The modern at sea surgeon should always be prepared for combat-related trauma, but it is important to recognize that even without naval warfare, the shipboard environment is potentially dangerous. Routine exercises, training missions, and even daily shipboard life can result in serious injuries and death. This chapter reviews shipboard and flight deck injuries occurring during routine operations as identified from Naval Safety Command data from 1970 to 2020 as well as injuries that can occur during modern naval warfare [1].

Non-flight Deck Injuries

A ship is a high-risk environment with millions of moving pieces and thousands of doors, hatches, and other locations that may cause injury to Sailors and Marines. Over the past 50 years, there have been 772 non-flight deck-related mishaps resulting in 1283 injuries and 803 fatalities [1]. **The most common mishap has been some type of extremity injury including amputations, crush injuries, or lacerations.** Of the 165 reported extremity injuries, the vast majority were soft tissue and orthopedic injuries and included digit (85%), foot (5%), and hand injuries (4%). Management of these injuries requires a basic understanding of both the principles of hand anatomy and injury management (Chap. 19) as well as damage control orthopedics (Chap. 24).

The most common event associated with mortality was drowning- or water-related injuries from personnel lost at sea or "man overboard" events. Anyone who has been out to sea for at least 24 h has undoubtedly experienced a "man overboard" drill for good reason. Since 1970, there have been 216 "man overboard" or drowning-related mishaps involving 435 personnel resulting in 115 injuries and 260 fatalities. This accounts for 28% of all identified mishaps and 32% of the fatalities [1]. The shipboard surgical team and medical department should be prepared to deal with drowning (Chap. 27), aspiration, and hypothermia (Chap. 28).

While they do not make up a large number of mishaps, ship collisions can cause profound damage to naval warships resulting in a significant number of injuries and fatalities. Not accounted for in the Naval Safety Command data are the civilian injuries and fatalities that have occurred aboard civilian vessels collaborating with naval forces, Military Sealift Command, or civilian commercial vessels involved in collisions with naval vessels. The recent 2017 collisions of the USS Fitzgerald (DDG-62) and the USS John S. McCain (DDG-56) with civilian commercial ships demonstrate the potentially devastating impact of collisions to both the ship and its crew. Both of these collisions resulted in significant holes below the waterline; ten Sailors died from drowning on the USS John S. McCain (DDG-56) and seven died from drowning on the USS Fitzgerald (DDG-62). In these two collisions, 51 total Sailors were injured. Three of the injured from the USS Fitzgerald (DDG-62) collision suffered some type of traumatic brain injury (TBI). Other injuries among survivors of these two events included seawater or fuel aspiration, extremity fractures, soft tissue lacerations, and chemical burns [2]. Fires can also occur after collisions. In 1989, the USS Kinkaid (DD-965) collided with a civilian vessel causing a berthing area to be flooded with seawater and a fire to break out in the starboard torpedo magazine [2]. Overall, there have been 14 at-sea collisions involving surface ships or submarines resulting in 164 injuries and 111 fatalities. Of these collisions involved ships with Role 1 medical departments led by Independent Duty Corpsmen (IDCs) performing the initial triage and care of these patients. There was no embarked surgical capability at the time of these mishaps, highlighting the importance of IDCs within the maritime trauma system and the crucial need for them to be well-trained, including ongoing clinical sustainment experiences relevant to injuries encountered in the deployed maritime environment.

Despite the proper check/tag-out requirements for working on energized circuits and equipment, electrocution injuries can still occur. These injuries can result in burns, ventricular fibrillation, and cardiac arrest. While most Sailors are not likely to report a minor shock, major electrocution injuries have occurred 32 times since 1970 and are usually fatal. Of the 32 recorded mishaps, there were 29 (91%) fatalities [1].

Depending on the type of naval warship, there are many types of industrial equipment and machinery aboard, including chains, heavy ropes, steel plates, forklifts, cranes, and smaller boats. Smaller warships such as surface destroyers (DDG) and cruisers (CG) have flight decks and usually deploy with helicopters on board. Amphibious warships are designed to transport and land an assault force ashore including tanks, trucks, and various armored vehicles via Landing Craft Air Cushion (LCAC). Aircraft carriers have flight decks with both rotary- and fixed-wing aircraft. Any piece of equipment, broken rope, or chain has the potential to cause blunt-force trauma to the body. The current United States (U.S.) Navy Fleet strength (Fiscal Year 2023) consists of 242 surface warships and submarines, including 11 aircraft and nine big-deck amphibious assault warships. Smaller surface warships (i.e., DDGs or CGs) have a complement of about 300 personnel, but an amphibious warship can carry up to 3000 Sailors and Marines, and a fully-loaded aircraft carrier can have between 5000 and 6000 personnel embarked. Thankfully, while a warship is a potentially dangerous environment, major blunt-force trauma remains a relatively infrequent occurrence. Over the last 50 years, there have been 95 major mishap events causing a blunt traumatic mechanism of injury resulting in 130 injuries and 65 fatalities. The most common was blunt torso trauma, accounting for 47% of the events, 85% of the injuries, and 46% of the fatalities. The second most common cause of death from blunt trauma was head injury, which occurred in 33% of events, accounted for only 4% of the injuries, but resulted in 40% of the fatalities. Chest trauma alone resulted in eight fatalities from nine mishaps. Even though there were an equal number of blunt trauma mishaps involving the lower extremity, they did not result in any fatalities.

Noncombat shipboard explosions have typically been associated with ammunition, ordnance, pressurized containers, and boilers. Ordnance-related mishaps are relatively infrequent but can be associated with structural damage and personnel injury. There have been eight such mishaps reported resulting in 27 injuries and 59 fatalities. The deadliest mishap occurred in 1989 when there was an ammunition explosion in the #2 16-in. gun aboard the USS Iowa (BB-61) resulting in 11 injuries and 47 fatalities [1]. Even though battleships are no longer a part of the current Fleet, all ships have a variety of weapons and ammunition. DDGs and CGs are both equipped with 5 in. guns and a variety of missiles. Littoral combat ships have a 57 mm forward gun and further weaponry depending on the combat package installed. Amphibious ships and aircraft carriers may not have offensive weapons but they are armed with several defensive weapons, including the 0.50 caliber machine guns, MK 44 machine guns, 20 mm Phalanx Close-in Weapon System (CIWS), Sea Sparrow, and Rolling Airframe Missile (RAM) launchers. Between 1970 and 2020 there have been 12 noncombat-related ordnance mishaps resulting in 18 injuries and 14 fatalities.

Similar to civilian trauma centers, falls and gunshot wounds happen both at sea and in port. The Naval Safety Command recorded 61 fall mishaps resulting in 25 injuries and 44 fatalities (72%). The majority of these patients had multisystem trauma requiring immediate surgical intervention. Gunshots have accounted for seven mishaps with six fatalities. All of these incidents involved accidental discharge while servicing weapons or their inappropriate use [1].

Fires can cause major damage to the ship and to the Sailors/Marines working to extinguish them. Metal alloys utilized in ship frame and equipment can perpetuate fires, making them difficult to control despite shipboard damage control measures. Sailors can receive severe burns and inhalation injuries despite appropriate protective equipment (see Chap. 25). Even though fire-related mishaps have only accounted for 10% (80) of the non-flight deck mishap events, they have been responsible for 40% of the injuries and 15% of the fatalities. A majority of fatalities were secondary to smoke inhalation. Related to inhalation injuries, poor preparation when working with toxic substances can cause chemical or inhalation injuries. Even though these types of mishaps tend to be rare with only 24 being identified over 50 years, they often result in mortality given rapid respiratory compromise.

While not part of the typical general surgery practice, eye trauma can be difficult to both identify and treat. Despite required eye protection by personnel in high-risk environments, there have been 13 reported eye mishaps resulting in 13 injuries since 1970 [1].

Beyond the high-risk shipboard environment for trauma, medical emergencies may also take place. Since 1970, there have been 11 reported suicides as well as four overdoses and 17 cardiac arrests associated with shipboard fatalities [1].

Flight Deck Injuries

The flight deck adds another level of danger while at sea. In addition to the shipboard risks discussed previously, ships with a flight deck have to contend with the potential injuries associated with aircraft mobilization in both the hangar bay and on the flight deck during both the launching and recovery of aircraft. Collisions between aircraft or mishaps related to flight deck equipment can also cause injury to personnel.

Landing or "trapping" a jet on an aircraft carrier with a pitching deck is a highly complex task and any small mishap can lead to a mass casualty incident (MCI). While a rare occurrence, a snapped arresting wire can cause significant injury including partial or complete traumatic lower extremity amputation [3]. Fortunately, ships with the largest flight decks, carriers, and large amphibious ships, typically have an embarked surgical team. Aircraft carriers have their own Ship's Surgeon and a Fleet Surgical Team (FST) is typically onboard landing helicopter assault (LHA) and landing helicopter dock (LHD) ships during flight operations while deployed. Over the past 50 years, there have been 191 documented aviation- and flight deck-related mishaps resulting in 421 injuries and 200 fatalities. Fifty-eight of these mishaps occurred specifically on flight decks resulting in 165 injuries and 60 fatalities [1].

In contrast, blunt trauma secondary to aircraft entering the water has occurred 71 times, responsible for 139 injuries and 120 fatalities. Contributing factors to high death rates in these flight crews were drowning and hypothermia.

Ejection seats are designed to save the pilot and flight crew during an aircraft emergency. An explosive charge is responsible for propelling the seat with the pilot/aircrew away from the aircraft. This associated force on the body can lead to a host of injuries, including vertebral compression fractures. Ejection-related mishaps are responsible for 59 incidents over the past 50 years resulting in 97 injuries and 10 fatalities according to Naval Safety Command data. A meta-analysis of 1710 aircrew ejections between 1971 and 2019 found an overall mortality of 10.5% and major injury rate of 29.8%. Of those with major injuries, the most common were spinal fractures (61.6%) and extremity trauma (27.3%). 8.9% suffered head trauma, although the head trauma tended to be relatively minor [4].

Noncombat-related midair aeronautical aircraft loss is rare and has only happened three times in the past 50 years. Two events involved aircraft striking each other and the third was an aircraft exploding after takeoff. In total, there have been 15 injuries and seven fatalities [1].

Injuries During Naval Warfare

As discussed in the introduction, between 1970 and 2020, there have been six attacks on U.S. Navy vessels causing injury or death. Table 4.1 describes the characteristics of these six attacks.

In the last months of the Vietnam War, the USS Goldsborough (DDG-20) was attacked by coastal artillery fire while deployed in the Vietnam area of operations, resulting in a 5-ft hole in the upper deck causing burn and inhalation injury casualties.

Towards the end of the Iran-Iraq War, the USS Stark (FFG-32) was attacked by two anti-ship Exocet air missiles in 1987, resulting in multiple explosions and flash fires. Of the 21 injured that survived, two suffered third-degree burns. Other documented injuries included contusions, shrapnel wounds, flash burns, and immersion-related injuries [5].

The three naval mine attacks occurred during the Iran-Iraq War (1980–1988) and Gulf War I (January–February 1991). In 1988, the USS Samuel B. Roberts (FFG-58) entered an Iranian minefield. Fortunately, a lookout spotted the mines, and the captain ordered all crew to their battle stations and all crew below decks topside. While attempting to back out of the minefield, it unfortunately hit a mine, lifting the entire ship out of the water, breaking the keel, and tearing a 21-ft hole into the port side of the ship, resulting in massive flooding and fires. Thanks to all Sailors wearing helmets (battle stations) and being topside, only ten Sailors were injured. All injuries were relatively minor, except for one severe burn [6]. During Gulf War I, both the USS Princeton (CG-59) and the USS Tripoli (LPH-10) were damaged by mines, resulting in seven injuries total.

The 2000 terrorist bombing of the USS Cole (DDG-67) caused 17 fatalities. In addition, 37 Sailors suffered the following injuries: long bone fractures (4 open, 2 closed), concussion (5), subdural hematoma (1), rib fracture (3), clavicle fracture (1), complex ligamentous knee injuries (3), first and second-degree burns of the face or extremity (4), tympanic membrane rupture (16), soft tissue injuries requiring antibiotics for cellulitis (25), inhalation injury (4), orbit fracture (1), mandible fracture (1), pulmonary contusion (1), and pulmonary blast injury (1) [7–9].

The last U.S. Navy Fleet engagement involving full-scale naval combat and one of the largest naval battles in history was during the World War II battle of Leyte Gulf near the Philippine Islands, during which the first ship with the namesake Samuel B. Roberts was sunk [10]. In the modern era, the most recent full-scale naval battle occurred in 1982 between Argentina and the United Kingdom during the Falklands War. In this 10-week war, 23 British ships were lost or damaged. The majority of injured Sailors were cared for on a nearby hospital ship. Common injury patterns included smoke inhalation, hypothermia, burns, and various penetrating injuries [11, 12]. Table 4.2 compares injury types from World War II, the Falklands War, and the attacks on the USS Stark and USS Cole. **In addition to penetrating injuries from explosions, burn injuries and burn-related asphyxiation and inhalation injuries are common during modern naval warfare.** Other common injuries include long bone fractures, TBI, and immersions/hypothermia.

Table 4.2 Comparison of World War II to Modern Naval Warfare injuries

Injury type	World War II [10] ($N = 4529$)	Falklands War [11, 12] ($N = 516$)	USS Stark and USS Cole [2] ($N = 58$)
Penetrating	39.2%	52.3%	6.9%
Burns	26.1%	21%	15.5%
Soft tissue injuries	7.6%	–	41.4%
Fractures	6.8%	–	24.1%
Concussion/traumatic brain injury (TBI)	4.5%	–	17.2%
Asphyxiation/inhalation	1.1%	15.5%	10.3%
Amputation	0.6%	–	0%
Immersions/hypothermia	0.2%	13.4%	8.6%

Conclusion

Despite the low number of combat-related mishaps over the past 50 years, the shipboard and flight deck environments continue to be a high-risk work environment for Sailors and Marines. Aircraft carrier surgical teams, FSTs, and Role 2 Light Maneuver/Expeditionary Resuscitative Surgical System (ERSS) teams should be aware of these potential injuries to prepare as much as possible prior to deployments, pre-deployment workups, or training exercises. It is equally as important to remember that these injuries may occur on vessels without surgical capability and may only have an IDC as the senior medical provider. It is important to prepare for these potential injuries as well as be prepared to talk and mentor someone through the management of the various potential injuries associated with routine naval operations and modern naval warfare.

Declaration of Interest The views expressed in this chapter are those of the authors and do not necessarily reflect the official policy or position of the Department of the Navy, Department of Defense, nor the US Government.

Funding This research did not receive any specific grant from funding agencies in the public, commercial, or not-for-profit sectors.

Conflict of Interest Statement The authors declare no conflict of interest.

References

1. Naval Safety Command. https://navalsafetycenter.navy.mil.
2. Tadlock MD, Gurney J, Tripp MS, et al. Between the devil and the deep blue sea: a review of 25 modern naval mass casualty incidents with implications for future Distributed Maritime Operations. J Trauma Acute Care Surg. 2021;91(2S Suppl 2):S46–55.
3. Chavez T, Cubano M, Hovijitra R. Mass casualty aboard USS Kitty Hawk (CV 63) January 2005--lessons learned. Mil Med. 2005;170(7):iii–vi.
4. Epstein D, Markovitz E, Nakdimon I, Guinzburg A, Aviram E, Gordon B, Shapira S, Sharon S, Steinfeld Y, Miller A, Lipsky AM. Injuries associated with the use of ejection seats: a systematic review, meta-analysis and the experience of the Israeli Air Force, 1990-2019. Injury. 2020;51(7):1489–96.
5. Pinkstaff CA, Sturtz DL, Bellamy RF. USS Franklin and the USS Stark--recurrent problems in the prevention and treatment of naval battle casualties. Mil Med. 1989;154(5):229–33.
6. Evans ML, Samuel B. Roberts III (FFG-58). Naval history and heritage command. 2020. https://www.history.navy.mil/research/histories/ship-histories/danfs/s/samuel-b%2D%2Droberts%2D%2Dffg-58%2D%2Diii.html.
7. Davis TP, Alexander BA, Lambert EW, Simpson RB, Unger DV, Lee J, Snyder ML, Liston WA. Distribution and care of shipboard blast injuries (USS Cole DDG-67). J Trauma. 2003;55(6):1022–7; discussion 7–8.
8. Lambert EW, Simpson RB, Marzouk A, Unger DV. Orthopaedic injuries among survivors of USS COLE attack. J Orthop Trauma. 2003;17(6):436–41.

9. Langworthy MJ, Sabra J, Gould M. Terrorism and blast phenomena: lessons learned from the attack on the USS Cole (DDG67). Clin Orthop Relat Res. 2004;422:82–7.
10. Gauker ED, Blood CG. Severity of battle injuries occurring aboard U.S. Naval Warships. Report No. 92-11. Medical Decisions Support Department, Naval Health Research Center; 1992.
11. Marsh AR. A short but distant war - the Falklands campaign. J R Soc Med. 1983;76(11):972–82.
12. Rylah OJ, Smith JJ. The early management of the burned patient in the Naval service. J R Nav Med Serv. 2015;101(1):55–62.

Chapter 5
I'm Deploying on a Ship, Now What?

Amy A. Hernandez

An ounce of prevention is worth a pound of cure.

Benjamin Franklin

Author deployment experience	
Amy A. Hernandez	Battalion Surgeon, 7th Engineer Support Battalion, Operation Enduring Freedom, Camp Leatherneck, Afghanistan, 2011
	Ship's Surgeon, USS Carl Vinson (CVN-70), WESTPAC, INDOPACOM Area of Responsibility, 2017
	Department Head, Federal Emergency Management Agency (FEMA) and Defense Support of Civilian Authorities (DSCA), COVID-19 Community Vaccination Center mission, St. Louis, MO, USA, 2021

BLUF (Bottom Line Up Front)

There are many methods for the surgical team to prepare for a shipboard deployment.

1. On ship, from a surgical perspective:
   (a) Get credentials and privileges established as soon as possible.
   (b) From the lowly sequential compression device machine to the backup anesthesia machine, catalog and trial all spaces, equipment, instruments, and consumables before deployment! Frequently follow-up on maintenance concerns.
   (c) Identify resources.

A. A. Hernandez (✉)
Department of Surgery, Naval Medical Center San Diego, San Diego, CA, USA
e-mail: Amyhern7@gmail.com

M. D. Tadlock, A. A. Hernandez (eds.), *Expeditionary Surgery at Sea*,
https://doi.org/10.1007/978-3-031-21893-4_5

   (d) Establish direction, capabilities, strengths, and limits of the surgical team, medical team, line leadership, both as individuals and as a whole system.
   (e) The most challenging aspect of shipboard medicine is the supply system and requires patience, persistence, and frequent follow-up.

2. On shore, from a surgical perspective:
   (a) Liaise early with local Medical Treatment Facility (MTF) at all levels of the team for surgical skill sustainment, supply requisition, equipment maintenance, and point of contact acquisition.
   (b) Ensure pertinent team members know how to and are registered to use resources, such as ADVISOR (Advanced Virtual Support for Operational Forces) for sub-specialty consultation.
   (c) Utilize regional military-civilian partnerships if available near the ship's home port to gain additional experience in burn, trauma, and critical care.
   (d) Seek out relevant training for the medical and surgical team to take together prior to deployment, such as Advanced Burn Life Support™ and Fundamentals of Critical Care Support-Resource Limited™; there is also surgeon-specific training available, such as the Advanced Surgical Skills for Exposure in Trauma (ASSET) course and the Emergency War Surgery course.

3. On ship, from a nonsurgical perspective:
   (a) Remember this is a unique experience - get a sponsor and maximize participation.
   (b) Pursue Surface Warfare qualifications early.
   (c) Formulate and plan for goals.

4. On shore, from a nonsurgical perspective:
   (a) Ensure professional career wickets are completed or arrangements made prior to departure.
   (b) Set expectations with loved ones about changes to communication. Ease the transition for children.
   (c) If an important family life event is scheduled to occur during a predeployment underway period, ask the chain of command for temporary coverage in order to attend—the worst they can say is no!
   (d) Make sure all affairs are in order prior to leaving.
   (e) Pack well.

Introduction

Preferably the maritime surgical team can meet and prepare prior to deployment, but sometimes that is not feasible. Any of these recommendations can be performed at any point during a deployment but have the most benefit preceding one. To successfully care for surgical patients on the ship, preparation on shore for professional and personal challenges prior to going out to sea can make a world of difference for the surgical team to combat the stresses of a maritime deployment.

Preparation: Ship/Surgical

The shipboard preparation of the surgical team involves a labor-intensive up-front inventory of the spaces, equipment, and personnel capabilities but proves invaluable. Each member of the surgical team needs to be acquainted with all the spaces, equipment, processes, and responsibilities of every part and person on the team, since the natural redundancies (e.g., personnel, equipment, supplies) of a Medical Treatment Facility (MTF) is not present in the middle of the ocean.

Credentials/Privileges

First and foremost, when the members of the maritime surgical team receive notice of going to a ship platform, they should initiate the credentialing and privileging process with the appropriate authorities in a timely manner as applicable. This process can be onerous, inefficient, and bureaucratic and frequently involves aggressive follow-up on the part of the service member. Medical leadership like the Senior Medical Officer (SMO) or Officer in Charge (OIC) can facilitate if problems arise.

Inventory, Supply, and Maintenance

On the ship, the most vital preparation for surgical patients starts with a thorough inventory of what the surgical team is responsible for—spaces, equipment, instruments, and consumables. These spaces include the Operating Room (OR) and substerile spaces like the Sterile Processing Department (SPD), but also potentially the biohazard spaces, Battle Dressing Stations (BDS), treatment rooms, storage areas, or other locations depending on how the medical department is organized. Do not neglect the non-OR areas if they are the responsibility of the surgical team. Of note, shipboard ORs have relatively high personnel turnover rates with long periods of disuse, putting them at high risk for expired, broken, or non-compatible gear. **Empty all the shelves and drawers, open every set, assemble each piece of gear, and trial run every piece of equipment – from the lowly Sequential Compression Device (SCD) machine to the backup anesthesia machine. Catalog the gear that is functioning, dispose of anything applicable, and reorder or resupply what is necessary for the mission.**

By far and away the most challenging aspect of shipboard medicine is the supply system and requires patience, persistence, and frequent follow-up. Take the normal complaints of any supply system, magnify them by being deployed in a resource-constrained environment, then exponentially multiply them by the ship's frequent restrictions in communication and physical unavailability so orders for items readily available on shore and necessary for surgery are frequently physically lost, held up in bureaucratic paperwork, or have no way to travel to the ship. Periodic checks of all gear are required so orders can be placed with sufficient cushion time to minimize disruption to surgical capabilities. Be aware of what is present, know what is needed, obtain what is possible ahead of time, and frequently follow-up on what is ordered or pending.

Finally, all equipment should be regularly maintained by the biomedical technicians (BMTs) on the ship. Check their schedule and be sure everything is safe prior to use. Some equipment or electrical issues may require more complex coordination of supply and maintenance or can only undergo annual maintenance on land, which is usually exclusively available during port time. Refer to Chap. 12 for a more thorough discussion of inventory, supply, and maintenance for the individual platforms.

Identify Resources

Surgery is surgery, but the ship environment makes it different and each ship has its own atmosphere. A good way to orient the team is for everyone to familiarize themselves with the same information. Instruction 6000.1, the Shipboard Medical Procedures Manual, which differs by region and platform (for example from San Diego: COMNAVAIRPACINST for CVN, COMNAVSURFPACINST/COMNAVSURFLANTINST for the other platforms) is the shipboard "Bible" with much of the necessary Navy-wide information. Many other resources are also available such as ship-specific instructions, Joint Trauma System (JTS) Clinical Practice Guidelines (CPGs), or textbooks. Review all of these resources with a focus on surgery-related topics upon arrival on the ship. Prior to deployment download the most current JTS CPGs as they are an excellent resource (available at https://jts.amedd.army.mil/index.cfm/pi_cpgs/cpgs). During deployments consider having team members review relevant high-yield CPGs during a regular "journal club" or CPG review. All members of the care team should participate. The OR should also have a Standard Operating Procedure (SOP) to be reviewed and updated when a new team checks in. Additionally, teams typically write an After-Action Report

(AAR) or cruise report that is compiled over time for a comprehensive and sequential experience of the lessons learned and experiences from past deployments. Find them and read them so as to not repeat history and reinvent the wheel.

Establish Capabilities

It is imperative to establish the capabilities, strengths, and limits of the surgical team, medical team, and line leadership as individuals and as a functioning system to care for complex patients. Start in the OR, spread to the ancillary services like Radiology and Lab (see Chap. 8), the medical evacuation/casualty evacuation (MEDEVAC/CASEVAC) personnel and system (see Chap. 31), and the guidance from leadership in any/all potential chains of command (see Chap. 6), which can change with each mission or even within a mission.

Preparation: Shore/Surgical

For many reasons, it is crucial for each member of the maritime surgical team to establish connection with their shore counterparts at the local MTF prior to deployment. Most importantly, workups and deployments may not have high case volumes. To maintain critical patient care skills, everyone should spend time working in their role during port at the MTF. For credentialed providers, this may involve an additional transfer of credentials/privileges, which can be a long process that should be initiated early, potentially at the time of initial credentialing/privileging. Utilize regional military-civilian partnerships if available near the ship's home port to gain additional experience in burn, trauma, and critical care. Additionally seek out and consider having the entire medical and surgical team take courses together such as Advanced Burn Life Support™ and Fundamentals of Critical Care Support-Resource Limited™; there is also surgeon-specific training available, such as the Advanced Surgical Skills for Exposure in Trauma (ASSET) course and the Emergency War Surgery course.

Next, the local MTF is an excellent resource for supply and maintenance concerns, in particular the consumables that expire and aren't part of the Authorized Medical Allowance Lists (AMALs) and the maintenance that can only occur in port.

Finally, having good points of contact for the different surgical subspecialties on shore is helpful, especially for the surgeon. Many times, for non-general surgery issues, it is advantageous to facilitate care or discuss cases with a specialist. Communication to and from the ship can sometimes be limited in both time and quality. Calling the correct person the first time is invaluable when time is of the essence. One option is to get a list of contacts from the local MTF. Additionally, the United States Army Institute of Surgical Research (USAISR) Burn Center is an excellent resource for the maritime surgical team and can be contacted both synchronously and asynchronously. Advanced Virtual Support for Operational Forces (ADVISOR) can also be an excellent resource for both synchronous and asynchronous sub-specialty consultation (see Fig. 5.1). At the time of publication, take note

Operational (Deployed) Virtual Health Consultation Resources

Step 1. Determine the nature of patient care:
Determine the type of consultation support required. Urgency/immediacy is determined by a combination of communications capabilities (i.e. limitations to communications "windows," network functionality/internet access), mission requirements and patient condition.

Routine	Urgent	Emergent
▪ Response within 24 hours. ▪ NORMAL vital signs ▪ Not going to deteriorate in 24hrs **SYNCHRONOUS SUPPORT** In some AORs GTPcan convert to a synchronous specialty care appointment via VTC. Landstuhl RMC VH: 42 Specialties available for direct care support of Operational Forces **Phone** Outside of Germany: 011-49-6371-9464-5890 (DSN: 314-590-5890)	▪ Urgent consults are all other cases that do not fall under the routine or emergent categories. ▪ Urgent consults usually require specialty medical advice (i.e. orthopedic surgery, cardiology, pediatrics, behavioral health, etc.) and would benefit for synchronous communication between the local caregiver and the remote consultant ▪ Mission requires rapid disposition of patient.	▪ Life threatening or potentially life threatening conditions like: o Shock o Respiratory failure o Renal failure o Liver failure o Complex wounds o Polytrauma o Burns o Severe infection/sepsis o Crush injuries o Severe electrolyte abnormalities o Encephalopathy/severe TBI o Abnormal vital signs o Complex arrhythmias. o Poisonings

Step 2. Accessing consultation support

Routine	Urgent+	Emergent+
To use GTPin its current form, you must have a username and password for GTP. To obtain a username/password for these systems, you must: - Have current HIPAA training. - For a GTPaccount, visit: https://path.tamc.amedd.army.mil ** Veterinary Care for MWDs currently not available through GTP please utilize ADVISOR line.	**833-ADVSRLN** **(833-238-7756)** **DSN (312) 429-9089** **Specialty Consults** ➢ General Surgery ➢ Orthopedic Surgery ➢ Pediatrics ➢ Toxicology ➢ Infectious Disease ➢ Hematology/Oncology ➢ OB/GYN ➢ Dental ➢ Ophthalmology ➢ Neonatology ➢ ER to request Specialty not listed ◊ **Emergency Department** ◊ **Burn Care (ISR)** ***** Training Option *****	**833-ADVSRLN** **(833-238-7756)** **DSN (312) 429-9089** ◊ **Critical Care Consultation** ◊ **Veterinary Care for MWDs** ▪ Europe/Atlantic ▪ Pacific ◊ **Chemical Casualty Care** **If you have video capability at your site:** **24/7 manned work station at NMCSD Tele-Critical Care:** **#1: 203651403@med.navy.mil** **#2: 203651404@med.navy.mil** **#3: 203651405@med.navy.mil**

+ If VTC needed for consultation, place phone call first, then establish VTC plan with remote consultant; NOTE, you must have VTC capability

****TRAINING***** **Training with ADVISOR must be pre-coordinated with dod.advissor_training@mail.mil**

ADVISOR
Advanced Virtual Support for Operational Forces

Fig. 5.1 Advanced Virtual Support for Operational Forces (ADVISOR) synchronous and asynchronous contact information and instructions. *AOR* area of responsibility, *GTP* Global Teleconsultation Portal, *VTC* video teleconferencing, *RMC* Regional Medical Center, *VH* virtual health, *TBI* traumatic brain injury, *HIPAA* Health Insurance Portability And Accountability Act, *MWD* military working dog, *ADVISOR* Advanced Virtual Support for Operational Forces, *OB/GYN* obstetrics and gynecology, *ER* emergency room, *ISR* Institute of Surgical Research; *NMCSD* Naval Medical Center San Diego. (Source: Military Health System (MHS) Virtual Medical Center, used with permission)

that ADVISOR utilizes GTP (Global Teleconsultation Portal), requiring the user to create an account, user name, and password at https://path.tamc.amedd.army.mil. Finally, the Military Health System (MHS) Virtual Medical Center also has an internal SharePoint site (which is Common Access Card (CAC)-enabled) at https://info.health.mil/army/VMC/Pages/VMC/OperationalMedicineAdvisor.aspx.

USAISR Burn Center

- DSN 312-429-2876 (429-BURN)
- Commercial (210) 916-2876 or (210) 222-2876
- Email to burntrauma.consult.army@mail.mil

Preparation: Ship/Nonsurgical

A shipboard deployment is anything but commonplace. Approaching it in this manner may help shine a positive light on a potentially challenging or unexpected situation. Take advantage of the time on the ship to soak up any unique opportunities and work toward achieving professional and personal aspirations.

Checking in/Sponsor

When checking in, go to all the places listed to help learn how to navigate the ship. If none is assigned, ask for a sponsor for orientation to the daily battle rhythm, language (refer to Appendix C for a list of common nautical terms), and expectations of shipboard life in general and specific to the platform and deployment.

Warfare Qualifications

Additionally, obtaining the Enlisted Surface Warfare Specialist (ESWS) or Surface Warfare Medical Department Officer (SWMDO) qualification early during deployment. This not only assists in learning about shipboard personnel, spaces, and equipment outside of the medical department unique to the maritime environment but it also aids in career progression. Talk to the SMO about the ESWS or SWMDO program if it is not introduced on arrival.

Goals

Finally, the author recommends setting up professional and personal goals for the duration of the deployment. Deployments usually have a fair amount of unscheduled time, and one can only go to the gym so much. This time away from normal professional and personal responsibilities can be used for taking courses, studying for exams, learning new skills, or even catching up on popular movies or books that were missed prior to deployment. Many of those goals require preparation prior to arrival (signing up for classes, bringing materials, downloading movies and books, etc.), so take that into consideration as well.

Preparation: Shore/Nonsurgical

One of the hardest aspects of a maritime platform is the shore responsibilities that remain behind, which are commonly not discussed since they are not "medical." However, they can be a significant contributing factor to stress and distraction. Onshore work on the front end can prevent personal trials during deployment that can detract from the mission.

Professional Requirements

The significant and sometimes prolonged delays and obstructions to communication makes the continuation of professional requirements and commitments difficult. Certifications (e.g., Basic Life Support) expiring during deployment should be renewed prior to departure. Many providers, in particular surgeons, can have board examinations to arrange during deployment, which now may additionally include arranging transportation to and from and coverage on the ship.

Expectations for Loved Ones

This communication gap also extends to family members, friends, and other loved ones left behind. For many people, this may be the first deployment away from their loved ones. **Setting expectations early over frequency and type of communication is essential**. In a society obsessed with instant gratification and 24/7 connection at the touch of a finger, the transition to shipboard life for both parties can be disconcerting and stressful. There may be no or limited WiFi/data services, text messages, or constant access to online social media platforms. Each environment is different, but snail mail and email (both government and civilian) delays email and telephone access restrictions, and frequent changes to schedules and plans are all common occurrences. Flexibility on both sides is encouraged.

If children are involved, there are many opportunities to ease this difficult transition for them, which include books (e.g., "Countdown 'til Mommy Comes Home" or "My Daddy is a Hero"), toys (e.g., "hug-a-hero" dolls or personalized teddy bears), incentive countdown activities (e.g., sticker calendars or candy jars), recordable picture frames, and pre-staged presents. Many ships offer opportunities for book reading on CD to mail home. There are also recordable books to purchase or alternately books can be recorded on a cell phone video prior to deployment and sent home on CD or flash drive at regular intervals during deployment. There are also usually other resources for families with the Family Readiness Officer (FRO), United Services Organization (USO), Fleet and Family Services, Chaplain, or Ombudsman.

Prior to a long deployment, there are often short, but frequent, underway periods. If an important family life event (e.g., birth of a child, graduation, funeral) is scheduled to occur during one of these periods then asking the chain of command for temporary coverage so a member of the surgical team can attend is reasonable. The answer will not always be "yes," but will be "no" 100% of the time when no one asks.

Affairs in Order

Another way to take care of the home is to ensure the loved ones left behind are prepared should deployed service members need administrative help while deployed. All affairs should be in order prior to departure since communication can be scarce. Bank accounts and other important information (e.g., rental agreement, insurance cards) along with legal documents like up-to-date wills, powers of attorney, and family care plans should be placed in secure known locations. Notify banks of deployment and port countries so expenditures aren't flagged and accounts frozen. Licenses, credit cards (both government and civilian), and passports (both government and civilian) should not expire on deployment or if they do, then preparations should already be in place to get the replacement to the deployed service member. Prepare instructions, emergency phone numbers, etc. as if the deployed service member will not be able to help at all in case of difficulty, as that is commonly the case.

Packing

Pack well. Packing differs for all people, deployments, missions, and situations. Refer to Appendix B for a sample packing list. Main things to remember: Bring uniform items. Plan for weather conditions. Bring technology and cords (and backup cords), including corded/non-Bluetooth options. Bring personal medical tools for the surgical mission like loupes, textbooks, etc. Bring hard copies of all relevant paperwork. Pre-download e-books and other media. Bring supplies/activities for non-scheduled time.

Conclusion

There are many ways to prepare on ship and shore in surgical and non-surgical ways to make a maritime surgical deployment as smooth as possible professionally and personally. Hopefully, this chapter and this book will get everyone on the team off to a great start!

Declaration of Interest The views expressed in this chapter are those of the authors and do not necessarily reflect the official policy or position of the Department of the Navy, Department of Defense, nor the US Government.

Funding This research did not receive any specific grant from funding agencies in the public, commercial, or not-for-profit sectors.

Conflict of Interest Statement The authors declare no conflict of interest.

Further Reading

Instruction 6000.1. The Shipboard medical procedures manual, which differs by region and platform (for example from San Diego: COMNAVAIRPACINST for CVN, COMNAVSURFPACINST/COMNAVSURFLANTINST for the other platforms). n.d.

Joint Trauma System (JTS). Clinical practice guidelines (CPGs). n.d. https://jts.amedd.army.mil/index.cfm/pi_cpgs/cpgs.

Military Health System (MHS). Virtual Medical Center internal SharePoint site (requires CAC Access). n.d. https://info.health.mil/army/VMC/Pages/VMC/OperationalMedicineAdvisor.aspx.

Chapter 6
Leadership and Communication 101

James G. Slotto, Kathleen A. Cannon, Katherine A. Wrenn-Maresh, and Theodore D. Edson

Leadership is the art of getting someone else to do something you want done because he wants to do it.

Dwight D. Eisenhower

Author deployment experience	
James G. Slotto	Officer in Charge, Expeditionary Resuscitative Surgical System Pacific, embarked on the USS McCampbell (DDG-85), 2019–2020; Provided embarked Role 2 Surgical Support, INDOPACOM Area of Responsibility, 2019–2020
	Anesthesiologist (COVID-19 Team), USS Theodore Roosevelt (CVN-71), WESTPAC, INDOPACOM Area of Responsibility, 2020–2021
Kathleen A. Cannon	Ship's Surgeon, USS Theodore Roosevelt (CVN-71), WESTPAC, INDOPACOM Area of Responsibility, 2020–2021
Katherine A. Wrenn-Maresh	Staff Surgeon, Fleet Surgical Team-9, embarked on the USS America (LHA-6), RIMPAC, INDOPACOM Area of Responsibility, 2016
	Staff Surgeon, NATO Role 3 Medical Unit, NATO Resolute Support and Operation Freedom's Sentinel, Kandahar Airfield, Afghanistan, 2019

J. G. Slotto (✉)
Navy Medicine Readiness and Training Command San Diego, San Diego, CA, USA
e-mail: james.g.slotto2.mil@health.mil

K. A. Cannon
Navy Medicine Readiness and Training Command Portsmouth, Portsmouth, VA, USA
e-mail: kathleen.a.cannon6.mil@health.mil

K. A. Wrenn-Maresh
Navy Medicine Readiness and Training Command Guam, Guam, USA
e-mail: katherine.a.wrenn-maresh.mil@health.mil

T. D. Edson
1st Medical Battalion, Camp Pendleton, CA, USA
e-mail: theodore.d.edson.mil@health.mil

M. D. Tadlock, A. A. Hernandez (eds.), *Expeditionary Surgery at Sea*,
https://doi.org/10.1007/978-3-031-21893-4_6

Author deployment experience	
Theodore D. Edson	Ship's Surgeon, USS Kitty Hawk (CV-63), Northern Pacific Cruise, INDOPACOM Area of Responsibility, 2003–2004
	Assistant Officer in Charge, Forward Resuscitative Surgical System/Shock Trauma Platoon, Operation Iraqi Freedom, Al Qaim, Iraq, 2005–2006
	Director Surgical Services, Surgical Shock Trauma Platoon, Operation Iraqi Freedom, Taqaddum, Iraq, 2006–2007
	Officer in Charge, Forward Surgical Team, Operation Enduring Freedom, Lagman, Qalat, Afghanistan, 2010–2011
	Staff Surgeon, Expeditionary Resuscitative Surgical System 11, 2013–2014; Provided embarked Role 2 Surgical Support, CENTCOM Area of Responsibility, 2013–2014
	Officer in Charge, Forward Resuscitative Surgical Trauma team, Operation Freedom Banner, INDOPACOM Area of Responsibility, 2021

BLUF (Bottom Line Up Front)

1. Aircraft Carrier (CVN) Ship's Surgeon

    (a) Keep your circle of communication tight to ensure efficiency of passing information, especially when time is of the essence. Communicate in clear, consistent, comprehensive, and coherent manner.
    (b) Set communication expectations early with your Senior Medical Officer (SMO). The SMO will communicate with the patient's chain of command (COC) and Commanding Officer (CO) when necessary, in particular preoperatively for urgent/emergent operations and postoperatively for all operations.
    (c) Know all of the people who need to be contacted in the event of a Medical Evacuation/Casualty Evacuation (MEDEVAC/CASEVAC) to assist your Medical Administrative Officer (MAO) with requirements and planning.
    (d) Notify SMO, Triage Officer, and person tracking casualties in event of a Mass Casualty Incident (MCI) to have situational awareness and when you will be operating and not available outside of the Operating Room (OR).

2. Fleet Surgical Team (FST) Staff Surgeon

    (a) Collaboration is the key to readiness. Build bridges to the ship's medical department of all ships you will be deploying with, not only the ship you will actually embark on. The Surgical Technologists (STs) assigned to those ships are critical for the readiness of the surgical spaces, and they need your support.

   (b) Some things never change! You will have two bosses; ensure there are clear expectations regarding communication with the SMO and Commander, Amphibious Task Force (CATF) surgeon while underway. Similar to your attendings in residency, you need to know what each of your bosses wants to be informed of in the moment and what can "wait until morning."
   (c) Maximize your resources. Engage all embarked medical units in MCI drills and other training regularly.
   (d) Trust but verify. Ensure all requirements involved in resuscitation (i.e., blood bank supplies and equipment) are functional and up to date. Ensure and exercise Walking Blood Bank (WBB) capability.

3. Expeditionary Resuscitative Surgical System (ERSS) Officer in Charge (OIC)

   (a) In a ship-based environment, the three players to be aware of are the co-located medical assets, the maritime platform leadership, and the customer requesting the support of a damage control surgery (DCS) team.
   (b) As the ERSS OIC, integrate yourself into mission operations and planning as early as possible to facilitate positive mission experience, prevent issues, and project competence to the non-medical chain of command.
   (c) No one outside of an ERSS team fully understands the capabilities, requirements, and limitations of an ERSS team. As the subject matter expert, you will need to inject realistic capabilities into planning. Many of the decisions may involve competing interests.
   (d) For most ship-based missions, donor blood availability and its lifespan will be the most significant logistical challenges to communicate and plan for.

4. Forward Resuscitative Surgical System (FRSS) Staff Surgeon

   (a) Be aware of capabilities/shortfalls of the FRSS in personnel, assets, and logistics.
   (b) Communicate and coordinate ahead of time with associated medical assets and supported unit(s).
   (c) Agree ahead of time upon delegation of triage and patient disposition authority and train for MCI events.
   (d) Perform team training as much as possible prior to real-world casualty events.

Introduction

While there are several different members of forward-deployed maritime surgical teams and every person in medicine is considered a leader, this chapter is predominantly focused and aimed at the person in the role that would be doing the most communicating up the chain of command for surgical patient care. Leadership and communication skills are just as essential for optimal patient outcomes as operative and airway management skills since the care of patients involves teams of people. This chapter shares the perspectives and recommendations of different surgical team leaders from different forward-deployed environments at different times in their careers.

In Depth: Aircraft Carrier (CVN) Ship's Surgeon

Team Personnel

The medical department on the carrier is meant to take care of the everyday needs and medical readiness of the embarked Sailors and Marines, and is also the main medical resource for the Carrier Strike Group (CSG). The medical department on an aircraft carrier (CVN) is large but those who actually partake in the surgical care of a patient can be counted on one hand. As the surgeon on a carrier, you will have an operating room (OR) team composed of two to three corpsmen trained as surgical technologists (STs) and an anesthesia provider. Postoperatively, the nursing care is provided by the Ship's nurse, who is a critical care registered nurse (CCRN). It is likely that your team has not trained together, but you can make up for this with efficient and constant communication, which can often be developed and practiced during the multiple medical training evolutions the ship is required to perform. What follows is an overview of how to communicate to effectively take care of surgical patients on an aircraft carrier.

The Senior Medical Officer (SMO) is a physician and the Department Head (DH) of the CVN's Medical Department and your immediate supervisor. On the carrier, each DH or "Head of Department," is commonly referred to as the HOD. The SMO is also the senior medical advisor to the CO, and any embarked or associated Commanders, including the Carrier Air Wing (CVW), the Destroyer Squadron (DESRON), and the Carrier Strike Group (CSG). See Chap. 1 for more details on the structure of a typical CSG, as the surgical team cares for any and all of the surgical patients in the entire strike group. The SMO should be kept abreast of the following scenarios: urgent/emergent operations, elective operations requiring general anesthesia, patients who require Medical Evacuation/Casualty Evacuation (MEDEVAC/CASEVAC), need for Walking Blood Bank (WBB) activation, and complex patients for clinical or social reasons that require chain of command (COC) involvement. All surgical cases requiring general anesthesia typically require commanding officer (CO) approval; SMO will obtain that approval for you. Additionally, the SMO can be a liaison between the medical department and the patient's COC, specifically their HOD/DH for Ship's company as well as leadership for embarked units and units within the strike group on other ships. This is particularly helpful when an urgent/emergent case comes in and your focus as the surgeon needs to be on assembling and preparing your team to take that patient to the OR. **Therefore, it is important to establish clear lines of communication between you and your SMO early so that in an urgent/emergent situation you are not wondering which one of you needs to contact whom in relation to the patient's pre- and postoperative care**.

Preoperative Communication

In the event you have an urgent/emergent case, you will need to assemble your team to include the two STs, anesthesia provider, and the Ship's nurse, who is a critical care registered nurse (CCRN). The following order of notifications prior to taking the patient to the OR are recommended:

1. Anesthesia Provider. The anesthesia provider, either a Certified Nurse Anesthetist (CRNA) or anesthesiologist, will need to evaluate the patient and develop their anesthetic plan. This also allows you to discuss with the anesthesia provider your operative strategy, including timeline, approach, and concerns.
2. Surgical Technologists. The OR is often staged in a semi-ready configuration. However, early notification of the STs not only allows them to prepare the OR, but also affords them an opportunity to go to the storeroom (often in another part of the ship–see Chap. 12) for equipment or supplies that are not stored in the medical department.
3. SMO. At this point, you'll have determined the operative plan and urgency of proceeding. Information that SMO needs in order to brief the COC includes the patient's name, patient's rank and rate, patient's department, planned operation, approximate start time, approximate duration, and your immediate and long-term postoperative plans, particularly if the patient will require a MEDEVAC/CASEVAC.
4. Ship's nurse. The nurse will need to be aware of the patient as they will oversee and arrange for the ward or Intensive Care Unit (ICU) corpsman to manage the patient postoperatively. The Ship's nurse can act as the OR circulating nurse, but not all nurses feel comfortable in this role or have availability if they have other patients they are caring for while the case is occurring.
5. Patient. Prior to the case, request that Sailors alert their immediate superiors personally to inform them of the situation even though SMO formally notifies their COC.

6. Oral maxillofacial surgeon (OMFS). They are an experienced surgical set of hands. Bringing them in on elective cases integrates them into your team, and will pay off later, especially for complex cases.

The same people will need to be alerted for elective cases. The only difference is the Sailor will route an approval sheet with your recommendations for surgery and postoperative expectations (sick-in-quarters (SIQ), light duty restrictions, etc.) through their COC to sign off on prior to surgery. That piece of paper is your communication with the COC and often no other communication with them is needed unless a complication were to arise. Do not proceed with an elective surgery without approval from the patient's COC.

Postoperative Communication

Following the surgical procedure, either urgent/emergent or elective, communication is largely with the same group of people. Depending on the arrangement between you and SMO, one of you will reach out to the COC to let them know the procedure is done and how it went. Ask your patients preoperatively who they want called after the case and if it is okay to discuss the surgery with their COC. Obviously, the COC needs to know that a Sailor is having surgery and what the postoperative expectations will be such as sick in quarters (SIQ), light duty, MEDEVAC/CASEVAC, etc. Remember, without the patient's explicit approval, details about the procedure should not be shared. Often, the COC will arrive in the medical department soon after it is decided the patient needs surgery and/or soon after the case is finished to check on their Sailor.

The Ship's nurse and ward/ICU corpsman will take care of patients postoperatively after the anesthesia provider has completed their portion of the postoperative care. Set expectations with the nurse for when to be notified about the patient and educate the ward corpsmen on how to care for that particular postoperative patient. Remember that this may be the first time the corpsmen have dealt with a postoperative surgical patient.

MEDEVAC/CASEVAC

In the event of a MEDEVAC/CASEVAC, an additional person you will need to communicate with is the Medical Administrative Officer (MAO). Alert the MAO and SMO *early* that a patient needs a MEDEVAC/CASEVAC. Once the location to which the patient will be transferred is identified, you will have to call the admitting hospital to identify an admitting physician. Once you discuss the patient with the on-call physician and get approval to transfer the patient to their institution, pass the accepting physician's name and phone number to your MAO. Do not forget to update the accepting physician with the expected MEDEVAC/CASEVAC timeline.

Lastly, be aware of all MEDEVAC/CASEVAC procedures as you cannot assume your MAO knows them and you may need to be the one arranging transport. Keeping the SMO in the loop should decrease the amount of communication you need to do. Ideally, in this case, you will only discuss the patient with SMO, MAO, and the accepting physician.

Trauma and Mass Casualty (MASCAL)

Lastly, preparing for trauma and non-trauma mass casualties (MASCAL) is a major focus of training aboard an aircraft carrier (see Chap. 7). A MASCAL obviously involves the entire medical department, in addition to many other departments around the ship. In the event of a MASCAL, you will need to communicate with your normal surgical team (anesthesia provider, STs, and CCRN) who are often already stationed down in the medical department. Additionally, you will need to communicate with three other people:

1. SMO. SMO is the one who would activate the WBB (See Chap. 23).
2. The Triage Officer. This role is often assigned to one of the Ship's dentists. The Triage Officer will work with the corpsman to triage patients and often need your assistance in determining the urgency of care in a resource-constrained environment. This allows you to get a "global perspective" on all of the casualties as corpsmen and other medical providers evaluate them and initiate treatment.
3. The person in charge of patient tracking at the scene of the event. Often this is performed by a chief petty officer. They are responsible for getting your surgical patients down to the OR by directing the stretcher-bearers to the surgical patient(s) first and securing the first spot on the elevators for transport of these patients.

The last communication piece in a MASCAL is making sure the SMO and Triage Officer understand that while you are operating, the remainder of the team will no longer have the surgeon available to assist in triage and initial treatment. You will obviously be available for questions, but you will not be able to help manage the remainder of patients. This is another reason why it is important to perform MASCAL drills and to develop as much situational awareness of other casualties and discuss interventions and contingency plans with the other providers delivering care at the scene.

Closing Thoughts

The surgeon typically has the most trauma knowledge and experience, so the shipboard trauma education commonly falls to you. Additionally, you are often the most experienced provider with respect to the care of any critically ill patient so you should collaborate with your colleagues on the care of non-surgical patients as well. Finally, don't forget that you have a vast amount of knowledge that many of the corpsmen are willing to absorb. After you have completed preparation for taking your patient to the OR, take the time to communicate with one or two of them, invite them into the OR, and discuss the case with them as it progresses. Before you know it, you will be writing multiple letters of recommendation to ST C-school!

The overall key to a successful deployment is to remember that your team is small and learning to communicate with each other is important. Work out any barriers to effective communication prior to deployment. Setting expectations for the flow of communication not only ensures that no one is left out when a case comes up, but also that communication is efficient and will not slow down the process of getting the patient to the OR. Always communicate any lessons learned in your cruise report and pass it on to your replacement when you are ready to move on.

In Depth: Fleet Surgical Team (FST) Staff Surgeon

Team Personnel

The Fleet Surgical Team (FST) is a relatively small unit with a focused mission set that gets integrated into the existing medical departments of ships with OR facilities. It provides the personnel and expertise for trauma resuscitation, surgical stabilization, critical care stabilization and holding, as well as en route care (ERC) for evacuating patients. However, it is reliant on the supplies and equipment of the ships on which it is deployed, as it does not have its own Authorized Medical Allowance List (AMAL). This symbiotic relationship is essential to the FST mission, and can make or break the deployment experience (see Chap. 12). The FSTs primarily embark on large- and medium-deck amphibious ships-Landing Helicopter Dock (LHD), Landing Helicopter Assault (LHA), and Landing Platform Dock (LPD)-because these ships house ORs and are generally designated as Casualty Receiving and Treatment Ships (CRTS).

The amphibious ships are organized into Amphibious Readiness Groups (ARGs), composed of multiple ships, including an LHD and an LPD. The primary FST will usually be embarked on the LHD, as the flagship, but is responsible for ensuring that the LPD is also ready to be used for surgical care should the need arise in disaggregate operations. The Officer in Charge (OIC) of the FST is a physician and is also the primary medical advisor to the Commander, Amphibious Task Force (CATF), holding the title of CATF surgeon and providing oversight of the medical departments of all ships in the ARG.

In addition to the core clinical teams, the FST includes clinical support and Command & Control (C2) elements. The OR team is led by the surgeon and manned by a Certified Perioperative Nurse (CNOR), two STs, and an anesthesia provider. The family practice or internal medicine physician heads resuscitative and intensive care efforts, along with a CCRN, a respiratory tech (RT), and two general duty corpsmen. The CCRN is also responsible for ERC, with the RT and/or a corpsman to assist. Clinical support members include two laboratory technicians, one radiology technician, a psychiatrist or psychologist, and a behavioral health technician. The C2 element includes the OIC, the Medical Regulating Control Officer (MRCO), and Senior Enlisted Leader (SEL), who together handle administrative functions.

As stated, the scope of responsibility for the FSTs extends beyond the large-deck ARG flagship they will likely deploy on, especially to the LPD because it also has an OR. There is nowhere near enough time for an FST to get both ships ready on their own, especially the more specialized areas like the OR, Sterile Processing Department (SPD), and the ICU, so leveraging your personnel assets is paramount. There is typically one ST assigned to an LHA or LHD and another assigned to an LPD, but because the surgical capabilities of the ship are not an emphasis when there is no FST embarked, it is easy for them to be burdened with multiple additional collateral duties (see Chap. 12). They usually welcome the arrival and support of the FST, as it empowers them to return to their "real job," and they can be a great asset for finding, inventorying, and organizing supplies and equipment. Be a resource for them and do what you can to protect their time, and they will be a force multiplier when you are occupied with other ships or tasks.

Chain of Command (COC)

As in many Navy medical situations, there are multiple chains of command to consider (i.e., medical, line/operational). Within the FST, and while ashore, you report to the FST OIC. However, once embarked on a ship, you and the other members of the FST integrate into the ship's medical department, falling under the ship's SMO for day-to-day functions. As the FST surgeon, you lead the FST in navigating this dynamic to preserve your mission integrity (surgical readiness!) while building the bridges essential to make sure the ship is prepared for any contingency the deployment might bring.

The CATF surgeon is focused on the bigger strategic picture for the ARG, while the SMO is solely responsible for the individual ship. However, as previously mentioned the CATF surgeon is still the OIC for the FST, so the lines of communication can get a little blurrier than in other operational situations. The SMO and CATF surgeon should work together to create expectations for how information moves up and down the COC. As the surgeon, you will be front and center in most urgent/emergent situations, requiring you to use these lines of communication efficiently and effectively. To do that, you need to understand this dynamic well, so it is incumbent on you to ask for clarification early if they have not been explicit.

As an FST surgeon, you are likely to find yourself in any number of organizational positions underway. Most of the time, you will likely be embarked on the large-deck ARG flagship (LHD or LHA) with your OIC functioning as CATF surgeon. However, at some point, you may find yourself on an LPD, either as a full FST or solely as a surgical detachment. You may be on that LPD with or without your

OIC; if they're with you, they may also be the CATF surgeon or they may be functioning solely as the OIC under another CATF surgeon. With the increase in disaggregated operations, it is impossible to predict exactly how an FST will be tasked, so building strong foundations of communication is essential to being flexible and efficient. **Similar to your attendings in residency, you need to know what each of your bosses wants to be contacted about in the moment and what can "wait until morning."**

Perioperative Communication

When surgical situations arise, much like on an aircraft carrier, you will have to notify the SMO, who will then notify the ship's CO. The SMO should also communicate with the patient's COC, whether that's their HOD/DH for ship's company or their OIC/unit medical personnel for embarked units. Whether or not you contact the CATF surgeon directly, or the SMO contacts them will depend on their expectations, but for more serious conditions, especially something requiring MEDEVAC/CASEVAC, it is likely best to contact the CATF surgeon directly to minimize the potential for message confusion and relay errors.

Once the decision to operate has been made, whether urgent/emergent or elective, the process is much the same as previously described for aircraft carriers. In addition to assembling the anesthesia provider and STs for a surgical case, notify the CNOR (a role that is not on the other platforms) and the CCRN to recover the patient following anesthesia and potentially admit them to the ward if inpatient care is necessary. There is no OMFS either, so if an extra pair of hands is needed in the OR besides the STs, potential options include the FST family practice or internal medicine physician, the general medical officer (GMO), or the dentist. Taking the time to bring them into the OR to orient them during simple, elective cases will pay dividends when you are faced with a big, emergent case and you really need the help.

MASCAL

In a MASCAL situation, the entire medical component on the ship will be involved, including ship's medical departement, the FST, and any embarked units' medical personnel. The amphibious mission is inherently tied into the Marine Expeditionary Unit (MEU) mission, so United States Marine Corps (USMC) medical assets will likely be on board. Frequently a USMC Shock Trauma Platoon (STP) led by an Emergency Medicine physician is embarked on the LHA/LHD or on another ship in the ARG. Potentially even a USMC Forward Resuscitative Surgical System (FRSS) team or an ERSS team could also be embarked depending on the situation. These assets can be a tremendous help if they are on board. Depending on the mission set, USMC assets may be ashore with the Marines feeding you patients. Therefore, the MASCAL bill should include provisions for how to organize the response if it is only the ship's medical and FST, as well as how to integrate these other embarked units to maximize capabilities and minimize confusion. Having the MASCAL bill on paper is not enough; it is essential to drill this when new units embark. You also need to ensure the protocols, equipment, and supplies for resuscitation are prepared, including your blood bank and WBB. You are the subject matter expert when it comes to trauma; take the lead on preparing the entire team, not only the FST.

As the surgeon, you should also have a good relationship with the Triage officer (usually the dentist) to ensure patients are arriving in the OR in the priority order you want them. If possible, survey all casualties up front and communicate priorities to the Triage officer, and then you have to trust that they've got it from there while you get to work in the OR. If you've done your part in training them well, they will.

In a MASCAL or other large event, the CATF surgeon and MRCO focus on the big picture, outside of the ship communications, while the MAO and SMO control the situation inside the ship. You will likely need to communicate with both because you need to know what your MEDEVAC/CASEVAC options are, if there are more casualties expected, status of blood products, and other variables will likely impact your operative decision-making. Make sure you read and understand the MASCAL bill, and don't be afraid to speak up during drills if it's not working well. That's the time to hash out the details, not during a real MASCAL.

Closing Thoughts

The FST fits into a larger medical system in unique and dynamic ways, with its influence and responsibility spread across multiple ships. Surgeons are natural leaders and our training to remain calm and decisive in emergencies means that the rest of the team will look to us for guidance and leadership no matter what the situation is. Take the time to cultivate those relationships, both within the FST and across the various medical units you will deploy with. Teach the corpsmen, mentor the general medical officers, advise your COC. Surgery is a team sport, but it's not a pick-up game.

In Depth: Expeditionary Resuscitative Surgical System (ERSS) OIC

Team Personnel

The ERSS consists of seven personnel including an emergency medicine physician, anesthesia provider (CRNA or anesthesiologist), general surgeon, critical care nurse (CCRN), ST, corpsman, and another advanced provider (usually a physician assistant or independent duty corpsman).

Chain of command (COC). Who serves in the OIC role is team dependent and is typically one of the three physicians or an operationally experienced physician assistant. Often surgeons act as the OIC for these types of austere resuscitative surgical teams. However, the surgeon may not be the best person for this role. In the event your team has to manage one or more operative casualties, the surgeon will often be task saturated and unable to perform time-sensitive and critical OIC tasks.

The primary role of the OIC of an ERSS team is to coordinate communication and actions between three fundamentally different entities. In a ship-based environment, the three players are the co-located medical assets, the maritime platform leadership, and the customer requesting the support of an austere resuscitative surgical team. The medical assets of a small ship are typically an E-6 or E-7 Independent Duty Corpsman (IDC) and 2–3 general duty corpsmen. The customer is often some variety of special operations forces (SOF) unit or occasionally a high-profile individual or group (such as a government official). **It is important to realize that the latter two groups (maritime platform and customer) likely know as much about trauma medicine as medical providers know about driving a ship or conducting state business. This means the ERSS team OIC needs to become involved as early as possible with planning and logistics to facilitate a positive mission experience and ensure unit/customer understanding of ERSS team capabilities. Additionally, the team (and especially the OIC) should have a base level of knowledge about ship design, manning, capabilities, and the basics of shipboard living.**

In many ways, the ship and customer will not understand things that a trauma medical team generally takes for granted, and there are many issues an ERSS team will encounter that a land-based surgical team (or even a large-deck FST) will not have had to deal with. Some examples include:

- Limited size (weight and cube) of an ERSS AMAL.
- Location, footprint, and flow of an OR setup.
- Fundamentals such as electrical supply, lighting, temperature control, oxygen, etc.
- Consequences of ship movement during surgery.
- Patient litter movement.
- Intensive Care Unit (ICU) level patient care and holding.
- Critical care transport and MEDEVAC/CASEVAC requirements.

For the non-medical communities that may employ or house an ERSS team, there is an expectation of a "plug and play" performance capability. Like any modern consumer, they purchase a product (damage control surgical resuscitation) and want that function to turn on, work as expected, and then turn off as required. While the ERSS team is built on a concept of adaptability and creative problem-solving, many issues can be addressed early on by proactive communication with the key players. This can mean the difference between mission success and failure. Perhaps equally as important, it can mean the difference between the appearance of skill versus the appearance of incompetence.

The most effective way to illustrate the points above is to walk through the important questions to ask following a mission assignment and discuss the pitfalls and opportunities for success throughout the process. One of the key features of the ERSS team is its rapid deployability. In the Pacific Area of Responsibility (AOR), the expectation was to have full operational capability (FOC) to perform missions within 72 h of notification. Whatever the lead time may be, there are multiple issues the OIC should be seeking clarification on for this unique maritime surgical mission.

1. Mission request

Often, customers will request an ERSS team for a specific task that does not require the maximum advertised team capability or even a surgical capability. It is important to ascertain the true need in terms of total likely patients and anticipated patient-holding requirements. There is a substantial difference in manning and gear for a two-patient scenario than a four-patient scenario. Likewise, there is a significant difference between 2-day and 5-day holding capacity. Is this a single dignitary, a small SOF team, or a larger element? The ability to get the first answer, expected number of patients, will likely depend on access to classified mission plans and/or planners. The answer to the second part, patient-holding time, will often come from the ship, and will depend on the specific AOR and anticipated MEDEVAC/CASEVAC ranges. Again, exact answers may require classified briefings. Often, you may only get answers like "plan for X patients for Y days" until the team is embarked on the ship for further details. Important considerations for the team will be "how many members of the team should go?" and "how much gear should be brought?" A mission request based on a submarine may specify to bring five people (i.e., a surgeon, emergency medicine physician, anesthesia provider, surgical technologist, and CCRN). A request for a high-level government official may require the entire seven-person team, plus potentially an orthopedic surgeon or an additional two-person ERC team. OICs should proactively discuss within the team various scenarios and "pre-plan" team compositions.

2. Gear requirements

Once the team composition is decided and the mission specifics are known to the greatest extent possible, the next decision is how much gear to bring. There are several obvious competing interests. The more gear, the greater the surgical and ICU capability. However, more gear packed is more gear to be carried, stored, and moved throughout the mission. As an example, a typical mission embarked on a small ship, such as a destroyer (DDG), could easily require 15 crates of gear, weighing between 2000 and 2100 pounds. It will be crucially important to identify the logistics contact on either the destination ship or the entity responsible for transporting the team to its final location. It is almost a guarantee that a surface warfare officer (SWO) will significantly underestimate the weight and cube of an ERSS team's gear. For smaller ship-based missions, the primary POC for the ERSS OIC will be the Operations Officer (OPSO), who will usually be a senior Lieutenant (O-3). This person should be identified as early as possible to begin planning and logistics discussions. Care will need to be taken regarding operational security (OPSEC) and modes of communication, but with appropriate thought, necessary information can usually be conveyed in a non-classified fashion until direct contact is made.

3. Blood product availability

There is no surgical capability without appropriate blood product availability and resuscitation. This cold surgical fact is often not understood by your potential customers, particularly in the non-SOF maritime environment. How much blood an ERSS team can carry and store will depend on proximity to a blood bank, feasibility of resupply, availability of a reliable refrigerator, and potentially the organic blood supply of the platform being used. Larger ships will often have either a frozen blood supply or a robust WBB program. Smaller ships, while theoretically capable of having a WBB, should not be assumed to have a functioning program without discussing with the ship's medical personnel.

An ERSS team may want to consider bringing a supply of blood donation kits in the event the ship has a roster of low-titer O blood donors. Throughout the duration of the mission, it is vitally important for the OIC to stay engaged with both ship leadership and any other operational command elements to keep the issue of blood supply at the forefront. With a maximum lifespan of 14 days once thawed, the mission timing may dictate the need for arranging blood resupply at sea or carefully timing a draw of whole blood donor units. If an ERSS OIC can properly convey the vital importance of donor blood, non-medical leadership is generally understanding and accommodating of the seriousness of those requests as they present some of the most significant logistical challenges.

4. Space setup

Space onboard a small ship, such as a DDG, is at a premium. Additionally, the design of these ships was not done with an eye towards "casualty receiving" logistics. The organic medical spaces are not typically located within a close proximity to the likely casualty receiving point (usually the aft helicopter deck). An ERSS team should conduct as many trial runs as needed to decide the most appropriate setup. Often, the optimum solution involves using the hangar bay for the patient receiving, trauma bay, and OR spaces. This will require communication with the ship and aircrew to allow sufficient time with an empty bay to set up, practice, troubleshoot, and train prior to a real-world operation. The air element on a DDG will have an assigned OIC, usually an O-4 or potentially an O-5.

The passageways on small ships are narrow, and have small, sharp corners that make litter movement challenging, especially with a critically injured patient. Planning with ship's company will be needed to organize and train litter teams for patient movement, as it is unwise to put the ERSS team members outside the skin of the ship and risk a one-of-one member to an accident or injury. The ship's Command Master Chief (CMC) is an excellent and mandatory resource when requesting to pull Sailors for ERSS purposes.

It is also critical to discuss with the ship how the MEDEVAC/CASEVAC plan will affect the hangar bay availability following mission completion. It may be necessary to bring helicopters back into the hangar bay prior to making the best speed to a higher level of care. In this case, following stabilization, plans should be in place to move patients for holding. The organic medical space is an option but on smaller ships is quite limited in size. Consider alternatives such as the crew's mess deck, Chief's mess, or other open areas to require as little patient movement as possible. The space will also require room for life-saving equipment such as intravenous (IV) pumps, drains, monitors, and potentially emergent re-exploration equipment.

5. MEDEVAC/CASEVAC

   Commonly, the mission parameters will include 2–4 days of patient holding to allow the ship to come into range of an appropriate MEDEVAC/CASEVAC site. Again, the logistics of this plan are often made without medical input, so an OIC should engage as early as possible. Options are often limited, and require a risk/benefit assessment between shorter holding on ship and sending to a non-United States (U.S.) facility versus holding onboard longer to return to a U.S. facility. These plans are often made by the SOF at the command level or via an office of the Executive branch of the government such as the State Department. The team must engage the process to know the capabilities of any MEDEVAC/CASEVAC site, ability to communicate with the said site, and methods of patient transport. Loading a patient litter onto a helicopter on the ship may be easy, but if there are no suitable landing facilities at the destination, the patient may need to be hoisted down. What type of transport capabilities does the patient require? What level of attendant should accompany the patient, and what is that person's return plan? It may be that the lowest risk plan is to continue to hold the patient despite the option to fly them off to a non-ideal facility. Furthermore, even the most reliable MEDEVAC/CASEVAC plan may not be available when you need it, so always plan for prolonged patient holding contingencies (Chap. 30).

Perioperative Communication and MASCAL

When augmenting a Role 1 platform there is no role for ERSS teams to perform elective surgical procedures, and patients requiring emergency general surgery should be transferred to a higher level of care (conventional Role 2 or higher) except for rare exceptions when your team is managing unstable patients who cannot be stabilized or transferred in a timely fashion. When augmenting platforms with formal OR spaces (e.g., LHD, LHA, LPD, CVN) the discussions in the FST and CVN in-depth sections hold true for the ERSS team as well. The ERSS team is designed to mitigate operational risk and be available for the unexpected. For the ERSS, one injured critically ill patient *is* a MASCAL. To successfully care for one or multiple patients during a MASCAL, dynamic subordination with fluid leadership of team members coupled with critical skill redundancy and open, effective communication are critical. To develop these team dynamic skills the OIC must encourage a culture of team trust, empowerment, and accountability.

Closing Thoughts

The greatest honor for an ERSS team is to allow our military special forces and government officials to conduct their business in remote and austere environments with the full confidence of a highly trained and adaptable surgical team standing by in case of emergency. Statistically, a successful ERSS mission does not involve an actual casualty, but this should never prevent the team from planning for and training for all worst-case scenarios. This planning *must* include the ship and customer to be maximally effective and ensure the highest chance for success should the worst-case scenario become reality.

In Depth: Forward Resuscitative Surgical System (FRSS) Staff Surgeon

The Forward Resuscitative Surgical System (FRSS) is the Damage Control Surgical Resuscitation unit deployed in support of USMC operations. A full description of the FRSS can be found in Chap. 1. There are currently discussions on changing how the FRSS is composed and deployed in the future, however, the discussion below is based on the current Statement of Need (SON).

The keys to successful FRSS deployment in the operational setting are: understanding how the FRSS is organized and awareness of capabilities/shortfalls, MASCAL communication, and coordination with associated medical assets and supported unit(s), agreed-upon delegation of triage and patient disposition authority, making the most of every CASEVAC, and team training as much as possible prior to casualty events.

Team Personnel

The FRSS is designed to address non-compressible hemorrhage and perform damage control surgery (DCS) as part of an overall resuscitation strategy. The FRSS is composed of two surgeons (usually two general surgeons), one anesthesiologist, one CCRN, one IDC, two STs, and one basic corpsman. The FRSS, in its current configuration, is deployed in support of either a Shock Trauma Platoon (STP) or Battalion Aid Station (BAS). The FRSS is most often coupled with a STP, combining to create a Surgical Platoon. The FRSS does not have the capability of self-sustainment, and is reliant on the unit it is supporting for Base Operating Support, otherwise known as BOS. BOS consists of electricity generation, climate control, water, etc.

As a surgeon assigned to FRSS, one of the first things you will notice is that the capabilities of the FRSS as advertised by non-surgeons do not necessarily match what your surgical intuition tells you. For this reason, it is important that you are actively involved in the medical planning for the utilization of the FRSS. Your understanding of MEDEVAC/CASEVAC capabilities, limitations, and considerations will be essential in your decision-making as to when to operate and when not to. Blood products available and the access to blood products whether components or stored whole blood and the status of a WBB is a critical baseline knowledge and should be part of your daily checklist. Cognizance of ongoing and prospective operations by the unit you are supporting may allow you time to develop and implement contingencies for dealing with sudden increases in number of patients. Finally, predeployment downloading and reading of the Joint Trauma System (JTS) Clinical Practice Guidelines (CPGs) is essential as these are a wealth of reference information based on actual experiences that have been condensed for easy reading and portability.

Perioperative Communication and MASCAL

Communication and coordination with all associated medical assets and supported units are vital in the care of any moderately to severely injured patients. Agreed-upon delegation of triage and patient disposition authority ahead of time is essential to management of rapidly changing operational environments and conditions. Most commonly, the FRSS will be coupled with an STP to create a Surgical Platoon as previously stated. It is imperative that the STP not be seen as an Emergency Room, with surgeons only participating when/after consulted by an Emergency Medicine physician. Both the STP and FRSS are undermanned to meet a sudden MASCAL event–either in complexity or severity of injured patients or the absolute number of patients. Two severely injured patients in class III or IV shock could stretch a Surgical Platoon's resources just as much as the sudden presentation of 10 moderately injured patients. For this reason, I advocate abandoning any recreation of the division of labor seen in the hospital setting. To maximize resources to meet rapidly evolving contingencies, there must be an agreed-upon delegation of triage and patient disposition authority prior to a Surgical Platoon deploying.

I have found it works best when there is a designated Medical Officer of the Day (MOOD) and Surgical Officer of the Day (SOOD). Overall triage of patients is the responsibility of the MOOD, but the SOOD should be actively scouring for and aware of potential surgical cases, to determine the best order of surgical intervention. Once initial triage is done, the MOOD can then transition to assuring ongoing Surgical Platoon throughput by arranging and optimizing MEDEVAC/CASEVAC patients, organizing resupply of CLASS VIII supplies (blood and bandages), and resetting of the Surgical Platoon while the FRSS performs DCS. The SOOD would also be responsible for coordinating patient disposition with the MOOD. While one surgeon is the SOOD, the second surgeon then can be the team lead for the most critically injured patient until it is time to take the first designated patient to the OR. Anesthesia providers being airway experts are best, in my experience, at rapidly evaluating the airways of all patients in the STP undergoing resuscitation, and should be utilized in this capacity until a decision has been made to bring a patient to the OR. One of the STs should prepare the OR for patient care, while the second ST assists with procedures in the STP.

MEDEVAC/CASEVAC

Do not hesitate to advocate for MEDEVAC/CASEVAC of your patients at the earliest opportunity, as the functionality of your unit is similar to the maxim of arterial repair from our training in vascular surgery, outflow is as vitally important as inflow to assure functionality.

Team Training

As a USMC Medical Battalion surgeon, it is important that you advocate for the participation of STs in clinical activities while in garrison. Make sure you reach out to the senior ST at the Medical Battalion every time you have a "big" case at the hospital. Hold training sessions with the STs on cases that they may not commonly do such as resuscitative thoracotomy, exploration of the trauma abdomen, central line placement, chest tube placement and pleurovac setup, etc. Coordinate and insist on ST participation with Medical Battalion surgeons in courses like Advanced Surgical Skills for Exposure in Trauma (ASSET (+)) and/or Combat Orthopedic Trauma Surgical skills (COTS (+)). When in the field for exercises and particularly once deployed: drill, drill, drill by running scenarios with your team allows you to think through cases while also getting everyone on the same page before a real world surgery.

Closing Thoughts: A Senior Surgeon's Perspective

My colleagues have elucidated many pertinent common points of taking on the role of an operational surgeon. Be realistic about your unit's true capabilities and capacity. Organize and train the team you belong to throughout the entirety of your deployment. Communication is key—establish and foster clean lines of communication within your unit and with the COC you report to. Prepare as much as you can prior to deployment–know your platform's capabilities, and potential pitfalls to become, as best you can, the subject matter expert for delivering surgical care in the operational environment. Especially in MASCAL situations. Be realistic about your unit's true capabilities and capacity. Finally, understand the unit/platform you are supporting, this can be done best by earning either your Surface Warfare Medical

Department Officer (SWMDO) Qualification or Fleet Marine Force (FMF) Warfare Qualification. Enjoy your tour, and remember there is only a small portion of American physicians and surgeons who will ever have the opportunity to have the experiences you will during your deployment.

Conclusion

While the different platforms vary in who their team is composed of, what their mission is, where their OR is located, and how their chain of command is structured, the basic tenets of leadership, communication, and preparation echo throughout the authors' recommendations for forward-deployed maritime surgical team leaders.

Declaration of Interest The views expressed in this chapter are those of the authors and do not necessarily reflect the official policy or position of the Department of the Navy, Department of Defense, nor the US Government.

Funding This research did not receive any specific grant from funding agencies in the public, commercial, or not-for-profit sectors.

Conflict of Interest Statement The authors declare no conflict of interest.

Further Reading

Instruction 6000.1, the Shipboard Medical Procedures Manual, which differs by region and platform (for example from San Diego: COMNAVAIRPACINST for CVN, COMNAVSURFPACINST/COMNAVSURFLANTINST for the other platforms).

Joint Trauma System (JTS) Clinical Practice Guidelines (CPGs).

OPNAVINST 3501.408, Required Operational Capabilities and Projected Operational Environment for the Role 2 Light Maneuver Expeditionary Resuscitative Surgical System. 14 June 2021. https://www.secnav.navy.mil/doni/Directives/03000%20Naval%20Operations%20and%20Readiness/03-500%20Training%20and%20Readiness%20Services/3501.408.pdf.

Part II
Before the Operating Room

Chapter 7
Shipboard Triage and Mass Casualty

Jesse Bandle and Miguel A. Cubano

By failing to prepare, you are preparing to fail.

Benjamin Franklin

Author deployment experience	
Jesse Bandle	Staff Surgeon, Fleet Surgical Team-7, embarked on the USS Bonhomme Richard (LHD-6), CERTEX, INDOPACOM Area of Responsibility, 2016–2017; Exercise Talisman Sabre, INDOPACOM Area of Responsibility, 2017
Miguel A. Cubano	Ship's Surgeon, USS Abraham Lincoln (CVN-72), WESTPAC, Operation Southern Watch, INDOPACOM and CENTCOM Areas of Responsibility, 1994–1995
	Task Force Surgeon (TFS), Commander, Amphibious Task Force (CATF) Surgeon, USS O'Bannon (DDG-987), UNITAS 40, SOUTHCOM Area of Responsibility, 1999–2000
	Ship's Surgeon, USS Kitty Hawk (CV-63), WESTPAC and Talisman Saber, INDOPACOM Area of Responsibility, 2004–2005
	Executive Officer, USNS Comfort (T-AH-20), Operation Continuing Promise, Caribbean, Central, and South America Areas of Responsibility, 2014–2016

BLUF (Bottom Line Up Front)

1. A shipboard mass casualty incident (MCI) can happen at any time. Sustained and frequent planning, training, and rehearsal are paramount to adequate preparation.
2. Early recognition of an MCI and activation of the Mass Casualty Bill are critical to an effective response.
3. Triage casualties, re-triage frequently, and document triage/changes.

J. Bandle (✉) · M. A. Cubano
Department of Surgery, Naval Medical Center San Diego, Navy Medicine Readiness and Training Command, San Diego, CA, USA
e-mail: jesse.bandle.mil@health.mil; miguel.a.cubano2.mil@health.mil

M. D. Tadlock, A. A. Hernandez (eds.), *Expeditionary Surgery at Sea*,
https://doi.org/10.1007/978-3-031-21893-4_7

4. Staffing of the immediate and delayed treatment areas should maximize the opportunity for the minimum number of staff to safely and efficiently care for the patients triaged to their area.
5. Resource constraints (personnel, physical places, and supplies/equipment including blood products) during a shipboard MCI must guide decision-making prior to, during, and following an MCI.
6. In the era of Distributed Maritime Operations (DMO), the distance between the ship and the next level of care may be great. Be prepared for prolonged stabilization of casualties on board.
7. Effective communication is both the best tool to overcome the chaos of an MCI and the most challenging aspect to achieve. Make efforts to simplify communication but have contingencies in place.
8. It is impossible to plan for every contingency, therefore be creative in team design and foster processes that can adapt to chaos.
9. Do everything possible to eliminate bottlenecks in the flow of patients. However, realize there is almost always a single resource limitation in the response process.
10. Drill, drill, then drill again! Learn from the drills to refine the process and provider triage skills at all levels.

Introduction

Mass casualty incidents (MCIs) occur when the number of patients or the severity of injuries exceeds the capabilities or resources of the facility and staff [1]. Therefore one or two severely injured patients can result in an MCI. The inherent limitations in personnel, supplies, and equipment of the shipboard medical department result in even relatively minor incidents having the potential to quickly become MCIs. Early recognition of an MCI at sea and rapid transition from routine to contingency operations are critical to the successful management of casualties.

Effective use of the principle of triage (sorting and prioritizing injured patients in the context of available resources, tactical situation, and mission) is paramount for combating the chaos of a shipboard MCI and providing the greatest benefit to the greatest number of patients [2]. **It is important to note that triage is NOT the same as patient assessment**; rather, it is an assignment of resources based on the initial patient assessment in the context of available resources. Triage is also not a singular event–it must be a dynamic, fluid, and repeated process throughout the MCI. Re-triage of patients and documentation of changes as they pass through every level of care, from first responder through evacuation to higher echelons of care, is essential to avoid missing changes in patient status during the chaos of an MCI. Triage categories, definitions, and examples of specific injury patterns are reviewed in Table 7.1 [2]. Changes in tactical circumstances, depletion (or addition)

Table 7.1 Triage categories, definitions, and examples of injury patterns [2]

Triage category	Definition	Examples of injuries/findings
Immediate	Attention/surgical intervention is urgently required to avoid death or major disability	• Airway obstruction/ compromise
	Interventions should be focused on patients with a good chance of survival if timely care is provided	• Tension pneumothorax
		• Uncontrolled hemorrhage
		• Pelvis, torso, or neck injuries with shock
		• Head injuries requiring decompression
		• Threatened loss of limb
Delayed	A procedure is indicated, but the injury/condition permits delay without endangering life, limb, or eye sight	• Abdominal or thoracic injuries without signs of shock
	Efficiently employed minor interventions (stabilizing fractures, fluid resuscitation, pain control, administration of antibiotics) may be required to allow for delay of definitive care	• Isolated long bone fractures
		• Soft tissue injuries without vascular involvement
		• Burns without immediate threat to airway or limb
Minimal	Minor injuries in patients who can effectively provide self-care or be treated with minimal medical involvement	• Minor lacerations
	Because of their mobility, these patients may be the first to arrive at the medical department in a mass casualty incident (MCI). Controls must be instituted to not allow these patients to divert resources/attention from the more critically-injured patients who could not self-transport to the medical spaces	• Abrasions
		• Small bone fractures
		• Minor burns
Expectant	Injuries are severe and would divert time and resources from patients who have a more realistic chance of survival	• Casualty arriving without vital signs
	Goals of care should include comfort measures and intermittent reassessment. If possible, segregation of the expectant triaged patients away from the view of other triage categories will help limit escalation of emotional chaos	• Penetrating head trauma
		• Open pelvic injuries with uncontrolled bleeding
		• Burns without reasonable chance for survival
		• High spinal cord injuries

of resources, or changes in patient status may all require shifting a patient from one triage Category to another over the course of an MCI.

Clinical Vignette 7.1

The USS Kitty Hawk (CV-63) was deployed off the southern coast of Japan in 2005 performing carrier qualification flight operations. An F/A-18F returning to the flight deck severed an arresting wire, which struck several flight deck personnel as the aircraft rolled off the port side angle deck into the ocean. Approximately 30 min after the incident, the six injured Sailors on the flight deck and the two involved aviators were transported to the ship's triage receiving stations and evaluated. Major injuries identified included:

1. *One patient had a left below-the-knee traumatic amputation, a right fibular fracture, and a left ulnar fracture.*
2. *One patient had a right patellar fracture and complete multi-ligament tear as well as a full-thickness scalp laceration.*
3. *One patient had a left shoulder dislocation and a left ankle sprain.*
4. *The remaining five injured air and deck crew had only minor injuries.*

The sailor with the traumatic amputation was taken to the Operating Room (OR) where three of the ship's six physicians participated in his operative care. The remaining seven patients were cared for by the flight surgeon and General Medical Officer (GMO) with the assistance of the Independent Duty Corpsman (IDC) and critical care registered nurse (CCRN). The ship's sole radiology technician was tasked with simultaneous requests for intraoperative and triage bay films, averaging three X-ray series per patient. Due to the ship's proximity to Japan, all patients with major injuries were able to get a medical evacuation (MEDEVAC) to Naval Hospital Yokosuka later that evening [3].

This vignette onboard the USS Kitty Hawk (CV-63) illustrates many of the key features of shipboard MCIs that will be detailed in this chapter. To facilitate planning, training, and drilling of MCIs, it is important for everyone on the team to familiarize themselves with historic examples and the lessons learned; suggested readings on the topic are available at the end of this chapter.

Initial Triage

Ship-specific triage areas are typically designated in each ship's Mass Casualty Bill. The exact area designated will vary depending on the location of casualties, the type of MCI causing the casualties (engineering versus flight deck versus off-ship mishap), as well as the tactical evolution of the ship at the time. Flexibility and creativity with the location of the initial triage are far better guiding principles than rigid adherence to dogmatic instruction. **Though it is impossible to predict every scenario a ship may encounter in an MCI, time and effort should be spent "war gaming" the likely presentation of patients from both on-ship and off-ship incidents in order to build a portfolio of contingency plans for triage and MCI operations**.

If possible, casualties should flow through a single triage area where rapid evaluation by the initial triage officer is accomplished. Once the casualty has been triaged to a specific Category, transportation to the designated (see Table 7.1: Immediate, Delayed, Minimal, and Expectant) treatment area should occur expeditiously. Staff in the triage area should not engage in extensive management of injuries, instead, they should focus on sorting into Categories, communication of findings, and quick transport of the casualty to the better staffed and equipped treatment areas. The goal of triage is to identify the minority of critically injured casualties requiring immediate treatment in order to provide care as soon as possible [4]. Ideally, the initial triage area should be in relative proximity to the treatment areas, provide for a one-way flow of patients, and have ample secondary staffing (litter bearers, recorders, and designated communication staff). The use of a color-coded triage tag can be helpful to transmit vital information about each patient and is especially helpful if radio/electronic communications are down. However, simply making a clearly visible notation with an indelible marker with triage Category assignment and numeric patient identifier can be sufficient.

Though an experienced surgeon may be the perfect triage officer, as is the case in many land-based Role 2–3–4 facilities, it is likely that their skills and training would be better utilized in the immediate treatment area/OR during a shipboard MCI. Furthermore, during routine operations, most maritime surgical teams (aircraft carrier (CVN), Fleet Surgical Team (FST), Expeditionary Resuscitative Surgical System (ERSS)) only have one surgeon (Chap. 1). A well-trained Dental officer can augment or assume the role of initial triage officer when personnel constraints and injury severity dictate the skills of trauma-trained providers (e.g., Emergency Medicine (EM) physician, anesthesiologist, surgeon) would be better utilized in the treatment area/OR.

Immediate/Delayed Treatment Areas

Distribution of providers is as critical, or more so, than the distribution of supplies in an MCI. Staffing of the immediate and delayed treatment areas should maximize the opportunity for the minimum number of staff to safely and efficiently care for the patients triaged in their area. For example, planning the layout of the immediate and delayed treatment areas to maximize the ability of limited staff to observe and participate in patient care is imperative. The commitment of too many personnel to a single critical casualty is dangerous when there are a significant number of injured patients and should be conscientiously avoided. Knowing the strengths and limitations of the team members will help to ensure appropriate treatment assignments. Assignment to the standing watch, quarter, and station bills should be made following an assessment of the individuals' training level, skills, and abilities. Realistic drills and simulation can be helpful to reveal deficits in training that need to be addressed for particular providers.

Special Considerations for Shipboard Triage: Limited Resources

MCIs can stretch the capabilities of shore-based hospital care, so it is no surprise that those effects are far more acute aboard a maritime vessel with enhanced resource vulnerabilities. Err on the side of over-triage, but be mindful of how this affects limited available resources. Specific constraints that require consideration before, during, and following a shipboard MCI include personnel, physical spaces, and equipment/supplies (including blood products).

Personnel: The capabilities, training background, and trauma management skills of individual providers must be critically analyzed in the planning and training phases in order to identify the most beneficial role they will play in an MCI. Additionally, remember that personnel must be considered a perishable resource. Fatigue will degrade the function of even the most highly skilled provider. This is especially important in the era of Distributed Maritime Operations (DMO), where Role 2 platforms are more geographically isolated. There is significant potential for prolonged stabilization/care of casualties far beyond the typical window of a shore-based Role 2 platform [5]. This highlights both the need for provider training in Intensive Care Unit (ICU) level critical care management as well as the importance for rest and crew rotation following the initial MCI response. MCI planning should include provisions and guidelines which ensure medical staff sustainment.

Physical spaces: Shipboard space is limited even during normal operations and the effect is amplified during an MCI. Coordination with non-medical units to utilize the needed space for triage areas (e.g., clearing the hangar bay of aircraft) is a vital part of the planning phases of MCI preparation. Consideration and planning for the loss of the primary medical spaces due to sustained damage or contamination is an important part of contingency planning. Identification of secondary and tertiary triage/treatment areas physically distant from the medical department should be well known to medical and non-medical crew.

Equipment/supplies-general: Effort should be taken to limit the overuse of equipment and supplies during an MCI. The pronounced logistic impediments to shipboard resupply in the era of DMO will impact the time one is required to work with "what's on hand." Re-sterilization of OR instrument sets may be limited, and consumables (e.g., medications, oxygen, dressings, sutures) will quickly run out if there isn't conscientious oversight and control of their use. Organizing supplies in the triage and treatment areas is also a way that simplifies their use and is a critical part of pre-MCI preparation.

Equipment/supplies-blood products: Another critical supply element to consider is the availability of blood and blood products. Casualty Receiving and Treatment Ships (CRTS) are equipped with frozen blood products and deglycerolization equipment. It is likely in an MCI there will be a need for hemostatic resuscitation with a balanced ratio of blood component therapy. Given the lack of platelets on naval warships, the finite stores of frozen blood products, and the time it takes to thaw/deglycerolize, preparations should also be made to collect warm fresh whole blood (FWB) from the Walking Blood Bank (WBB). On many other maritime platforms, the WBB is the only source of blood for resuscitation. The United States (U.S.) Department of Defense (DoD) Committee on Tactical Combat Casualty Care (TCCC) has recommended whole blood over component therapy for resuscitation in hemorrhagic shock [6, 7]. Activation of the WBB during MCI drills and pre-identification of suitable donors will greatly accelerate the availability of blood for hemostatic resuscitation. During an actual MCI aboard the USS Bataan (LHD-5) in 2017, the crew was able to generate 12 units of warm FWB from the WBB in 30 min [6], far outpacing what would have been available from thawing the stored frozen blood products.

Communication

"What Do I Know? Who Needs to Know? Have I Told Them?"

This United States Marine Corps (USMC) leadership principle is especially poignant during a shipboard MCI. Even face-to-face communication during the chaos of an MCI can be challenging. Efforts should be made to limit loud talking during the care of patients. As providers and treatment teams direct the care of patients, the volume invariably escalates to the point where communication can become impossible. Focus the teams, maintain auditory discipline, and discourage any side commentary from medical and non-medical crew.

Ensure leaders have a dedicated liaison for communication with ship line leadership (see Chap. 6). Communication of patient status, supply status, and casualty numbers will be critical for command-level decision-making. Coordination of patient movement, equipment, and ship personnel during an MCI typically goes through Damage Control Central, and the medical representative assigned there should communicate the needs of the medical response. Likewise, command-down communication of tactical situations, logistics of re-supply, and capability of evacuation will be valuable information for medical personnel during triage and re-triage of ongoing MCI casualties.

Training and Drills

Planning for a wide variety of scenarios is critical to shipboard MCI preparation. Any new arrivals to the ship should review the current Mass Casualty Bill and familiarize themselves with the spaces and processes. Evaluate the plan for potential bottlenecks in triage, patient movement, and patient evaluation/treatment. Don't be attached to ship dogma, what worked for the previous crew may not be ideal for the current team. Planning for different MCI scenarios should begin with the core treatment team conducting contingency 'war games.' Review the likely injury patterns from onboard MCI (e.g., engineering mishap, flight deck mishap, ballistic attack) as well as the possible casualties that may be received from mission-related transport to the ship. See Chap. 4 for a discussion of mechanisms of injury in modern naval operations. Progressing from tabletop discussion to a walk-through review of MCI/triage response and critical inspection of the physical spaces is an important step in the identification of weak spots in the process design. Once the team is confident in the overall efficiency of patient flow through triage and treatment areas, concentrate on staffing assignments with deference to particular provider strengths and weaknesses.

Now is the time to start drilling, there is no way to predict if the next MCI will happen today, tomorrow, or next week. Start drills with individual treatment teams (stretcher-bearers, triage, immediate/delayed treatment, OR team) and progress to a full medical department run-through. Time department-specific drills in the lead-up to scheduled mandatory mass casualty drills. Of note, the majority of litter bearers are non-medical ship personnel, so they need to be drilled as well even if they do not work in the medical spaces. They participate in the mass casualty drills but most importantly, they play a critical role in patient care: getting the patient safely to the surgical team. See Chap. 11 for more information about litters and Chap. 31 for patient movement.

Each drill is an opportunity to identify weaknesses in both the process and in individual team members so that additional, preferably on-the-spot, training can fill in the gaps. It's easy to push the department into drill fatigue, but the time spent training and drilling is the only way to minimize the chaos of a true MCI. Maritime MCI can be even more difficult to manage than land-based MCI and present unique challenges to the medical team, but with focused preparation, planning, and training everyone can ensure the best possible care for the greatest number of casualties when the worst-case scenario becomes reality.

Conclusion

Triage, re-triage, and always document. Recognize and plan for resource constraints, including the possibility of DMO operations and extending onboard care of casualties when applicable. Communication is vital and challenging; always ask "What do I know? Who needs to know? Have I told them?" Examine the process and flow for potential bottlenecks and mitigate where feasible. Plan for the worst-case scenario, develop robust contingency plans, and train for the best outcomes. Creativity and ingenuity trump instruction and dogma. Then drill like everyone's lives depend on it. Semper Gumby!

Declaration of Interest The views expressed in this chapter are those of the authors and do not necessarily reflect the official policy or position of the Department of the Navy, Department of Defense, nor the US Government.

Funding This research did not receive any specific grant from funding agencies in the public, commercial, or not-for-profit sectors.

Conflict of Interest Statement The authors declare no conflict of interest.

References

1. American College of Surgeons Committee on Trauma. Advanced trauma life support student course manual. Chicago: American College of Surgeons; 2012. p. 6.
2. U.S. Department of Defense. Emergency war surgery. Fort Sam Huston: Borden Institute, US Army Medical Department Center and School Health Readiness Center of Excellence. Fifth United States Revision; 2018. p. 23–39.
3. Chavez T, Cubano M, Hovijitra R. Mass casualty aboard USS Kitty Hawk (CV 63) January 2005 –lessons learned. Mil Med. 2005;170:iii–vi.
4. Frykberg E, Tepas J. Terrorist bombings – lessons learned from Belfast to Beirut. Ann Surg. 1988;5:569–76.
5. Day W, Cooper E, Phung K, et al. Prolonged stabilization during a mass casualty incident at sea in the era of distributed maritime operations. Mil Med. 2020;11–12:2192–7.
6. Miller B, Lin A, Clark S, et al. Red tides: mass casualty and whole blood at sea. J Trauma Acute Care Surg. 2018;85(1 Suppl 1):S134–9.
7. Butler F, Holcomb J, Schreiber M, et al. Fluid resuscitation for hemorrhagic shock in tactical combat casualty care: TCCC guidelines change 14-01. J Spec Oper Med. 2014;14(3):13–38.

Further Reading

COMNAVAIRFORINST 6000.1 (Section 5) 13501. Mass Casualty Planning. 13-15–13-19.

Hoang T, Kang J, Siriratsivawong K, et al. Hyper-realistic, team centered fleet surgical team training provides sustained improvements in performance. J Surg Educ. 2016;73(4):668–74.

Hubbard Z, Henderson F, Armonda R, et al. The shipboard Beirut terrorist bombing experience: a historical account and recommendations for preparedness in events of mass neurological injuries. Neurosurg Focus. 2018;45:1–7.

Jankosky J. Mass casualty in an isolated environment: medical response to a submarine collision. Mil Med. 2008;173:734–7.

Lambert E, Simpson B, Marzouk A, et al. Orthopaedic injuries among survivors of USS COLE attack. J Orthop Trauma. 2003;17(6):436–41.

Netzer I, Weiss A, Hoppenstein D. Naval casualty management training using human patient simulators. Disast Mil Med. 2015;1:1–7.

Tactical Combat Casualty Care – quick reference guide. https://emsa.ca.gov/wp-content/uploads/sites/71/2017/07/TCCC_Quick_Reference_Guide_2017.pdf.

Tadlock M, Gurney J, Tripp M, et al. Between the devil and the deep blue sea: a review of 25 modern naval mass casualty incidents with implications for future distributed maritime operations. J Trauma Acute Care Surg. 2021 Aug 1;91(2S Suppl 2):S46-S55.

Chapter 8
Shipboard Diagnostics: Laboratory and Radiology

Roderick C. Borgie and Clara A. Pangco

A scientist in his laboratory is not a mere technician: he is also a child confronting natural phenomena that impress him as though they were fairy tales.

Marie Curie

Author deployment experience	
Roderick C. Borgie	Flight Surgeon, Carrier Air Wing Nine (CVW-9), embarked on the USS John C. Stennis (CVN-74), Operation Desert Shield, Persian Gulf, 2000
	Force Surgeon/Deputy Force Surgeon, Commander Naval Air Forces, 2015–2019
	Staff Neuroradiologist, Naval Medical Center San Diego, 2015–2022
	Force Surgeon, Commander Naval Air Forces Reserve, 2019–2022
Clara A. Pangco	Laboratory Technician, USNS Mercy (T-AH-19), Pacific Partnership, Indonesia, Philippines, Vietnam, Cambodia, 2012
	Laboratory Department Head, NATO Role 3 Multinational Medical Unit, NATO Resolute Support and Operation Freedom's Sentinel, Kandahar Airfield, Afghanistan, 2017–2018
	Laboratory Officer, 3rd Medical Battalion, Okinawa, 2018–2020; Deployed in support of Korean Marine Exchange Program, Korea, 2019; Dragon Lift, Korea, 2019; Task Force Medical in response to the USS Theodore Roosevelt (CVN-71) COVID-19 Outbreak, Guam, 2020

R. C. Borgie (✉) · C. A. Pangco
Navy Medicine Readiness and Training Command San Diego, San Diego, CA, USA
e-mail: Roderick@BorgieMD.com; clara.a.pangco.mil@health.mil

M. D. Tadlock, A. A. Hernandez (eds.), *Expeditionary Surgery at Sea*,
https://doi.org/10.1007/978-3-031-21893-4_8

BLUF (Bottom Line Up Front)

1. Laboratory testing on ship and shore greatly assists providers in making informed decisions when evaluating their patients.
2. Strict monitoring of staff training, safety, Standard Operating Procedures (SOPs), and quality assurance of all laboratory equipment is important to ensure accurate patient results.
3. Tests designated as Clinical Laboratory Improvement Amendments (CLIA)-waived are simple complexity, low risk, and can be performed by any sufficiently trained personnel, including non-laboratory technicians on smaller ships. Nonwaived tests are higher complexity tests that must be performed by a trained laboratory technician with specific qualifications and educational requirements and are typically limited to the larger platforms (e.g., hospital ships, aircraft carriers (CVNs), and large deck amphibious assault ships).
4. The availability and CLIA status of laboratory tests are ever-changing. As of 2021, the common tests available on most platforms are Complete Blood Count (CBC), Urinalysis, Urine human chorionic gonadotropin (HCG), Occult Blood, Rapid Flu, and Rapid Blood Glucose. Tests that typically are only available on larger platforms with designated laboratory technicians are Basic Metabolic Panel (BMP), Comprehensive Metabolic Panel (CMP), Liver Function Test (LFT), and Prothrombin Time/Partial Thromboplastin Time (PT/PTT).
5. X-rays are the mainstay of diagnostic imaging at sea and are available on the hospital ships, CVNs, and large deck amphibious assault ships. Their technology has advanced to computed radiography (CR) for most platforms and digital radiography (DR) for others.
6. With advances in technology, radiographic information can be initially interpreted immediately by onboard staff with near real-time backup final interpretation provided by a board-certified radiologist remotely.
7. Point-of-Care Ultrasound (POCUS) is available and can be particularly useful, although operator technique and experience in this area can be variable.
8. The most common studies performed are of the chest, extremities, and abdomen. It is important to obtain two views if possible to maximize the information used to diagnose and treat patients.
9. Surgical team members should familiarize themselves with the diagnostic capabilities of the laboratory and radiography suites for the ships on which they deploy.
10. Medical departments of larger ships typically do not stock contrast for procedures such as intraoperative cholangiogram or retrograde urethrogram. While performing these imaging procedures is rarely required at sea, surgeons should consider acquiring appropriate contrast prior to deployment.

Introduction

Surgical team members may not realize how reliant they are on the advances medicine has made in ancillary services until they are floating in the middle of the ocean with a sick patient. Laboratory and radiographic testing with readily available results ubiquitous at a medical treatment facility (MTF) may not be available immediately or offered at all on a naval warship. Surgical team members should familiarize themselves with the diagnostic capabilities of the laboratory and radiography suites for the ships on which they deploy prior to caring for patients to maximize their ability to plan for and deliver patient care.

Shipboard Laboratory: Historical Perspective

Medical diagnosis through clinical laboratory testing has drastically evolved throughout the years. Ancient physicians would evaluate body fluids (like urine) and expose them to environmental elements to observe certain reactions. Depending on their findings, they would then formulate their diagnosis. Tasting of the urine was even the norm to look for evidence of diabetes.

The invention of the microscope in the 1600s opened up a whole new world in medicine. In the 1800s, the field of laboratory science exploded with discoveries in hematology, blood chemistry, coagulation, and microbiology. In the 1900s, the field expanded on those discoveries and formalized much of what is known and practiced today. Over the years, manufacturers have been able to produce sophisticated yet compact instruments and kits that are more fitting for shipboard testing, which is important because modern medicine uses laboratory tests to arrive at a majority of their diagnoses.

Shipboard Laboratory: Current Overview

Laboratory Suite

On ships, the laboratory spaces can vary in size and configuration (see Fig. 8.1 for a sample space), as can the equipment, depending on the platform, ship, and medical capabilities. The surface Fleet Type Commander (TYCOM) is responsible for approving and checking which equipment should be on the platform to be inspected. Table 8.1 is a list of typical fleet laboratory equipment that would be inspected on a Technical Assist Visit (TAV). Prior to use for patient testing, a complete instrument validation must be performed to ensure that the personnel, installation, and operational qualification requirements are met and approved by the Senior Medical Officer (SMO).

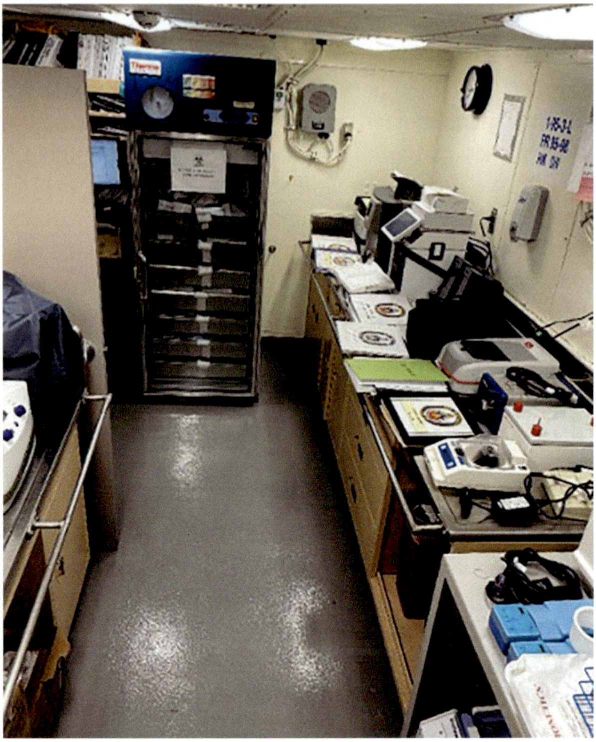

Fig. 8.1 The laboratory space of Portland class cruiser, the USS Portland (LPD-27), 2021. (Source: Photo courtesy of Clara A. Pangco, MLS)

Table 8.1 Fleet Technical Assist Visit (TAV) checklist equipment list for laboratory spaces

LABORATORY SECTION	EQUIPMENT
Hematology	☐ Act T 2 Diff ☐ QBC Star ☐ Sysmex
Chemistry	☐ Piccolo ☐ Vitros
Blood Gas	☐ i-Stat
General Lab	☐ Centrifuge ☐ Microscope ☐ Rotator ☐ AccuCheck ☐ Refrigerator ☐ Freezer ☐ Incubator ☐ Thermometer
Urinalysis	☐ Status ☐ Advantus ☐ Refractometer
Blood Bank	☐ ACP 215 ☐ Plasma Thawer ☐ Tubing Stripper ☐ Sealer ☐ Donor Scale
Coagulation	☐ i-Stat
Waived Tests	☐ Rapid Strep ☐ Rapid HIV ☐ HCG ☐ Malaria ☐ MonoSpot ☐ Occult Blood ☐ Rapid Flu ☐ RPR ☐ Rapid Chlamydia ☐ Rapid Hepatitis C
Microbiology	☐ Gram Stains

Source: Fleet Laboratory Technical Assist Visit Checklist, Section: Current Fleet Equipment, developed by the Navy Clinical Laboratory Improvement Program, not in copyright

HIV human immunodeficiency virus, *HCG* human chorionic gonadotropin, *RPR* rapid plasma reagin

Regulation

For over 30 years, the fleet laboratories operated under an exempt status that did not require any regulatory oversight. In 2018, a memorandum of understanding (MOU) was signed which requires all fleet individual laboratory sites to register for compliance, biennial inspection, and re-certification. The inspection is contingent upon the ship's approved Authorized Medical Allowance List (AMAL). Ships must reach out to the laboratory officer of the nearest military MTF in their homeport to complete this.

The Centers for Medicare and Medicaid Services (CMS) regulates all human laboratory tests through the Clinical Laboratory Improvement Amendments (CLIA). Tests are assigned a category based on a number of criteria set forth by CLIA. The category dictates the complexity of the test, who can perform it, and any inspection requirements. The two broad categories are:

1. Waived testing,
2. Nonwaived testing.

Waived tests are considered simple complexity tests with low risk for an incorrect result and can be performed by any sufficiently trained personnel. These are commonly point-of-care (POC) tests. Nonwaived testing (either moderate or high complexity) must be performed by trained and tested personnel and has to meet certain industry-measured quality system standards, such as proficiency testing, quality control and assessment, and testing personnel requirements.

The complexity of the tests available is based on the testing personnel. For smaller ships like destroyers or cruisers with only an Independent Duty Corpsman (IDC) and zero laboratory technicians, only waived tests can be performed for standardization. Microscopes are no longer available on these ships. Ships with dedicated laboratory technicians (Navy Enlisted Classification (NEC) L31A) can have more testing capabilities and complex instruments.

Shipboard Laboratory: Common Technology and Tests

As stated previously, the technology and capability for laboratory testing vary by platform and mission. **A surgical team should be aware of what tests are and are not available and the basic timeline required for results to prepare for the work-up and perioperative care of patients.** The availability and CLIA status of laboratory tests are ever changing. As of 2021, the most common tests available on most platforms are Complete Blood Count (CBC), Urinalysis, Urine human chorionic gonadotropin (HCG), Occult Blood, Rapid Flu, and Rapid Blood Glucose. Tests that typically are only available on larger platforms with designated laboratory technicians are Basic Metabolic Panel (BMP), Comprehensive Metabolic Panel (CMP), Liver Function Test (LFT), and Prothrombin Time/Partial Thromboplastin Time (PT/PTT).

Hematology

The QBC Star (Fig. 8.2) is a standard hematology system on most deployed platforms. It can perform a CBC within a matter of minutes, which is a CLIA-waived test. It can measure or calculate the following results:

- Hematocrit (%).
- Hemoglobin (g/dL).
- Mean Corpuscular Hemoglobin Concentration (MCHC) (g/dL).
- White Blood Cell (WBC) Count ($\times 10^9$/L).
- Granulocyte ($\times 10^9$/L).
- Granulocyte (%).
- Lymphocyte/Monocyte Count ($\times 10^9$/L).
- Lymphocyte/Monocyte (%).
- Platelet Count ($\times 10^9$/L).

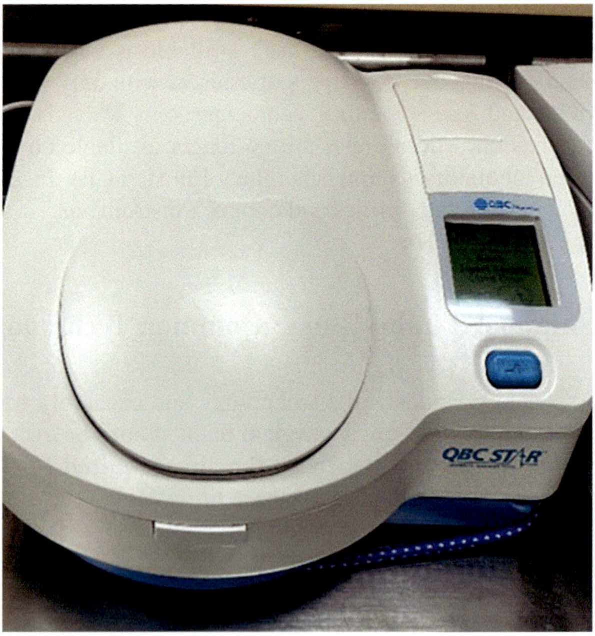

Fig. 8.2 Standard hematology system on deployed platforms: the QBC Star. (Source: Photo courtesy of Clara A. Pangco, MLS)

Chemistry

The Piccolo Xpress Chemistry analyzer (Fig. 8.3) is an example of a system offered on some deployed platforms that delivers blood chemistry diagnostic information. It offers predominantly CLIA-waived test panels such as Basic Metabolic Panel (BMP), Electrolyte Panel, Renal Function Panel, Comprehensive Metabolic Panel (CMP), Liver Function Testing (LFT), and Lipid Panel.

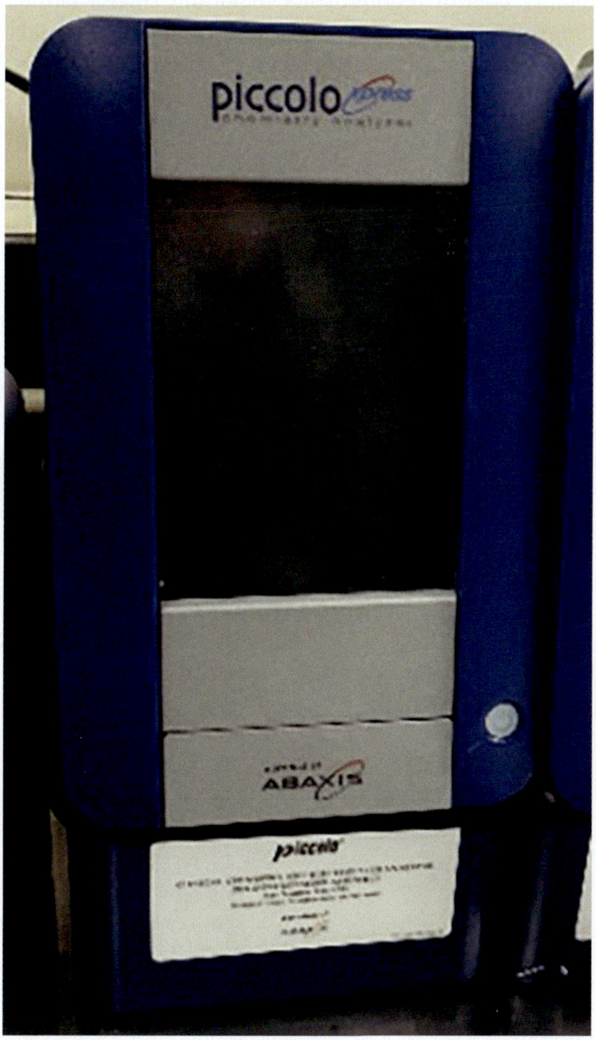

Fig. 8.3 Sample chemistry analyzer for deployed platforms: the Piccolo Xpress. (Source: Photo courtesy of Clara A. Pangco, MLS)

Blood Gases

The i-STAT system is a lightweight, portable, and easy-to-use blood analyzer. It is widely used by most hospitals as a POC medical diagnostic tool that can deliver results within 2–15 min. It can also be found on deployed platforms, in particular larger platforms that provide critical care like hospital ships, CVNs, and large deck amphibious assault ships. It has a broad menu of test panels, including a variety of CLIA-waived and nonwaived panels, each with its own specific calibration and quality control requirements including BMP/Chem8, cardiac Troponin I (cTnI), pregnancy tests, blood gases, and coagulation panels. Table 8.2 shows the wide array of diagnostic tests that can be run with the i-STAT System.

Additional Tests

Table 8.3 shows additional tests that may be performed on the ship depending on availability. The turnaround time is based on the manufacturer's package insert; however, actual turnaround time from the time the specimen is submitted may vary, depending on the technician's current workload.

Table 8.2 The i-STAT system range of diagnostic tests

THE i-STAT SYSTEM RANGE OF DIAGNOSTIC TESTS	
Lactate	$CG4^+$
Hematology	$EC8^+$, $CG8^+$, $EG7^+$, $CHEM8^+$, $EG6^+$,
Chemistries and electrolytes	$EC8^+$, $CG8^+$, $EG7^+$, $CHEM8^+$, $EG6^+$,G, Crea, $CG4^+$
Cardiac markers	cTnl, CK-MB, BNP
Endocrinology	Total β-hCG
Blood gases	$EG7^+$, $CG8^+$, $EG6^+$, $CG4^+$
Coagulation	PT/INR, ACT Kaolin, ACT Celite®
Traumatic brain injury	TBI Plasma*

Source: Public domain image, not in copyright. Available at: https://www.globalpointofcare.abbott/en/product-details/apoc/i-stat-system.html

cTnI cardiac troponin I, *CK-MB* creatine kinase myocardial band, *BNP* B-type natriuretic peptide, *B-hCG* beta-human chorionic gonadotropin, *PT* prothrombin time, *INR* international normalized ratio, *ACT* activated clotting time, *TBI* traumatic brain injury

Table 8.3 Additional testing kits that may be available on deployed maritime platforms

Test	Sample type	Time from test to results
Rapid Strep	Throat swab	5 min
HCG	Urine	3 min
Rapid Flu	Nasal/nasopharyngeal Swab	10 min or less
Occult Blood	Stool	About 7 min
MonoSpot	Whole blood, serum, or plasma	About 5 min
Malaria[a]	Whole blood EDTA	15 min
Rapid HIV[a]	Whole blood	About 20 min
Rapid Hepatitis C[a]	Whole blood	About 20 min
Rapid Hepatitis B surface antigen[a]	Whole blood, serum, or plasma	30 min

HCG human chorionic gonadotropin, *EDTA* ethylenediamine tetraacetic acid, *HIV* human immunodeficiency virus
[a]Used for the screening of Walking Blood Bank (WBB) donors during activation

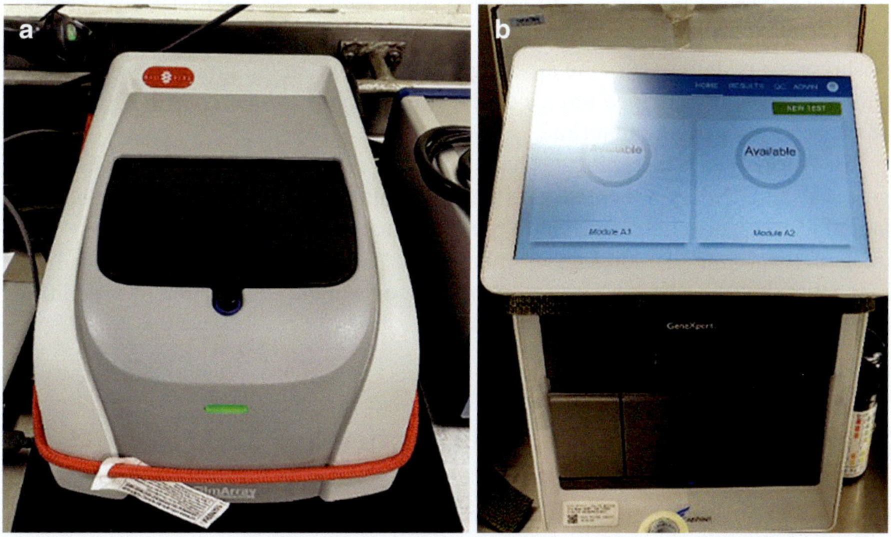

Fig. 8.4 Systems for detection of common viral pathogens, only found on larger deployed maritime platforms (**a**) Biofire FilmArray (**b**) Cepheid GeneXpert. (Source: Photos courtesy of Clara A. Pangco, MLS)

Additional testing platforms have been added due to the recent coronavirus disease 2019 (COVID-19) pandemic. A bigger surface ship with dedicated laboratory technicians, such as a hospital ship, CVN, or large deck amphibious assault ship, may now have the BioFire FilmArray and/or the Cepheid GeneXpert (Fig. 8.4a, b, respectively). These platforms can deliver results for various viruses and pathogens via the detection of nucleic acid (e.g., Influenza A/B, SARS-COV-2 or COVID-19, RSV).

Tests that are not available onboard may be pre-arranged by the SMO and/or the laboratory technician with the local MTF or if pulling into a port. It is important to get guidance on proper collection, packaging, shipping, and stability requirements.

Finally, the laboratory is involved in many other aspects of medical care at sea. This chapter focuses on what the surgical team would need to know. Additionally, Chap. 12 touches on specimen processing and preparation prior to submission to the lab, and Chap. 23 discusses blood products, resuscitation, and the Walking Blood Bank (WBB) in depth.

Shipboard Radiology: Historical Perspective

The discovery of X-rays by Wilhelm Roentgen in 1895 set in motion a remarkable series of scientific discoveries and development for this tool in medicine. As necessity can accelerate the maturation and improvement of technology, wartime around the turn of the century fostered the use and acceptance of X-rays as a viable tool for patient care.

One of the first instances of radiology use onboard ships was during the Spanish-American War. At this time only hospital ships had X-ray machines, but surgeons realized their value as a helpful tool in their preoperative assessment. Localization of shrapnel and bullets was the most significant benefit at the time. The information gained from X-rays helped reduce exploratory surgery, which contributed to much of the morbidity during that time.

By World War I, the ability to have an X-ray machine became somewhat more practical and widely accepted as a supplemental tool in military medicine. The famed Marie Curie helped develop portable imaging with X-rays by having them integrated into small radiological cars called "little Curies" near the front lines. Since that time, shipboard X-ray machines have been the cornerstone of expeditionary diagnostic imaging and remain so today.

Shipboard Radiology: Current Overview and Technology

Radiology capabilities at sea remain relegated to the hospital ships, CVNs, and large deck amphibious assault ships. The large-deck amphibious ships are outfitted with radiologic equipment as they are designated as casualty receiving and treatment ships (CRTS). Although they are not a CRTS, a CVN primarily has this capability because of the sheer number of personnel in a carrier strike group (CSG) for which their medical department is responsible.

Radiology Suite

The single-room shipboard radiology suite is like a hospital imaging center, although much smaller (Fig. 8.5). In the center of the room, there is the main X-ray production unit, table, Bucky tray and grid, and the image receptor. Immediately adjacent

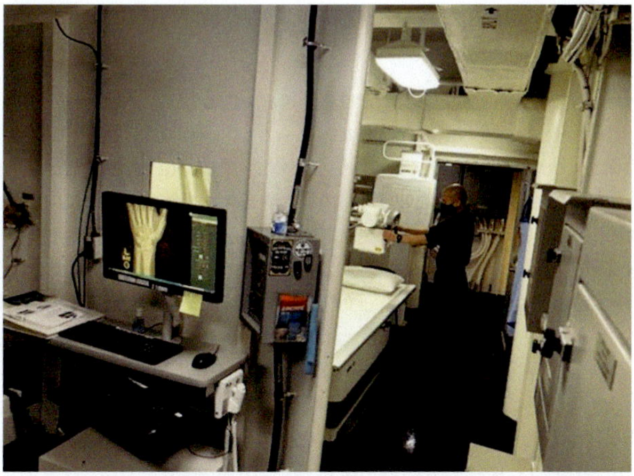

Fig. 8.5 Typical set up of shipboard radiology suite with HM2 Sen Ung preparing equipment for the next patient on board Nimitz class aircraft carrier, the USS Theodore Roosevelt (CVN-71), 2021. (Source: Photo courtesy of Roderick C. Borgie, MD)

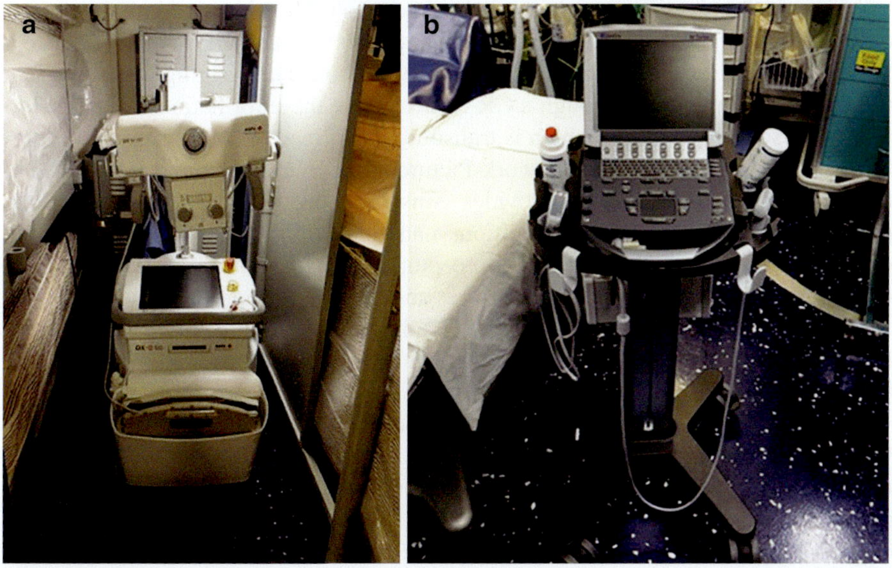

Fig. 8.6 (**a**) Portable X-ray unit with digital radiography (DR) (**b**) Portable Sonosite ultrasound. (Source: Photos courtesy of Roderick C. Borgie, MD)

to the table is a small room with a shielded wall to protect the technician performing the studies. This room also houses the computer on which the images are processed and initially interpreted. This machine also can transfer images to a remote location to be read by consulting specialists.

As seen in Fig. 8.6a, these ships also carry a portable X-ray unit, which can be used on patients unable to access the suite or during certain medical or surgical procedures. However, it is most commonly utilized as a backup machine when the main machine is not operating or is under repair.

Radiography Technology Advances

In the past, ships obtained radiographic images on film, which consisted of an emulsion of silver halide, usually silver bromide (silver halide is a compound that can form between the element silver and one of several halogens: bromide, chlorine, iodine, and fluorine) that could produce an image when exposed to X-rays. However, the hard copy film could not be transmitted, and only medical providers on the ship could read the images. These images would be transported to a radiology department in an MTF to be read by a radiologist once the ship was back in port. However, it was not unusual for a radiology department to take several weeks to read images accumulated from a 6-month or longer deployment. This delay presented challenges for patient follow-up and quality assurance of interpretation of findings.

As digital imaging became available, ships' systems updated to computed radiography (CR). This technology allowed the digitization of imaging while still using a conventional X-ray machine (digital detectors still use conventional X-ray machines; the main difference is the image receptor). The film used in "film-screen cassettes"had to be developed through a film processor in a darkroom to produce a hard copy of the image, which is read from a view box. The imaging plate used in a CR cassette is processed through a CR reader where the information is digitized to produce a soft copy image, which is transmitted and read off of workstation monitors, via the Digital Imaging Network-Picture Archiving Communications System (DINPACS). This digitization provides considerable efficiency and convenience over plain film development. In addition, many platforms have upgraded further to digital radiography (DR). The image receptor consists of a flat panel detector that can instantly register computerized images and remove the intermediate processing step of a CR reader. **These images, like CR, have the potential to be transmitted in real-time to telemedicine sub-specialists who can interpret and help direct forward-deployed medical providers' care.**

There are several benefits to DR. First, post-processing corrections can be made, which limits the number of errors that can be caused by under- or overexposure to create more consistent quality. As a side note, medical readiness and quality assuredness inspections onboard ships look at rates of retakes for images among technicians. This number has substantially declined in the digital era. Another benefit of DR is rapid image production. For instance, if a surgeon wished to do a modified fluoroscopic study (e.g., intraoperative cholangiogram) utilizing CR technique, the radiology technician would have to take the X-ray, remove the cassette to be read by the CR reader (likely in a different location), and convert it to an image readable by the surgeon. With the DR technique, the X-ray images are processed on the spot and taken in relatively rapid succession if needed, which minimizes operative time. A final major advantage is the elimination of filing & storage space for hard copy films and increased capacity for archiving a large number of images in electronic files. Overall, DR benefits patients, radiology technicians, surgeons, and the medical system alike.

Before deployment, a surgical team should assess whether their assigned ship has CR or DR. As mentioned previously, the difference in technology can have ramifications in planning modified fluoroscopic procedures with the different time delays in processing images. As of this publication, most of the CVNs already have DR equipment, while most large-deck amphibious ships have CR equipment while awaiting the planned upgrade. Surgical teams on CVN's and large amphibious assault ships should also determine if and what type of contrast is available on the ship. Most ships do not have the contrast needed to perform cholangiograms or retrograde urethrograms.

While some French Navy and Royal Navy (United Kingdom) warships (Chapter 2) have Computed Tomography (CT) machines, in the U.S. Navy they are currently utilized on hospital ships only, and not yet available on any other expeditionary ships (e.g., CVN or amphibious warships).

Shipboard Ultrasound

Ultrasound capability nicely supplements shipboard diagnostic tests and is typically available on larger ships (e.g., CVN and amphibious warships). Although a board-certified radiologist's presence is limited to the hospital ships, many other specialties have supplemental training in Point-of-Care Ultrasound (POCUS), making it a valuable tool on forward-deployed ships.

The Sonosite is an example of a portable ultrasound machine (Fig. 8.6b) commonly utilized by forward-deployed medical providers. Workup of acute pelvic pathology or early pregnancy issues often utilizes the Sonosite, but ultrasound imaging can also assist in trauma evaluation, limited echocardiography, assessment for gallstones and other intra-abdominal or scrotal pathology, deep venous evaluation, musculoskeletal injuries, and localized fluid collections. See Chap. 9 for a discussion of the techniques and clinical pearls for common POCUS applications.

Ultrasound images remain on the portable device for viewing without the shipboard capability to transmit the images to a central computer or picture archiving and communication system (PACS). The leading utility of POCUS is in troubleshooting diagnostic questions in real-time scenarios. If there was a need to send images somewhere for communicating results or consultation, then a digital picture taken of the screen could be sent via email or uploaded for use in a remote location.

The benefit derived from ultrasound is related to the experience and skill of the operator. A major training gap is formal ultrasound training for shipboard medical providers including Independent Duty Corpsman, surgeons, and shipboard medical officers. While ultrasound is a useful tool, shipboard providers have to seek out training experiences individually or rely on previous experience. Fortunately, in Navy Medicine, the saying is "one team, one fight," and providers come together to share experiences for the benefit of the patient.

Shipboard Radiology: Common Exams

Most shipboard imaging is for relatively routine primary and urgent care concerns. The most performed studies are chest radiographs looking for pneumonia and other acute pathology (Figs. 8.7 and 8.8). Extremity radiographs are also commonly looking for fractures, dislocations, and foreign bodies (Figs. 8.9 and 8.10). Abdominal radiographs can also assist surgical decision-making even if they do not yield a final diagnosis. For example, Fig. 8.11 shows an example of an abdominal radiograph with an obstructive bowel gas pattern; ultimately, the patient was found to have a cecal volvulus.

Several artifacts can occur with radiologic imaging whose discussion is beyond the scope of this text. Fortunately, many artifacts are due to film technique and are not factors with CR or DR technique. Postprocessing in the digital era can somewhat correct under- or overexposure. Motion artifacts can blur images and sometimes make intact bones look fractured. However, some of the most notorious artifacts are objects external to the patient that a provider cannot discern as external on a single view. **The importance of multiple views should be stressed when imaging is done to problem-solve a diagnosis** (Figs. 8.7, 8.8, and 8.9).

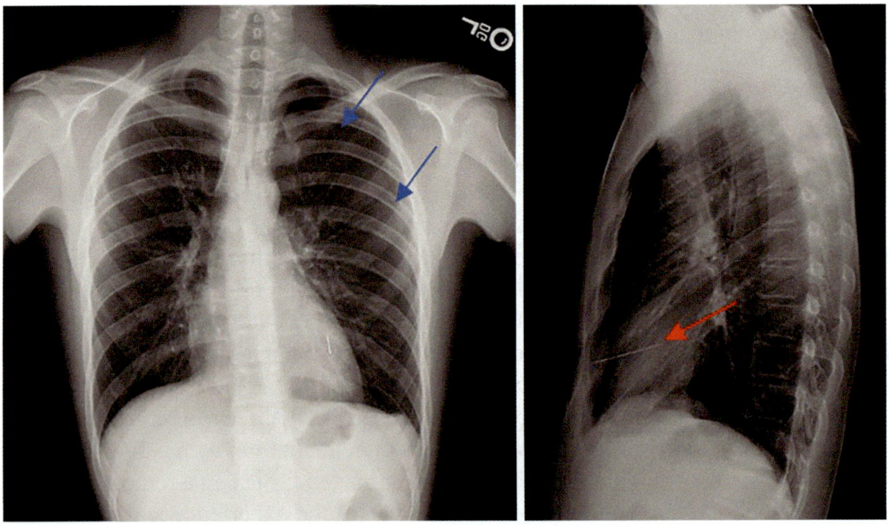

Fig. 8.7 Radiographs of the chest and extremities are the most common exams performed onboard a ship. Two or more views can be particularly important in assessing the full clinical picture, seen here where this sewing needle pierced the heart (red arrow points to needle) and caused a left pneumothorax (blue arrows point to pleural line). (Source: Images courtesy of Amy Condos, MD)

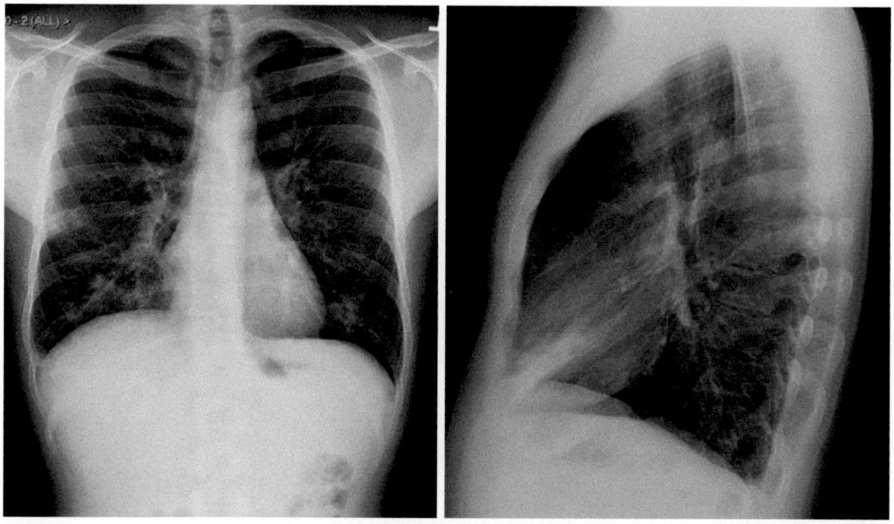

Fig. 8.8 Chest radiographs are commonly used to screen for acute disease. These images demonstrate multi-focal pneumonia where the right middle lobe infiltrate obscures the well-defined right heart border on frontal view, which is corroborated on lateral view. (Source: Images courtesy of Gil Boswell, MD)

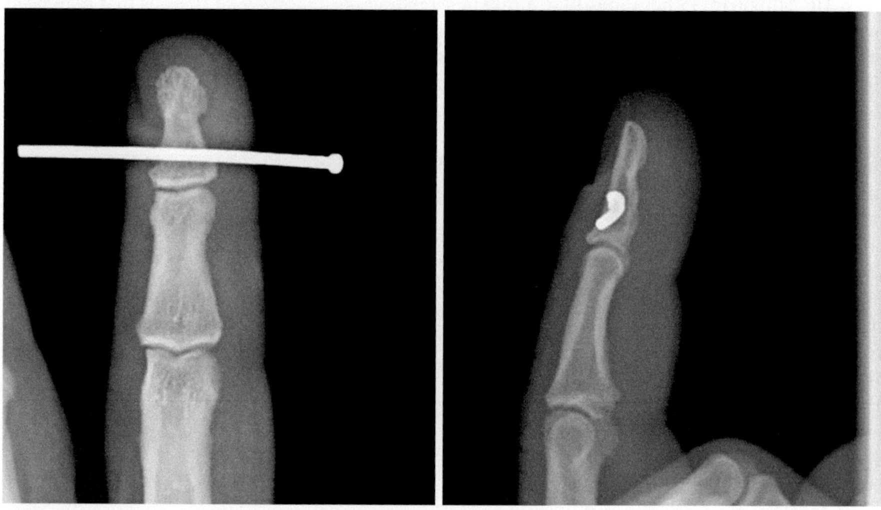

Fig. 8.9 Is this nail through the bone? This figure illustrates the importance of multiple views to better assess the clinical situation. (Source: Images courtesy of Roderick C. Borgie, MD)

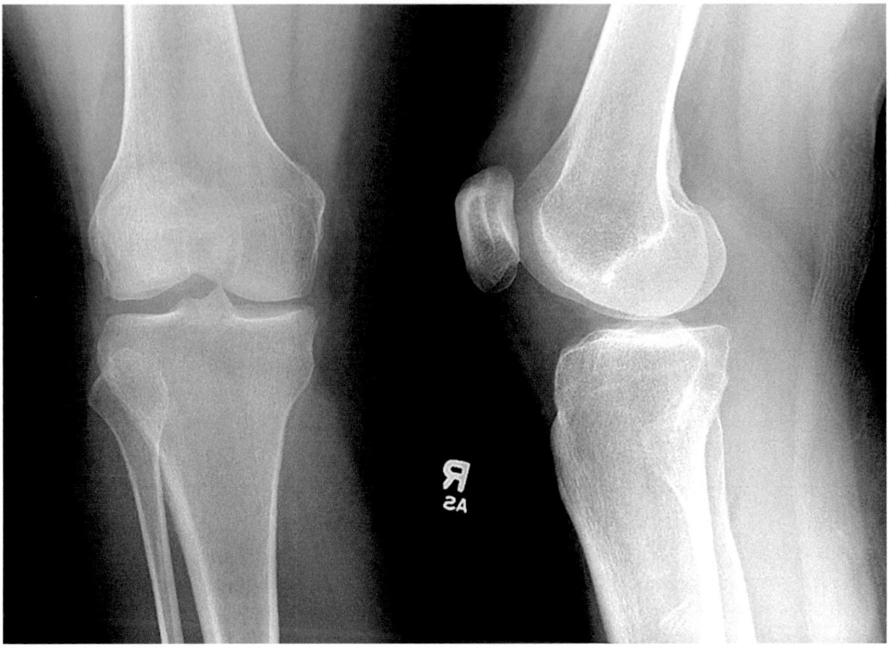

Fig. 8.10 Shipboard radiographs play a role in screening musculoskeletal injuries that may need further imaging. Shown here a subtle fracture of the medial tibial plateau (reverse Segond's fracture) was associated with disruption of the posterior cruciate ligament found on subsequent Magnetic Resonance Imaging (MRI). (Source: Images courtesy of Gil Boswell, MD)

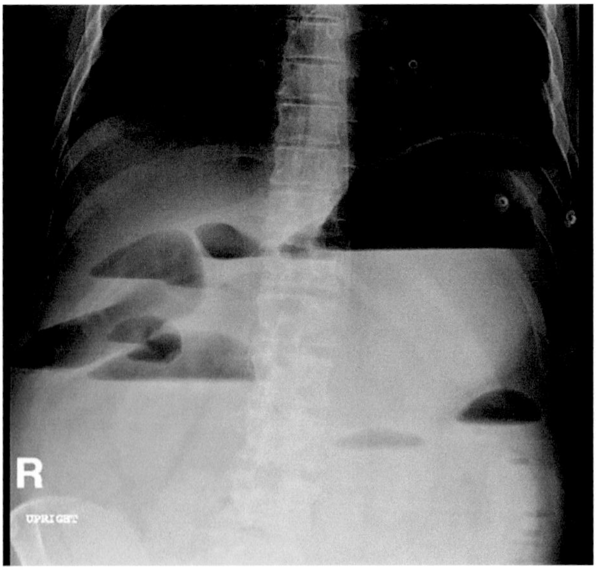

Fig. 8.11 Abdomen radiographs are many times used as a screening tool for forward-deployed surgeons to assist in decision-making on whether to perform or not an exploratory surgery. In this example, an obstructive bowel pattern is noted, which was eventually found to be a cecal volvulus. (Source: Image courtesy of Roderick C. Borgie, MD)

Conclusion

Shipboard diagnostic tools are essential supplements to clinical acumen and judgment. The surgical team needs to be familiar with their platform's laboratory and radiology capabilities to maximize their ability to plan and care for patients.

Declaration of Interest The views expressed in this chapter are those of the authors and do not necessarily reflect the official policy or position of the Department of the Navy, Department of Defense, nor the US Government.

Funding This research did not receive any specific grant from funding agencies in the public, commercial, or not-for-profit sectors.

Conflict of Interest Statement The authors declare no conflict of interest.

Chapter 9
Principles of Shipboard Ultrasound

Matthew V. Speicher, Christopher H. Frederick, Michael T. LaRoy, Lawrence C. Decker, and John A. Siefert

It is essential to have good tools, but it is also essential that the tools should be used in the right way.

Wallace D. Wattles

Author deployment experience	
Matthew V. Speicher	F-14 Radar Intercept Officer, Fighter Squadron-213, embarked on the USS Theodore Roosevelt (CVN-71), Operation Iraqi Freedom, Persian Gulf, 2005–2006
	Staff Emergency Physician, Role 2 Light Maneuver team, Air Base 201, Agadez, Niger, Operation Juniper Shield, West Africa, 2020; Provided embarked Role 2 damage control surgery and resuscitation capability, AFRICOM Area of Responsibility, 2020
Christopher H. Frederick	Resident Emergency Medicine Physician, Naval Medical Center San Diego, 2018–present
Michael T. LaRoy	Force Surgeon, Special Purpose Marine Air-Ground Task Force, Operation Northern Viper, INDOPACOM Area of Responsibility, 2019
Lawrence C. Decker	General Medical Officer, 15th Marine Expeditionary Unit, embarked on the USS Pearl Harbor (LSD-52), contingency operations, INDOPACOM Area of Responsibility, 2008
	Assistant Director of Medical Services, USNS Comfort (T-AH-20), Operation Continuing Promise, Haiti, Dominican Republic, Guatemala, Honduras, El Salvador, Nicaragua, Panama, Columbia, Dominica, Jamaica, and Belize, 2015
	Staff Emergency Physician, Special Purpose Marine Air-Ground Task Force, Operation Inherent Resolve, Kuwait and Syria, 2019

M. V. Speicher (✉) · C. H. Frederick · M. T. LaRoy · L. C. Decker · J. A. Siefert
Navy Medicine Readiness and Training Command San Diego, San Diego, CA, USA
e-mail: matthew.v.speicher.mil@health.mil; christopher.h.frederick4.mil@health.mil; michael.t.laroy.mil@health.mil; lawrence.c.decker.mil@health.mil; john.a.siefert4.civ@health.mil

M. D. Tadlock, A. A. Hernandez (eds.), *Expeditionary Surgery at Sea*,
https://doi.org/10.1007/978-3-031-21893-4_9

Author deployment experience	
John A. Siefert	Flight Surgeon, VP-49/45, Naval Air Station Sigonella, Sigonella, Italy, 1986–1989
	Senior Medical Officer, USS Essex (LHD-2), WESTPAC, Sasebo, Japan, 2000
	Chief of Professional Services/Staff Emergency Physician, Bravo Surgical Company, 1st Medical Battalion, Operation Iraqi Freedom, Fallujah, Iraq, 2004

BLUF (Bottom Line Up Front)

1. Point-of-Care Ultrasound (POCUS): Shipboard units equipped with ultrasound imaging devices can provide life-saving diagnoses and advantageous information to the medical team. However, POCUS is more frequently utilized to confirm, or rule in, a disease process rather than to rule it out.
2. Extended Focused Assessment with Sonography in Trauma (eFAST): POCUS allows for the expeditious identification of free fluid in the abdomen, thorax, or pericardium in the trauma patient. Repeat exams can increase the sensitivity of the eFAST exam, in particular, if there is a change in vital signs or clinical status.
3. Limited echocardiography: In addition to detection of pericardial fluid, POCUS assessment of the heart allows the provider to evaluate for global cardiac function, cardiac tamponade, right-sided heart strain, cardiogenic shock, and cardiac arrest.
4. Right Upper Quadrant (RUQ) Ultrasound: While not as robust as a formal radiology department-obtained RUQ ultrasound, POCUS can detect significant hepatobiliary pathology including cholelithiasis, cholecystitis, and choledocholithiasis.
5. Appendicitis: POCUS can detect acute appendicitis with high specificity and prompt urgent surgical evaluation and/or medical evacuation (MEDEVAC).
6. Testicular torsion: Utilizing POCUS to compare blood flow to each testicle can aid in the diagnosis of testicular torsion and uncover the need for rapid surgical intervention.
7. Lower extremity deep vein thrombosis (DVT): In the setting of lower extremity pain or shortness of breath, POCUS evaluation for thrombus in the proximal veins of the lower extremity may indicate the need for anticoagulation.
8. Intrauterine pregnancy (IUP) and ectopic pregnancy: Lower abdominal pain and abnormal vaginal bleeding should prompt evaluation for ectopic pregnancy. POCUS provides the means to do so and can provide prompt diagnosis of this life-threatening condition.

9. Ovarian torsion: While not a definitive study, POCUS can provide evidence of ovarian torsion through the comparison of each ovary's size and blood flow.
10. Central venous catheter (CVC) placement: POCUS can provide real-time visualization of venous cannulation, as well as decrease the likelihood of complication of misplacement or damage to surrounding structures.

Introduction

Imaging modalities are often limited in the deployed setting, and shipboard medical departments are no exception. Depending on the size of the vessel, X-ray capabilities may be present, but Point-of-Care Ultrasound (POCUS) is likely to be part of any shipboard medical unit's arsenal. An understanding of the capabilities and limitations of POCUS is extremely important to physicians and medical providers at sea.

It is imperative to understand that ultrasound studies performed at the bedside are limited in nature. Typically, POCUS should be used to answer a specific clinical question. For instance, in trauma, a provider might perform an exam to evaluate for the presence of intraabdominal free fluid. The goals of limited ultrasound studies do not often include full measurements of solid organs, such as the liver or kidneys.

In general, POCUS is more frequently utilized to confirm, or rule in, a disease process rather than to rule it out. This means that pathology noted by the provider, such as intraabdominal free fluid or an enlarged appendix, is likely to be a true positive. Conversely, if there is no pathology appreciated, there is a higher chance of a false negative. This should not discourage the shipboard medical provider from incorporating POCUS into their practice because a positive finding can expedite treatment or medical evacuation (MEDEVAC).

Most shipboard medical teams, especially those formed for trauma and resuscitative care, will often include a provider comfortable with the basics of POCUS. While this individual should be considered the ultrasound subject matter expert for the team, there are applications, such as the Extended Focused Assessment with Sonography in Trauma (eFAST), which most members of the team should be proficient in performing. It is advisable that the individual most comfortable with POCUS train and support other members of the team in their use of ultrasound.

POCUS has many applications spanning multiple fields of medicine. It is not the goal of this chapter to familiarize the reader with all of those applications. Rather, this chapter will familiarize the reader with certain indications, techniques, and keys to success that may aid in detecting life-threatening pathology that could require emergent surgical (or nonsurgical) treatment and/or MEDEVAC.

Extended Focused Assessment with Sonography in Trauma (eFAST)

Introduction and Indications

In the setting of blunt or penetrating trauma to the chest or abdomen, eFAST is used to rapidly identify injuries during the primary survey of trauma patients and should only take a few minutes to complete. It is a modern adjunct to the Advanced Trauma Life Support (ATLS) algorithm as well as in the Tactical Combat Casualty Care (TCCC) Advanced Resuscitative Care Clinical Practice Guideline (CPG). The eFAST is only a single data point and should be repeated whenever there is a clinical or vital sign change as part of the patient reassessment.

The eFAST exam consists of six views, assessing multiple areas for free fluid in the abdomen or thorax, as well as for free thoracic air. These views include cardiac, right and left upper quadrant, pelvic/bladder, and anterior right and left chest.

The cardiac views are used to assess for evidence of hemopericardium in the setting of trauma, as well as evaluate for evidence of cardiac tamponade. While hypotension in the setting of trauma is often due to hypovolemia and blood loss, tamponade from hemopericardium or tension pneumothorax must also be considered.

The right and left upper quadrant views are generally intended to identify free fluid within the peritoneal cavity. The eFAST exam can detect volumes of fluid as low as 100 mL in the peritoneal cavity in the hands of an experienced operator [1]. It is also important to identify the diaphragm in these views to assess the area superior to the diaphragm for hemothorax.

The pelvic/bladder views assess for free fluid within the pelvis. The most dependent location for free fluid to collect in the supine position is either the rectouterine pouch in women or the retrovesicular pouch in men.

The anterior right and left chest views are used to evaluate lung sliding along the pleural line between two ribs using M-mode. No movement will appear more like a "bar code" and is concerning pneumothorax.

Technique

The eFAST exam can be accomplished with either the curvilinear or phased array probes. The curvilinear probe may offer higher fidelity images, while the phased array probe will provide a smaller footprint that may improve images that are hindered by rib shadows. The shipboard medical team should train with both probes to determine their individual preference.

The entire exam, including cardiac and lung windows, can be done with the abdominal mode selected on the machine. If time permits, the phased array probe in the cardiac setting can be utilized for cardiac views and the linear probe can be used for lung windows, but often one probe in one mode will be used.

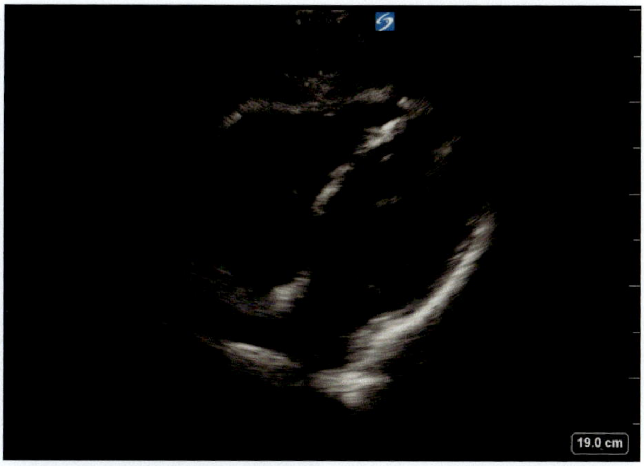

Fig. 9.1 Normal subxiphoid cardiac view seen on Extended Focused Assessment with Sonography in Trauma (eFAST). (Source: Image courtesy of Matthew V. Speicher, DO)

Subxiphoid Cardiac Views (Fig. 9.1)

This is often the first view obtained in performing an eFAST due to the significant mortality associated with traumatic cardiac injury. To obtain the subxiphoid view, hold the probe with the hand on top and the probe marker pointed toward the patient's right side. Place the probe on the skin inferior to the xiphoid process and offset slightly to the patient's right. This placement uses the liver as an "acoustic window" through which the provider can visualize the heart. Point the probe toward the patient's left shoulder and observe for cardiac motion. Increasing the depth of the monitor may improve visualization. In the subxiphoid view, pericardial fluid would appear as an anechoic (dark) stripe between the pericardium and myocardium. This view is also discussed in multiple sections of the Limited Echocardiography section of this chapter.

Right Upper Quadrant (RUQ) Views (Fig. 9.2)

Place the probe on the right posterior axillary line below the costal margin with the probe marker cephalad. Visualize the kidney and the liver. The interface between the two is known as Morrison's pouch or the hepatorenal recess. "Fan" through this area by keeping the probe in the same place on the skin, but moving the handle of the probe posteriorly and anteriorly to view the entire space from anterior to posterior. Ensure that the caudal edge of the liver is also visualized, as this is often a site of free fluid accumulation. Finally, note the pleural space above the diaphragm, which will normally be a hyperechoic (bright) stripe overlying the liver. The pleural space should appear as a mirror image of the liver. If this area is hypoechoic, and the spine can be seen extending past the diaphragm, this is indicative of a pleural effusion or hemothorax.

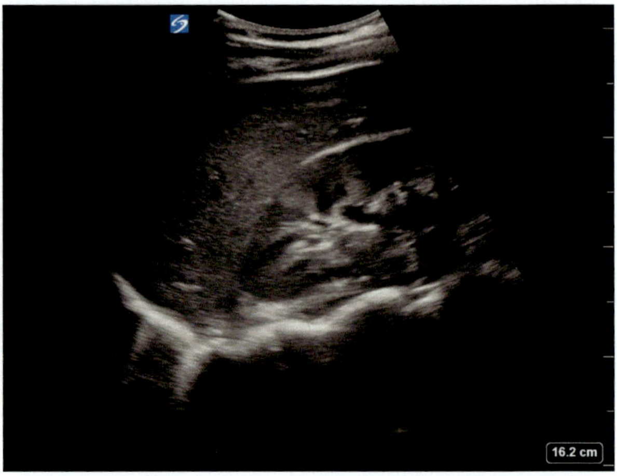

Fig. 9.2 Normal right upper quadrant (RUQ) view seen on Extended Focused Assessment with Sonography in Trauma (eFAST). (Source: Image courtesy of Matthew V. Speicher, DO)

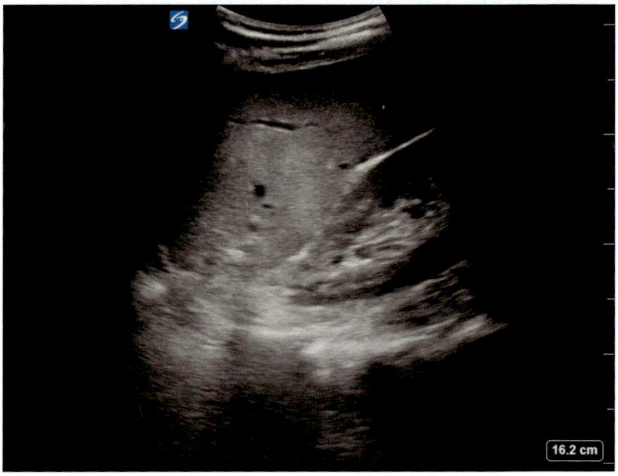

Fig. 9.3 Normal left upper quadrant (LUQ) view seen on Extended Focused Assessment with Sonography in Trauma (eFAST). (Source: Image courtesy of Matthew V. Speicher, DO)

Left Upper Quadrant (LUQ) Views (Fig. 9.3)

Place the probe with the probe marker cephalad, posterior to the posterior axillary line, and above the costal margin. This view will most often be obtained in the rib spaces and is more difficult to obtain as the spleen and left kidney are more posterior and superior than the liver and right kidney were on the Right Upper Quadrant (RUQ) view. Often the back of the hand holding the probe will be on the bed or gurney. Visualize the spleen, kidney, and diaphragm on the left side and fan through the area as done in the RUQ view. Free fluid or blood will most often accumulate in the space between the spleen and the diaphragm. Again, make note of the pleural space above the diaphragm, which should again show a mirror image of the spleen and other structures beneath it.

Pelvic/Bladder Views (Figs. 9.4 and 9.5)

Place the probe in the transverse plane above the pubic symphysis and point the probe down to obtain a view of the bladder. Fan through the bladder as described above to visualize the entire area from the superior to inferior bladder. For improved sensitivity, both transverse and sagittal views should be obtained. Rotate the probe 90° so the probe marker is cephalad and again fan through the bladder from left to right looking for fluid posterior to the bladder wall. In this view, free fluid posterior to the uterus in women or posterior to the bladder in men is considered a positive exam.

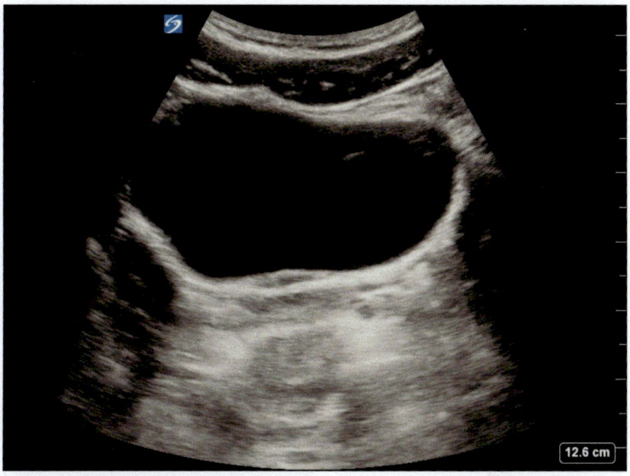

Fig. 9.4 Normal pelvic/bladder transverse view seen on Extended Focused Assessment with Sonography in Trauma (eFAST). (Source: Image courtesy of Matthew V. Speicher, DO)

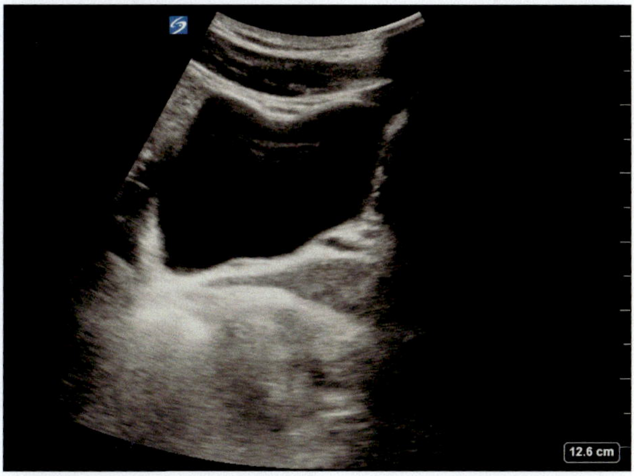

Fig. 9.5 Normal pelvic/bladder sagittal view seen on Extended Focused Assessment with Sonography in Trauma (eFAST). (Source: Image courtesy of Matthew V. Speicher, DO)

Anterior Right and Left Chest Views

To assess for pneumothorax, place the probe in the sagittal plane with the probe marker cephalad on the most anterior portion of the chest, cephalad to the breast in women. Assess for lung sliding along the pleural line between two ribs. This appears as a back-and-forth motion of the hyperechoic stripe between the two ribs. Figure 9.6 illustrates a normal lung view. M-mode can be used to confirm the presence or absence of lung slide by selecting M-mode and placing the vertical line on the screen between the two ribs. Motion below the pleural line will appear as a "sandy beach" that indicates normal lung slide (Fig. 9.7). No movement will appear more

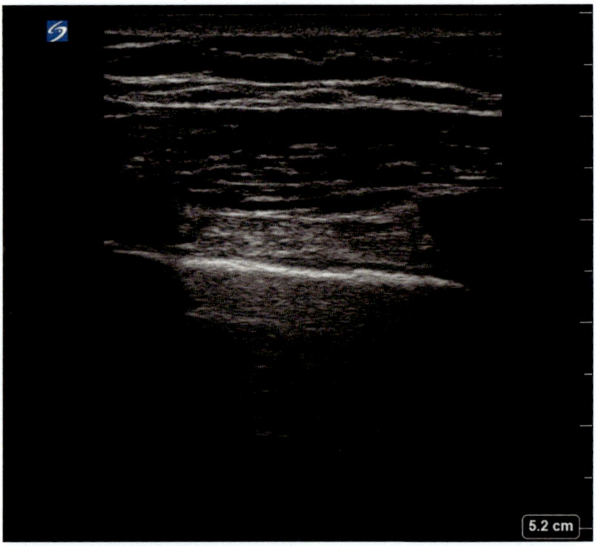

Fig. 9.6 Normal lung view seen on Extended Focused Assessment with Sonography in Trauma (eFAST). (Source: Image courtesy of Matthew V. Speicher, DO)

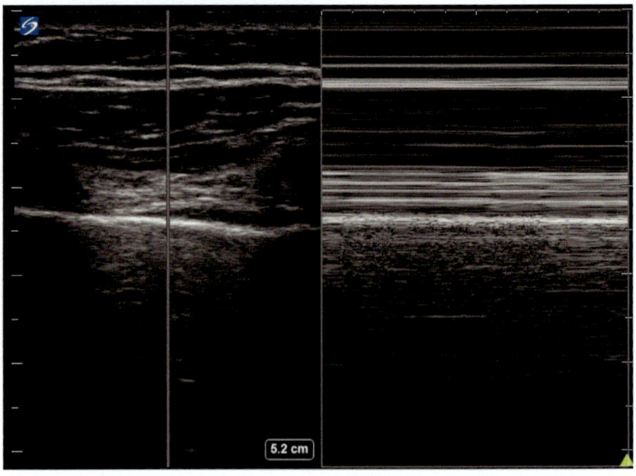

Fig. 9.7 Normal lung slide present appears like a "sandy beach" on M-mode seen on Extended Focused Assessment with Sonography in Trauma (eFAST). (Source: Image courtesy of Matthew V. Speicher, DO)

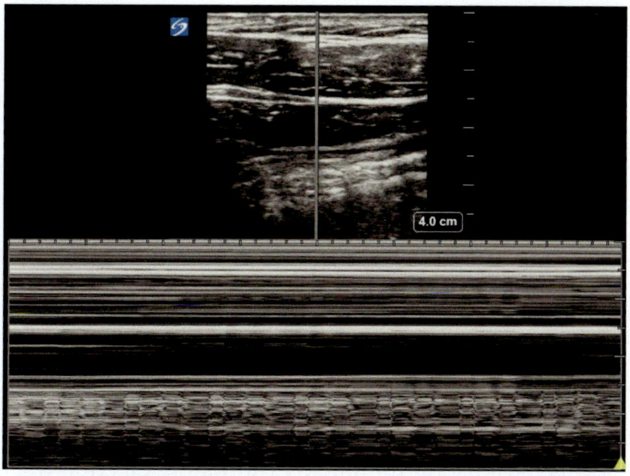

Fig. 9.8 Lung slide absent appears like a "bar code" on M-mode, concerning pneumothorax, seen on Extended Focused Assessment with Sonography in Trauma (eFAST). (Source: Image courtesy of Matthew V. Speicher, DO)

like a "bar code" and is concerning pneumothorax (Fig. 9.8). If no lung slide is appreciated, move the probe laterally to assess for a lung point, which is where lung slide is intermittently present, indicating the edge of the lung that is still moving with respiration. This is pathognomonic for a pneumothorax.

Keys to Success

- **Repeat exams can increase the sensitivity of the eFAST exam, in particular, if there is a change in vital signs or clinical status.**
- If the subxiphoid cardiac view is difficult to obtain, the parasternal long axis (PLAX) view (as discussed in the Limited Echocardiography section of this chapter) can be a valid substitute and will allow for good detection of a pericardial effusion or hemopericardium.

Limited Echocardiography

Introduction and Indications

POCUS limited echocardiography is most useful in patients with undifferentiated shock, chest pain, or shortness of breath. Specifically, evidence of cardiac tamponade, massive pulmonary embolism (PE), decompensated heart failure, and depleted intravascular volume can be found. It can also be used to guide Advanced Cardiovascular Life Support (ACLS) resuscitation and address some reversible causes of cardiac arrest.

Technique

POCUS evaluation of the heart is typically performed utilizing four cardiac views and one of the inferior vena cava.

Parasternal Long Axis (PLAX) View (Fig. 9.9)

Place the probe on the left parasternal border in the fourth or fifth intercostal area. Have the probe marker aimed at the patient's right shoulder. Scan until mitral valve (MV) is in the center of the screen and the right ventricle (RV), aortic outlet, and left atrium (LA) are lined up vertically towards the right side of the screen. The PLAX view is most useful for quickly estimating ejection fraction (EF) and overall cardiac contractility. The vertical heights of the RV, aortic outlet, and LA should have a 1:1:1 ratio. An enlarged RV suggests right heart strain (PE or chronic pulmonary hypertension).

Parasternal Short Axis (PSAX) View (Fig. 9.10)

From the PLAX view, twist the probe 90° clockwise so that the probe marker is aimed at the left shoulder. This should provide a view of the full cross-section of the left ventricle (LV), septum, and at least part of the RV. The parasternal short axis (PSAX) view is best for assessing right heart strain as discussed later in this section.

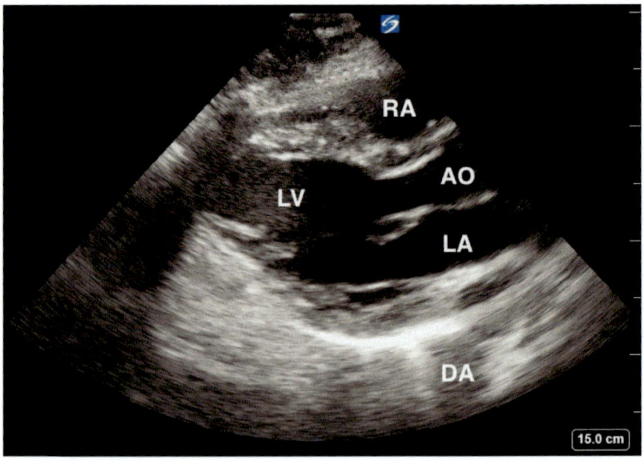

Fig. 9.9 Normal parasternal long axis (PLAX) view seen on limited echocardiography. *RA* right atrium, *LV* left ventricle, *LA* left atrium, *AO* aorta, *DA* descending aorta. (Source: Image courtesy of Matthew V. Speicher, DO)

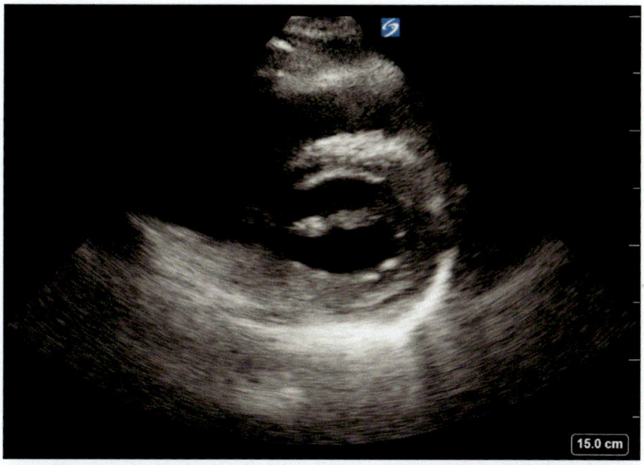

Fig. 9.10 Normal parasternal short axis (PSAX) view seen on limited echocardiography. (Source: Image courtesy of Matthew V. Speicher, DO)

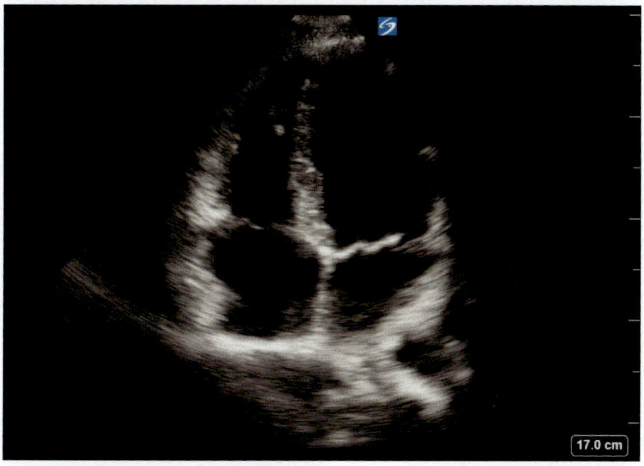

Fig. 9.11 Normal apical four-chamber (A4Ch) view seen on limited echocardiography. (Source: Image courtesy of Matthew V. Speicher, DO)

Apical 4 Chamber (A4Ch) View (Fig. 9.11)

Place the probe under the nipple or along the inframammary fold with the probe marker aimed toward the patient's left. Scan left and right until a view of all four chambers of the heart is seen. Tilt the probe until the septum is nearly vertical on the screen with equal views of the LV and RV. The apical 4 chamber (A4Ch) view is generally the most intuitive view of the heart and is useful for all echocardiography indications.

Subxiphoid View

Place the probe in the epigastrium with the probe marker aimed towards the patient's left and the probe angled upwards towards the patient's left shoulder. Ideally, the user should be able to visualize all four chambers with the heart lying in a near-horizontal orientation on-screen, the RV being the most superficial chamber. If the view is inadequate, slide the probe to the right of the epigastrium until a portion of the liver is seen between the probe and the heart. This provides an "acoustic window" that will improve the view of the heart. Moderate downward force on the probe may be required to obtain an adequate view. This view is also discussed in the eFAST section of this chapter and visualized in Fig. 9.1.

Inferior Vena Cava (IVC) View (Fig. 9.12)

From the subxiphoid view, twist the probe so the probe marker is cephalad. Angle the probe so that the probe is now oriented midline. Tilt the probe cephalad until the heart comes into view, then fan left/right until an anechoic tubular structure that communicates with the right atrium is seen. This structure is the inferior vena cava (IVC). To ensure this structure is not the aorta, look for pulsatility and respiratory variation. The IVC will communicate with the right atrium, is typically non-pulsatile, and may have respiratory variation with respect to diameter. The aorta will be pulsatile with no respiratory variation in diameter. Measure the IVC diameter 3 cm from the right atrium and assess the degree of collapsibility. This can be used to estimate intravascular volume status. An IVC <1 cm in diameter at its largest during the respiratory cycle and collapsing more than 50% with inspiration suggests hypovolemia. An IVC >2.5 cm in diameter with no respiratory variation suggests hypervolemia. Measurements between those two values are less useful for predicting volume status [2].

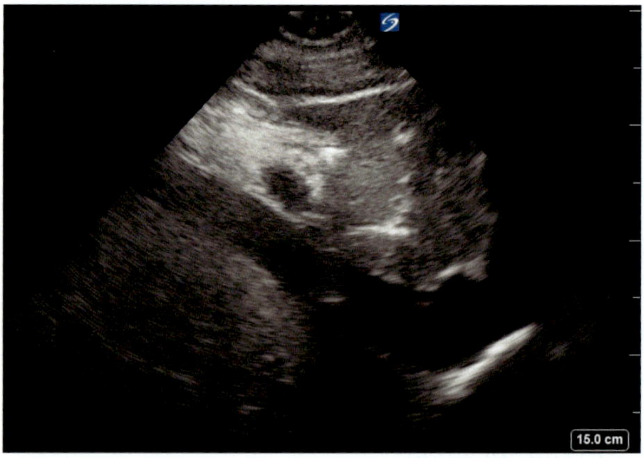

Fig. 9.12 Normal inferior vena cava (IVC) seen on limited echocardiography. (Source: Image courtesy of Matthew V. Speicher, DO)

Cardiac Tamponade

While all four cardiac views can identify a pericardial effusion, the subxiphoid view is often the most rapidly obtainable making it the preferred view during eFAST and cardiac arrest to rule out tamponade. A pericardial effusion will appear as an anechoic stripe within the pericardium, often layering in the most dependent portion of the pericardial sac. The likelihood of cardiac tamponade in the setting of pericardial effusion depends on the hemodynamic stability of the patient and/or echocardiographic findings. If the effusion develops rapidly, as little as 150 mL of blood can cause tamponade whereas chronic effusions can hold over 1000 mL without tamponade [2]. Tamponade is generally associated with a large and non-collapsible IVC, RV diastolic collapse, or right atrium (RA) systolic collapse.

Right Heart Strain

Right heart strain in an otherwise healthy individual with hemodynamic or respiratory compromise is highly concerning massive PE. **The simplest way to diagnose right heart strain on limited echocardiography is to evaluate the RV in relation to the LV in any of the four cardiac views.** In normal physiology, the LV should be larger in diameter than the RV. RV dilation can be seen in either acute pulmonary hypertension (e.g., PE) or chronic pulmonary hypertension (e.g., chronic obstructive pulmonary disease (COPD) or cor pulmonale). In the PSAX view, the LV should appear as a near-perfect circular structure with no intrusion of the RV into the LV. If the RV appears to be pushing into the LV, this is a sign of right heart strain and is termed "D Sign" as the septum will appear to be a linear structure dividing a mirror image of two "Ds" as seen in Fig. 9.13. If the RV is the circular structure and the LV appears smaller than the RV, this is considered severely abnormal and would be concerning a massive PE.

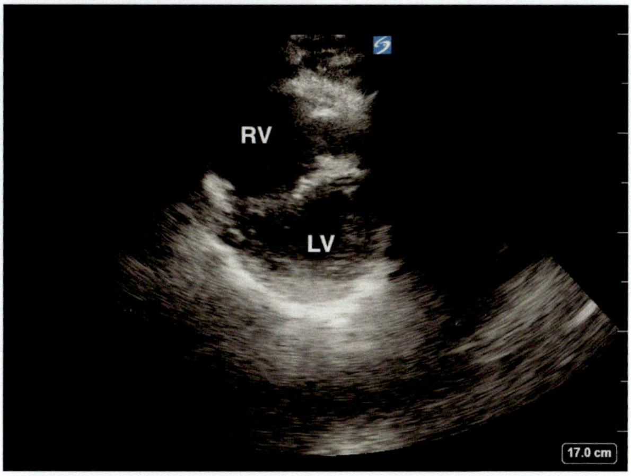

Fig. 9.13 Cardiac "D-sign," concerning right heart strain, seen on limited echocardiography. *RV* right ventricle, *LV* left ventricle. (Source: Image courtesy of Matthew V. Speicher, DO)

Cardiac Contractility and Ejection Fraction (EF) Estimation

Decreased EF in a patient with undifferentiated shock is concerning acute decompensated heart failure, myocarditis, or massive acute myocardial infarction. Increased EF, or a hyperdynamic heart, suggests hypovolemia. There are two methods to estimate EF with POCUS:

1. Eyeball Method.
2. E-Point Septal Separation (EPSS).

The Eyeball Method is a quick visual estimation of EF based on the kinetic motion of the LV. The LV can either appear as normal, hyperkinetic, or hypokinetic. This method requires some degree of familiarity with what is normal and abnormal. While this method can be used in any of the four cardiac views, it is usually easiest to assess in the PLAX view. If the anterior MV leaflet is rapidly moving towards and appears to be "slapping the septum," this would indicate a hyperdynamic heart and suggests hypovolemia. On the other hand, a slowly moving or hypodynamic LV with little MV excursion is indicative of a decreased EF.

EPSS is a quantitative estimate of EF which can only be obtained in the PLAX view. Orient the probe so the septum is horizontal on the screen and the anterior valve of the mitral leaflet is visualized throughout the entire cardiac cycle. Select M-Mode and drag the vertical cursor so that it overlies the tip of the anterior leaflet of the MV. Select "Start" and the ensuing image will display the structures through which that line passes versus time. After 3–5 s click "Freeze Image." Use calipers to measure the distance between the tip of the MV leaflet and the septum when it is at the shortest distance between the two. A reduced EF will have an EPSS >7 mm [2]. Figure 9.14 is an example of a normal EPSS.

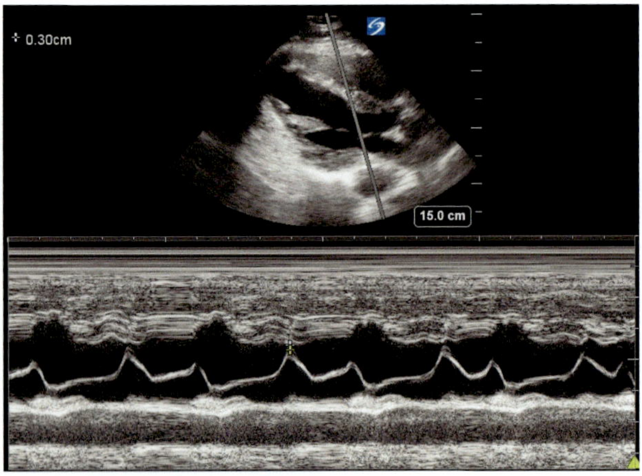

Fig. 9.14 Normal E-point septal separation (EPSS) seen on limited echocardiography. (Source: Image courtesy of Matthew V. Speicher, DO)

Cardiac Arrest

POCUS can help guide the management of cardiac arrest by diagnosing reversible causes, identifying return of spontaneous circulation (ROSC) at pulse checks, and prognosticating for termination versus continuation of Advanced Cardiac Life Support (ACLS). Adequate cardiac views are usually only attainable during pulse checks. Multiple studies have shown that bedside ultrasound significantly prolongs the length of time for pulse checks, so it is imperative to limit pulse check scans to 10 s. There are three reversible causes of cardiac arrest that can be easily and immediately identified on ultrasound: cardiac tamponade, tension pneumothorax, and hypovolemia. Any significant amount of pericardial effusion, usually seen on a subxiphoid view, should be presumed to be the cause of cardiac arrest. Evidence of a tension pneumothorax can be with a lack of lung sliding on anterior chest views while the patient is being ventilated. Hypovolemia/hemorrhage can be suspected with a small collapsible IVC. Poor forward flow during cardiac arrest typically results in a large non-collapsible IVC. Therefore, a small collapsible IVC during pulse checks should be considered abnormal and the team should strongly consider an intravenous fluid bolus or blood transfusion.

Keys to Success

- Do not confuse pleural effusion for pericardial effusion. Find the circular pulsatile descending aorta in the PLAX view posterior to the heart. Fluid between the heart and the aorta is a pericardial effusion. Fluid posterior to the aorta is a pleural effusion.
- Do not use mid-arrest RV dilation as the only sign to diagnose massive PE. Due to the equalization of RV and LV pressures from poor forward flow during cardiac arrest, RV dilation is non-specific for right heart strain. The decision to use thrombolytics during cardiac arrest should not be made based an isolated finding of mid-arrest RV dilation.

Right Upper Quadrant (RUQ) Ultrasound

Introduction and Indications

Consider RUQ ultrasound in patients presenting with RUQ pain, epigastric pain, sepsis from a suspected unknown abdominal source, or jaundice. The purpose of RUQ ultrasound is to evaluate for biliary colic, cholecystitis, choledocholithiasis, and/or cholangitis.

Biliary colic classically presents as recurrent colicky RUQ pain caused by mechanical stimulation of the gallbladder contracting against a gallstone temporarily in its neck. The diagnosis of biliary colic can be made by the clinical picture along with isolated ultrasound findings of gallstones without the later described findings of cholecystitis.

Cholecystitis classically presents as prolonged RUQ pain, fever, and leukocytosis. It is often caused by a gallstone lodged in the gallbladder neck causing proximal obstruction, inflammation, and subsequent infection.

Choledocholithiasis refers to a gallstone obstructing one of the extrahepatic biliary ducts, typically the common bile duct (CBD). Cholangitis is the subsequent life-threatening infection that can occur secondary to that obstruction with concomitant infection, "pus under pressure." Cholangitis classically presents as RUQ pain, fever, jaundice or elevated bilirubin, hypotension, and mental status changes. If clinically suspected, a dilated CBD with wall thickening on ultrasound can confirm the diagnosis. Due to low sensitivity, if suspicion for choledocholithiasis still remains with a negative RUQ ultrasound, then additional workup may be warranted with magnetic resonance cholangiopancreatography (MRCP) and/or endoscopic retrograde cholangiopancreatography (ERCP) and thus MEDEVAC from the ship should be considered. Alternatively, if clinical suspicion for choledocholithiasis or cholangitis is low (nontoxic appearing patient and normal bilirubin) and POCUS is otherwise negative for cholecystitis, there is an exceedingly low chance of missing choledocholithiasis if the CBD is normal in diameter or even if not visualized [3, 4].

Technique

The gallbladder is not a fixed organ, so adequate views often require patient repositioning, switching probe types and probe position, and patient inspiration and breath-holding. The curvilinear probe should be attempted first, but the phased array probe may be superior in obese patients or with intercostal views. There are two main views to obtain in evaluating the gallbladder: longitudinal (Fig. 9.15) and

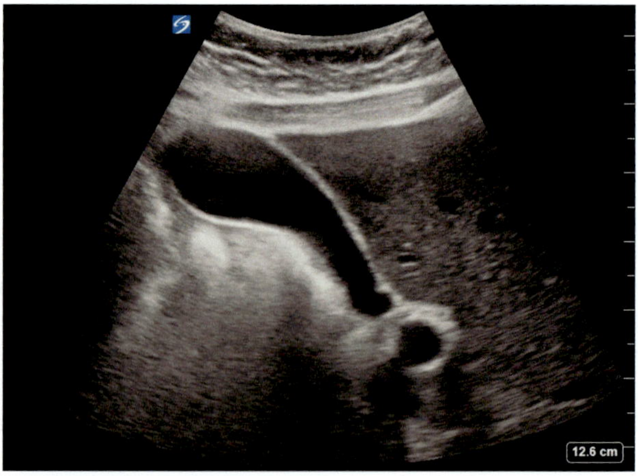

Fig. 9.15 Normal gallbladder longitudinal view is seen on right upper quadrant (RUQ) ultrasound. (Source: Image courtesy of Matthew V. Speicher, DO)

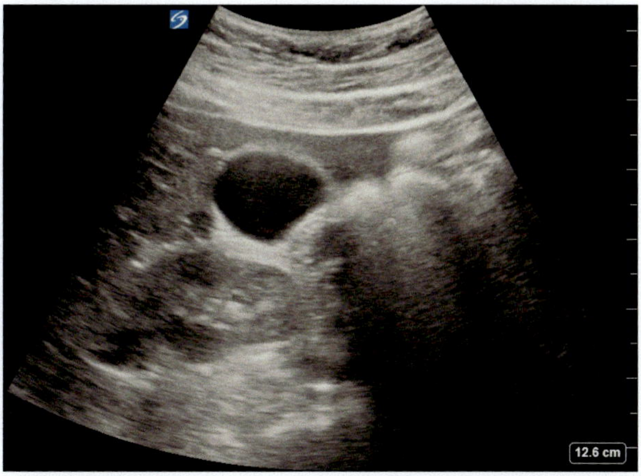

Fig. 9.16 Normal gallbladder transverse view is seen on right upper quadrant (RUQ) ultrasound. (Source: Image courtesy of Matthew V. Speicher, DO)

transverse (Fig. 9.16). Start with the patient in a supine position. Place the probe in the epigastrium with the probe marker cephalad. Slide the probe underneath the costal margin towards the patient's right. The gallbladder should appear around the midclavicular line. If the view is inadequate, have the patient take a deep breath and hold, then repeat the scan. If the view is still inadequate, roll the patient to the left lateral decubitus position and repeat the scan. If the view is still inadequate, attempt an intercostal view. Start in the right posterior axillary line using a phased array probe with the probe marker cephalad as if performing the RUQ view on an eFAST. Find liver/kidney interface then slide the probe anterior until gallbladder appears. Once an adequate view of the gallbladder is obtained, twist the probe to first find an optimal longitudinal view, then twist the probe 90° to obtain a transverse view.

Abnormal Findings: The four sonographic findings of calculous cholecystitis are cholelithiasis, sonographic Murphy's sign, gallbladder wall thickening (>3 mm), and pericholecystic fluid. The sonographic finding concerning choledocholithiasis is CBD diameter > 6 mm up to the age of 60, then an additional 1 mm for each decade of life after (i.e., normal can be up to 7 mm in a 70-year-old patient).

- Gallstones will appear as hyperechoic round structures within the gallbladder lumen. They will have "acoustic shadowing," which will appear as hypoechoic vertical shadows emanating from directly behind the stone (Fig. 9.17). Lack of gallstones on POCUS with visualization of the entire gallbladder in longitudinal and transverse views significantly decreases the odds of cholecystitis or biliary colic.
- To assess for sonographic Murphy's sign, obtain a subcostal view of the gallbladder and center it on the screen. Apply downward pressure directly over the gallbladder. This sign is present when the point of maximal tenderness is directly over the gallbladder. Unlike the non-sonographic Murphy's Sign, this does not require patient respiration.

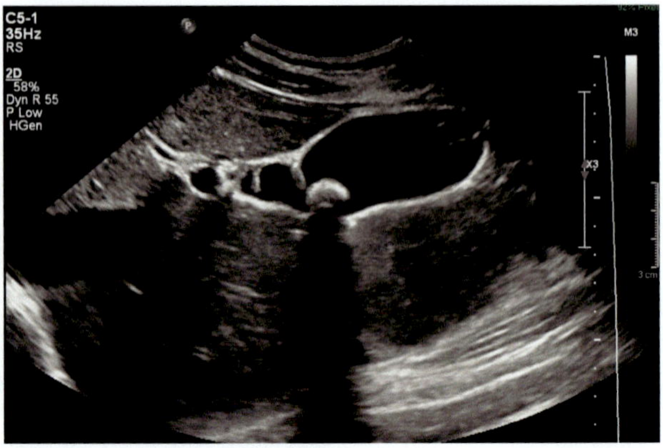

Fig. 9.17 Cholelithiasis with single cholelith and posterior shadowing is seen on right upper quadrant (RUQ) ultrasound. (Source: Image courtesy of Navy Medicine Readiness and Training Command San Diego Radiology Department, used with permission)

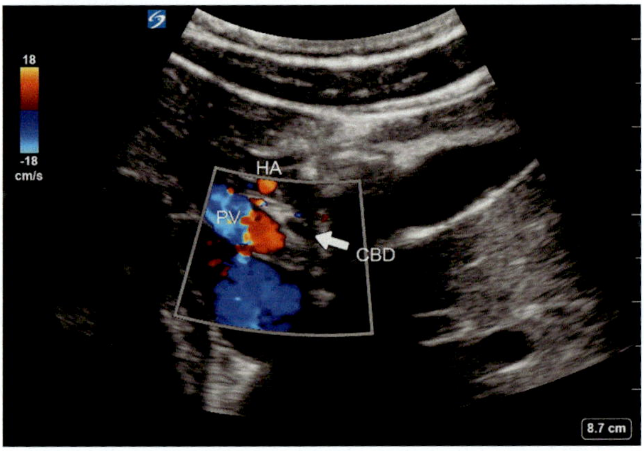

Fig. 9.18 Normal "Mickey Mouse" sign of the portal triad is seen on right upper quadrant (RUQ) ultrasound. The lack of flow on color mode can be used to identify the common bile duct (CBD). *HA* hepatic artery, *PV* portal vein, *CBD* common bile duct. (Source: Image courtesy of Matthew V. Speicher, DO)

- Gallbladder wall thickness should be measured on the anterior wall (most superficial wall) in the transverse view. A thickness > 3 mm is abnormal and 92% sensitive to cholecystitis [3]. However, it is non-specific as it can also occur in other conditions such as ascites, congestive heart failure, renal failure or nephrotic syndrome, an acquired immunodeficiency syndrome (AIDS), or postprandial contraction.
- Pericholecystic fluid will appear as hypoechoic edema surrounding the gallbladder.

Choledocholithiasis: The first step is identifying the CBD. Follow the gallbladder in the longitudinal view to where it tapers at the neck and locate the anechoic circular "exclamation point" distal to where it ends. This will be the portal vein (PV) and is the easiest structure to identify within the portal triad. There are two structures that abut the PV making up the remainder of the portal triad: the hepatic artery (HA) and CBD. Together, they will make the ears of the "Mickey Mouse" sign that can be seen in Fig. 9.18. Once all three structures are identified, color can be used to detect blood flow in the HA and PV, but not in the CBD. The CBD should then be measured from inner wall to inner wall in the anterior to posterior dimension. A diameter of >6 mm up to the age of 60, with 1 mm for each decade thereafter, indicates dilation from possible choledocholithiasis.

Keys to Success

- Measure the gallbladder wall in transverse view at the section of the wall which has the crispest and most easily identifiable borders.
- Posterior shadowing can be easier to identify than gallstones themselves. This is especially true for stones lodged in the neck, which are the most important stones to identify. If no obvious gallstones, rescan through the gallbladder and look for shadowing only.
- The gallbladder can be confused for the small intestine, dilated hepatic vein, or IVC. Obtain a good longitudinal view as the transverse view is more prone to this confusion. Look for peristalsis to make sure it isn't the small intestine. Use color flow to rule out a vascular structure.
- If the patient recently ate, the gallbladder may be contracted to the point of being difficult to find. Rescan in 1–2 h to gain better images.
- Gallbladder polyps are typically benign but can be mistaken for gallstones. Polyps will not have posterior acoustic shadowing.
- The absence of gallbladder wall thickening or pericholecystic fluid does not rule out the diagnosis of cholecystitis in a patient with a clinical history and physical exam.
- The absence of gallstones does not rule out biliary disease in a patient with biliary colic or cholecystitis symptoms from microlithiasis (which cannot be seen on POCUS) or thick sludge (can be seen on POCUS). See Chap. 15 and Fig. 15.1 for an example of a gallbladder filled with sludge on ultrasound.

Appendicitis

Introduction and Indications

Appendicitis is a significant concern in patients presenting with right lower quadrant abdominal pain and significant tenderness on exam. They may have associated nausea, vomiting, fevers, chills, or anorexia. POCUS can be used at the bedside to evaluate for the presence of a dilated and hyperemic appendix. Due to low sensitivity, it can only be used to rule in appendicitis. It is most useful for patients with below-average body mass index (BMI).

Technique

Start with the curvilinear probe. However, a linear probe may be superior for patients with a low BMI. Start at the point of maximum pain and tenderness and use a "lawn-mower" technique to scan up and down the abdomen; sliding the probe left or right upon reaching the inguinal ligament or costal margin. The iliac crest should be the lateral border; the psoas muscle should be the posterior border. Locate the iliac artery and vein, as these are important landmarks. The appendix often lies adjacent to this area.

The appendix should appear as a hypoechoic tubular structure, ending in a blind pouch, and without peristalsis. A normal appendix is oval-shaped (horizontal diameter > anteroposterior (AP) height), compressible, and <6 mm in diameter. An abnormal appendix is circular, non-compressible, and >6 mm in diameter. A perforated appendix may be difficult to identify. Secondary signs of free fluid or abscess (a complex, ill-defined, mixed echogenic area) and a concerning clinical picture should prompt a surgical evaluation. Figure 9.19 shows a large appendix with surrounding edema concerning appendicitis. It can be common to find the appendix in the transverse orientation first, at which point the probe should be rotated to appreciate the blind pouch on a longitudinal view. Figure 9.20 shows the same appendix in the transverse view with an appendicolith in the center.

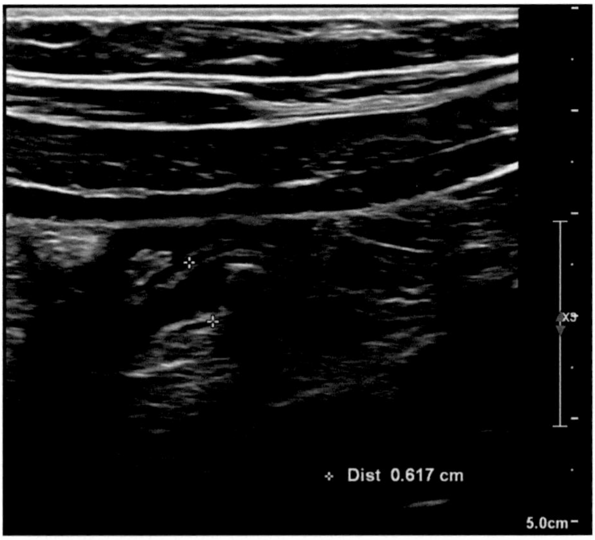

Fig. 9.19 Dilated appendix with edema on longitudinal view, concerning appendicitis, seen on Point-of-Care Ultrasound (POCUS). (Source: Image courtesy of Navy Medicine Readiness and Training Command San Diego Radiology Department, used with permission)

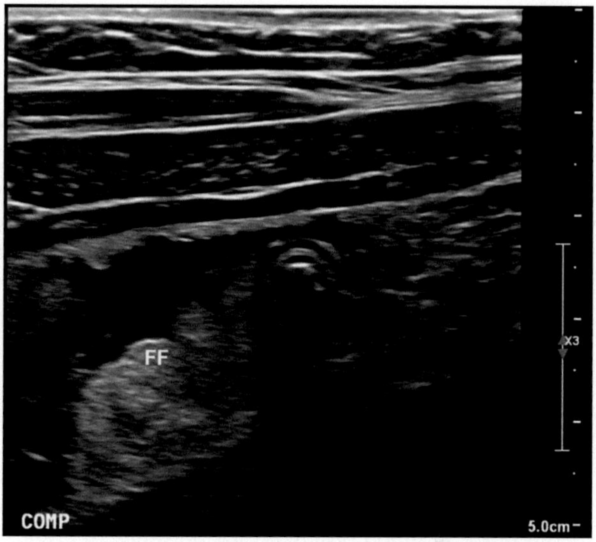

Fig. 9.20 Appendix with intraluminal appendicolith on transverse view, concerning appendicitis, seen on Point-of-Care Ultrasound (POCUS). *FF* free fluid. (Source: Image courtesy of Navy Medicine Readiness and Training Command San Diego Radiology Department, used with permission)

Keys to Success

- Have the patient point with one finger to the most painful section of their abdomen and start scanning that area.
- Use a graded compression technique to push bowel gas out of the way. This may require analgesia due to peritoneal irritation.
- An appendicolith will appear similar in appearance to gallstones with a hyperechoic foci and posterior acoustic shadowing. In a patient with high clinical suspicion, its presence is near pathognomonic for appendicitis.
- Confusion of the ileum with the appendix can cause false positives. Scan through in the transverse view then obtain an adequate longitudinal view to ensure the structure ends in a blind pouch.

Testicular Torsion

Introduction and Indications

Torsion of the testicle classically presents as severe, sudden onset, unilateral testicular pain, although the presentation can vary. Ultrasonography can be a valuable tool to aid in the diagnosis of testicular torsion. Through the utilization of color doppler, the presence or absence of blood flow to the testicle can be established.

Technique

It should be noted that once the color mode is selected on the ultrasound machine, the gain switch is often then used to change the sensitivity, or gain, of the color. If turned up too high, the slightest hand movements could result in the presence of color on the screen; if it's too low, the presence of blood flow may not be detected. Therefore, it is important to evaluate the unaffected testicle first to establish the proper level of color gain that demonstrates blood flow then proceed to evaluate the affected testicle.

The probe of choice is the high-frequency linear array probe. The patient should be positioned in the supine position with legs spread apart. The probe is placed on the inferior portion of the scrotum in the transverse plane with the probe horizontal or parallel to the floor. The testicles can be evaluated individually or at the same time in a side-by-side "buddy" view. A view of a single normal testicle can be seen in Fig. 9.21.

Once the unaffected testicle is identified, color doppler is selected. Evaluate for the presence of blood flow with the presence of color within the color doppler box on the ultrasound display. As mentioned previously, the gain may have to be set in order to avoid the false presence or false absence of flow. Blood flow should appear as consistent color returns on the display. Color flow is blue or red and does not indicate arterial or venous flow; it only indicates the direction of flow in relation to the probe.

After establishing the appearance of "normal" on the unaffected side, the provider should then place the probe in the same position to evaluate the affected testicle. With the same gain setting that was used to evaluate blood flow on the unaffected testicle, the presence or absence of flow should become apparent. Lack of blood flow is highly concerning testicular torsion (Fig. 9.22). While the presence of blood flow is reassuring that complete torsion is not present, decreased flow may indicate partial torsion.

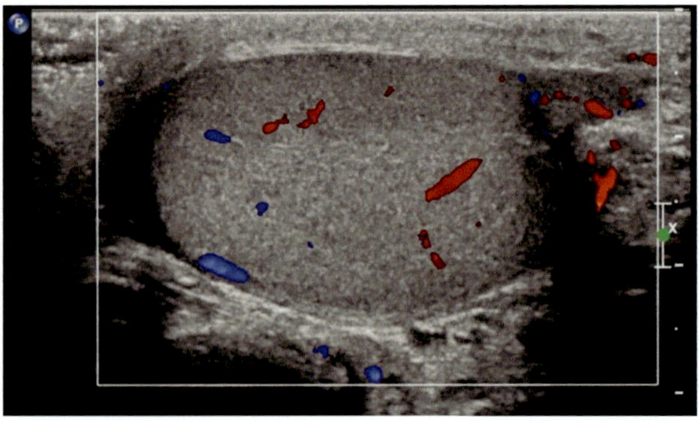

Fig. 9.21 Normal testicle seen on Point-of-Care Ultrasound (POCUS). (Source: Image courtesy of Navy Medicine Readiness and Training Command San Diego Radiology Department, used with permission)

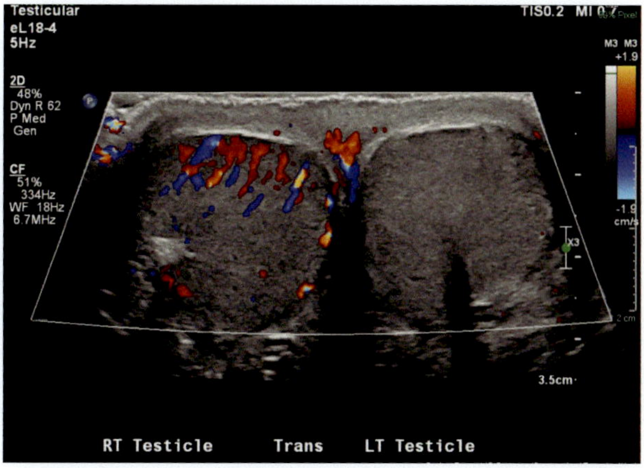

Fig. 9.22 Bilateral testicles with no flow to left testicle, concerning testicular torsion, seen on Point-of-Care Ultrasound (POCUS). (Source: Image courtesy of Navy Medicine Readiness and Training Command San Diego Radiology Department, used with permission)

Keys to Success

- If a proper "buddy view" can be obtained, asymmetric blood flow is concerning torsion.
- Even if pulsatile blood flow is present, torsion is not excluded as venous flow will usually be compromised prior to arterial flow. Rely on clinical gestalt.

Lower Extremity Deep Vein Thrombosis (DVT)

Introduction and Indications

In a patient presenting with nontraumatic unilateral lower extremity swelling and pain, deep vein thrombosis (DVT) must be considered. The Well's score for lower extremity DVT may be helpful in risk-stratifying patients for the probability of DVT. Ultrasound is a useful tool to evaluate lower extremity DVT utilizing a three-point compression technique. The exam can be performed in 5–7 min and has a sensitivity and specificity of 90% and 98%, respectively, for proximal DVT [5].

This exam will evaluate the proximal portion of the lower extremity. Distal, or calf, DVT has a lower incidence of propagation to the lungs, and treatment with anticoagulation is controversial. Most can be managed conservatively with repeat scanning of the proximal veins in 5–7 days to ensure the clot has not propagated.

Technique

The linear probe offers high resolution in more superficial structures, making it the probe of choice for this exam. However, in a larger patient, the curvilinear probe may be needed. Place the patient in the supine position and raise the head of the bed to 45°. Have the patient abduct and externally rotate the lower extremity of interest and slightly flex at the knee in a "frog leg" position.

The probe should be placed near the inguinal ligament to identify the common femoral vein (CFV), which is typically medial to the femoral artery (FA). Find the branch of the great saphenous vein (GSV) emanating from the CFV, as seen in Fig. 9.23. This will be the first area of compression. Compress the area until the superficial and deep walls of the veins collapse completely. Continue to follow the CFV inferiorly for 10 cm below the inguinal crease, compressing every 2 cm. The femoral vein should course deep to the FA as seen in Fig. 9.24.

Next, the popliteal vein is evaluated. This is achieved by placing the probe in the popliteal fossa of the posterior knee. The popliteal vein will lie superficial to the popliteal artery (Fig. 9.25). Following this vein inferiorly, the provider should appreciate the trifurcation of the popliteal vein. Return the probe to above this trifurcation and apply moderate pressure and ensure complete compressibility of the popliteal vein.

If at any point, the walls of the vein do not fully compress under moderate pressure, this is concerning a DVT, and generally treatment should be initiated.

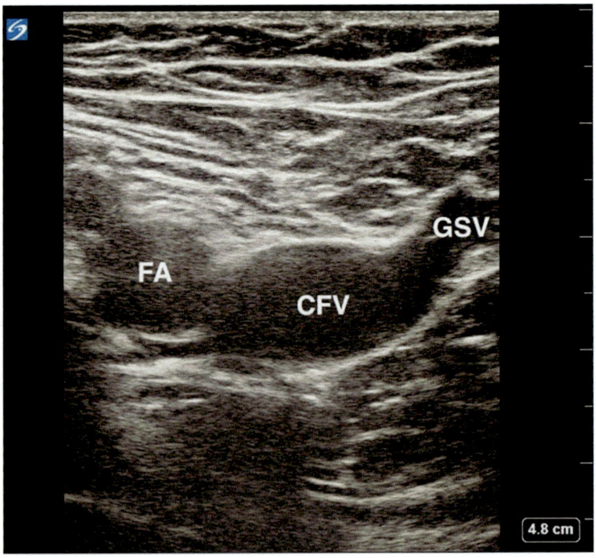

Fig. 9.23 Normal common femoral vein (CFV) at the great saphenous vein (GSV) junction seen on Point-of-Care Ultrasound (POCUS). *FA* femoral artery, *CFV* common femoral vein, *GSV* great saphenous vein. (Source: Image courtesy of Matthew V. Speicher, DO)

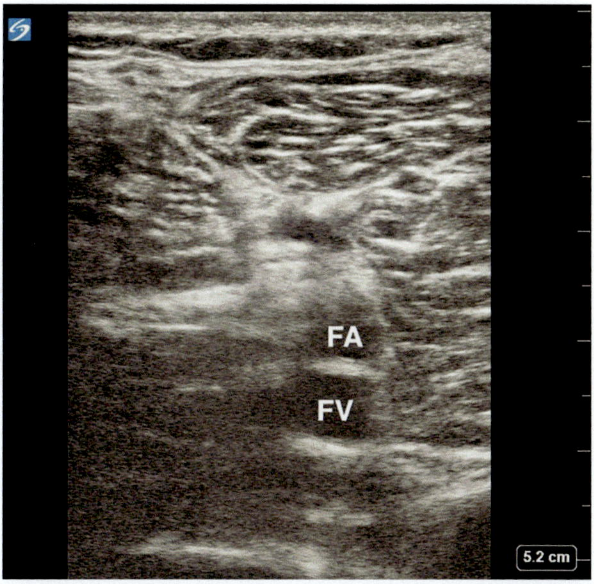

Fig. 9.24 Normal superficial femoral vein (SFV) deep to the femoral artery (FA) seen on Point-of-Care Ultrasound (POCUS). *FA* femoral artery, *FV* femoral vein. (Source: Image courtesy of Matthew V. Speicher, DO)

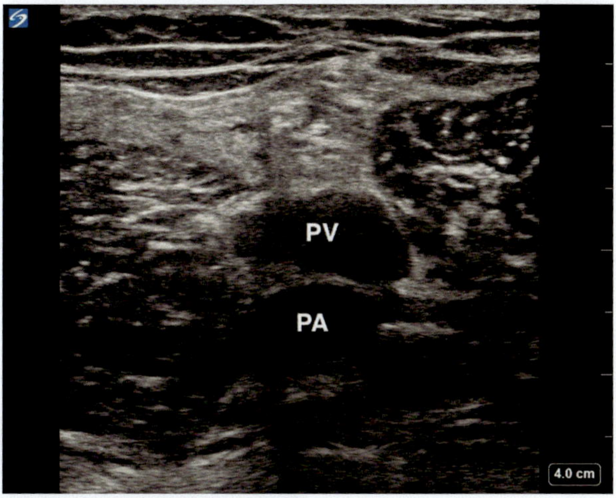

Fig. 9.25 Normal popliteal vein superficial to the popliteal artery seen on Point-of-Care Ultrasound (POCUS). *PA* popliteal artery, *PV* popliteal vein. (Source: Image courtesy of Matthew V. Speicher, DO)

Keys to Success

- Do not mistake a lymph node for a non-compressible vein. If there is concern, evaluate in the sagittal plane, as the lymph node will have a discreet beginning and end, unlike a venous tubular structure.
- Ensure that the FA or the popliteal artery is appreciated when compressing the veins, as deep veins will almost always run adjacent to an artery.

Pregnancy

Introduction and Indications

In the shipboard patient with a newly diagnosed pregnancy, the pregnancy can generally be assumed intrauterine and does not necessitate ultrasound evaluation if there are no complications. In that same patient with lower abdominal pain, pelvic pain, vaginal bleeding, or other concern for an extrauterine or ectopic pregnancy, POCUS should be utilized to confirm an intrauterine pregnancy (IUP). POCUS is used to rule in an IUP. It does not rule out an ectopic pregnancy. POCUS relies on the low incidence of heterotopic pregnancy to do this. If the patient has any risk for a heterotopic pregnancy, she needs a formal radiologic study.

Technique

Evaluation for the presence of an IUP begins with a transabdominal study utilizing the curvilinear probe. Choose the obstetric menu setting for the exam. The probe is placed on the abdomen above the pubic symphysis in the transverse orientation. Using the bladder as a landmark, the probe should then be manipulated to evaluate the uterus, which will be located superior to the bladder.

Within the uterus, findings can range from a normal-appearing, non-gravid uterus to a full gravid uterus containing a fetus. The first potential indicator of a pregnancy is a gestational sac, which will be a hypoechoic region within the uterus. Unfortunately, this hypoechoic finding can also be a pseudo-gestational sac sometimes seen in the setting of ectopic pregnancy. Therefore, the presence of an intrauterine yolk sac is the first evidence that can be used to confirm that the pregnancy is intrauterine (Fig. 9.26). At this stage of evaluation if there are signs of hemodynamic instability the curvilinear probe can be used to do an eFAST exam looking for

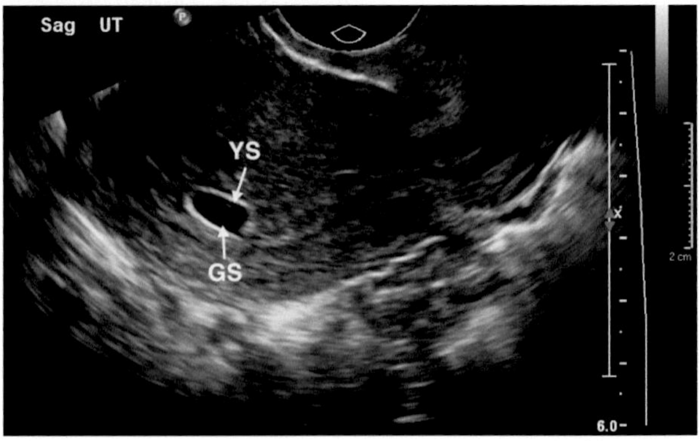

Fig. 9.26 Normal intrauterine pregnancy (IUP) with yolk sac seen on Point-of-Care Ultrasound (POCUS). *YS* yolk sac, *GS* gestational sac. (Source: Image courtesy of Navy Medicine Readiness and Training Command San Diego Radiology Department, used with permission)

free abdominal fluid. The presence of free fluid, a documented positive pregnancy test, and no clearly identified IUP warrant management as a ruptured ectopic pregnancy until proven otherwise.

If there is no evidence of an IUP with a transabdominal approach, the intracavitary probe should be used. After placing gel over the probe, followed by a protective sheath, sterile gel or lubricant is applied to the outside of the covered probe. The probe is then inserted into the vagina with the patient in the supine position. The probe should be in the sagittal orientation initially. The clinician should then fan the probe from left to right to evaluate the entire uterus. The findings of an IUP remain the same as in the transabdominal approach. A yolk sac remains the initial confirmation of an IUP. If no evidence of an IUP is noted, the adnexa should be evaluated for evidence of an ectopic pregnancy, which may include an extrauterine structure that could be a gestational sac with or without a yolk sac, fetal pole, or fetus located within it. Figure 9.27 shows an ectopic pregnancy located in the adnexa.

If there is no evidence of an intrauterine or extrauterine pregnancy, but the patient has a positive pregnancy test, then it is a pregnancy of unknown location. While it is possible that the pregnancy is too early to be visualized on ultrasound, emergent surgical evaluation and/or MEDEVAC should be considered in the symptomatic patient.

If an IUP is identified, a fetal heart rate (FHR) can offer additional reassurance. It is recommended to avoid the use of doppler to measure the heart rate at these early stages of pregnancy. Instead, M-mode can be used with the M-mode cursor placed over the observed heartbeat. The repetitive rhythmic waves in the area of the heart will be seen on the M-mode graph. A freeze button on the machine acquires the still image of this heart tracing. This allows the user to measure the FHR using embedded machine software. This is a menu setting on the machine. It is most easily activated by choosing the obstetrics setting at the start of the exam. The cursors can be placed to contain one cardiac cycle, which will then display the FHR on the monitor as seen in Fig. 9.28.

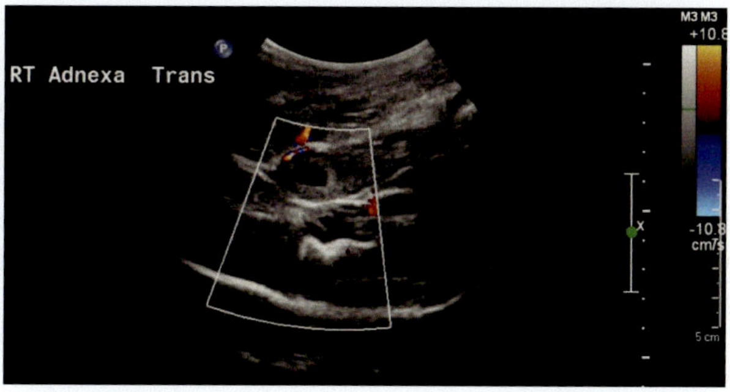

Fig. 9.27 Ectopic pregnancy in the adnexa seen on Point-of-Care Ultrasound (POCUS). (Source: Image courtesy of Navy Medicine Readiness and Training Command San Diego Radiology Department, used with permission)

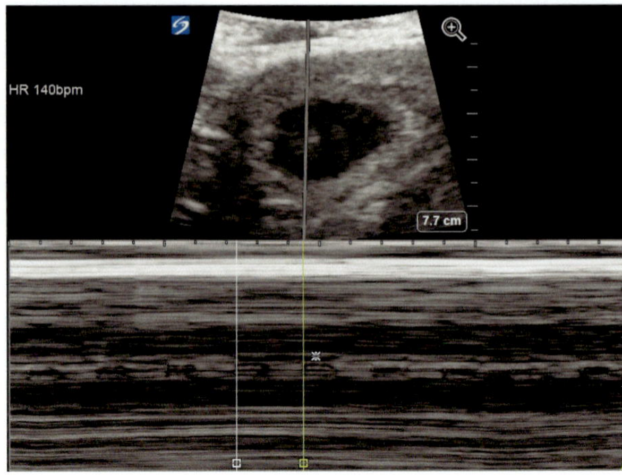

Fig. 9.28 Normal fetal heart rate (FHR) by M-mode seen on Point-of-Care Ultrasound (POCUS). (Source: Image courtesy of Matthew V. Speicher, DO)

Keys to Success

- In the deployed environment, if an IUP cannot be confirmed in a newly diagnosed pregnancy with significant pelvic pain and/or vaginal bleeding, ectopic pregnancy is of the utmost concern. The patient will require an expeditious surgical evaluation and/or MEDEVAC.
- Without a history of assisted reproductive technologies, such as in-vitro fertilization or intrauterine insemination, the likelihood of heterotopic pregnancy is exceedingly rare.

Ovarian Torsion

Introduction and Indications

Female patients experiencing sudden onset, severe, unilateral pelvic pain pose a concern for ovarian torsion. The presentation can vary, but risk factors include pregnancy (10–22% of all ovarian torsions) and ovarian cysts or masses, often 5 cm or greater, which are present in over 80% of patients with ovarian torsion [6]. In the shipboard setting, the clinical concern based on history and physical should prompt expeditious surgical evaluation and/or MEDEVAC, but POCUS can help to confirm the diagnosis.

The ovaries are mobile structures and visualization can pose a challenge to the novice sonographer. Transabdominal views can at times allow the sonographer to evaluate the ovaries, but a transvaginal view utilizing the intracavitary probe is recommended.

Technique

The intracavitary probe is set up as noted previously for the pregnancy exam. With the patient lying in the supine position with legs abducted, the probe is placed into the vagina in the sagittal or vertical orientation, until resistance is met at the cervix or the posterior fornix. Once the uterus is visualized, the probe should be rotated 90° counterclockwise giving a transverse view of the uterus. The probe should then be pointed toward the adnexa of the unaffected side to evaluate the normal ovary (Fig. 9.29).

Once the ovary of the unaffected side is seen, it should be evaluated for size and blood flow using color doppler. A normal ovary will typically measure <4 cm in diameter and will have color present indicating blood flow. Once color doppler is selected, the gain knob on the ultrasound machine will now change the sensitivity or gain of the color. If it is set too high, any slight movement by the operator or patient can result in false color returns. If the gain is set too low, blood flow will not be detected. The operator may have to adjust the gain to appreciate normal blood flow throughout the ovary. This process is similar to the evaluation of testicular torsion in the prior section.

Once a "normal" ovary is appreciated on the side without pain, the other ovary is then evaluated in the same method using the set gain. An enlarged ovary, at times up to eight times the size of a normal ovary, and a complete lack of blood flow can aid in the diagnosis (Fig. 9.30) [7]. Multiple angles should be evaluated for the presence of blood flow to lower the chance of a false-positive result.

Keys to Success

- Similar to testicular torsion, the presence of blood flow does not rule out intermittent torsion. Therefore, a negative study with a high clinical suspicion of ovarian torsion should not exclude the diagnosis.
- Large hypoechoic ovarian cysts can be seen and are often the source of the patient's pain. Ensure that blood flow is present prior to attributing pain to a cyst.

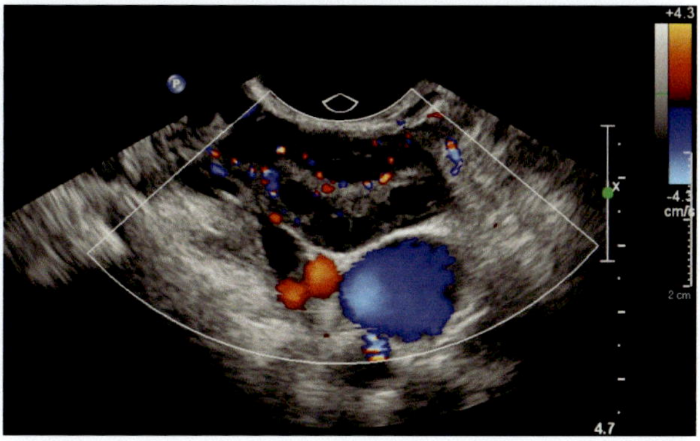

Fig. 9.29 Normal ovary seen on Point-of-Care Ultrasound (POCUS). (Source: Image courtesy of Navy Medicine Readiness and Training Command San Diego Radiology Department, used with permission)

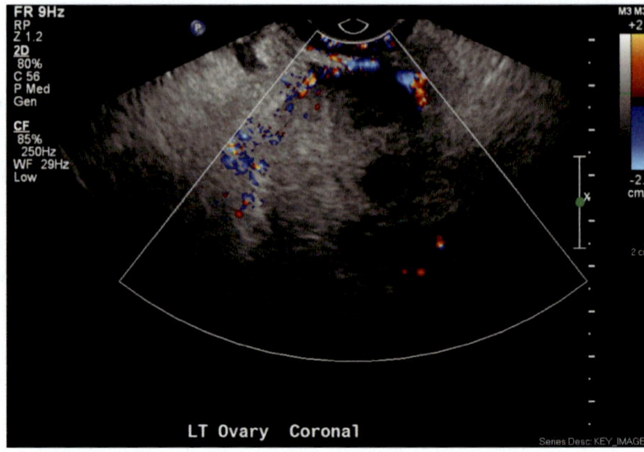

Fig. 9.30 Left ovary with lack of blood flow, concerning ovarian torsion, seen on Point-of-Care Ultrasound (POCUS). (Source: Image courtesy of Navy Medicine Readiness and Training Command San Diego Radiology Department, used with permission)

Central Venous Catheter (CVC) Placement

Introduction and Indications

Over the past several years, utilization of POCUS for central venous catheter (CVC) placement has become commonplace if not standard of care. As ultrasound has been shown to decrease the number of attempts for cannulation as well as decrease complications, the Agency for Healthcare Research and Quality has recommended its use for 20 years [8]. POCUS can be used in all three major sites for CVC placement: internal jugular vein (IJV), subclavian vein, and femoral vein.

For example, for the IJV both transverse (Fig. 9.31) and longitudinal (Fig. 9.32) views of the vein should be obtained, and cannulation should be attempted using the longitudinal view which allows for direct visualization of the needle through the soft tissue to the lumen of the vein.

Technique

Begin with placing the probe over the vessel to be cannulated in the transverse plane. Evaluate the surrounding structures, and find an area where the vessel can be distinguished from the accompanying pulsatile and less-compressible artery. Find an area of approach that lessens the chance of violating the artery. Once a favorable site has been determined, prepare to perform the procedure under sterile conditions by donning appropriate personal protective equipment (PPE), preparing the patient, and placing a sterile probe cover.

Once sterility has been achieved, place the probe on the skin using sterile gel to again identify and confirm the vessel to be cannulated in the transverse plane. Bring the vein to the center of the screen and rotate the probe 90° about its center axis,

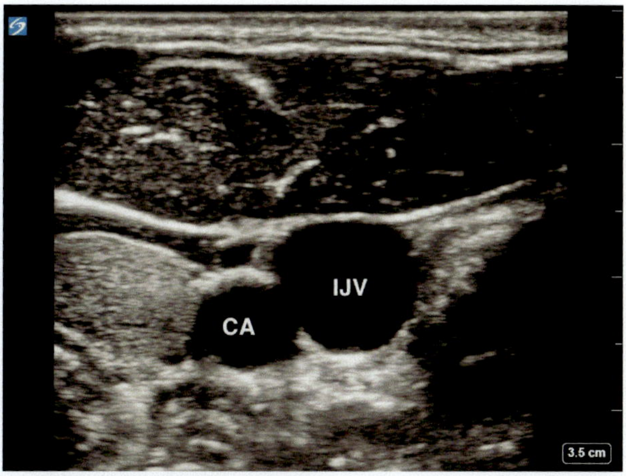

Fig. 9.31 Normal internal jugular vein (IJV) to the right of the carotid artery in the transverse plane seen on Point-of-Care Ultrasound (POCUS) for placement of an IJV central venous catheter (CVC). *CA* carotid artery, *IJV* internal jugular vein. (Source: Image courtesy of Matthew V. Speicher, DO)

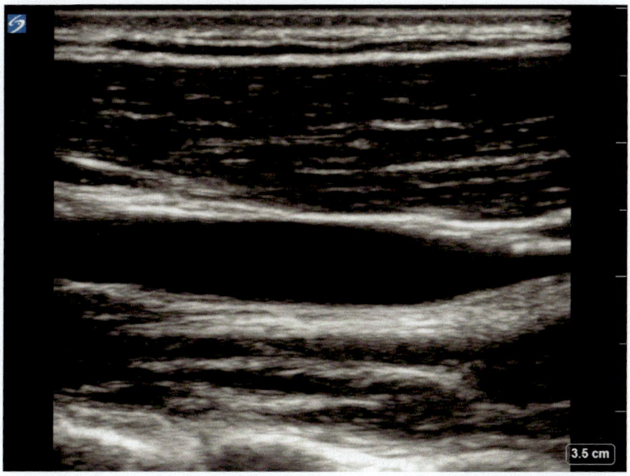

Fig. 9.32 Normal internal jugular vein (IJV) in the longitudinal plane seen on Point-of-Care Ultrasound (POCUS) for placement of an IJV central venous catheter (CVC). (Source: Image courtesy of Matthew V. Speicher, DO)

providing a longitudinal view of the vein. Insert the needle at a 45° angle just under the probe (Fig. 9.33). Once the needle is in the skin, ensure that the needle tip is seen and can be followed through the soft tissues as it is advanced into the lumen of the vein in plane with the probe.

Upon entering the vein, shallow the needle's angle of approach to the vein while slightly advancing the needle into the lumen. Aspirate and ensure venous blood return. At this point, the probe can be laid on the field. This allows the provider to use both hands to insert the wire via the Seldinger technique. Once the wire is in, it is recommended to place the probe again over the vessel in the longitudinal plane to visualize and document that the wire lies within the vein. The procedure can then be completed with dilating of the tract, placing of the catheter, and proper securing and dressing of the site. These portions of the procedure do not require ongoing ultrasound visualization.

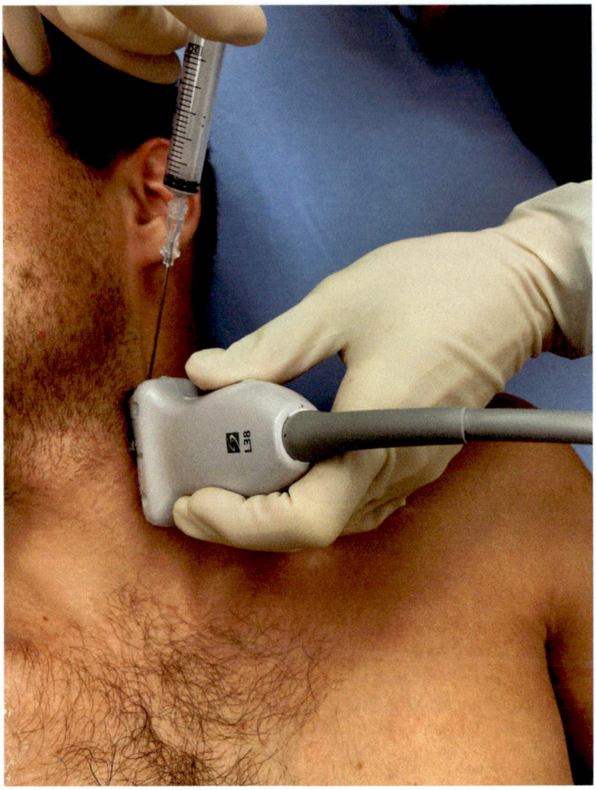

Fig. 9.33 Introducer needle placement using the longitudinal plane approach seen on Point-of-Care Ultrasound (POCUS) for placement of a left internal jugular vein (IJV) central venous catheter (CVC). (Source: Photo courtesy of Matthew V. Speicher, DO)

While it is likely that at least one member of the shipboard medical team has experience in the placement of an IJV or femoral vein CVC under ultrasound guidance, subclavian vein CVC placement has historically been performed utilizing landmarks only. To use ultrasound for this site, place the probe lateral to the clavicle as shown in Fig. 9.34. The view will show the subclavian vein and artery as well as the pleural line (Fig. 9.35). Once the vein is appreciated, place it in the center of the image and rotate 90° and cannulate as described above using the longitudinal plane approach.

Keys to Success

- Position the POCUS machine so that it is directly in line with the line being placed. The provider should only have to use minimal head movement to look at the screen during the procedure.
- Evaluate bilateral veins to select the vein that offers the best approach with the least concern for surrounding structures or potential complications.

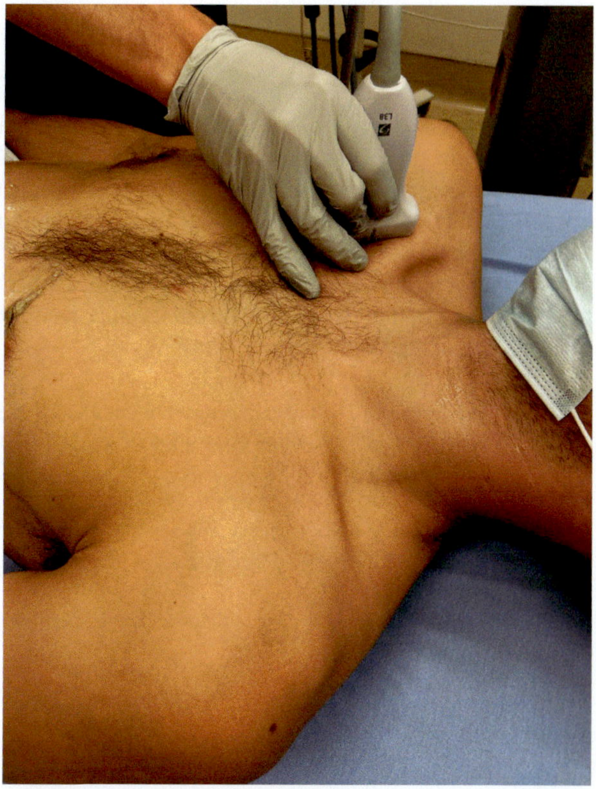

Fig. 9.34 Probe placement for Point-of-Care Ultrasound (POCUS) for placement of a right subclavian vein central venous catheter (CVC). (Source: Photo courtesy of Matthew V. Speicher, DO)

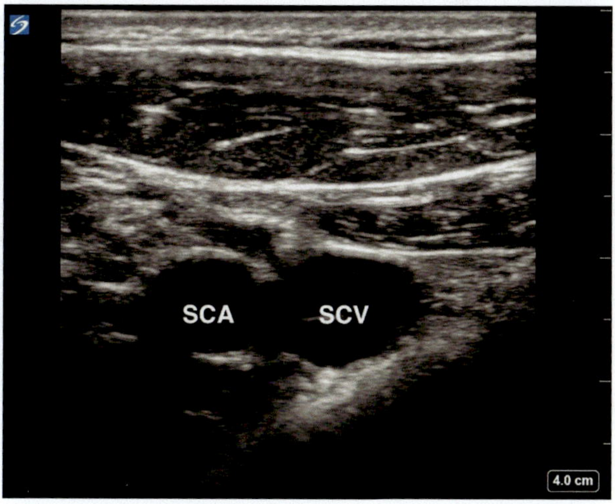

Fig. 9.35 Normal subclavian vein on the right of the subclavian artery transverse view seen on Point-of-Care Ultrasound (POCUS) for placement of a right subclavian vein central venous catheter (CVC). *SCA* subclavian artery, *SCV* subclavian vein. (Source: Image courtesy of Matthew V. Speicher, DO)

Conclusion

As described above, POCUS has several applications that can improve the diagnostic capabilities of the shipboard medical team. While at least one provider should be comfortable in performing the above studies, all members of the team should be aware of their existence and be able to perform some of them, such as the eFAST. Without the ability to obtain advanced imaging, POCUS may act as an adjunct to the physical exam and provide a wealth of information that can aid in the disposition of a patient to the operating room, to MEDEVAC, or return to duty. Understanding both the capabilities and limitations of POCUS can lead to improved survivability of the warfighter.

Declaration of Interest The views expressed in this chapter are those of the authors and do not necessarily reflect the official policy or position of the Department of the Navy, Department of Defense, nor the US Government.

Funding This research did not receive any specific grant from funding agencies in the public, commercial, or not-for-profit sectors.

Conflict of Interest Statement The authors declare no conflict of interest.

References

1. Sisson C, Solis-McCarthy J. Chapter 24: peritoneal free fluid. In: Soni NJ, editor. Point of care ultrasound. 2nd ed. Amsterdam: Elsevier; 2020. p. 219–28.
2. Reardon RF, Laudenbach AP, Heller KM, Barnes R, Reardon L, Pahl TJ, Weekes A. Chapter 5: transthoracic echocardiography. In: Ma O, Mateer JR, Reardon RF, Byars DV, Knapp BJ, Laudenbach AP, editors. Ma and Mateer's emergency ultrasound. 4th ed. New York: McGraw-Hill; 2020.
3. Murray D, Mailhot T. Chapter 12: hepatobiliary, clinical indications, jaundice and biliary duct dilation. In: Ma O, Mateer JR, Reardon RF, Byars DV, Knapp BJ, Laudenbach AP, editors. Ma and Mateer's emergency ultrasound. 4th ed. New York: McGraw-Hill; 2020.
4. Lahham S, Becker BA, Gari A, Bunch S, Alvarado M, Anderson CL, Viquez E, Spann SC, Fox JC. Utility of common bile duct measurement in ED point of care ultrasound: a prospective study. Am J Emerg Med. 2018;36(6):962–6. https://doi.org/10.1016/j.ajem.2017.10.064. Epub 2017 Nov 20. PMID: 29162442.
5. Zuker Herman R, et al. Comparison between two-point and three-point compression ultrasound for the diagnosis of deep vein thrombosis. Prehosp Disaster Med. 2017;32(S1):S45. https://doi.org/10.1017/s1049023x17001339.
6. Huang C, Hong MK, Ding DC. A review of ovary torsion. Ci Ji Yi Xue Za Zhi. 2017;29(3):143–7. https://doi.org/10.4103/tcmj.tcmj_55_17.
7. Mynatt I. Chapter 18: gynecologic concepts. In: Ma O, Mateer JR, Reardon RF, Byars DV, Knapp BJ, Laudenbach AP, editors. Ma and Mateer's emergency ultrasound. 4th ed. New York: McGraw-Hill; 2020.
8. Moore CL. Ultrasound first, second, and last for vascular access. J Ultrasound Med. 2014;33(7):1135–42. https://doi.org/10.7863/ultra.33.7.1135.

Chapter 10
Practical Nursing Principles Afloat

Shawn M. Harris, Darcy R. Guerricagoitia, and Heather A. Hernandez

I attribute my success to this: I never gave or took any excuse.

Florence Nightingale

Author deployment experience	
Shawn M. Harris	Critical Care Registered Nurse, Fleet Hospital 8, Operation Iraqi Freedom/ Operation Enduring Freedom, Rota, Spain, 2003
	Critical Care Registered Nurse, Fleet Surgical Team-5, Global War on Terror, Joint Operations Area, Philippines, 2004–2005
	Certified Registered Nurse Anesthetist, first Medical Battalion, Bravo Surgical Company, Operation Enduring Freedom, Southern Helmand Province, Afghanistan, 2010
	Officer In Charge, Expeditionary Resuscitative Surgical System Pacific, 2016–2017; Provided embarked Role 2 Surgical Support on the USS Ohio (SSGN-726), 2016–2017
	Commander, Naval Surface Force, U.S. Pacific Fleet (CNSP) Force Nurse, San Diego, CA, USA, 2018–2021

S. M. Harris
Naval Surface Force, U.S. Pacific Fleet, San Diego, CA, USA

D. R. Guerricagoitia (✉)
Navy Medicine Readiness and Training Command Portsmouth, Portsmouth, VA, USA
e-mail: darcy.r.guerricagoitia.mil@health.mil

H. A. Hernandez
Navy Medicine Readiness and Training Command Yokosuka, Yokosuka, Japan
e-mail: heather.a.hernandez8.mil@health.mil

M. D. Tadlock, A. A. Hernandez (eds.), *Expeditionary Surgery at Sea*,
https://doi.org/10.1007/978-3-031-21893-4_10

Author deployment experience	
Darcy R. Guerricagoitia	Critical Care Registered Nurse, Camp Bastion Role 3, Operation Enduring Freedom, Southern Helmand Province, Afghanistan, 2010
	Ship's Nurse, USS Enterprise (CVN-65), 2011–2013; 2 deployments in support of Operation Enduring Freedom, Persian Gulf, 2011–2013
	Critical Care Registered Nurse, Damage Control Surgery Team, Joint Special Operations Task Force, Operation Freedom's Sentinel, Operation Inherent Resolve, AFRICOM Area of Responsibility, 2016–2017
	Officer in Charge, 2nd Medical Battalion, 2nd Marine Logistics Group, Task Force Southwest Camp Shorab Role 2, Operation Freedom's Sentinel and Resolute Support, Southern Helmand Province, Afghanistan, 2019–2020
	Deputy Group Surgeon, 2nd Marine Logistics Group, II Marine Expeditionary Force, Camp Lejeune, NC, 2020–2021
Heather A. Hernandez	Individual Augmentee, Troop Medical Clinic, Operation Iraqi Freedom, Camp Virginia, Kuwait, 2007
	Squadron Lead Corpsman, Marine Fighter Attack Squadron-211 (VMA-211), Marine Aircraft Group-13, 13th Marine Expeditionary Unit, embarked on the USS Boxer (LHD-4), Operation Enduring Freedom, CENTCOM Area of Responsibility, 2010
	Squadron Lead Corpsman, Marine Fighter Attack Squadron-211 (VMA-211), Marine Aircraft Group-13, Operation Enduring Freedom, Camp Bastion, Helmand Province, Afghanistan, 2012
	Ship's Nurse, USS Nimitz (CVN-68), Operation Inherent Resolve and Operation Freedom's Sentinel, CENTCOM and INDOPACOM Areas of Responsibility, 2020–2021

BLUF (Bottom Line Up Front)

1. Seek out skills sustainment opportunities prior to deployment, not only in the areas of nursing that are typical for a critical care registered nurse (CCRN) like an Intensive Care Unit (ICU), but also in trauma bays and operating rooms (ORs).
2. The nurse on a maritime surgical team commonly holds administrative leadership positions such as Nursing Supervisor, Division Officer (DIVO), or Training Officer, with many additional responsibilities across the platform.
3. Pre-deployment Role 2 Team-based training is essential in preparing the team for receiving casualties. The preparation, planning, and organization of training are often the responsibilities of the nurse on the maritime surgical team and are critical for the team's success and preparedness.
4. Train the corpsmen. They are a force multiplier and an invaluable asset to the team! Corpsmen who are efficient and competent in basic nursing functions can allow rest and decrease burnout for everyone on the team.
5. The main reason for medical evacuation (MEDEVAC) off the ship was lack of supplies and resources; patient packaging and transport for MEDEVAC is essential and may require additional training prior to deployment.

6. As many experienced during the coronavirus disease 2019 (COVID-19) pandemic and will experience in the future with Distributed Maritime Operations (DMO), prolonged patient holding prior to MEDEVAC may be required. For critically ill patients is a nursing-heavy exercise and requires preparation and a team approach for good patient outcomes.
7. Doing the inspection as a team and ensuring the team is familiar with all equipment, instruments, and consumables and that they are all compatible and functional and well-supplied is essential for team success in austere environments.

Introduction

Nurses have a long history serving in the military and a longer history serving in wartime efforts, from Florence Nightingale's selfless dedication in the Crimean war to those women who volunteered under anonymity during the early American Revolutionary and Civil Wars. On May 13, 1908, President Theodore Roosevelt signed the Naval Appropriations Bill, authorizing the establishment of the United States (U.S.) Navy Nurse Corps. This establishment produced the "Sacred Twenty," the first official Nurse Corps candidates. Today, U.S. Navy Nurses continue to be instrumental serving as members of Navy Medicine dedicated to the wartime efforts ashore and at sea during times of peace and wartime.

This chapter will review the roles and responsibilities of the nurse serving as Ship's Nurse on an aircraft carrier (CVN), onboard a large deck amphibious assault ship with a Fleet Surgical Team (FST), or as a team member of an Expeditionary Resuscitative Surgical System (ERSS) or United States Marine Corps (USMC) Forward Resuscitative Surgical System (FRSS), providing austere resuscitative surgical care. The objective is to convey expectations of roles and responsibilities, clinically relevant and practical information to nurses interested in or chosen to support these operational platforms including leadership information, lessons learned, and "pearls of wisdom." Roles that nurses fill on these platforms include Certified Registered Nurse Anesthetist (CRNA), Critical Care Registered Nurse (CCRN), and Certified Perioperative Nurse (CNOR). The Secretary of Defense designated these wartime nursing specialists as critical to meet a Military Service's healthcare wartime mission, thus it is imperative nurses serving in these operational roles have and sustain the clinical competancy and operational skillsets required to perform and excel when serving on these platforms, both in the roles they have been trained in but also in roles they do not commonly play. Oftentimes, operational nurses carry a large leadership and administrative burden that may not reflect their responsibilities onshore. The intent of this chapter is to add content to the operational "toolbox" with the goal to produce competent nurses bound to practical principles afloat.

Aircraft Carrier (CVN) Nursing

The Ship's Nurse on an aircraft carrier must have specialty training and experience in critical care nursing (subspecialty code 1960). Their most important job is to provide nursing care and assist other health care providers in the medical treatment and care of thousands of Sailors and Marines aboard the ship itself and deployed on various warships of the Carrier Strike Group (CSG). However, they typically also play many other roles within the department.

Nursing Supervisor and Medical Training Team (MTT) Leader

They also serve as nursing supervisor for the inpatient medical department at both the Intensive Care Unit (ICU) and ward levels of care, overseeing all nursing functions within the department regardless of location and ensuring appropriate nursing care is both carried out and documented. The nurse reports directly to the Senior Medical Officer (SMO) in this role and directly supervises the corpsmen who work in the ICU and on the ward. The nurse also trains corpsmen to be functional nursing assistants with education, training, and testing on administration of medication, electrocardiograms (EKG), and basic nursing care. When there are truly sick patients that require 24/7 nursing care, having well-trained corpsmen is key to providing excellent patient care while allowing rest and preventing burnout for all members of the medical team.

The nurse is also the medical training team (MTT) leader as set forth in COMNAVAIRFORINST 3500.20E and COMNAVAIRFORINST 6000.1B 4–9. Not only does the nurse provide training to corpsmen throughout the medical department, but the nurse is also responsible for the medical education of thousands of Sailors and Marines aboard including:

- Basic Life Support (BLS) qualifications.
- BLS instructor qualifications.
- Basic shipboard first aid and rescue (SFAR) injury education.
- Buddy aid training.
- Stretcher-bearer training.
- Health education promotion.
- Maintenance of the Watch Quarter Station Bill and Stretcher Bearer Watch bill to support 10 Repair lockers and six Battle Dressing Stations (BDS).

At the time of publication, tiered mandatory Tactical Combat Casualty Care (TCCC) training for all Sailors in the Fleet is being implemented and the exact roles and responsibilities of this rollout for each platform have not been clearly defined. However, it is quite likely that the nurse will play a major role on the CVN platform.

The nurse has many other important administrative roles on the carrier. This includes working with the corpsmen in the various areas to ensure that all supplies are stocked, all equipment is functioning, and all resupply is followed up on. The nurse also typically serves as the crash cart coordinator, quality assurance coordinator, and patient safety manager; in general, the nurse is responsible for all quality assurance and risk management matters. The Ship's Nurse truly plays one of the most important roles in the CVN medical department!

Aircraft Carrier (CVN) Medical and Surgical Capabilities

The CVN has a 52-bed ICU/Ward, including three ICU beds and 49 ward beds. However, approximately one-half of these beds are essentially bunk beds and only capable of serving patients with minimal care requirements. Therefore, depending on patient type and acuity as well as corpsmen manning and training, ACTUAL ward capacity could be half that, particularly for high acuity patients. The ward has a main ward and two separate isolation rooms that have a four-bed capability each with a private restroom. Of note, they are not negative pressure isolation rooms.

The major equipment generally includes three ZOLL EMV+® ventilators, two mini-ventilators, four ZOLL M® monitors, five ZOLL MD® defibrillators, one Belmont® rapid infuser, one Hotline® blood and fluid warmer, nine Braun® single channel intravenous (IV) pumps, six portable and three bedside suction machines, three ICU beds, three crash carts, one gurney, and one stair chair. Figure 10.1 shows a critically ill patient on a 2021 CVN deployment who required 24/7 nursing care in the ICU.

A wide range of admission diagnoses with varying levels of acuity and complexity from a recent CVN deployment is demonstrated in Table 10.1. **Interestingly, nearly 70% of inpatient ward/ICU admissions required surgical consultation during that deployment.** Being able to manage inpatients can be complex when balancing supply constraints, operational missions, and limited personnel, none of which would be nursing concerns in a land-based hospital.

A suggestion for team preparation is doing hypothetical ICU rounds, where the inpatient team discusses hypothetical patients to review potential treatment plans, medication management, required equipment, and hospital stay duration. This exercise can be extremely useful from a training perspective but also from a supply and equipment management perspective. It prompts the team to ensure the ancillary services on the ship have the capability and non-expired equipment and consumables to support patient care for both an acute short-term patient but also in a potential prolonged patient holding situation, either because of a global constraint (such as the coronavirus disease 2019 (COVID-19) pandemic) or because of mission constraints in distributed maritime operations (DMO).

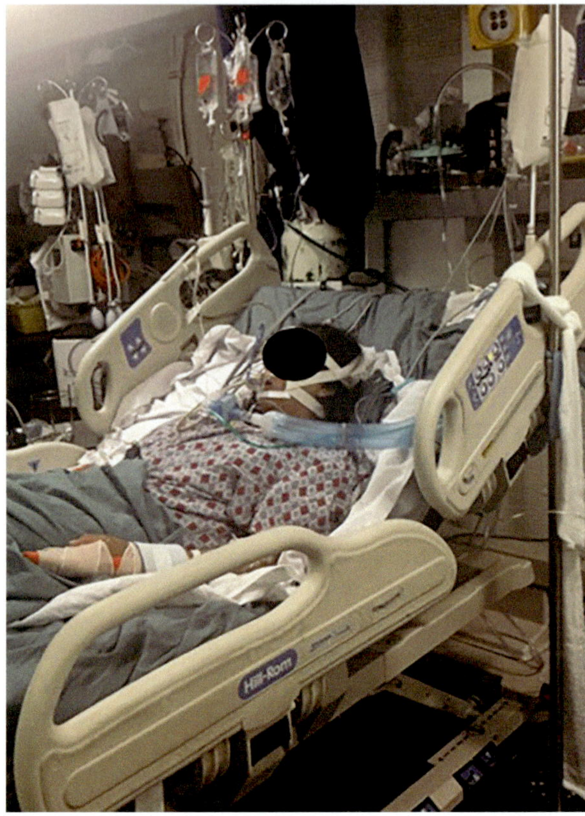

Fig. 10.1 Intensive Care Unit (ICU) admission on Nimitz class aircraft carrier, the USS Nimitz (CVN-68), 2021. Woman presented with tonic-clonic seizures refractory to benzodiazepines. She is intubated, sedated on propofol and ketamine drips, and has had central and arterial lines placed (Source: Photo courtesy of Heather A. Hernandez, CCRN)

Medical Evacuation (MEDEVAC)

The discussion needs to be had early and often about what needs to happen if a truly sick patient needs a medical evacuation (MEDEVAC) off the ship. Many times, the other personnel on a CVN with varying levels of critical care training outside of the CCRN include the SMO (potentially, as their specialty training is variable), the general surgeon, the family medicine physician, the CRNA, a few flight surgeons (who have only completed an internship), the physician assistant (PA), two Independent Duty Corpsmen (IDC), and two Search and Rescue Medical Technician (SMT) trained corpsmen. One option is to have the SMT and the flight surgeon fly on a MEDEVAC flight with the patient. However, if the patient is on drips, intubated, and/or paralyzed, the CCRN would go as well to monitor and manage the patient and the equipment. The CRNA would fill the role of the CCRN on board the ship if this ever needed to happen. Additional MEDEVAC training for the CCRN is discussed in the ERSS portion of this chapter (Fig. 10.2).

Table 10.1 Total Ward and Intensive Care Unit (ICU) inpatient admissions by diagnosis during an 11-month aircraft carrier (CVN) deployment

Diagnosis	Number of admissions
Hand injury*	11
Appendicitis*	9
Rash/cellulitis*	8
Suicidal ideation	7
Colitis/enteritis*	5
Perioral abscess*	5
Seizure	4
Abscess*	3
Fracture*	3
Other mental health	2
Abdominal pain*	2
Burn*	2
Deep vein thrombosis*	2
Other menstrual health	2
Pyelonephritis	2
Urolithiasis	2
Small bowel obstruction*	1
Spontaneous pneumothorax*	1
Pancreatitis*	1
Diabetes	1
Gastrointestinal bleeding*	1
Hernia repair*	1
Hypokalemia	1
Mononucleosis	1
Otitis media	1
Palpitations	1
Paraspinal compartment syndrome*	1
Penile edema*	1
Pheochromocytoma*	1
Stroke	1
Syncope	1
Thigh contusion*	**1**
Thrombophlebitis*	**1**
Total inpatient admissions	*86*
Total requiring surgical consultation* (%)	**60 (69.8%)**

Clinical Pearls

The nurse should consider cross-training in the operating room (OR) during routine and emergency operations. Knowing equipment location, being familiar with patient preparation procedures, and understanding the sterilization process will

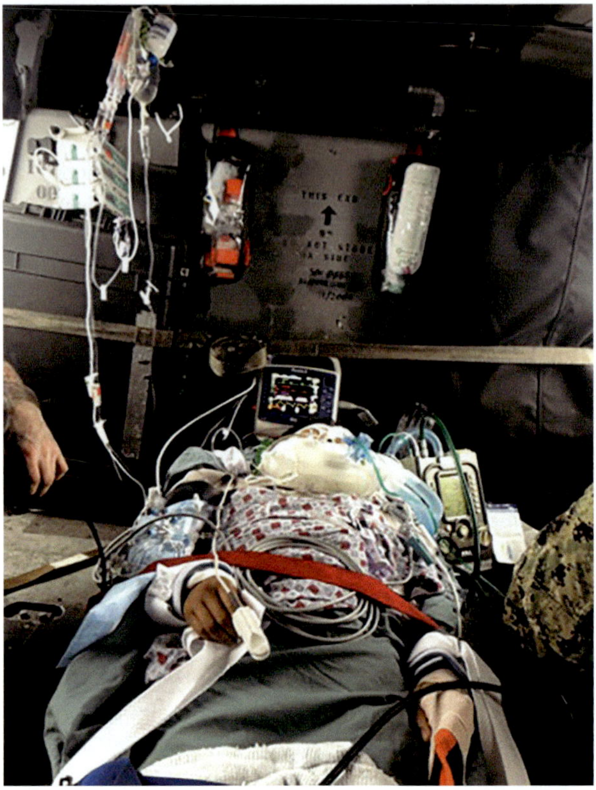

Fig. 10.2 Medical Evacuation (MEDEVAC) from Nimitz class aircraft carrier, the USS Nimitz (CVN-68), 2021. Patient is intubated and paralyzed for transport and being cared for by the Critical Care Registered Nurse (CCRN) and Search and Rescue Medical Technician (SMT) (Source: Photo courtesy of Kimberly Gerber, CRNA)

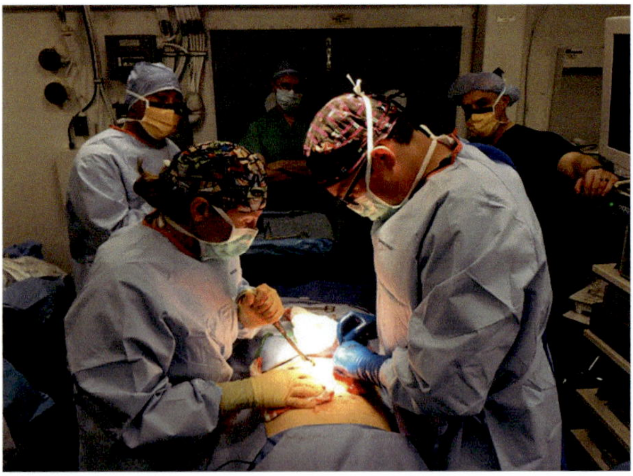

Fig. 10.3 General surgeon and Critical Care Registered Nurse (CCRN) operating together on board Nimitz class aircraft carrier, the USS Nimitz (CVN-68), 2021 (Source: Photo courtesy of Heather A. Hernandez, CCRN)

potentially help out the surgical team during a mass casualty incident (MCI) requiring one or more surgical operations. Consider scrubbing with Ship's Surgeon as well (Fig. 10.3).

There is a requirement for three crash carts–one each in the ICU, Main BDS (treatment room in the medical department), and dental clinic. Create Advanced Cardiac Life Support (ACLS) go bags; no shipboard medical emergency ever starts in the medical department. There are over 5000 personnel on the ship during deployment; while the majority are young and healthy, there are always a few people with undiagnosed chronic medical problems aboard too. Not to mention the fact that the ship is a dangerous place in general, with many possibilities for injury in both daily activities and in the workplace. Medical and trauma emergencies will likely happen somewhere on the ship where maneuvering is extremely difficult. Be prepared and learn the ship. Know the best routes and escape plans for every space. Networking with the ship's Fire Marshall is key; they also know the ship inside and out as well as all the equipment and resources available to get someone out of a space.

Fleet Surgical Team (FST) Nursing

The primary mission of a large deck amphibious assault ship and its associated Amphibious Readiness Group (ARG) is to support the United States Marine Corps (USMC) mission to launch a landing force from sea to land. The secondary mission is to provide a medical capability as a Casualty Receiving Treatment Ship (CRTS). To serve this function, an FST typically embarks, augmenting the ship's medical department. The execution of the CRTS capability may occur during a peer-to-peer fight, or during the full range of military operations ranging from disaster relief to foreign humanitarian assistance to noncombatant evacuation operations. Similar to a CVN medical department, the FST may also help provide routine and emergency medical and surgical care for the Sailors and Marines of the ship's company and also deployed on the various warships in the ARG. Therefore, the medical and surgical teams onboard need to be ready to respond anytime, anywhere, to any type of casualty. Depending on the mission, the FST may split and the surgical element may augment other smaller CRTS-qualified and equipped platforms within the ARG. See Chaps. 1, 6, and 12 for discussion of how the FST integrates with the ARG.

The FST is composed of eight Officers and 10 corpsmen. Among the officers, nursing services are rendered by the CRNA, CCRN, and CNOR, the only maritime expeditionary team to have all three roles. They provide a spectrum of clinical knowledge, skills, and abilities to the nursing care assets of an FST. Leadership roles may be split between them, including Walking Blood Bank (WBB) officer, Division Officer (DIVO), training officer, infection control officer, quality assurance coordinator, narcotic custodian, moderate sedation program manager, and/or safety manager, some of which are discussed below. In the end, preparation is key and is the best remedy to prevent poor performance resulting in a poor outcome.

Certified Registered Nurse Anesthetist (CRNA)

CRNAs are highly trained advanced practice registered nurses clinically privileged to work independently as the sole anesthesia provider within many expeditionary maritime surgical teams, including an FST. The CRNA's primary role is to render a full scope of anesthesia services to patients requiring anesthesia care management (see Chap. 13). Along with routine anesthesia delivery care, the CRNA also potentially can be expected to assist with critical care coverage and participate in MEDEVACs.

In trauma, the CRNA needs to be competent to care for casualties at multiple points in their care. This encompasses a spectrum of Advanced Trauma Life Support (ATLS) interventions from initial triage, resuscitation, and postoperative critical care.

Naturally, airway management is the primary skill of the CRNA, but the ability to perform damage control resuscitation (DCR) is of equal importance. In extremis, the casualty will warrant hemostatic resuscitation with a balanced component therapy or fresh whole blood (FWB) delivery. The CRTS platform is equipped with a large supply of frozen component blood including packed red blood cells (PRBCs) and Fresh Frozen Plasma (FFP), although it lacks platelets and cryoprecipitate. Furthermore, deglycerolizing takes time, thus it is crucial to understand how to execute the WBB for immediate delivery of FWB (see Chap. 23 for discussion of DCR). Often the ship's medical department may not take the time to practice and refine this process prior to deployment. **As one of the most experienced providers on the platform, it is imperative to be actively involved in both the execution and training of the WBB for both FST and ship's company medical personnel.** This will include ensuring a percentage of the ship is prescreened per instruction prior to deployment, providing assistance in the procurement of the allotted blood supply for the platform, and supervising the drills for the medical teams.

Critical Care Registered Nurse (CCRN)

The CCRN is in charge of the ICU, ward, and post-anesthesia care unit (PACU). A CCRN is a board-certified critical care registered nurse with an advanced clinical background in critical care and/or emergency nursing. Their primary responsibility is to render critical care nursing services to the patient in all health statuses from minimal to critical for time frames ranging from acute to prolonged care. It is highly recommended the maritime CCRN receive additional training in critical care air transport to effectively participate in a casualty MEDEVAC off the ship to shore when needed, see ERSS portion of this chapter for more details. During transport, be ready to provide life-saving interventions, manage mechanical ventilation, and administer medications to control hemodynamic stability and analgesia (see Chap. 31). Upon arrival to the next echelon of care, the team should be able to efficiently and thoroughly report a patient's condition to the accepting medical facility.

A common leadership role the CCRN assumes is the role of the DIVO because that person is already involved in many areas of patient care and readiness because of their job description. The DIVO is directly responsible to the ship's SMO for inpatient area operational readiness. The DIVO ensures personnel working with patients are present, maintain good orderly discipline, and most importantly are sufficiently trained to provide safe patient care. It is imperative that the personnel working in the medical spaces are cross-trained to assist in performing basic nursing care including assessments, interventions, documentation, and evaluations. Enhancing the team's core competencies will enable the corpsmen to work independently to maximize efficiency and safety. The DIVO also supervises that all equipment, supplies, and consumables are available, functioning, and in sufficient supply for the duration of the deployment across all the ships on the CRTS platform.

Another common collateral duty is the training officer, who is responsible to plan, organize, and execute individual and team training. Part of this role is ensuring all members of the medical team maintain mandatory qualifications like BLS, ACLS, ATLS, Trauma Nurse Core Course (TNCC), and/or TCCC. The training officer often organizes various drills and verifies the crash carts are fully equipped, functional, and meeting medical inspection criteria.

Certified Perioperative Nurse (CNOR)

Certified Perioperative Nurses (CNORs) are board-certified perioperative registered nurses with experience in the intraoperative clinical setting, infection prevention, and sterilization. The CNOR executes the role and responsibility to provide perioperative care to patients before, during, and after surgery. Duties include verification of surgical instrument sterility, preparation of equipment for surgical procedures, and maintenance of OR readiness. For the FST platform, the CNOR ensures OR integrity across all associated ships on the platform prior to deployment. Furthermore, they should work closely with the ship's company and FST surgical technologists (STs) and the FST surgeon to verify all equipment, instruments, and consumable supplies are available and functional (see Chap. 12). While embarked, the CNOR takes responsibility for the ORs, manages the STs, and ensures all staff members abide by perioperative nursing standards encompassing the preoperative, intraoperative, and postoperative phases of care. These standards include preoperative patient assessment, room readiness, patient transport to OR, patient safety, intraoperative patient positioning, final count completion, and postoperative transport to the recovery unit. The CNOR should also assist with the postoperative recovery of the patient and assist with medical ward duties if needed.

Expeditionary Resuscitative Surgical System (ERSS) Nursing

As a CCRN on a small ERSS team, it is imperative to be clinically competent and have a bank of resources to access when needed. The CCRN will likely be involved and/or responsible for many parts of patient care including trauma resuscitation, preoperative care, surgical resuscitation, OR circulation, assisting the anesthesia provider, postoperative assessment and care, patient packaging for MEDEVAC, and prolonged patient care if MEDEVAC capabilities are limited. The name of this role is “flexibility,” as it is ever changing, fast-paced, and extremely demanding.

Preoperative: Trauma Resuscitation

CCRNs are typically adept at using multiple pieces of equipment such as rapid infusing and warming devices, ventilators, multiple IV pumps, and suction machines while managing the lines and tubes required of the typical trauma/surgical patient. Therefore, they are well-suited to work in the resuscitation/trauma bay area of the ERSS, assisting with DCR and potentially preparing for the OR. Tips for preparing for this responsibility are to be intimately familiar with equipment, current resuscitation guidelines including medications and emergency interventions, TCCC, Joint Trauma System (JTS) Clinical Practice Guidelines (CPGs), and TNCC or ATLS trauma assessments. Any time spent in an emergency department or trauma bay prior to deployment is time well spent.

Current doctrine states that typical ERSS team size is seven personnel, with only one CCRN. However, sometimes nine-person teams have been deployed (see Chap. 1), usually with an emergency/trauma nurse (CEN) as one of the additional team members. If present, having open and clear communication with this person and developing a strong working relationship is critical for mission success in these small austere teams as oftentimes they will both be asked to be interchangeable. The authors recommend cross-training in each other’s key clinical competencies and sharing role insights. This also applies to the corpsman on the team–any time training and educating is time well spent. Ensuring everyone on the team has insight into the roles/responsibilities and clinical knowledge a CCRN brings to the team only enhances the team and its response and capabilities.

Intraoperative: Operating Room (OR)

This role is likely the most outside of the realm of a typical CCRN. Any time spent in the OR prior to deployment learning sterile draping, opening of instruments, and names of basic instruments is also time well spent for any CCRN and their deployed OR team, particularly in the seven-person ERSS team where there is only one nurse.

It is also a good idea to be familiar with how to set up electrocautery, prep the patient before the surgeon cuts, insert a foley catheter, and obtain additional IV access. Sometimes the CCRN assists the surgeon scrubbed in or the OR in a nonsterile way, "running" for supplies, equipment, or medications. Most likely, the CCRN will be assisting the anesthesia provider with blood product administration via rapid infusing and warming devices (i.e., the Belmont ® and Hotline ®), drip titration, medication administration, and interventions to aid in managing the patient's hemodynamic status.

Tips for this area to best prepare prior to deployment are to know and practice using the rapid infusing/warming devices available and to go to the OR with the surgical team to tailor the skills and knowledge a CCRN has that would complement and accommodate the needs of the team.

Postoperative: Intensive Care Unit (ICU) & Medical Evacuation (MEDEVAC)

The ICU is the realm of a CCRN and their place to shine; therefore, it is essential to get plenty of skills-sustainment experience in the ICU ensuring clinical competence prior to deployment if a CCRN has not been actively practicing their skills. Many times, the CCRN is working independently on a patient postoperatively while the rest of the team is managing the next patient, therefore a CCRN needs to be mentally and physically prepared.

One of the benefits of being in the OR with the patient intraoperatively is the intimate knowledge of the surgical procedures, interventions, and the patient's hemodynamic status. The teamwork and constant communication with the surgeon and anesthesia provider make follow-on care a smooth transition. Additionally, there is ample time to do a thorough full body assessment and reassess all interventions performed in the OR.

Given the austere environments ERSS teams operate in, be familiar with current JTS CPGs. Cross-train the team on how to help monitor critical patients for prolonged periods of time when rapid MEDEVAC is not available. In an austere environment postoperative and patient care during prolonged holding periods must be a team sport to ensure patients get the best care possible while all team members are able to get rest.

Patient packaging for MEDEVAC is paramount. Depending on location this may be a fixed or rotary wing asset, which have different requirements. Any formal training prior to deployment is time well spent to help in the postoperative and transport care of patients while on deployment. Critical Care Air Transport (CCATT) is the fixed-wing course provided by the U.S. Air Force and is a wealth of knowledge about how altitude, time, and equipment affect patient transportation. Joint EnRoute Care Course (JECC) is a rotary wing course to prepare to package and transport in that environment. Proper and careful packaging of the patient will ensure successful transport and improve patient survival.

General Practical Tips

No matter the platform, maintenance and supply will be a constant struggle (see Chap. 12)! Prior to deployment, the entire surgical team should participate in an inspection of each piece of gear to ensure all is in working order/compatible and to take inventory of what is needed. Know and test equipment for form, fit, and function prior to deployment. Read instruction manuals, speak to equipment representatives, and cross-train all team members in equipment familiarization. Ensure all equipment, supplies, and consumables are stocked PRIOR to deployment and ordered in a timely fashion when resupply is required. There are often discrepancies between equipment and consumables being compatible and having awareness to these issues prior to deployment or as soon as possible will help to troubleshoot and find ways around these issues. Nurses may be involved in or even responsible for this process in departments or with gear that is both familiar and unfamiliar to their normal workflow.

To maintain some sense of normalcy during long austere deployments with high levels of clinical and administrative responsibility, the authors recommend bringing creature comforts as described in Chap. 5 and Appendix B. Plan ahead and find out what has to be brought, what can be brought, and how to get resupply of personal care items. The more austere the deployed environment, the more unreliable the mail system, so bring at least 3–6 months of personal care items if possible.

Conclusion

Flexibility, teamwork, and clinical competence are the keys to being an effective member of a small surgical team. Often the training pipelines are complex with dynamic schedules; being flexible with a positive attitude can go a long way. Cross-train in different roles and train the corpsmen to do the same. Get comfortable being uncomfortable. Truly a jack-of-all-trades, a nurse can play a variety of roles on any expeditionary maritime medical platform, usually with clinical and administrative roles and responsibilities that are different from what is expected in a land-based facility. Preparation prior to deployment, training during deployment, and communication constantly are essential to foster a cohesive team.

Declaration of Interest The views expressed in this chapter are those of the authors and do not necessarily reflect the official policy or position of the Department of the Navy, Department of Defense, nor the US Government.

Funding This research did not receive any specific grant from funding agencies in the public, commercial, or not-for-profit sectors.

Conflict of Interest Statement The authors declare no conflict of interest.

Further Reading

Instruction 6000.1. The Shipboard Medical Procedures Manual, which differs by region and platform (for example from San Diego: COMNAVAIRPACINST for CVN, COMNAVSURFPACINST/ COMNAVSURFLANTINST for the other platforms).

Joint Trauma System. Clinical practice guidelines. n.d.-a. https://jts.amedd.army.mil/index.cfm/PI_CPGs/cpgs.

Joint Trauma System. Prolonged casualty care clinical practice guidelines. n.d.-b. https://jts.amedd.army.mil/assets/docs/cpgs/Prolonged_Casualty_Care_Guidelines_21_Dec_2021_ID91.pdf.

Chapter 11
Alone and Unafraid: The Independent Duty Corpsman at Sea

Todd Burkholder

> *We must never forget why we have, and why we need our military. Our armed forces exist solely to ensure our nation is safe, so that each and every one of us can sleep soundly at night, knowing we have "guardians at the gate."*
>
> *Allen West*

Author deployment experience	
Todd Burkholder	Fleet Marine Force Corpsman, Joint Task Force-Special Operations Command, Operation Iraqi Freedom, multiple locations, 2003–2004
	Fleet Marine Force Corpsman, Quick Reaction Force Marine ForcesSecurity Command, Operation Enduring Freedom, Guantanamo Bay, 2005
	Leading Petty Officer, Fleet Surgical Team-3, embarked on the USS Tarawa (LHA-1), Operation Enduring Freedom, Iraq and CENTCOM Area of Responsibility, 2007–2009
	Fleet Marine Force Corpsman, Explosive Ordnance Disposal Mobile Unit 8 (EODMU-8), Operation Enduring Freedom, AFRICOM Area of Responsibility, 2011
	Senior Medical Department Representative/Independent Duty Corpsman, USS Preble (DDG-88), Operation Enduring Freedom, Fifth and Seventh Fleet Areas of Responsibility, 2012–2015
	Medical Department Leading Chief, USS Makin Island (LHD-8), Operation Octave Quartz, Somalia and CENTCOM Area of Responsibility, 2017–2021

T. Burkholder (✉)
USS Makin Island (LHD-8), San Diego, CA, USA
e-mail: todd.burkholder222@gmail.com

M. D. Tadlock, A. A. Hernandez (eds.), *Expeditionary Surgery at Sea*,
https://doi.org/10.1007/978-3-031-21893-4_11

BLUF (Bottom Line Up Front)

1. The crew of your ship is depending on you to save their lives, so treat your education like your lifeline. Make it a priority prior to deployment. Taking personal responsibility for your education and skillset acquisition is a crucial step in being ready to deploy on a Role 1 platform.
2. If you don't know something or have a question, call a specialist or your physician supervisor for advice. It might save a life.
3. The majority of laboratory, radiology, and pharmacology ancillary services don't exist on a Role 1 platform. You are limited on personnel, equipment, resources, and medical evacuation (MEDEVAC) options. You can't always be a hero. Know when you have done enough to get the patient on to the next level of care and do it as quickly as possible as the mission allows.
4. Train your junior corpsmen like your life and the lives of the crew depend on it because they very well might!
5. Patient transport on the ship when a patient is not ambulatory is dangerous and must be done methodically and safely for optimal outcomes. Train litter bearers regularly and prepare for worst-case scenarios.
6. Be a master communicator with everyone including your junior corpsmen, Commanding Officer (CO) and Triad, physician supervisor, and most importantly, your patients.
7. Earning your CO's trust and respect is vital for you to care for your patients. Be competent, confident, and concise when you discuss the risks and benefits of the CO's options, and keep them informed on patient statuses.
8. Know how to MEDEVAC a patient; it is a complex process that varies by region. With the limited resources you have, it is vital and essential for your patients' outcomes to get them expeditiously to platforms with more resources.
9. Build a good working relationship with your physician supervisor. Knowing how and being able to contact them at any time is critical to your success onboard a Role 1 platform. They should be a sounding board and training resource for you and your corpsmen.
10. You will have a Medical Readiness Inspection within a 90-day window prior to your deployment. Preparation for this important inspection starts as soon as you check in to the ship. There are many resources available to prepare you and your team. Do things by reference, not preference.
11. Know your AMAL and ensure all of your supplies will be at 100% through your projected deployment period. This process starts at least 6 months prior to deployment and often requires communication and acquisition of supplies outside of the formal U.S. Navy Supply System, which is fraught with issues at every level.

Introduction

For an Independent Duty Corpsman (IDC), being both the solo independent medical provider and the senior medical department representative (SMDR) at sea is one of the most complex and challenging assignments out there. Typical first platforms for an IDC coming out of IDC School are Role 1 medical platforms, including Destroyers (DDG), Cruisers (CG), Minesweepers, or a United States Marine Corps (USMC) field unit.

As stated in many other chapters of this book, one of the biggest challenges of the shipboard medical environment for any level of provider is the lack of medical technology commonly found in shore-based facilities. For an IDC in a Role 1 shipboard environment, many of the resources found on the larger ships (e.g., aircraft carriers (CVNs), and amphibious assault ships) will not be available to you. For example, as the IDC on a DDG, you must predominantly rely on what you can see, hear, feel, and think when it comes to practicing medicine. There are no basic X-ray or Ultrasound capabilities. Your laboratory capability is limited to a Complete Blood Count (CBC) and minimal rapid point-of-care (POC) testing that you must personally analyze, essentially functioning as your own laboratory technician. There are minimal medications and no blood products available.

Warships are industrial and dangerous environments during both peace and wartime postures. The potential injuries any provider could need to manage are endless. It is even more difficult as the solo independent provider with minimal resources available on a Role 1 platform. Here are two clinical vignettes to demonstrate what could happen and how to optimize patient outcomes.

Clinical Vignette 11.1

Several years ago while pier-side, I was in the conference room of a large naval warship when "Man Down" was called over the 1-MC (1-Main Circuit, the standard United States (U.S.) Navy shipboard public address circuit). Normally our ship had a robust Role 2 medical capability when fully staffed. However, because of ongoing construction aboard the ship, we did not have access to our medical spaces so our configuration and supply set were similar to that of a DDG Role 1 medical department. When I arrived at the berthing area (not on the main decks) where the man down was, I found two of my corpsmen assessing an unresponsive Sailor on the ground. I immediately recognized him; he was a male in his late 20s with no known medical history, however, he was on restriction to the ship for a positive drug test. He was not breathing, cyanotic, and pulseless.

One of my corpsmen began chest compressions while I assessed the airway and began ventilating the patient with a Bag-Valve-Mask (BVM). I sent the other corpsman to retrieve the Automated External Defibrillator (AED), medication bag, and portable oxygen. I also asked the security personnel who responded to the scene to do an emergency search and seizure of his locker nearby to determine if he had ingested anything. During the resuscitation, his initial oxygen saturation was 70%, and he required 100% oxygen with BVM. Presuming an opioid overdose, I instructed my team to administer naloxone without improvement. After 17 min of cardiopulmonary resuscitation (CPR), the patient regained a pulse but continued to require constant assisted BVM ventilation.

It took the Federal Fire Department nearly 20 min to respond. Had our team not recognized a likely opioid overdose and initiated prompt high-quality CPR, he likely would have died. Fortunately, he was able to make a full recovery after being admitted to a local hospital for a week where he required a naloxone drip and other interventions before he was able to breathe on his own. The etiology of his condition was found to be an overdose of heroin and fentanyl from a street drug called White China.

Clinical Vignette 11.2

While forward deployed on my first ship as an IDC in the Seventh Fleet Area of Responsibility (AOR), I was called to the engineering spaces where a Sailor sustained a witnessed fall down a vertical ladder of three decks (approximately 35 feet). When I looked down the ladder, all I saw was the Sailor's feet but no movement. Thankfully when I arrived, I found an alert and breathing, albeit disoriented and immobile Sailor. Somehow, he managed to miss all the safety nets on the way down and had visible lacerations down his forearms; presumably from grasping for something to break his fall. He had struck the ground on his feet and crumpled to the deck according to a watch-stander in the space. His acute complaints were severe pain in his lower spine and neck. He wasn't sure where he was but was able to follow commands and move his upper extremities but not lower extremities.

My junior corpsman and I placed him in a cervical spine collar, positioned him on a spine board, and maintained full spine precautions, utilizing stretcher-bearers for assistance. While palpating, I felt an obvious deformity over his lower lumbar spine while the rest of his exam was otherwise unremarkable. At this point, we knew we had a spinal injury and at a minimum a concussion, but there was the potential for a more severe traumatic brain injury (TBI).

After our primary and secondary surveys, we assessed that he was stable but critical. We also recognized that his condition could change at any moment because we had no capability to assess for internal bleeding; a real possibility given his injury pattern. On a Role 1 platform without the ability to obtain imaging or any meaningful laboratory data, monitoring, reassessment, and support was the most we could do. Therefore, the priorities for this patient were to safely transport him out of the engineering spaces, arrange for a medical evacuation (MEDEVAC) to a higher level of care, and closely monitor him for changes in vital signs and mental status/consciousness while in our care.

Our Commanding Officer (CO) quickly arrived on the scene, as it is common for the CO of a Role 1 platform to respond to emergencies. When he saw that I was working on the patient, he asked what I needed. I asked him to arrange helicopter

MEDEVAC transport to a nearby CVN as fast as possible. He rushed back up the ladder, and by the time we had vertically extricated the patient up the shaft using the Reeves Sleeve, the helicopter was ready and our CO had spoken to the CO and Senior Medical Officer (SMO) onboard the CVN.

We had the patient loaded onto the helicopter within 30 min from the time of our response to the call. Ultimately, this Sailor was diagnosed with a lumbar spine fracture and was able to return to full duty within 6 months of injury.

These two real-life clinical vignettes illustrate the importance of being prepared in every way for the unique role of a shipboard Role 1 IDC. Both of these patients were critically ill and required immediate treatment and urgent transport to a higher level of care, which occurred without delay, contributing to their good outcomes. Having the knowledge to think through a patient's condition, the wisdom not to get tunnel vision and consider all the possible outcomes, the foresight to practice and prepare as a team, the leadership to direct and guide both the junior corpsmen on the medical team and the non-medical personnel who respond, and the communication skills to relay information about patient status and MEDEVAC requirements with ship leadership are all essential to save a patient's life as a forward-deployed maritime IDC. This chapter is not only to guide the new shipboard IDC on how to best care for all patients, including surgical ones, but also to provide insight for the surgical teams receiving patients from a shipboard Role 1 medical department led by an IDC.

Being Prepared with Medical Knowledge

As demonstrated in the previous vignettes, an IDC should know the initial treatment of a wide range of illnesses and injuries in an austere shipboard environment without any special equipment. They must be able to recognize concerning clinical changes based on frequent reassessment, and when to ask for a timely MEDEVAC. There is no substitute for sound complex decision-making.

Despite improvements in medicine over the past several decades, the shipboard Role 1 environment is still relatively austere in its medical capability compared to garrison military medical treatment facilities (MTF) or even larger maritime platforms. This is not due to a lack of technology in the military or availability, but the configuration of smaller U.S. Navy warships. There is simply no physical space for advanced equipment such as fixed or portable X-ray or ultrasound machines, laboratory processing equipment, or any other typical medical resources found in any stateside hospital. Therefore, when managing patients, IDCs must rely on what they can see, hear, and feel to problem-solve based on their individual knowledge, clinical experience, and prior training. The better prepared you are, the better outcome for your patients.

Basic skill sets that IDCs are expected to be experienced and competent in include Basic Life Support (BLS), Advanced Cardiac Life Support (ACLS), and Provider-level Tactical Combat Casualty Care (TCCC). It is also highly recommended that all IDCs become qualified in Advanced Trauma Life Support (ATLS). But certification alone is not sufficient. Not only do you have to practice your skillset, but you must also ensure your team of corpsmen and non-medical Sailors are trained and ready to help you respond to any emergency. This requires multiple ACLS- and TCCC-related drills to ensure the entire ship is ready to respond. However, this important training can be logistically difficult to accomplish due to the sheer volume of patient care and administrative responsibilities you have onboard.

Navy medical personnel are routinely required to have TCCC training at various points during their careers, however, it was not routinely required while assigned to a shipboard medical platform prior to April 2021. While there are some differences in casualty care in the maritime environment, the core principles of TCCC are the same no matter the deployed environment. The TCCC responder levels are listed in Table 11.1. Prior to deployment, a shipboard IDC should be a Tier 4 and a corpsman should be a Tier 3 TCCC provider. Furthermore, prior to deployment, you should develop a plan to train the entire ship's crew to be Tier 1 and Tier 2 responders as appropriate. This is a new requirement that the IDC will be responsible for, as well as the culture change required to successfully implement it.

While proficiency in BLS, ACLS, and TCCC are critical skills to have, evaluating and resuscitating injured patients, including managing a Walking Blood Bank (WBB), are also critical skill sets in the distributed maritime environment. While taught in IDC School, these skills must be refined and practiced to ensure optimal patient outcomes. For example, the establishment and management of an operational WBB program takes a great deal of pre-deployment work (discussed thoroughly in Chap. 23). Personnel have to be screened and properly identified to establish a pool of eligible participants. To be proficient in this skill, you must be able to have a unit of blood out of one person and into your patient in less than 30 min, all while still providing emergent care to a critically ill patient. If you ever

Table 11.1 Tactical Combat Casualty Care (TCCC) Responder Levels

Responder level	Provider type	TCCC task/skill examples
Tier 1	All service members	• TCCC • Care under fire/threat • Tactical field care
Tier 2	Combat lifesaver	• All tier 1 skills • Tactical evacuation care
Tier 3	Combat medic hospital corpsman	• All tier 2 skills • Life-saving interventions including triage, junctional tourniquet application, airway adjunct use, cricothyroidotomy, oxygen administration, shock and burn resuscitation, fracture management
Tier 4	Combat paramedic provider (including physicians and IDC)	• All tier 3 skills • Advanced life-saving interventions such as endotracheal intubation and tube or finger thoracostomy

TCCC tactical combat casualty care, *IDC* independent duty corpsman

experience a shipboard mass casualty incident (MCI) with multiple patients, some of which require blood, knowing how to run an efficient WBB will be a necessary skill.

Finally, in today's maritime environment the U.S. Navy is forward-projecting power across the globe and developing concepts like Distributed Maritime Operations (DMO), making the possibility that a critically ill patient may not be able to MEDEVAC for several days on any platform. While this unique situation has rarely occurred since World War II, being prepared to treat trauma and manage sick patients for several days is something a shipboard IDC must be ready to encounter.

Being prepared to accomplish this set of complex tasks means you have taken the time to learn the medical knowledge required to perform the skillset and relied on the local MTF and Medical Readiness Division (MRD) to train and prepare you and your team. That being said, being prepared is ultimately a personal choice that requires significant effort and dedication to your education. This is easier said than done when assigned to a shipboard Role 1 platform because your day-to-day routine includes evaluating patients each morning and ensuring multiple administrative programs important to overall crew readiness are running smoothly and efficiently in the afternoon. The needs of the ship and her crew never cease. But you must find the time for your own personal education not solely for you, but for your patients. **It's not a matter of *if* you will care for Sailors with medical emergencies or traumatic injuries while in a remote forward-deployed maritime environment, it's a matter of *when*.**

Training Your Junior Corpsmen

The first responders in both introductory clinical vignettes were junior corpsmen. Typical shipboard Role 1 platforms have only two junior corpsmen (one male, one female) to assist the IDC in everything medical. They represent the medical department to the crew; showing that they are competent and can perform in trauma/emergencies as well as day-to-day medical care strengthens your department and rapport with the crew. Having two well-trained corpsmen who can care for patients independently also allows for efficient healthcare to occur and optimally prepares your team for a possible MCI. As such, they play a key role in the success of a medical department on a Role 1 platform and your success as the leader of that department.

Corpsmen are like plants: water them with knowledge and they will grow, give them nothing and they will wither away. It is your responsibility to ensure they are well-trained in medical knowledge and well-versed in medical logistics so that you are comfortable with their healthcare delivery in your absence. Challenge them and ensure your physician supervisor is training and challenging them as well. Perform high-fidelity medical drills and invest time in training prior to deployment. Train them like everyone's life depends on it, because it may!

Safe Patient Movement Throughout the Ship

As both prior clinical vignettes illustrate, ships are not only dangerous environments but injury and illness can occur in locations that are physically challenging to access. Patient transport throughout the ship when a patient is not ambulatory is dangerous and must be done methodically and safely for optimal outcomes. These skills are not taught during BLS, ACLS, or TCCC. While they are taught in IDC School, safe patient movement is so crucial that some basic principles will be reviewed here.

Military personnel are taught how to carry casualties in a field environment during TCCC, but that type of transport is not feasible on a ship because the environment is completely different: narrow passageways, frequent hatches, vertical ladders, etc. Therefore, there are two main types of litters utilized for casualty transport onboard a ship:

1. Stokes Litter.
2. Reeves Sleeve.

The Stokes Litter (also called a Stokes Stretcher or Stokes Basket, depicted in Fig. 11.1) is found on all Navy surface ships. It can *only* be used for same-level transport, not up or down ladder wells, as a patient cannot be adequately secured. It was created by and named after the 14th Surgeon General of the U.S. Navy after his experiences as an assistant surgeon during the Spanish-American War in 1898 transporting patients off the hospital ship USS Solace (AH-2) using canvas litters that provided no stability for long-bone fractures. It is made of a metal wire frame with a wooden understructure for support. While used infrequently, it is useful if you have a patient with no spine precautions. The transport of patients in this type of litter is typically on the main decks where the main medical space is located or on the flight deck where it will not melt in the event of a fire; you can quickly egress

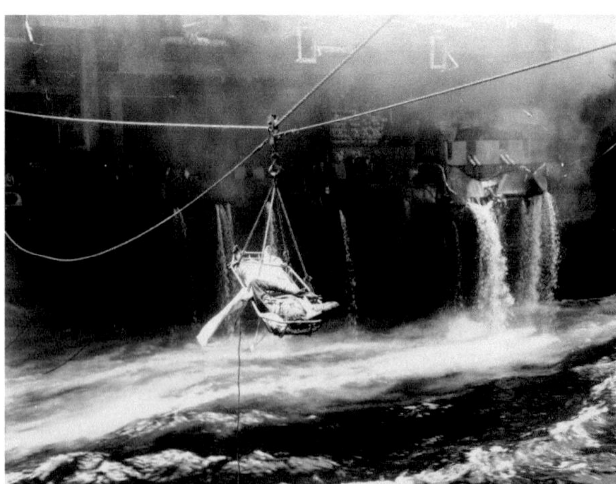

Fig. 11.1 Ship-to-ship transfer of a casualty using the Stokes Litter during World War II (May 11, 1945). The casualty is being transferred from the USS Bunker Hill (CV-17) to the USS Wilkes-Barre (CL-103) near Okinawa, Japan. (Source: Government publication, not in copyright. Available at: https://catalog.archives.gov/id/520682)

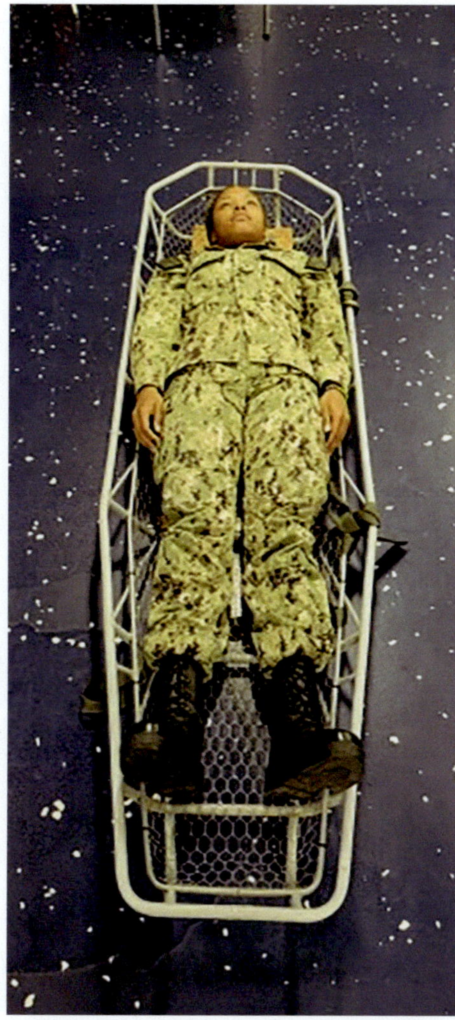

Fig. 11.2 Stokes Litter. On the main decks and in the medical department, it will contain straps as depicted here. On the flight deck, the straps will be removed. It is for routine transports on the main decks and medical department or urgent transport away from dangerous areas by crash and salvage teams on flight decks. It does not provide full spine precautions. (Source: Photo courtesy of Senior Chief Hospital Corpsman Barryon Starks)

a casualty into safety using this litter. On the main decks, it will contain straps as seen in Fig. 11.2, and on flight decks, the straps will be removed.

The main type of patient transport device used onboard U.S. Navy maritime vessels is a Reeves Sleeve (highlighted in Clinical Vignette 11.2, depicted in Fig. 11.3). It cocoons the patient to allow for complete immobilization, and it has a removable spine board that slides into the back to provide full spine precautions. Therefore, it can be used for both transport on the same level and vertical transport up or down ladder wells. Used in almost any emergency situation, they can be found throughout ships mounted on bulkheads for easy access. Patients can quickly be secured with cervical spine precautions into the litter; an experienced stretcher bearer team can secure a patient to the litter in less than 1 min. They are also used to transport patients between ships and ship-to-shore (see Chap. 31). The Reeves Sleeve can

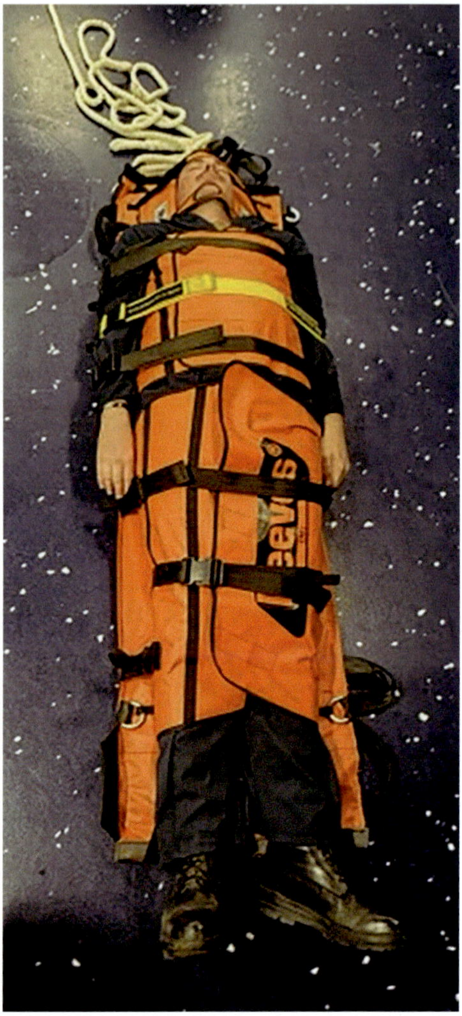

Fig. 11.3 Reeves Sleeve. It is the most commonly used litter on board modern Navy maritime vessels. Once secured, the patient is completely immobilized and in full spine precautions. In the Figure, the securing straps are not in their final position; they go under and over the boots and ankles to secure the feet. The bright yellow strap goes over the arms. On the top, a tending line is attached with a locking carabiner to aid in pulling patients up ladders and to secure them with a safety line when going down ladders. (Source: Photo courtesy of Senior Chief Hospital Corpsman Barryon Starks)

also fit inside the Absorbent Patient Litter System (see Chap. 28) to allow for patient warming with all leads and monitors placed over the torso and between the legs. The main body straps secure the legs and torso. Securing straps go under and over the boots and ankles to secure the feet, and a bright yellow strap goes over the arms and main body straps, completely immobilizing the patient. The tending line seen at the top of the stretcher is attached with a locking carabiner and will be secured to the litter and to a hard fixed post or ladder post onboard the ship with a minimum of three turns to utilize as a safety line when traversing ladders.

The tending line should be as long as the longest vertical ladder onboard your ship. A tip you won't find anywhere is to contact your Boatswain's Mates (BMs), bring some line, measure the longest ladder or shaft on board your ship, and make all your tending lines that long. Have the BMs splice in the carabiner for you, and you will have the best tending lines that are guaranteed to reach the bottom of your longest ladder or shaft.

Of note, most stretcher-bearers are non-medical ship personnel. Practicing litter drills with your stretcher-bearer teams is required quarterly as part of basic training requirements for the medical department. Challenge them during these evolutions so they are prepared. Emphasize their **VITAL** role in patient care: if patients cannot safely get to the medical department and/or the flight deck in a timely manner, they will not be able to receive the life-saving care they need.

Building a Relationship of Trust and Mutual Respect with Your Commanding Officer (CO)

In Clinical Vignette 11.2, the great working relationship with the CO was the primary reason the patient was able to obtain a MEDEVAC so rapidly. A major key to your success as an IDC on a Role 1 platform at sea is building a relationship of trust and mutual respect with your Commanding Officer. **The COs of Role 1 platforms are Surface Warfare Officers (SWOs); their job is to take a warship to sea and project power across the globe safely. They rely on their IDC to provide timely, honest, competent advice when it comes to the health and wellness of the Sailors under their command.**

Building a relationship of trust with the CO requires that you be a master of communication. Communicate in terms that the CO will understand, and avoid throwing medical jargon at them as it is not helpful. Be concise. Explain the risks and benefits involved for all options. COs operate and make decisions based on risk. For example, you must be able to explain to the CO the risk involved with keeping a patient onboard with an emergent medical condition versus sending them to a higher echelon of care. There are times when the mission will come first, but the CO makes that choice after you arm them with the information necessary to make a sound decision.

Communicate frequently with your CO. Keep them in the know all of the time when it comes to the status of their Sailors; if they get blindsided by information, it erodes their trust in you.

Foster the same trust, mutual respect, and open honest communication with the other members of the Triad as well: the Executive Officer (XO) and Command Master Chief (CMC). The XO and CMC are the day-to-day leaders of the crew, and they can typically help you resolve any issues that come up within the crew or reach out to external entities to obtain assistance if you need it. It takes a team to run a ship, and they are crucial members.

Finally, if you want to gain trust from the onset, ensure you do extremely well on all of your inspections so the CO does not have to worry about the medical department. If you have good communication, pass inspections, and take excellent care of Sailors while balancing the needs of the mission…trust will begin to grow, as demonstrated in the following vignette.

Clinical Vignette 11.3

I was a brand-new IDC on my first platform, a DDG. We were operating a few hundred miles off of the southern California coast conducting our Anti-Submarine Warfare Certification, a qualification required for the ship to deploy on time later that year. I knew the CO had trust issues with IDCs because he had detached my predecessor due to lack of confidence in their skills and judgment to run the medical department safely. So not only was I fresh out of IDC School and underway with a new command, but I also had received absolutely no turnover.

Fast forward to 2 weeks on the ship when a 28-year-old Lieutenant entered the medical department complaining of severe pain and vision loss in his left eye. He had no medical history and no history of trauma to his eye. When I examined him, I saw a protruding eyeball that came to a point like a pyramid from the corneal view. Immediately I thought back to my IDC School ophthalmology rotations and thought to myself, "This can't be acute angle glaucoma, this guy is too young." That being said, he had all the signs and symptoms of it, so I immediately ran to combat and contacted the duty ophthalmologist at Naval Medical Center San Diego (NMCSD), a Navy Captain. He wasn't sure my diagnosis was correct but agreed that the patient needed to be evaluated emergently given such a protrusion and vision loss coupled with severe pain.

I brought this information to my new CO. He initially declined my request for MEDEVAC. He wasn't sure I was right and wanted to finish the certification, which was scheduled for another 8 h. Furthermore, landing a helicopter on the back of a moving DDG is an extremely dangerous evolution. I respectfully informed the CO that if he chose that course of action that it would be his responsibility to explain to the patient, one of his officers, why he lost his eyesight if I was right. When I put it that way to the CO, he immediately changed his course of action and contacted the Fleet Commander's office to get a helicopter out to the ship. I balanced the needs of the mission and of the Sailor, presented him with the risks and benefits associated with his options, and enabled him to make an informed choice.

The patient underwent emergent eye surgery for acute angle glaucoma caused by a rare hereditary condition. He did not lose his vision and returned to full duty as a nuclear officer because of his expedited MEDEVAC and evaluation by a surgical sub-specialist.

This event established a great deal of trust with the CO, which was a good start for me. When our department passed our Medical Readiness Inspection with perfect scores, our relationship further solidified. It was also reinforced with constant, concise, and honest communication.

The facts are simple: to be successful as an IDC at sea you have to be a master of your craft and a master of communication. Having a good working relationship with your CO and Triad takes a lot of hard work, but pays off in the care of your patients.

Principles of Medical Evacuation (MEDEVAC)

The patients of all three clinical vignettes so far have required transport off the ship to higher echelons of care. A shipboard IDC must master the MEDEVAC process. Larger platforms have Medical Service Corps (MSC) officers whose responsibilities include the arrangement and tracking of patient movement in the MEDEVAC system. However, this is yet another job that an IDC absorbs on a Role 1 platform.

Each Fleet AOR has established MEDEVAC requirements, operation orders (OPORD), and an Annex Q. Fleet Commander orders dictate how and where to MEDEVAC personnel and have all the necessary resources to contact and assist you in the movement of patients. You must thoroughly understand this complex process for each Fleet you operate in; failure to adhere to these requirements and orders may hinder your ability to successfully move patients, thus putting them and your unit as a whole at risk.

Working with Your Physician Supervisor

Every IDC in the U.S. Navy has a physician supervisor, assigned from the local MRD. The professional relationship between an IDC and physician supervisor is outlined in Navy Medicine instructions; the personal relationship, putting aside the requirements of the instructions, is also a critical one.

Their responsibilities include peer-reviewing your patient care, being your sounding board for medical decision-making, and ensuring you have appropriate training and preparation to perform a full spectrum of patient care including primary care, medical emergencies, and trauma management.

Physician supervisors should be the person you reach out to with any and all questions regarding patients that you are not 100% comfortable treating. By instruction, you are also required to contact them for certain complex patient presentations outside the scope of your care. They are your lifeline in caring for difficult patients, and they will evaluate your patients after you have tried interventions without success. Building a good working relationship with your physician supervisor and having the ability to contact them at any time is critical to your success. Have the wisdom to admit when you are out of your comfort zone and need either assistance or a second set of eyes, especially in your first year onboard a new platform or fresh out of IDC School.

Work with your physician supervisor to ensure you and your team get the appropriate training. Ask them to run drills with you and your team. Take advantage of their medical knowledge to maximize the educational benefit of this important relationship, especially prior to deployment.

While pier-side, a physician supervisor should routinely visit monthly to execute their responsibilities. On a forward-deployed Role 1 platform, while your supervisor is not physically located onboard, remember they are always a phone call, email, or in-person visit away for any questions or concerns. Finally, if you are deployed independently and cross from one Fleet to another, the Fleet IDC and Fleet Surgeon for that AOR act as your physician supervisor. If you are in a battle group such as a Carrier Strike Group (CSG), the SMO onboard the CVN is your physician supervisor. These people are also your local lifelines with the largest wealth of working knowledge of the medical assets and infrastructure in that AOR. Ensure you are in early and constant contact with them. Finally, when operating with larger platforms, leverage their increased capabilities and provider specialties to your patients' benefit.

Clinical Vignette 11.4

While deployed, I evaluated a 25-year-old male with a rash all over his body, including on his palms and soles of his feet. During the patient interview, I learned he was recently evaluated at the local MTF for this issue a few months ago and was diagnosed and treated for scabies. Upon physical exam, I did not agree with this assessment and was concerned that the rash was far more consistent with Stage 2 syphilis.

I did not have the capability to run the appropriate laboratory testing, but a nearby large deck amphibious assault ship did. I called my physician supervisor and presented the case to get their opinion. My supervisor agreed and advised me to get the patient's laboratory tests to the nearby ship. The results confirmed syphilis.

I contacted the Infectious Disease (ID) clinic at the nearest MTF and developed a treatment plan that involved high doses of antibiotics. They also gave me warning signs for adverse effects of the treatment. I then notified my physician supervisor and provided the email documentation from the ID physician. After a prolonged treatment course and follow-up with the ID clinic, the patient did well, had no adverse effects, and made a full recovery.

This diagnosis in Clinical Vignette 11.4 is typically out of an IDC's scope of care, but being deployed there is no one else to see the patient, so you have to figure it out. With strong and regular communication with your physician supervisor and appropriate specialists, you can ensure excellent care for the Sailors in your care while keeping them in the fight and avoid any potential miscommunication.

Administration at Sea

There are many requirements to ensure a warship safely deploys. Not only do you bear the full weight of responsibility for the safe medical care of the ship's personnel and full training of your corpsmen, but you also have administrative duties to attend to. Not knowing and not performing them correctly can negatively impact not only your department's morale and success but can destroy your relationship with your CO and can even result in you being relieved of duty, as demonstrated in Clinical Vignette 11.3.

How do you prevent this from happening? First, know your requirements; all Navy medicine at sea requirements can be found in Instruction 6000.1 (COMNAVSURFPACINST or COMNAVSURFLANTINST). Not only does it lay out everything required of an IDC for each platform, but its enclosures and sister instructions provide you with the checklists that you need to prepare for your inspections.

The best advice I have is to build your inspection binders upon arrival to your platform and update them periodically (every 2 weeks). If you have a question on how an inspectable checklist item should look, contact the Senior Medical Inspector (SMI) from the local MRD that is assigned to your Fleet Commander's office. The Fleet Surgeon's Office and MRD are there to answer your questions, assist you, and ensure you succeed when they inspect you. It can be an overwhelming and daunting task, so pick their brains. Take your Quarterly Assessments with your SMI seriously. Schedule a Medical Readiness Assessment Technical Assist Visit (TAV) with your SMI as well. Have them review your administrative requirements *prior to your inspections* so they can find discrepancies so that you can fix them *prior* to your formal inspection. If you prepare correctly the first time and build your administrative requirements upon check-in, it will be much easier to keep things updated as you go, rather than to recreate the wheel every time you have an inspection.

Utilize the "waterfront" as well; your fellow IDCs have gone through these same inspections, so get their pearls of wisdom! Network and communicate, but above all use the reference. I like to say, "Reference not preference will never steer you wrong." Know your references and instructions so you can adequately prepare and ensure you are doing things by the letter of the law!

You will have a Medical Readiness Inspection within a 90-day window prior to your deployment. Inspect your Authorized Medical Allowance Lists (AMAL) at least 6 months before deployment to ensure all of your supplies are at 100% and will be *through your projected deployment period.* Inspect everything within your AMAL to determine safety and resupply levels. Then bring extra! Deployments can be unpredictable, and resupply is often troublesome. Bring extra medications, trauma supplies, and general medical supplies so you are prepared for anything. Role 1 platforms will not always be with a CSG or Amphibious Readiness Group (ARG). They also deploy independently, which may make a Role 1 IDC the only independent medical provider for hundreds, if not thousands, of miles. Ensure you have enough supplies to cover holding a patient for a few days to weeks in the event a MEDEVAC is not possible.

As outlined in several chapters (Chaps. 5, 10, 12), the U.S. Navy Supply System onboard ships can be finicky. Items are often on backorder due to government contractual obligations or mismatched supply and demand. If you are having trouble procuring supplies through formal channels, communicate early and often with your local MRD and SMI if pier-side, and work with the Fleet Surgeon's office if deployed. They will assist you at the Type Commander (TYCOM)/Fleet level to get you what you need. Think outside of the box as well; there is a waterfront full of ships so communicate with the ships sailing in the same AOR, returning from deployment, or heading into a maintenance period to see if they can send you supplies that may be hard to come by if they will not be needing them for the foreseeable future.

Conclusion

It is not a secret that one of the most difficult jobs in the U.S. Navy is being an IDC in the Role 1 environment at sea. The amount of responsibility that you have is unheard of in practically any other environment. Leverage the knowledge of the IDCs who have succeeded before you, your physician supervisor, and the SMIs and Fleet Surgeon. Remember that although you may feel alone and physically be the only independent provider for thousands of miles, you are never truly alone if you use all of the resources available to you that have been outlined in this chapter. If you can master your craft and communication skills, you will succeed. Always prepare like your life and the lives of all the personnel onboard depend on it, because they do.

It is not easy. The hours are long but taking care of a crew and building that lasting bond with your fellow Sailors is priceless. Impacting ONE person's life positively makes everything worth it! **Bottom Line: Being an IDC on a Role 1 platform puts you in a position of extreme responsibility. Prepare for it! You cannot wing it…you ARE it!**

Declaration of Interest The views expressed in this chapter are those of the authors and do not necessarily reflect the official policy or position of the Department of the Navy, Department of Defense, nor the US Government.

Funding This research did not receive any specific grant from funding agencies in the public, commercial, or not-for-profit sectors.

Conflict of Interest Statement The authors declare no conflict of interest.

Part III
Elective and Emergency Surgical Care

Chapter 12
Mess Deck, Hangar Bay, or Operating Room? The Shipboard Operating Theater

Alexis Torres, Angela F. Harris, Justin Yabut, and Amy A. Hernandez

Whenever your preparations for the sea are poor; the sea worms its way in and finds the problems.

Francis C. Stokes Jr., American trans-oceanic solo sailor (1926–2008)

Author deployment experience	
Alexis Torres	Surgical Technologist, Expeditionary Medical Facility-Kuwait, Operation Iraqi Freedom and Operation Enduring Freedom, Camp Patriot and Camp Arifjan, Kuwait, 2008–2009
	Surgical Technologist, Fleet Surgical Team-9, in support of Pacific Partnership, Tonga, Vanuatu, Papua New Guinea, Timor Leste, Federated States of Micronesia, 2011
	Trauma Lead Surgical Technologist, NATO Role 3 Medical Unit, NATO Resolute Support and Operation Freedom's Sentinel, Kandahar Airfield, Afghanistan, 2015–2016
	Lead Surgical Technologist, USS Carl Vinson (CVN-70), WESTPAC, INDOPACOM Area of Responsibility, 2017–2018
Angela F. Harris	Lead Surgical Technologist, USNS Mercy (T-AH-19), Pacific Partnership, Indonesia, Malaysia, Singapore, Vietnam, 2018
	Surgical Technologist, Fleet Surgical Team-9, embarked on the USS Tripoli (LHA-7), maiden voyage, from yards to San Diego homeport, 2020

A. Torres · A. A. Hernandez (✉)
Navy Medicine Readiness and Training Command San Diego, San Diego, CA, USA
e-mail: alexis.torres24.mil@navy.mil; Amyhern7@gmail.com

A. F. Harris
Fleet Surgical Team-9, San Diego, CA, USA
e-mail: angela.f.harris@navy.mil

J. Yabut
Fleet Surgical Team-5, San Diego, CA, USA
e-mail: justin.yabut@navy.mil

M. D. Tadlock, A. A. Hernandez (eds.), *Expeditionary Surgery at Sea*,
https://doi.org/10.1007/978-3-031-21893-4_12

Author deployment experience	
Justin Yabut	Surgical Technologist, Expeditionary Resuscitative Surgical System
	Pacific, 2019–2020; provided embarked Role 2 Surgical
	Support, INDOPACOM Area of Responsibility, 2020
Amy A. Hernandez	Battalion Surgeon, 7th Engineer Support Battalion, Operation Enduring Freedom, Camp Leatherneck, Afghanistan, 2011
	Ship's Surgeon, USS Carl Vinson (CVN-70), WESTPAC, INDOPACOM Area of Responsibility, 2017
	Department Head, Federal Emergency Management Agency (FEMA) and Defense Support of Civilian Authorities (DSCA), COVID-19 Community Vaccination Center mission, St. Louis, MO, USA, 2021

BLUF (Bottom Line Up Front)

1. In general, the maritime surgical team will have a general surgeon, an anesthesia provider, and one or two surgical technologists (STs). Only Fleet Surgical Teams (FSTs) have a Certified Perioperative Nurse (CNOR), so this role for other platforms needs to be covered by other members of the surgical team.
2. A thorough inventory of all Authorized Medical Allowance List (AMAL) and supplemental equipment, instrument sets, and medical consumables prior to, during, and following deployment is essential. This process differs by platform.
3. The supply system is fraught with barriers on all the platforms from deficient or outdated equipment, expired or near expired consumables, and significant lags in delivery of ordered supplies, frequently forcing teams to "tactically acquire" equipment and consumables prior to deployments.
4. Maintenance of the complex equipment required for a functioning Operating Room (OR) can be difficult without the robust biomedical technical support system available on land. Much of the repair and the annual maintenance can only be done during port and thus needs to be scheduled ahead of time.
5. The OR should be the cleanest place on the entire ship, which requires a substantial amount of dedication to execute because of issues ranging from limited space and lack of pressure/temperature/humidity control to damage of the autoclaves by the water created using reverse osmosis.
6. The autoclaves on aircraft carrier (CVN) and Fleet Surgical Team (FST) platforms are finicky pieces of equipment and often break down. Prepare for this contingency and have a backup plan.
7. The maritime OR is usually located in the medical department but occasionally will be in a Battle Dressing Station (BDS), hangar bay, mess deck, or wherever a makeshift one can be safely created. This is more typical of Expeditionary Resuscitative Surgical System (ERSS) missions but can be necessary during a Mass Casualty Incident (MCI) on other platforms.

8. STs' OR responsibilities often are considered secondary to their primary general duty corpsmen responsibilities. The maintenance and upkeep of a maritime OR is a time-consuming, detail-oriented, constantly challenging process and is the responsibility of the whole surgical team.

Introduction

Each member of the maritime surgical team plays a vital role in the preparedness of the maritime Operating Room (OR). Flexibility and the ability to think outside the box are the best ways to approach maintaining a ready maritime OR since challenges are as ever-present and unpredictable as the waves in the ocean. This chapter details, compares, and contrasts the team members, equipment, supply chain, maintenance responsibilities, sterility processing, and non-standard OR locations of the different surgical maritime platforms: aircraft carrier (CVN), Fleet Surgical Team (FST), and Expeditionary Resuscitative Surgical System (ERSS).

Surgical Team Members (Table 12.1)

On each platform, the responsibilities of the surgical team members are relatively similar but with one key difference in nursing capability.

- The general surgeon performs the procedure/surgery with the assistance of the surgical technologists (STs), and the surgeon's responsibilities include overseeing and guiding the pre/postoperative care.

Table 12.1 Comparison of the three platforms' surgical team members

	# total officers	# total enlisted	Members of the surgical team
CVN	10/13 (with carrier air wing embarked)	30/40 (with carrier air wing embarked)	1 general surgeon 2 STs 1 anesthesia provider 1 CCRN
FST	8 *not accounting for additional ship medical staff, # depends on platform	10 *not accounting for additional ship medical staff, # depends on platform	1 general surgeon 2 STs 1 anesthesia provider 1 CCRN 1 CNOR
ERSS	5	2	1 general surgeon 1 ST 1 anesthesia provider 1 CCRN

CVN aircraft carrier, *ST* surgical technologist, *CCRN* critical care registered nurse, *FST* Fleet Surgical Team, *CNOR* certified perioperative nurse, *ERSS* Expeditionary Resuscitative Surgical System

- The ST's responsibilities additionally include preparing the OR for surgery, cleaning the OR post-surgery, regularly checking on and ordering supplies, maintaining equipment, and decontaminating and sterilizing instruments.
- The anesthesia provider can be an anesthesiologist or a Certified Registered Nurse Anesthetist (CRNA); their responsibilities include administering general anesthesia, sedation, and/or nerve blocks prior to surgery and helping with immediate postoperative pain management. See Chap. 13 for a discussion of Anesthesia at sea.

On the Fleet Surgical Team (FST), the Certified Perioperative Nurse (CNOR) advocates for the patients and their belongings, initiates pre/postoperative timeouts, charts in the patient's record, collects, labels, and turns over specimens for processing, oversees the room readiness, and monitors the patient until turn over with the Critical Care Registered Nurse (CCRN) in recovery. On Expeditionary Resuscitative Surgical System (ERSS) and aircraft carrier (CVN) platforms, those responsibilities are absorbed by other members of the team.

CVN

Although CVNs are the largest platform in the Navy, they are not slated to be Casualty Receiving and Treatment Ships (CRTS) from a manning and equipment perspective, so there may be a misconception of their surgical capabilities. A CVN is billeted for one general surgeon and two STs. The anesthesia provider is usually sent on Temporary Assigned Duty (TAD) from a supporting military Medical Treatment Facility (MTF). A CVN is also billeted for one CCRN, who provides pre/postoperative care of the patient.

Specimens from the OR are placed in a sterile container, logged in a logbook maintained by the OR staff, and both the specimen request form and the container are labeled appropriately with patient demographics by the ST. The surgeon signs the form, and both are sent to the laboratory and logged into their logbook. The laboratory technician ensures the specimen is processed properly, whether that is processing on the ship or preparing for the specimen to be flown off to a supporting lab. The surgeon should follow-up the results if a supporting laboratory processes them, and it is their responsibility to communicate results to patients.

FST

Each FST is composed of eight officers and ten enlisted members that supplement the medical capabilities onboard CRTS, typically operating within an Amphibious Readiness Group (ARG), described more in Chaps. 1 and 6. This support is used to establish Role 2 Forward Resuscitative Capability on board the platform they are assigned. The OR team is typical of a hospital setting: general surgeon, anesthesia provider, CNOR, and two STs. One CCRN provides pre/postoperative care for patients.

Specimens from the OR are processed similarly to the CVN, except the CNOR typically does the initial processing of the specimen.

ERSS

Historically, there were up to nine members of an ERSS team, however, the newest doctrine has seven members. Often there will only be three people in the OR: general surgeon, anesthesia provider, and ST. The role of CNOR may need to be covered by any member of the team; other members of the team, including the CCRN, are typically busy with the trauma bay and pre/postoperative care of patients.

As surgery usually is damage control in nature and occurs in unpredictable locations, there isn't a laboratory to receive any specimens that may be made. If any specimens are removed, they would be placed in a clean container, clearly labeled with patient demographics, and transported with the patient for processing at a future facility.

Equipment/Sets/Inspections

Item requirements for each platform are found in the appropriate INSTRUCTION 6000.1, the Shipboard Medical Procedures Manual, which differs by region and platform (for example from San Diego: COMNAVAIRPACINST for CVN, COMNAVSURFPACINST/COMNAVSURFLANTINST for the other platforms). There are appendices detailing types of instrument sets and their contents for each Fleet platform. These instructions additionally hold a scoring matrix for inspections with a checklist of required critical items, associated Authorized Medical Allowance Lists (AMALs) for each section of medical, fleet instrument sets by platform, as well as their associated set lists. Ships must pass these inspections with a C-2 grade or higher prior to any deployment or underway exercises.

As soon as the maritime OR team is assembled, it is recommended they all do a full "wall to wall" inventory of all the OR and Sterile Processing Department (SPD) spaces right away to determine if everything required and desired is present, functional, not expired, cohesive, and maintained, including all the major equipment as applicable (anesthesia machines, laparoscopy towers, endoscopy machines, autoclaves), minor equipment, surgical AMALs and sets, consumables, etc.

Reprocessing is quite time-consuming due to limited equipment and capabilities, so it is crucial to know the inventory of sets and instruments, particularly in mass casualty incidents (MCIs), as this could be a limiting factor in a number of cases.

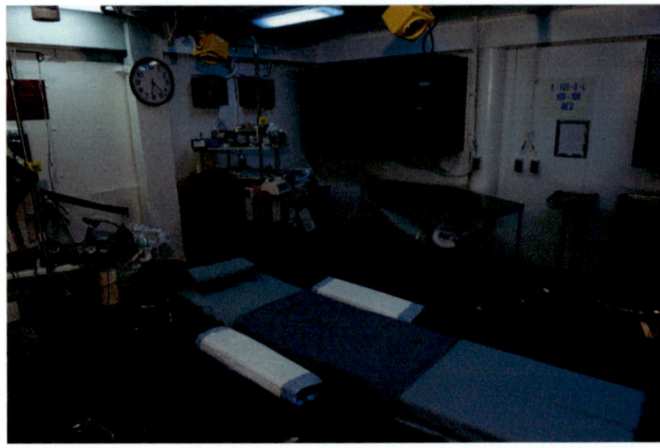

Fig. 12.1 The Operating Room (OR) of Nimitz class aircraft carrier, the USS Carl Vinson (CVN-70), on deployment in the Pacific Ocean, 2012 (Source: Photo courtesy of Mass Communication Specialist James Evans)

CVN

A typical CVN has one OR with two anesthesia machines (one as backup), one laparoscopy tower, one endoscopy machine, and two autoclaves (one as backup). Figure 12.1 shows a sample CVN OR.

CVN ORs typically contain sets for basic emergent cases to include laparoscopic cases (e.g., appendectomy, cholecystectomy) and open sets for emergent laparotomy, thoracotomy, and craniotomy. There are also vascular and head/neck sets. Surgical sets are frequently checked to ensure packaging is kept intact; they are also required to be opened, inspected, and reprocessed for sterilization at a minimum once a year or whenever sterility is compromised.

Inspections of CVNs happen annually at a minimum, however, prior to deployment, there is an initial inspection and a final Medical Readiness Assessment (MRA), which must be passed prior to leaving the dock. This covers all areas of the medical department from staff training/certifications to AMAL and equipment deficiencies, including the OR and SPD areas. The CVN medical staff are responsible for the correction of identified discrepancies.

FST

FST teams do not travel with their own equipment, instrument sets, or medical consumables; rather, they rely on the platform they are supporting to supply what will be needed. Typically, they are assigned to an ARG, typically composed of at least two CRTS, each having at least one ST attached to them (see Chap. 6). However, these STs often experience barriers to being responsible for the supply, maintenance, and inspection of the OR and SPD areas, as this is often considered their secondary duty and they will often be pulled away to perform as a general duty corpsman. Therefore, it is even more imperative for the FST OR team to check on their spaces as soon as possible and partner with the CRTS medical staff to make sure the ORs are ready.

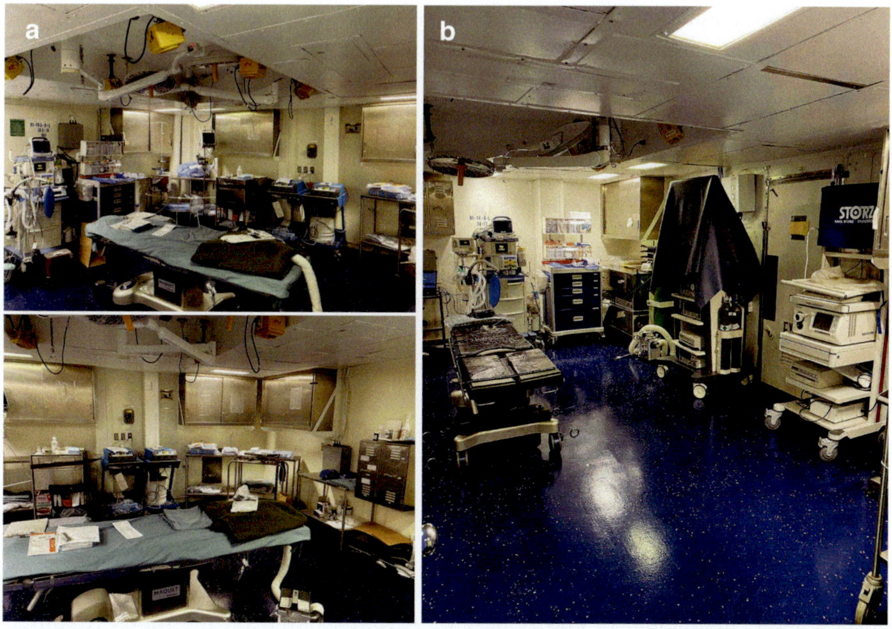

Fig. 12.2 The Operating Room (OR) spaces of Wasp class amphibious assault ship, the USS Essex (LHD-2), on deployment in the Indian Ocean, 2022. (**a**) Main OR (**b**) OR with laparoscopic capabilities (Source: Photos courtesy of Lara H. Spence, MD)

The larger CRTS may have several ORs, each equipped with its own anesthesia machine and possibly laparoscopy tower and/or endoscopy machine, depending on the platform. The smaller CRTS may only have a main OR with an adjacent OR that functions as a Battle Dressing Station (BDS) but is fully equipped and can easily be converted into an OR. Figure 12.2 shows the OR spaces utilized by a typical FST. Usually, two autoclaves are available, but the smaller CRTS may have less.

Sets are determined by platform. Typical set lists are outlined in the CVN portion of this section, however, there are higher quantities of them because it is a CRTS. Unlike CVNs, CRTS typically have sets and consumables available for external fixation cases.

The frequency of inspections is similar to a CVN. The FST personnel that are assigned to the platform are actively engaged in this process and work side by side with CRTS medical staff to prepare and ensure discrepancies are corrected; however, only the CRTS medical staff are responsible to correct the discrepancies. To be noted, this process is true for ALL ships with OR capabilities within the ARG.

ERSS

The ERSS team travels with all the gear they need. As such, there is no anesthesia machine, only portable ventilators (see Chap. 13).

An ERSS team typically carries 3–4 surgical sets created from the AMAL, including one craniotomy set, 1–2 major laparotomy sets, a thoracotomy set, and external fixation kits. Depending on the surgeon's preferences, additional surgical sets can be made from the remaining instruments left in the AMAL (i.e., creating multiple chest tube sets). For the most part, the AMAL contains the essential consumables needed to operate in a Role 2 environment, but it is not unheard of to be short of required gear or gear that is not required could potentially be useful (e.g., Resuscitative Endovascular Balloon Occlusion of the Aorta (REBOA)).

The ERSS team members perform Limited Technical Inspection (LTI) every 6 months lasting 4–5 days. They go through the AMAL making sure everything that is within 6–9 months of expiration is tagged and re-ordered to arrive in time for the next LTI, ensuring all missions are fully equipped.

Supply

BUMEDINST INSTRUCTION 6700.13, Management and Procurement of Authorized Medical and Dental Allowance Lists, establishes responsibilities for development, maintenance, and review of AMALs based on the unit's Required Operational Capabilities and the Projected Operational Environment (ROC/POE). Consumables and supplies should at a minimum cover a 60-day period.

Deletions or additions to AMALs must be done through an ACR (Allowance Change Request) with a valid justification for the change. The ACR is then submitted through Navy Medical Logistics Command (NMLC) to be approved through the Fleet chain of command. NMLC will then initiate administrative change based on commodity management efforts in the Defense Medical Logistics Item Identification System (DMLIIS). The process is often long and tedious and changes are slow to happen, especially since it usually requires consensus of multiple providers on the same platform, all limited in communication, with a system that has multiple steps for review and approval. That being said…PAY IT FORWARD! If the AMAL needs to be changed, work through the system to change it! Don't only change it for the current ship/team but work to make it better for all ships/teams. There are several methods to do this:

- Submit a formal AMAL change request (see above).
- Request to participate in the biennial AMAL review for the maritime platform.
- Utilize the recently created Maritime Surgery Quality Improvement (MSQI) program (part of the Bureau of Medicine and Surgery Clinical Communities) to gain consensus across the fleet and change AMALs Fleetwide.

In addition to the difficulty with updating AMALs to reflect current OR requirements, there are also several difficulties with the supply chain itself including lost orders, late shipments, lost shipments (either because of incorrect paperwork or they literally cannot catch up to the ship), shipments of expired or near expired consumables, and shipments of items out of date for current surgical conditions. It is strongly recommended to maintain a database of all equipment sales representatives available for at-sea underway periods. Orders should be proactively created with some buffer time based on knowledge of expiring items and frequently followed up to minimize delays.

Despite best efforts many times it is necessary to "tactically acquire" equipment, instruments, or consumables from an outside source such as a local MTF or another ship/team with or without formal paperwork. This is not the best practice, but the aforementioned barriers within the supply system can force maritime OR teams into it to ensure smooth operations and a ready OR during deployment. See Appendix A for a summary of items to tactically acquire or MacGyver.

CVN/FST

CVN medical staff are responsible for the inventory of AMAL items, consumables, and other equipment along with the appropriate supply ordering and follow-up to maintain a ready OR. As stated previously for FSTs embarked within an ARG, the CRTS medical staff (in particular the STs) are responsible for this process for all CRTS within the ARG, so the FST personnel should work closely with them in preparation for deployment.

ERSS

The medical portion of the mission will only go on as long as there are supplies. Once all sets have been used, if the mission continues then any remaining resources are used to resuscitate patients. Any resupply of items occurs after the mission is completed and before the next one begins.

Maintenance

Unlike hospitals on land, there are limited BioMedical Technicians (BMTs) on ships, and they commonly do not have the experience, knowledge, or capability to troubleshoot the specialized and complex equipment in the OR. Occasionally, they are not even tracking the OR equipment in the shipboard scheduled maintenance systems (3M, SKED, etc.), so the responsibility for ensuring everything is being maintained on schedule falls on the OR team.

Keep all equipment manuals and Instructions for Use (IFU) accessible for troubleshooting problems easily, processing instrumentation properly, and having potential repair/replacement parts readily available.

Autoclaves must be tested daily and weekly and undergo testing by BMTs biannually to verify functionality. If all manufacturer parameters are met, maintain and save documentation for 2 years.

Many of the large equipment items require annual inspections and maintenance, which are only available in port (e.g., endoscopy machine, anesthesia machine). Because the maintenance is often contracted out, it needs to be scheduled far in advance; this can be challenging with constantly changing operational commitments and schedules of the ship.

CVN/FST

As with equipment and supply, the CVN medical staff are responsible for the annual or biannual maintenance of large equipment items. Again, for FST deploying with an ARG, the CRTS medical staff (in particular the STs) are responsible for all equipment in all ORs in all ships of the ARG, and the FST personnel should work closely with them in preparation for deployment.

ERSS

During the LTI every 6 months, the team will look at all their equipment and send anything defective or requiring maintenance to the BMT department at their home port command, where all their gear is stored.

Decontamination, Sterile Processing, and Storage

Sterility is a concept and one of the greatest challenges of the maritime OR. Follow all sterile surgical processing protocols but know that there are many hurdles to overcome, including limited space, lack of positive/negative pressure control, temperature/humidity extremes, and reprocessed seawater that is not optimal for sterile processing. For all these reasons, prior to deployment or 1 year after initial sterilization, STs should coordinate with local MTF SPD to take all sets for mass sterilization to ensure all sterility protocols have been completely met.

CVN/FST

Once on deployment, STs should separate all cleaning supplies from the rest of the medical department to ensure there is no cross-contamination. Space is limited since the SPD on a ship is small, so organization and flow (dirty to clean) for reprocessing instruments is critical, although not always possible.

Decontamination starts on the back table by flushing lumens, wiping down instruments, and removing as much bioburden as possible before the breakdown of the room. Instruments are then taken to the decontamination area of SPD and placed in a small sink to soak. They are then cleaned first with manual washing. Next enzymatic cleanser is used which comes in capsules and must be mixed in proper ratios with water prior to use. Finally, some ships may have an exceedingly small tabletop ultrasonic machine to agitate bioburden off the instruments; because of its size, it can only handle a handful of instruments at a time.

Once the instruments are cleaned, they are placed in a washer, usually placed either between the dirty and clean side of SPD or on the clean side of the room. Cabinetry may be the only thing separating the dirty and clean sides of the room.

Once items are cleaned and dried, there should be a designated clean space for assembling and blue-wrapping instrument sets with needed supplies in the same area to minimize traffic. Setlists are then used to put them back together; they are found in an Appendix of INSTRUCTION 6000.1, the Shipboard Medical Procedures Manual, which differs by region and platform (for example from San Diego: COMNAVAIRPACINST for CVN, COMNAVSURFPACINST/ COMNAVSURFLANTINST for the other platforms. Instruments should be checked for any remaining bioburden; if found, they should be washed again. In a hospital setting, instruments would be inspected under a magnifying glass. This is not something that is accounted for on the AMAL, leaving room for potential contamination when instruments are used on patients the next time. Once the sets are blue-wrapped, they are placed into the autoclave for sterilization.

Once sterilization is complete, the sets are cooled slowly. Cooling starts by opening the autoclave in stages and then bringing out the instrument sets out in stages to reduce the chance of a wet load. Once the sets are cooled and verification of sterility parameters are documented, the surgical sets should be placed within a plastic wrap–a roll of plastic and a heat sealer used to create custom sizes. Plastic wrapping has a threefold purpose, acting as a dust cover, a barrier to protect the blue wrap from water damage or tears, and an additional sterile barrier.

Plastic-wrapped instruments are then stored in secured OR cupboards for next use. Organization and labeling are critical when storing instruments, sets, and consumables to assist with inventory and easy localization in emergencies. Storage is limited in the OR and SPD areas. While there are dedicated storage areas scattered below the main deck, storing sterile consumables and other supplies there is problematic as these spaces lack temperature and humidity controls that meet manufacturer recommendations. Therefore, it is advisable to store any sterilized items and consumables in the medical spaces as much as possible to maintain sterility and functionality.

Finally, the water used for sterilization is seawater processed by reverse osmosis. It is hard on the sterilizers, causes spotting on the blue wrap, and leads to sediment build-up on pipes and inside the autoclave. Make sure to clean autoclaves at least once a week or more to prevent this accumulation. At sea when the autoclaves go down, it is imperative to contact the BMT immediately to figure out what is going on. **If the OR loses sterile processing capability, then it limits ongoing surgical capability.** It is not unheard of for these instruments to go down for long periods of time. In this situation, Appendix B of the Joint Trauma System Clinical Practice Guideline "Acute Traumatic Wound Management in the Prolonged Field Care Setting (CPG IG: 62) cited in Chap. 1 is a useful reference.

Additionally, most CVN and FST platforms have endoscopy equipment and capabilities (see Chap. 18). Surgical technologists (STs) should ensure they are familiar with high-level disinfection (HLD), especially if they have not been responsible for this process previously during their career. The exact process depends on the brand, model, and type of scopes or other heat-sensitive medical devices on the platform; however, the basic tenets are discussed here. As stated previously, find, download, and store the IFU from the internet prior to going underway due to limited internet access at sea. The IFU provides guidance for decontaminating and reprocessing to ensure no damage is done to the medical equipment as well as the frequency that these processes should be performed if the devices sit for prolonged periods of time. A common source is the manufacturer's website. Additionally, there are different instructions depending on whether the platform has a functioning (i.e., up to date on preventative maintenance, all required attachments and consumables are in supply) automatic endoscope reprocessor or if none is available and manually reprocessing is necessary. If manual reprocessing for HLD is necessary, it is important to establish and maintain a dirty and clean area and keep them separate and labeled correctly to prevent cross-contamination between the two sides. Set timers to ensure the minimum exposure time is being met when flushing or exposing the equipment to the chemical disinfectors. Proper storage of medical equipment requiring HLD is also essential, particularly in the shipboard environment where temperature and humidity control is difficult. Proper personal protective equipment (PPE) is required when conducting HLD. Finally, it is a requirement and an inspectable item to keep a log of the HLD that is conducted, containing all information with dates and signatures.

ERSS

Depending on the location and platform of the ERSS mission, there may not be an SPD available. This limits the patient count to the number of sets brought on the mission. After the mission, pack used instruments in a pelican case separate from the rest of the clean gear. The AMAL contains cleaning wipes and solutions like Glutaraldehyde to clean soiled instruments while they get stowed away until the team arrives at an MTF or another ship to drop off the gear for sterile processing. Chap. 1 cites standard and non-standard methods of sterilization in Appendix B of the Joint Trauma System Clinical Practice Guideline "Acute Traumatic Wound Management in the Prolonged Field Care Setting (CPG IG: 62).

OR Capabilities Outside of Primary OR

INSTRUCTION 6000.1, the Shipboard Medical Procedures Manual, which differs by region and platform (for example from San Diego: COMNAVAIRPACINST for CVN, COMNAVSURFPACINST/COMNAVSURFLANTINST for the other platforms), standardizes patient care, documentation, laboratory test collection, sterility practices, operating room protocols, sterile processing functionality, and much more. These practices correlate with the Association of Perioperative Registered Nurses (AORN), the Joint Commission (TJC), and the Association for the Advancement of Medical Instrumentation (AAMI) guidelines and help to maintain the same standard of care across the waterfront. That being said, the maritime OR has a much higher likelihood of the need to adjust and relocate, particularly for ERSS teams or during a MCI. In this case, the OR team should have a set plan to work with the medical department even when they are not physically there.

CVN

The main BDS is located in the medical department, adjacent to the primary OR, and it has the capability to be converted into a basic OR if anesthesia equipment is moved. There are also multiple BDS strategically placed throughout the ship that can be set up for a basic case to stabilize in an emergency but are not meant to sustain anything major or long-term. The main limitation is the number of surgical staff onboard. In a true emergency, they would all be in the primary OR where they have the most resources, so it is best to move patients needing surgical capabilities there.

FST

While there can be several functioning ORs available, there is typically only one surgical team available to support surgery. As one surgery is completed the surgeon can then head to the next room where another ST can assist in the next surgery, leaving the CNOR and the first ST to complete care of the first patient. However, it is not unheard of to have multiple teams on board at the same time; in Chap. 22 the authors describe three surgical teams all on the same ship with two teams operating in tandem during an MCI.

Although highly unlikely, there is also the capability to set up an OR outside the medical department in one of the many BDS on the ship. Similar to a CVN, the main limitation is the numbers of surgical staff onboard.

ERSS

ERSS missions are unpredictable and can be located just about anywhere, including on ships that do not have any surgical capabilities. In that case, the OR can be set up in the hangar bay (Fig. 12.3), mess deck/galley (Fig. 12.4), or anywhere that benefits the ship. The maritime surgical team communicates with ship leadership on the best plan for a trauma bay and OR in the same area, see Chap. 6 for more about this discussion. Space and light are usually limited, so having a mobile OR light is beneficial.

Prepare to be as light and mobile as possible. In case the location of the OR becomes "unsafe," the team has to quickly pack everything back up and move to the next location. These missions can be high profile and quite physical, as the OR is literally carried in and out on the team members' backs.

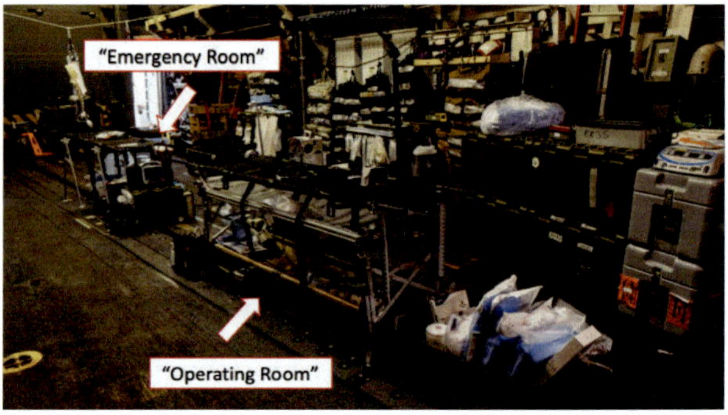

Fig. 12.3 Expeditionary Resuscitative Surgical System (ERSS) resuscitation/postoperative care area adjacent to the Operating Room (OR) area in a Destroyer (DDG) hangar bay, 2020 (Source: Photo courtesy of Matthew D. Tadlock, MD)

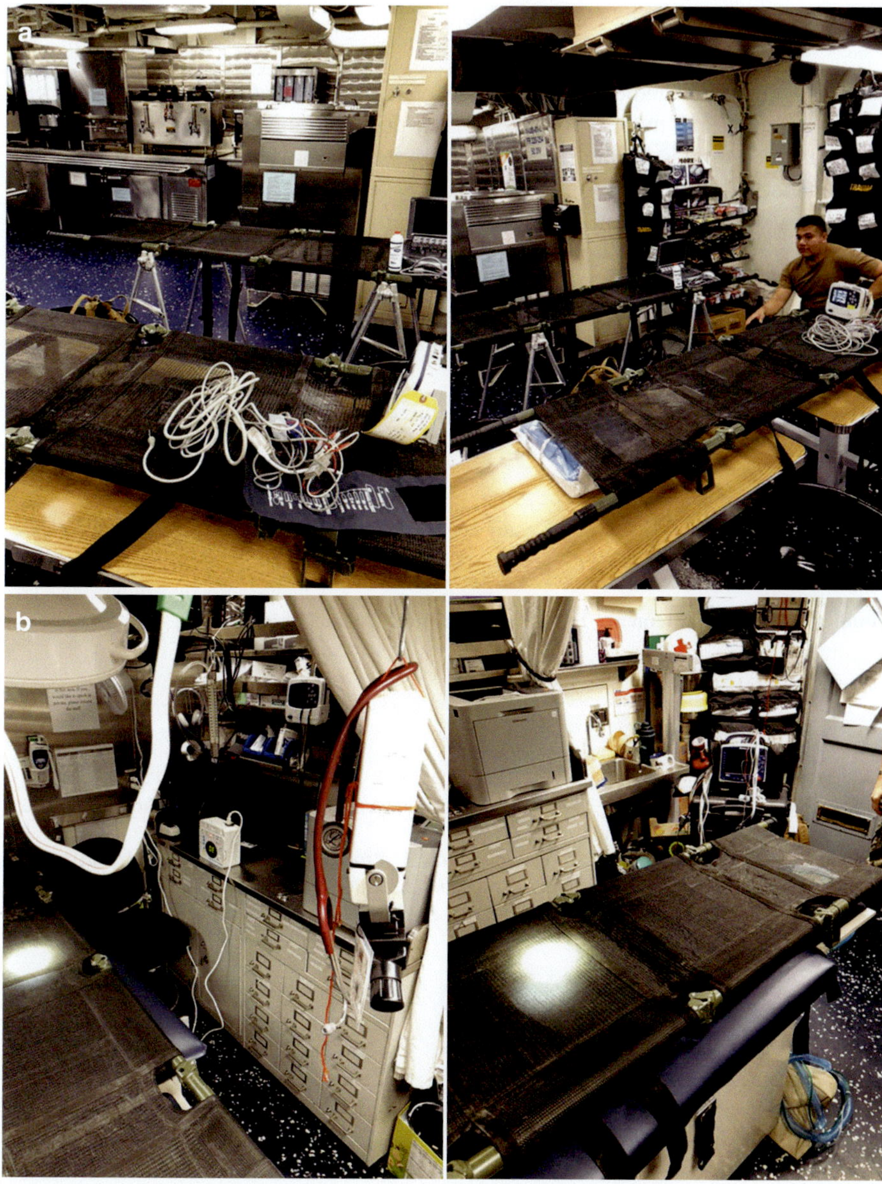

Fig. 12.4 Expeditionary Resuscitative Surgical System (ERSS) set up on a Destroyer (DDG), 2019. (**a**) Resuscitation/postoperative care area in the galley (**b**) Operating Room (OR) located in the adjacent medical space, separated by a door (Source: Photos courtesy of Jay A. Yelon, DO)

Conclusion

For STs, shipboard medical departments commonly consider their OR duties secondary and place far more emphasis on their primary duties as general duty corpsmen despite copious limitations of personnel, equipment sets, supply chains, maintenance requirements, and sterile processing. Close regular communication with the surgeon, OR team, and medical department leadership is essential as the readiness of the OR is a requirement for the ship to be able to deploy. The surgeon should be an advocate if STs encounter any obstacles regarding the upkeep of the OR. **Think two steps ahead, have solutions to problems before they happen, and above all do not procrastinate – always be ready!**

Declaration of Interest The views expressed in this chapter are those of the authors and do not necessarily reflect the official policy or position of the Department of the Navy, Department of Defense, nor the US Government.

Funding This research did not receive any specific grant from funding agencies in the public, commercial, or not-for-profit sectors.

Conflict of Interest Statement The authors declare no conflict of interest.

Further Reading

BUMEDINST INSTRUCTION 6700.13. Management and procurement of authorized medical and dental allowance lists; n.d.

INSTRUCTION 6000.1. The Shipboard Medical Procedures Manual, which differs by region and platform (for example from San Diego: COMNAVAIRPACINST for CVN, COMNAVSURFPACINST/COMNAVSURFLANTINST for the other platforms); n.d.

Chapter 13
Principles of Maritime Expeditionary Anesthesiology

Jeffrey M. Carness, Jonathan D. Hamrick, Shane E. Lawson, and Mark J. Lenart

It is not genius where reveals to me suddenly and secretly what I should do in circumstances unexpected by others; it is thought and preparation.

Napoléon Bonaparte

Author deployment experience	
Jeffrey M. Carness	Staff Anesthesiologist, Expeditionary Resuscitative Surgical System, 2017–2018; Provided embarked Role 2 Surgical Support, INDOPACOM Area of Responsibility, 2017–2018
	Staff Anesthesiologist, Damage Control Surgical Team, Special Operations Joint Task Force, AFRICOM Area of Responsibility, 2018–2019
	Staff Anesthesiologist, USNS Mercy (T-AH 19), Pacific Partnership, 2022
Jonathan D. Hamrick	Critical Care Registered Nurse, Bravo Surgical Company, I Marine Expeditionary Force, Operation Enduring Freedom, Helmand Province, Afghanistan, 2010
	Certified Registered Nurse Anesthetist, Fleet Surgical Team-6, embarked on the USS Bataan (LHD-5), Operation Inherent Resolve, CENTCOM Area of Responsibility, 2017
	Certified Registered Nurse Anesthetist, Fleet Surgical Team-6, embarked on the USS New York (LPD-21), Operation Odyssey Resolve, AFRICOM Area of Responsibility, 2018
	Certified Registered Nurse Anesthetist, Fleet Surgical Team-6, embarked on the USS Arlington (LPD-24), Operation Odyssey Resolve, CENTCOM and AFRICOM Areas of Responsibility, 2019

J. M. Carness
Navy Medicine Readiness and Training Command San Diego, San Diego, CA, USA
e-mail: jeffrey.m.carness.mil@health.mil

J. D. Hamrick · S. E. Lawson
Navy Medicine Readiness and Training Command Portsmouth, Portsmouth, VA, USA
e-mail: jonathan.d.hamrick.mil@health.mil; shane.e.lawson2.mil@health.mil

M. J. Lenart (✉)
U.S. Navy Bureau of Medicine and Surgery, Falls Church, VA, USA
e-mail: mark.j.lenart.mil@health.mil

M. D. Tadlock, A. A. Hernandez (eds.), *Expeditionary Surgery at Sea*,
https://doi.org/10.1007/978-3-031-21893-4_13

Author deployment experience	
	Certified Registered Nurse Anesthetist, Surgical Resuscitation Team, US Special Operations Command, Operation Inherent Resolve, CENTCOM Area of Responsibility, 2020–2021
	Certified Registered Nurse Anesthetist, Surgical Resuscitation Team, US Special Operations Command, CENTCOM Area of Responsibility, 2022–2023
Shane E. Lawson	Critical Care Registered Nurse, I Marine Expeditionary Force, Operation Iraqi Freedom, Iraq, 2003
	Critical Care Registered Nurse, II Marine Expeditionary Force, Operation Iraqi Freedom II, Kuwait, 2004
	Certified Registered Nurse Anesthetist, Army Forward Surgical Team, Operation Enduring Freedom, Qalat, Afghanistan, 2010
	Certified Registered Nurse Anesthetist, Fleet Surgical Team-8, embarked on the USS Bataan (LHD-5), Contingency operations, fifth Fleet Area of Responsibility, 2011–2012
	Certified Registered Nurse Anesthetist, Fleet Surgical Team-8, embarked on the USS Wasp (LHD-1), supporting Humanitarian Assistance and Disaster Relief (HADR) operations following Hurricane Sandy, Eastern Seaboard, USA, 2012
	Certified Registered Nurse Anesthetist, USS Gerald R Ford (CVN-78), Sea Trials, Norfolk, VA, USA, 2015–2017
	Executive Officer, Expeditionary Medical Facility Juliet, 2020–2022; Defense Support of Civilian Authorities (DSCA), COVID-19 response mission, Navajo Nation and Texas, USA, 2020–2021; Operation Allies Welcome, Virginia, USA, 2021; Expeditionary Medical Unit 10G Rotation 11, Iraq, 2021–2022
Mark J. Lenart	Staff Anesthesiologist, Director Acute Pain Service, NATO Role 3
	Multinational Medical Unit, Operation Enduring Freedom/International Security Assistance Force, Kandahar, Afghanistan, 2012–2013
	Joint Force Maritime Component Commander Surgeon & Officer in Charge, Fleet Surgical Team-4, embarked on the USS Kearsarge (LHD-3), supporting Humanitarian Assistance and Disaster Relief (HADR) operations following Hurricane Maria, Puerto Rico, 2017
	Branch Head, Surface Medicine, U.S. Navy Bureau of Medicine and Surgery, Falls Church, VA, USA, 2019–2023

BLUF (Bottom Line Up Front)

1. Thorough pre-deployment administrative and logistic preparation enhances deployment performance.
2. The importance of robust, high-quality medical team training that incorporates all aspects of care (point-of-injury (POI), triage, resuscitation, surgical procedures, and medical evacuation (MEDEVAC)) cannot be overstated.
3. Within small, single-surgeon teams, it is paramount that all members gain familiarity with each piece of medical equipment that may be used in order to optimize team effectiveness.
4. Principles of airway management in expeditionary environments should include preparation for fewer adjuncts, fewer experienced personnel, and an increased likelihood of surgical airway intervention.

5. Maritime expeditionary anesthesia principles largely mirror the basic tenets of trauma anesthesia. However, resource constraints mandate familiarity with total intravenous anesthesia (TIVA), volatile anesthesia, and regional anesthesia.
6. As anesthesia providers play a critical role in resuscitation efforts, they need to be intimately familiar with what blood products are available and how the ship's walking blood bank (WBB) functions.
7. Intravenous (IV) calcium should be administered early when patients are being resuscitated with large volumes of blood products.
8. Everyone on the team should know where the emergency surgical airway kit is and ensure it is stocked at all times.
9. Anesthesia providers must collaborate closely with both the surgeon and the line commander to ensure all anesthesia treatments are supported by the operational security posture of the tactical environment.
10. Anesthesia providers should be familiar with and prepare for prolonged holding of critically ill patients prior to deployment.

Introduction

The first anesthetic was performed in Massachusetts General Hospital's surgical amphitheater on October 16, 1846. Since then, the practice, method, and setting of anesthesia care have expanded across the globe, to include military casualties as well. Early historical accounts report the use of various tinctures and anodynes to treat the suffering of injured military personnel [1]. As early as 1864 in the United States (U.S.) Navy, surgeon John M. Browne performed an upper extremity amputation on an injured quarter gunner utilizing chloroform (Chap. 3). In the Royal Navy, an early recorded formal account of anesthesia administration aboard a naval vessel came in late 1847 when a medical officer used chloroform to extract a tooth onboard the HMS Columbine. Within 5 years, chloroform had become a naval store item onboard all Royal Navy vessels [2]. In September 1942, a corpsman, Pharmacist's Mate First Class (PhM1/c) Wheeler B. Lipes, performed a life-saving appendectomy using ether anesthesia onboard the USS Seadragon (SS-194) while underway and in enemy waters [3]. The discovery of spinal anesthesia in 1898, combined with the discovery of local anesthetics such as tetracaine and procaine, yielded the addition of spinal anesthesia to the World War II anesthetic arsenal of ether, nitrous oxide, and sodium thiopental [4].

In modern maritime settings, anesthesia providers face a myriad challenges in the preparation and delivery of anesthesia for surgical care. Thankfully, the contemporary maritime anesthesia arsenal now includes general anesthesia, both inhalation and intravenous (IV), as well as regional anesthesia, including neuraxial and advanced peripheral nerve block techniques. As a matter of importance, the spectrum of anesthetic tools must be carefully considered when planning for contemporary maritime expeditionary anesthesia. This chapter aims to discuss the challenges facing maritime anesthesia providers and contrast the differences between the different platforms.

Pre-deployment Considerations

An expeditionary unit, by definition, is one prepared to execute a mission abroad. The maturation of modern military doctrine has developed this definition to include one that is mobile, flexible, and capable of conducting operations during a crisis. In a maritime environment, a small expeditionary surgical team provides the commander with a sea-based medical capability, enabling greater participation in crisis response, contingency operations, and theater warfare whether maritime, amphibious, or land-based. Due to expeditionary anesthesia's isolated nature, Anesthesiologists and Certified Registered Nurse Anesthetists (CRNAs) perform their duties autonomously and usually without support, functioning self-sufficiently. Thus, pre-deployment preparation requires an understanding of the mission with the aim to aptly respond within the expected environment while simultaneously achieving superior patient outcomes.

Factors influencing mission success include leadership, administration, logistics, and preparation. The expected mission environment determines the pre-deployment workup. Teamwork and proficiency are essential to the development of esprit-de-corps. Cohesion challenges include ambiguous transportation details, excessive pre-deployment administrative burdens, and logistic shortfalls. Uncertainty associated with these factors and others increases stress and erodes solidarity. See Chap. 5 for some ways to both prepare as a team and individually prior to deployment to minimize the fallout from these challenges.

Leadership and Administration

As discussed in Chap. 6, maritime surgical teams should carefully consider who will be designated as the leader, as a solitary spokesperson for the team will enhance team dynamics and will improve communication flow with operational line leaders.

When possible, delay deployment training until all team members can complete it together. While military medical personnel are typically flexible and adapt, inserting or replacing a new team member at the completion of pre-deployment training can disrupt a team's cohesion, resulting in poor outcomes.

Team members should also maintain their administrative requirements and informally document their performance, beginning during the pre-deployment period and continuing through re-deployment. Anesthesia providers may be required to provide documentation of their clinical and non-clinical activities for use in after-action reports (AARs), fitness reports, and award write-ups.

Logistics and Preparation

As discussed in several other chapters, especially Chaps. 5 and 12, the inventory of equipment, instruments, and consumables is essential in the time leading up to deployment. If anesthesia machines are available, they usually need maintenance and repair, which can exclusively be provided in port by contractors that need to be arranged ahead of time. Anesthesia providers must inventory their equipment as soon as possible after receiving an assignment to a surgical team, whether it is based on an aircraft Carrier, Volplane, Nuclear (CVN), a fleet surgical team (FST), or a damage control surgical team (e.g., Expeditionary Resuscitative Surgical System (ERSS)). The equipment list should be inventoried in light of the unit mission and the expected resource limitations.

The Joint Trauma System (JTS) Clinical Practice Guidelines (CPG) [5] describe a ruck-truck-house model to describe expeditionary anesthesia. Using this model, providers must consider whether they will be using a mobile pack-out model (i.e., ruck on land, ERSS at sea) in which providers will carry all of their equipment and consumables for the duration of the mission, being transported to a fixed facility (i.e., truck on land, FST at sea), or operating out of a fixed facility (i.e., house on land, CVN or FST at sea). This model assists in setting expectations for the supplies and equipment that will be used. Great effort has been made to standardize and update Authorized Medical Allowance Lists (AMALs) on all ship types, promoting resuscitation equipment familiarity if providers must move between platforms. The modern shipboard AMAL may contain point-of-care ultrasound (POCUS), video laryngoscope, oxygen cylinder(s), suction canister(s), vital signs monitors, invasive hemodynamic monitoring, portable mechanical ventilators, defibrillators, anesthetic gases, and many of the types of medications commonly found in most hospitals. Additional resuscitation equipment that providers should consider obtaining includes a rapid infusing/warming machine and airway/resuscitation adjuncts. It is imperative that providers make specific notation of and review the accessories attached to their equipment and ensure they are compatible with the ones that have been supplied (e.g., invasive blood pressure cables, temperature cables, defibrillator pads).

Additionally, providers must also have a plan for narcotic medications, including acquisition, security, dispensing, and return. The anesthesia provider may be a natural choice to be the narcotic custodian for the platform or have to work closely with whoever is playing that role.

Finally, as discussed below, anesthesia providers must also formulate a plan with their team for acquiring, transporting, utilizing, and replenishing blood products. Planning for these issues during the pre-deployment period, especially establishing a donor pool for the walking blood bank (WBB), will reduce stress and will promote team effectiveness.

Deployment Considerations

Maritime expeditionary anesthesia, though nuanced with regard to environment, largely follows the basic tenets of trauma anesthesia. Treatment considerations include mechanism of injury, degree of expected prehospital treatment, triage, the extent of resuscitation, airway management, general versus regional anesthesia, and the likelihood of providing prolonged patient holding and austere critical care.

Mechanism of Injury

The early phases of Operation Iraqi Freedom (OIF) and Operation Enduring Freedom (OEF) witnessed higher rates of combat-related fatality associated with thoracic and extremity injuries. Holcomb et al. reported an 85% non-survivable injury rate among Special Operations Forces with gunshot wounds, but a lower incidence of blast trauma, a potentially survivable injury associated with hemorrhage amenable to a tourniquet [6]. As a result, there was a marked improvement in body armor and a rise in the use of extremity tourniquets. With the development and widespread use of tactical combat casualty care (TCCC) and associated tourniquet implementation, extremity hemorrhage decreased significantly [7]. Additionally, as improved body armor became more ubiquitous, the predominant injury pattern shifted toward blast injuries with shrapnel penetration.

Prehospital Treatment (i.e., Tactical Combat Casualty Care (TCCC))

Prehospital treatment while aboard a maritime platform may occur during amphibious/ground operations, following waterborne rescue (downed aircraft or maritime vessel rescue), or amidst internal shipboard casualties, and it includes all treatments that occur prior to the patient arriving at the designated medical triage location. TCCC training is the Department of Defense (DoD) standard for treating traumatic, life-threatening injuries. Based on data collected during OIF and OEF, TCCC-trained personnel made a significant impact on survival rates for those casualties moving to the next echelon of care [8].

For anesthetic planning, it is important that every anesthesia provider has an understanding of what prehospital care, if any, is likely (Fig. 13.1) and should also be prepared to teach others. Military prehospital care personnel are typically an audience eager to be trained in how to intervene when faced with massive

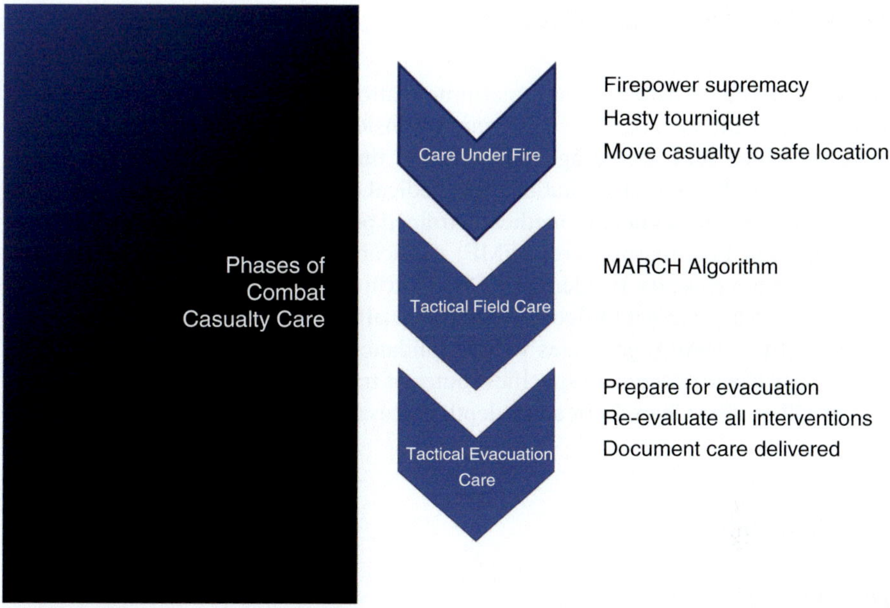

Fig. 13.1 Phases of combat casualty care

Table 13.1 The Joint Trauma Service (JTS) Tactical Combat Casualty Care (TCCC) algorithm of interventions

Algorithm	Assessment	Possible Interventions in Response to Injury
M	Massive hemorrhage	Wound packing, pressure dressing, TXA, tourniquet(s)
A	Airway	Oral/nasal pharyngeal airway, supraglottic airway, cricothyrotomy
R	Respirations	Needle decompression, finger thoracostomy, chest tube placement
C	Circulation	IV/IO placement, blood products, calcium
H	Hypothermia	Active warming measures: "ready heat," hypothermia prevention management kit (HPMK), advanced patient litter system (APLS)

TXA tranexamic acid, *IV* intravenous, *IO* intraosseous

hemorrhage, airway, respiration, and circulation compromise, as well as hypothermia (MARCH algorithm). Teams must know how to apply appropriate interventions to life-threatening injuries, such as placing a tourniquet, performing cricothyrotomy (when appropriate), needle decompressing a pneumothorax, establishing intraosseous access, and minimizing hypothermia. The JTS provides a TCCC algorithm of interventions (Table 13.1).

Triage/Receiving Casualties

When receiving casualties aboard maritime platforms, the medical team must consider whether the incoming casualties are intrinsic or extrinsic to the vessel and the route by which they are being transported to the ship (i.e., air, surface, or well-deck). One of the biggest limitations for medical care in maritime austere environments is usually the number of medically trained personnel. In many cases, maritime platforms and fleet marine force (FMF) medical units are co-located with dental units; for mass casualty incidents (MCIs), maritime medical platforms commonly utilize U.S. Navy Dental Officers as the triage officer. However, each ship's senior medical officer (SMO) generates written guidance that designates an individual as the primary triage officer and specifies routes of transport as well as collection areas for casualties. See Chap. 7 for an in-depth discussion of MCIs and triage.

Resuscitation

Intravenous (IV) Access

Adequate IV access is as essential for patients in the maritime environment as it is during hospital-based anesthesia. Though IV access is critical, intraosseous (IO) access is far more common during wartime damage control surgery (DCS) and is regularly utilized for blood product resuscitation until more definitive access can be obtained [9].

Blood Products

The maritime setting does not permit the robust blood bank services of shore facilities. Surgical teams on ships with a designated surgical capability (CVN, FST, and hospital ships (T-AH)) may be equipped with cold and frozen storage of blood products that meet Armed Services Blood Program (ASBP) requirements. However, even if these resources are available, they are limited by the logistic challenges of space and time. The WBB helps solve this problem by collecting units of fresh whole blood (FWB) from pre-screened type-matched donors for resuscitation. Where balanced component transfusion is not available, FWB represents an alternative and superior replacement in hemorrhage [10]. However, military resuscitation guidance also supports balanced blood product resuscitation using fractionated blood products. In the absence of a functional WBB, smaller operational platforms often choose low-titer O-whole blood (LTOWB) transfusion programs in which donors with low-titer A/B antibody levels (<1:256) are utilized as donors. Recent investigation suggests better patient outcomes with the administration of FWB, particularly in a setting with limited platelet availability [10, 11]. See Chap. 23 for a more in-depth discussion of damage control resuscitation (DCR) capabilities on the different platforms.

Hemostatic Pharmacologic Adjuncts

Additional pharmacologic adjuncts like the anti-fibrinolytic tranexamic acid (TXA) may improve outcomes in trauma resuscitation. The CRASH-2 study demonstrated a reduction in all-cause mortality and risk of death due to bleeding when tranexamic acid was administered to bleeding trauma patients [12]. Current TCCC guidelines also recommend the administration of TXA to all combat-injured personnel deemed likely to receive a blood product transfusion [13]. Importantly, this potential mortality benefit decreases with time from the initial injury and is lost completely after approximately 3 hours.

The Lethal Triad

Adequately mitigating the lethal triad (hypothermia, coagulopathy, and acidosis) can be difficult in the modern hospital setting. In the maritime environment, it can be nearly impossible. The prevention of hypothermia is often an insurmountable task when at sea. Modern ships are equipped with zone-specific, central temperature monitoring systems, but are not designed to selectively heat/cool specific spaces such as intrinsic trauma bays or operating rooms (ORs). In older ships, environmental monitoring includes the use of chilled water systems for cooling and steam systems for heating. Operating these systems requires a technical understanding of the location and function of system components. Thus, increasing the ambient temperature to greater than 30 °C is not likely, even with active warming devices such as forced air warmers or warm water circulating blankets. The entire medical department must focus on the management of hypothermia while in the operating environment (see Chaps. 22, 23, 28).

In trauma with associated hemorrhage, coagulopathy and acidosis quickly become life-threatening. Rapid implementation of transfusion protocols is necessary to counteract these effects. However, while transfusion of FWB collected from the WBB has been shown to be an excellent buffer in acidosis, the anesthesia provider must be cognizant of the deleterious effects of citrate preservative on circulating calcium. Careful monitoring of blood calcium levels in a trauma patient is nearly impossible in the maritime expeditionary environment. **Calcium administration (in either chloride or gluconate form) should be given early, with consideration of administering it even prior to the initiation of large volumes of blood products** [14, 15].

Airway Management

Non-surgical Airway Management

Trauma patient airway management in the expeditionary setting may be additionally impacted by the austere environment. Importantly, there may be limited availability of additional adjuncts to facilitate airway intervention. Initial airway evaluation should include external and intraoral evaluation when possible. Trauma patients may arrive with a cervical spine collar in place, complicating airway management techniques for a solo anesthesia provider. External examination may demonstrate maxillofacial trauma and/or oral bleeding. Airway preparation should include verification of induction agents, direct laryngoscopy, video laryngoscopy (if available), airway adjuncts (e.g., gum elastic bougie, nasopharyngeal airway, oral airway), laryngeal mask airway (LMA), suction, bag valve mask (BVM), instruments for a surgical airway, and supplemental oxygen.

In the trauma setting, a definitive airway with an endotracheal tube is nearly always preferred. Generally, a rapid-sequence induction is indicated. Typical induction agents include ketamine, etomidate, or propofol.

If unable to intubate, consider the placement of an LMA. If unable to mask-ventilate or obtain adequate ventilation with an LMA, an emergent surgical airway is indicated.

Surgical Airway Management

In the setting of significant maxillofacial trauma or during a difficult airway in which oxygenation/ventilation is unsuccessful, a surgical airway is critical. One should consider whether to prepare their own cricothyrotomy kit ahead of time, customizing it to the unique expeditionary setting. These kits usually include a topical antiseptic, scalpel, bougie-type device, forceps, tracheostomy tube (6-0 ID, cuffed), 10 mL syringe, and appropriate means of securing the tracheostomy/modified-endotracheal tube in place to prevent dislodgement. **Everyone on the team should know where the kit is and ensure it is stocked at all times.**

Anesthesia in the Deployed Setting

It is likely that both the environment and extent of the patient's injuries will determine the method of anesthesia. Isolated extremity injuries may be amenable to regional anesthesia through either peripheral nerve blockade or neuraxial anesthesia, but polytrauma patients will likely require general anesthesia.

As discussed in other chapters, the decision to proceed with maritime surgery should not be taken lightly. Discussion about the risks and benefits for the patient as well as the risk to the mission must include the surgeon, anesthesia provider, SMO, and the commanding officer (CO); even a simple, straightforward procedure has the potential for complication, requiring an emergent medical evacuation (MEDEVAC) that could force the ship to move out of the designated area of operation. **Therefore, a risk-benefit analysis must be done prior to commencing any maritime expeditionary surgical procedure to discuss both the surgical procedure and the level of anesthesia that is required.** This analysis would not prohibit minor surgical procedures nor emergency surgery where a safe and reasonable capability exists. However, it requires the procedure to be performed to be consistent with the highest standard of surgical care. The minimum standards that apply under emergency circumstances are insufficient for elective surgery.

General Anesthesia

Standard anesthesia machines are available on CVNs and large deck amphibious assault ships. Small, portable anesthesia machines may be the only option in the expeditionary setting on board smaller vessels such as cruisers and destroyers. Any decision to utilize these devices will largely depend upon logistic considerations, transportation feasibility, and provider familiarity. Small team-based expeditionary anesthesia, such as on an ERSS team, often forgo the use of these portable machines due to an operational requirement for a small footprint and mobility. Therefore, many of these teams have portable ventilators and nothing else.

Invasive monitoring is a luxury feature not often available in expeditionary anesthesia. Safety issues surrounding patient transport while using these devices often prohibit their use. Similarly, an increased technical knowledge about their operation, a requirement for compatible monitor couplings, and a risk of dislodgement often overwhelms the benefits of additional physiological data and/or central venous access. One specific deviation from this principle involves femoral line access that enables resuscitative endovascular balloon occlusion of the aorta (REBOA). In traumatic arrest and hemorrhagic shock, a REBOA may control hemorrhage and augment cardiac afterload. This feature should be discussed by the surgical team prior to deployment so that roles, techniques, and usage are well-understood by all team members. See Chap. 22 to discuss REBOA in the context of DCS.

Regional Anesthesia

Regional and neuraxial anesthesia in the deployed setting is a topic with some associated controversy. Because the supplies for neuraxial and regional anesthesia are often pre-packaged, the logistic and supply burden is heavy, often prohibitively so.

In contrast, depending on the setting, regional anesthesia can be viewed as a resource-conservation measure, reducing the need for additional pain medications and facilitating a more basic and safer patient-transport scenario.

Unfortunately, the value of regional anesthesia is often thoughtlessly disregarded in light of the regional anesthesia guidelines from various anesthesia societies. For example, the practice of placing regional or neuraxial blocks in adults while under general anesthesia is a controversial topic, yet has been endorsed as acceptably safe and as the standard of care for pediatrics [16]. Expeditionary anesthesia providers must consider whether the use of regional or neuraxial anesthesia in the combat setting may be a means of providing the best care for injured personnel in the maritime combat setting.

Prolonged Patient Holding and Austere Critical Care

Current military doctrine has placed DCS assets closer to the point of injury (POI) than ever before. For example, ERSS teams are often far forward-deployed in order to provide DCS close to the POI. Naval vessels performing operations at sea are unlikely to be in close proximity to an established medical facility. As a result, anesthesia providers operating on a shipboard platform may find themselves in a remote location and in increasingly austere conditions. Though past conflicts have enjoyed the benefit of sea and air superiority and MEDEVAC systems, future conflicts almost assuredly will not. When these capabilities/resources are unavailable, anesthesia providers must be prepared to provide austere critical care. Once stabilized, critically ill patients must be continuously monitored. This will inevitably strain the resources of a small team.

In addition to continuous monitoring, additional considerations include antibiotic therapy, venous thromboembolic (VTE) prophylaxis, stress ulcer prophylaxis, and intensive nursing to include wound care, dressing changes, routine skincare, oral hygiene, indwelling Foley catheter and other drain surveillance and care, and intravenous catheter maintenance. Though a thorough discussion of critical care is beyond the scope of this chapter, Chap. 20 discusses principles of critical care in the shipboard environment, Chap. 21 discusses ventilator management and respiratory failure, and Chap. 30 discusses the principles of Prolonged Casualty Care. Anesthesia providers preparing for deployment should consider the provision of prolonged patient holding and austere critical care as part of their assessment of team preparedness. As an example, IV catheter maintenance, which is routinely accomplished by nursing staff in modern hospitals, must be given intentional consideration by the surgical team in an austere expeditionary environment. As such, "rules" for catheter/tubing replacement every 3 days must be weighed against the realities of material limitations, expected time to evacuation, as well as operational considerations. However, the team must check IV catheters daily to monitor for thrombophlebitis and infection.

Platform-Based Considerations for Maritime Expeditionary Anesthesia

CVN

The mission of the modern CVN is to operate offensively in a high-density, multi-threat environment as a fundamental member of a carrier strike group (CSG) or expeditionary strike group (ESG), providing credible, sustained forward presence, conventional deterrence, and air support during sustained operations of war (Navy Operational Medicine Capabilities Handbook - 2020). See Chap. 1. On board a deploying warship, an intensive industrial complex, the elevated risk of traumatic injury and severe illness makes surgical services an essential inherent capability.

Surgery conducted aboard a CVN, while of the highest quality, can be limited when compared to the capabilities and resources of shore-based facilities. There is one OR with one anesthesia machine (and one backup machine), which both should be inspected and undergo annual maintenance while in port. CVNs have modern anesthesia machines with isoflurane and/or sevoflurane vaporizers. The scavenging system is generally ad hoc and vacuumed into the ship's exhaust ventilation system. Oxygen, medical-grade air, and nitrous oxide are supplied in the form of large H-cylinders stored throughout the medical spaces. These cylinders are normally marked as full, partial, or empty, but the nitrous oxide cylinders are not weighed, and thus usage time cannot be determined. Once emptied, the oxygen H-cylinders cannot be refilled, so oxygen should be treated as a valuable commodity. However, a common struggle concerns the performance of oxygen sensors in shipboard anesthesia machines, as they often malfunction or are found to be expired. As a result, clinical anesthesia delivery is often modified so that 100% fraction of inhaled oxygen (FiO2) is used, eliminating the risk of a hypoxic gas mixture for the patient.

The anesthesia provider should perform an assessment of anesthesia-specific inventory and ensure maintenance has been performed and supplies procured. Understandably, general anesthesia administered aboard CVNs is administered only by anesthesia providers, unless there is an emergency situation to save life and limb (as determined by the SMO), in which case the oral maxillofacial surgeon (OMFS) may do it.

There are traditionally no frozen blood capabilities, therefore FWB transfusions from the WBB are the only available blood product source if necessary. See Chap. 23 for more details on the planning and execution of the WBB.

Fleet Surgical Team (FST)

Traditionally, an FST is employed as the afloat Role 2 surgical team for an amphibious ready group (ARG) in support of United States Marine Corps (USMC) combat operations. An FST is a single-surgeon team with a single anesthesia provider that adds the capability of Role 2 care in support of peacetime, forward presence missions, and contingency operations. FSTs provide surgical support, expanded lab and blood bank services, as well as an intensive care and ward care capability. For a more robust surgical capability, the FST complement of 18 personnel may be supplemented with an adaptive force package so that additional surgical and medical specialties can be added on board a casualty receiving and treatment ship (CRTS).

In a normal deployment scenario, an FST will be embarked aboard a landing dock helicopter (LHD) or landing helicopter assault (LHA) class ship. These platforms are configured for four fully equipped ORs with the capacity to potentially surge an additional two rooms in support of large-scale operations. In recent years, an increase in the distributed maritime operations (DMO) of ships has resulted in a disaggregated ARG, with ships operating significant distances apart, in some cases reporting to different geographical combatant commanders. This has often resulted in the deployment of a second FST, scaled-down in personnel, to be embarked upon the landing platform dock (LPD) class ships to add an increased surgical, holding, and laboratory capability. LPDs are configured with two ORs but generally only dedicate one of them for surgery, using the second space as a treatment or triage room. The LHD/LHA and LPD class ships typically have the same anesthesia machines, scavenging systems, and gas cylinders (oxygen and otherwise), along with the same limitations in their capabilities to the CVN platform. The difference is that there may be one for each functioning OR – more machines requiring inspection, maintenance, and supplies.

The anesthesia providers assigned to FSTs usually belong to the team. However, unlike other platforms, FSTs do not have an organic capability but rely on the medical departments that are part of Ship's Company for each ship with OR capability in the ARG to monitor the AMAL for consumables and durable equipment, order necessary supplies, and maintain equipment (see Chaps. 5, 6, and 12 for more recommendations about this relationship). FSTs should regularly review, assist, and advise shipboard medical departments to ensure medical and surgical readiness and to establish a strong collegial relationship with the crews. Gaps in AMAL levels and/or non-functional equipment must be addressed prior to deployment. The anesthesia provider should pay particular attention to all the anesthesia-specific requirements for all the ships on the platform.

LHD/LHA class ships possess a robust refrigeration system with redundancy for cold and frozen storage of blood products. However, the ship has the ability to initiate a WBB for the collection of FWB as well. When all equipment is fully functional, three units of Packed Red Blood Cells (PRBCs) can be thawed and deglycerolized simultaneously, but it takes 45 minutes. During an emergent need for significant transfusion, activation of the WBB should be considered. LPDs have the same limitations in blood product processing as the LHD/LHA class ships, but have a significantly reduced storage and thawing capability. For patients requiring a massive transfusion, a balanced blood product resuscitation is required. As there are no platelets on board, a WBB needs to be activated for effective damage control resuscitation during a massive transfusion situation; refer to Chap. 23 for discussion of DCR for all platforms.

Expeditionary Resuscitative Surgical System (ERSS) or Role 2 Light Maneuver (R2LM)

The purpose of the ERSS or Role 2 Light Maneuver (R2LM) team is to provide emergency resuscitative surgery, capable of functioning in support of forward operations from a small maritime or shore-based platform. These teams trade large size and capability for flexibility and proximity. Small teams necessarily have limited redundancy, so that specialty cross-training is a necessity. In preparation for this, teams must execute mission-specific, team-centric training to optimize the team's capabilities. Equipment must either be prepositioned (i.e., aboard a naval vessel) or will be part of an expeditionary package.

Oxygen sources may not be readily available, as they are often only available as large, cumbersome oxygen cylinders. Portable oxygen concentrators have relatively short battery life and require electricity for continuous use. In these settings, and in order to maintain a small medical footprint, total intravenous anesthesia (TIVA) may be required. Regional anesthesia, with inherent minimal airway management, can provide postoperative pain management during MEDEVAC and may require minimal equipment. As such, it may be an attractive alternative to general anesthesia. Small, lightweight, portable POCUS machines are ubiquitous and may be useful for patient triage, line placement, and regional techniques.

The team is designed with a single surgeon, anesthesia provider, and surgical technologist (ST) performing the surgeries with no resupply (see Chaps. 1 and 12), so it can provide significant surgical intervention for only one or two patients. Caring for additional patients requires resupply and MEDEVAC. Depending on the location, providing austere critical care is a real possibility for ERSS teams.

In the increasingly austere surgical environment where these teams often operate, fractionated blood products are similarly unavailable. Surgical teams will likely only have whatever blood products they can carry. If available on the platform the ERSS is supporting, FWB administration from the WBB may be necessary (Chap. 23).

Conclusion

Though the principles of quality medical care are critical, resource limitations, reduced personnel availability, and constraints imposed by the operational environment can significantly impact care delivery and vary by platform; preparation prior to deployment is paramount. Anesthesia providers must be intimately familiar with the available equipment and resources prior to expeditionary maritime deployment to ensure they can execute the mission safely. Delivering anesthesia in a maritime expeditionary environment can be challenging but can be successful with a teamwork-based approach.

Declaration of Interest The views expressed in this chapter are those of the authors and do not necessarily reflect the official policy or position of the Department of the Navy, Department of Defense, nor the US Government.

Funding This research did not receive any specific grant from funding agencies in the public, commercial, or not-for-profit sectors.

Conflict of Interest Statement The authors declare no conflict of interest.

References

1. Houghton IT. Some observations on early military anaesthesia. Anaesth Intensive Care. 2006;34(Suppl 1):6–15. https://doi.org/10.1177/0310057X0603401S01.
2. Shepherd J. The Crimean doctors: a history of the British medical Services in the Crimean War, vol. 1. Liverpool: Liverpool University Press; 1991.
3. U.S. Naval Institute. World War II submarine appendectomy. Naval history blog. https://www.navalhistory.org/2010/09/02/world-war-ii-submarineappendectomy. Accessed 20 July 2017.
4. Falciola V, Waisel DB. Surgical and anesthetic challenges aboard non-hospital ships in the Pacific during World War II. J Anesth Hist. 2018;4(4):214–21. https://doi.org/10.1016/j.janh.2018.07.007; Epub 2018 Aug 1.
5. Anonymous Anonymous. Joint trauma system clinical practice guideline: austere resuscitative and surgical care - 30 October 2019. J Spec Oper Med. 2020;20(2):25–42.
6. Holcomb JB, McMullin NR, Pearse L, et al. Causes of death in U.S. Special Operation Forces in the Global War on terrorism 2001-2004. Ann Surg. 2007;245(6):986–91.
7. Eastridge BJ, Mabry RL, Seguin P, et al. Death on the battlefield (2001–2011): implications for the future of combat casualty care. J Trauma Acute Care Surg. 2012;73(6):S431–7. https://doi.org/10.1097/TA.0b013e3182755dcc.
8. Butler FK. Two decades of saving lives on the battlefield: tactical combat casualty care turns 20. Mil Med. 2017;182(3):e1563–8. https://doi.org/10.7205/MILMED-D-16-00214.
9. Tyler JA, Perkins Z, De'Ath HD. Intraosseous access in the resuscitation of trauma patients: a literature review. Eur J Trauma Emerg Surg. 2021;47(1):47–55. https://doi.org/10.1007/s00068-020-01327-y; Epub 2020 Feb 20.
10. Nessen SC, Eastridge BJ, Cronk D, Craig RM, Berséus O, Ellison R, Remick K, Seery J, Shah A, Spinella PC. Fresh whole blood use by forward surgical teams in Afghanistan is associated with improved survival compared to component therapy without platelets. Transfusion. 2013;53(Suppl 1):107S–13S. https://doi.org/10.1111/trf.12044.

11. Shea SM, Staudt AM, Thomas KA, Schuerer D, Mielke JE, Folkerts D, Lowder E, Martin C, Bochicchio GV, Spinella PC. The use of low-titer group O whole blood is independently associated with improved survival compared to component therapy in adults with severe traumatic hemorrhage. Transfusion. 2020;60(Suppl 3):S2–9. https://doi.org/10.1111/trf.15696; Epub 2020 Jun 1.
12. CRASH-2 trial collaborators, Shakur H, Roberts I, Bautista R, Caballero J, Coats T, Dewan Y, El-Sayed H, Gogichaishvili T, Gupta S, Herrera J, Hunt B, Iribhogbe P, Izurieta M, Khamis H, Komolafe E, Marrero MA, Mejía-Mantilla J, Miranda J, Morales C, Olaomi O, Olldashi F, Perel P, Peto R, Ramana PV, Ravi RR, Yutthakasemsunt S. Effects of tranexamic acid on death, vascular occlusive events, and blood transfusion in trauma patients with significant haemorrhage (CRASH-2): a randomised, placebo-controlled trial. Lancet. 2010;376(9734):23–32. https://doi.org/10.1016/S0140-6736(10)60835-5; Epub 2010 Jun 14.
13. Drew B, Auten JD, Cap AP, Deaton TG, Donham B, Dorlac WC, DuBose JJ, Fisher AD, Ginn AJ, Hancock J, Holcomb JB, Knight J, Koerner AK, Littlejohn LF, Martin MJ, Morey JK, Morrison J, Schreiber MA, Spinella PC, Walrath B, Butler FK Jr. The use of tranexamic acid in tactical combat casualty care: TCCC proposed change 20-02. J Spec Oper Med. 2020;20(3):36–43.
14. Ditzel RM Jr, Anderson JL, Eisenhart WJ, Rankin CJ, DeFeo DR, Oak S, Siegler J. A review of transfusion- and trauma-induced hypocalcemia: is it time to change the lethal triad to the lethal diamond? J Trauma Acute Care Surg. 2020;88(3):434–9. https://doi.org/10.1097/TA.0000000000002570.
15. Wray JP, Bridwell RE, Schauer SG, Shackelford SA, Bebarta VS, Wright FL, Bynum J, Long B. The diamond of death: hypocalcemia in trauma and resuscitation. Am J Emerg Med. 2021;41:104–9. https://doi.org/10.1016/j.ajem.2020.12.065; Epub 2020 Dec 28.
16. Lönnqvist PA, Ecoffey C, Bosenberg A, Suresh S, Ivani G. The European society of regional anesthesia and pain therapy and the American society of regional anesthesia and pain medicine joint committee practice advisory on controversial topics in pediatric regional anesthesia I and II: what do they tell us? Curr Opin Anaesthesiol. 2017;30(5):613–20.

Chapter 14
Elective and Emergency Surgery: Operate, Observe, or Transfer? (If You Can)

Craig Shepps

Should I stay or should I go now?
If I go, there will be trouble
And if I stay it will be double …

The Clash

Author deployment experience	
Craig Shepps	Battalion Surgeon, 2nd Battalion, 8th Marines, 22nd Marine Expeditionary Unit, embarked on the USS Gunston Hall (LSD-44), Mediterranean Sea Deployment, Liberia, Albania, North African countries, 1996
	Staff Surgeon, Fleet Surgical Team-8, embarked on the USS Wasp (LHD-1), Operation Enduring Freedom, Arabian Gulf, 2002
	Staff Surgeon, Fleet Surgical Team-8, embarked on the USS Bataan (LHD-5) and the USS Kearsarge (LHD-3), Operation Iraqi Freedom, Arabian Gulf, 2003
	Chief of Medical Staff, Expeditionary Medical Facility Kuwait, Operation Iraqi Freedom, Kuwait, 2008–2009
	Chief of Professional Services, Bravo Surgical Company, 1st Marine Logistics Group, Forward Operating Base Edinburgh, Operation Enduring Freedom, Helmand Province, Afghanistan, 2012
	Ship's Surgeon, USS Dwight D. Eisenhower (CVN-69), Operation Freedom's Sentinel, North Arabian Sea, 2020

BLUF (Bottom Line Up Front)

1. The shipboard decision to operate, observe, or transfer is a complex multifactorial decision, only a part of which is clinical decision-making, including but not limited to the location of ship, location and capability of transfer facilities, weather, overall ship's mission execution, mission con-

C. Shepps (✉)
Navy Medicine Readiness and Training Command Portsmouth, Portsmouth, VA, USA
e-mail: craig.d.shepps.mil@health.mil

M. D. Tadlock, A. A. Hernandez (eds.), *Expeditionary Surgery at Sea*, https://doi.org/10.1007/978-3-031-21893-4_14

tributions of the patient, expected and worst-case convalescence needs, and timing during the mission.
2. The decision is not actually that of the surgeon but ultimately that of the ship's Commanding Officer (CO).
3. Open and frequent communication between surgeon, the medical department's Senior Medical Officer (SMO) or Officer in Charge (OIC), and the line chain of command (CoC) are necessary for optimal patient outcomes and simultaneous mission support.
4. The shipboard surgeon must be prepared to diagnose and treat conditions they may have never encountered in training or practice. Garrison subspecialists are always available for expert consultation, though timely communication can be a challenge.
5. Conditions of suspected ongoing hemorrhage, tissue ischemia, or uncontrolled inflection almost always warrant immediate surgical intervention. Severe pain and/or pain preceding other symptoms like nausea and vomiting is always a sign for concern.
6. Non-urgent conditions can be managed on board, delayed, or transferred (via routine medical evacuation (MEDEVAC)) depending on the clinical condition. Elective procedures can also be performed on board or delayed until return to port, depending on multiple variables.
7. In the absence of a definitive diagnosis, observation is a valuable initial management strategy for potential surgical conditions. Never trust a negative study.
8. Laparoscopic equipment is available on most ships with surgical capability and should be used liberally as a diagnostic tool. On a ship, a negative laparoscopy is not a failure, but a victory.
9. Anoscopy should also be used liberally as a diagnostic tool; if no anoscope is on board then it should be brought.
10. If after surgical specimen removal the surgeon has concerns for malignancy (or any other reason the histology is critical) divide the specimen and retain a portion on board in formalin until the diagnosis is complete or until the specimen is confirmed to have reached the laboratory.

Introduction

The Clash posed a question in their 1983 album, appropriately entitled "Combat Rock:" Should I Stay or Should I Go? Throughout the song, they never really answered the question. It is probably not because they were not capable of making a decision. It is more likely that the answer was "It depends."

It seems as if surgeons are regularly faced with such a dilemma, and this dilemma is even more frequent at sea. Not only does the decision to "Stay or Go" (or observe) depend on the patient's presentation, but equally, or often more so, on the situation.

There are innumerable combinations of shipboard capabilities with regard to equipment and resources. There is a wide range of comfort and capabilities among medical personnel and a wide variety of command attitudes regarding the acceptance or avoidance of risk. Perhaps the greatest situational determinant is similar to the greatest "three" variables in the value of real estate: Location, Location, Location. **The location of the ship and the current mission play an enormous role in decision-making regarding the urgency and location of the management of medical and surgical conditions.** The management of these conditions is usually secondary to the mission, much to the surprise and shock of some medical professionals.

Prior to shipboard assignment, a surgeon has had years of training and is generally capable of determining who needs an operation and who does not, as well as the urgency of treatment. However, the answer is not always perfectly clear. At sea, the patient's symptoms and signs are only a small part of the challenge.

The most critical aspect of surgical decision-making on board a ship is COMMUNICATION. Surgeons are accustomed to coming to a conclusion regarding management then INFORMING others regarding what follows. Surgeons are used to telling the facility and adjunct staff when a patient requires admission, operation, and/or transfer. On board a ship, the actual decision comes from the Commanding Officer (CO); therefore, regular, complete, and timely communication between medical department personnel and the operational chain of command (CoC) is essential (see Chaps. 6 and 11). The surgeon must incorporate knowledge of the ship's situation into their RECOMMENDATIONS in order to aid the ship's Senior Medical Officer (SMO) and/or team Officer in Charge (OIC) in making a judgment to operate, observe, or transfer. This recommendation must be presented to the ship's CO for the ultimate decision.

As previously mentioned, location is critical. A ship transiting the Red Sea has few options for transfer via medical evacuation (MEDEVAC) to a more optimal facility, even less when transiting across the Atlantic or the Pacific Ocean, and none around Cape Horn and the Antarctic Peninsula. Often MEDEVAC to a more optimal facility will require a delay, and typically more than one would like, which can be a significant factor in determining whether to operate, observe, or transfer. An additional critical element of communication is ideally to and from the potential receiving provider on land. The actual capabilities of that facility may not be certain nor whether the intended management will actually take place.

There exists no text or rule book to use as a go-by for managing a surgical patient at sea [1]. This text is an attempt to provide guidelines rather than rules.

Clinical Vignette 14.1

One day near midnight while making "gator squares" on a ship in the Arabian Gulf, I received a phone call from the ship's SMO inviting me to see a patient in the morning. The patient was pregnant with right lower quadrant (RLQ) pain. I responded, "Morning is in 3 min, so I'll be right there." The patient was tachycardic, remained so despite resuscitation, and had significant RLQ tenderness. The SMO could not confidently identify an intrauterine pregnancy (IUP).

I was concerned for ectopic pregnancy and the need for emergent surgical intervention. I had never seen this operation before, let alone done it. However, we determined that there was little choice (i.e., none) as we were concerned for rupture and ongoing hemorrhage.

Though we had to get creative in fashioning a suction device, a laparoscopic salpingectomy proved not to be terribly difficult. Fortunately, the patient recovered fully and stayed on board for the remainder of the deployment. Even in the best of circumstances, MEDEVAC of such a patient would be ill-advised.

There are clear reasons to operate in nearly any circumstance while deployed: hemorrhage, uncontrolled sepsis, or tissue necrosis [2]. *Even off the coast of Norfolk or San Diego, the time delay to transfer to expert care may pose a serious life-threatening risk. It was rather anxiety-provoking to be faced with a condition I had not encountered before, but it may be necessary. There were many potential options I may not have considered at the time. What if she responded immediately to resuscitation or did not even require it, and the concern for active ongoing bleeding was not great? Should I have considered MEDEVAC to expert care?*

Clinical Vignette 14.2

A year later I encountered the same condition but under quite different circumstances. Six weeks into deployment transiting the Mediterranean Sea, a senior enlisted leader presented with a non-perforated ectopic pregnancy. It would likely have been reasonable, and even expected, to evacuate the patient to the next available European civilian or military medical treatment facility (MTF) since there was not likely ongoing hemorrhage (or sepsis or necrosis).

However, both she and her CoC had a strong desire that this "1 of 1" senior leader remain onboard since it was so early in deployment. We performed salpingotomy and evacuation of products of conception, which was her preference (and at the time I had presumed equivalent or even preferred to salpingectomy). The SMO personally oversaw shipment of quantitative human chorionic gonadotropin (hCG) laboratory tests to confirm completion. While I am confident this management was reasonable, I would discourage salpingostomy for current readers. See Chap. 17 *for an in-depth discussion of the diagnosis and management of ectopic pregnancy. The logistic issues with the laboratory are potentially significant, the risk of incomplete treatment is real, and the risk of recurrent ectopic pregnancy is higher than with salpingectomy. However, as this was before the immediate availability of the Internet at sea and immediate communications to specialty care were also less than readily accessible, I was not privy to this information prior to operating.*

These vignettes from the author's personal deployment experiences are particularly clear illustrations of the importance of communication. In Clinical Vignette 14.2, a more aggressive attempt at specialty consultation prior to a non-emergent procedure may have led to a different management course. They also highlight how different presentations of the same condition, in different patients, on different missions may lead to different decisions of whether to operate, observe, or transfer.

Logistical decision-making may be the most challenging issue, but surgical decision-making is still critical and strongly influenced by shipboard factors (especially LOCATION, LOCATION, LOCATION). This chapter will focus on the shipboard management considerations for the common surgical conditions encountered at sea by the general surgeon (outside of trauma). The word "general" was purposefully left off before "surgical" because, as demonstrated throughout this book, the general surgeon carries a much broader definition at sea than at a typical civilian or even military MTF.

Operate, Observe, or Transfer: Factors to Consider

Communication and Mission

Thankfully with modern technology, the surgeon does not typically need to make decisions alone. Having direct contacts for various specialists and communication with potential receiving facilities can be a great anxiety relief. The Global Teleconsultation Portal (GLP) has also been developed (formerly Health Experts onLine at Portsmouth (HELP) and Pacific Asynchronous Telehealth (PATH)) to provide deployed providers regular access to specialist advice, though it may not always provide emergent feedback. The Advanced Virtual Support for Operational Forces (ADVISOR) system is a 24/7 consultative service for deployed units, where the shipboard surgical team can seek advice from many different surgical and non-surgical subspecialists (Chap. 5 for more information).

Open communication between the surgeon, SMO, OIC, patient, CoC, and potential receiving facility/specialists is critical for determining whether and how a patient should get an operation and recover on board (see Chap. 6). Additionally, the patient's specific role in the mission and the ability of the command to perform the mission in his or her absence also plays a role in the decision-making.

Finally, even in an ideal location for transfer via MEDEVAC, the weather frequently does not cooperate. Rough seas, poor visibility, and other factors put the transport team at risk and must be considered in any MEDEVAC, potentially causing delays or even precluding transfer as an option altogether.

Quality of Life/Quality of Work

True surgical emergencies, for which the decision to operate may be unequivocal, are much less typically encountered than urgent or more routine conditions. However, delaying treatment for some elective interventions may impact a Sailor's performance of his or her duties and must be weighed against the impact of "elective" (non-emergent) surgery with its required convalescence, including the possibility of complications that may delay recovery further.

Berthing and messing accommodations may also play a factor, especially if they must be modified for a long period of time. A Sailor who bunks on the third rack (above two others) and who has to travel up and down four ladders several times each day to get to the mess decks, berthing, and workspaces may have difficulty simply traversing the ship for weeks after hernia repair, let alone doing their job. Prolonged ward recovery (i.e., a patient living in the medical department without receiving ongoing medical care) may be necessary.

Training

Some consideration should likely also go toward ensuring the surgical team is prepared in the event they must act. This may call for the performance of some non-urgent cases on board, in order to serve as real-life, though not as hectic, training opportunities. Only one-third of all surgical procedures performed aboard ship are urgent, and fewer still actually require a surgeon specifically [3]. Therefore, there are few actual practice opportunities during which to train the entire surgical team.

The team may be unfamiliar with the supplies and equipment available on board. Staplers, retractors, and other instruments may not be the same as what the surgeon or surgical technologists (STs) have become accustomed to using. A particularly frequent issue is difficulty in troubleshooting laparoscopic and endoscopic equipment [4]. Doing at least a few elective cases can alert the surgical team regarding potential shortcomings before they are more dangerous in an emergency.

Pathology

An often-overlooked factor is the challenge of specimen handling and histopathologic diagnosis. See Chap. 12 for a discussion of surgical pathology initial preparation and processing. Any procedure with a pathology specimen carries a risk of delay in diagnosis. Further, potential loss of a specimen in transport (e.g., bags have been known to be dropped from helicopters) should be considered a possibility. For this reason, it is not unreasonable to divide the surgical specimen and retain a portion on board until the final diagnosis is received or until the specimen is confirmed to have reached the laboratory. This suggestion is particularly applicable if there is consideration of malignancy.

Inactivity

There isn't much of a surgical workload on board ship, so there may be a tendency for a surgeon to become complacent and presume low acuity conditions, rather than presuming disaster. However, NEVER FORGET—bad things can happen, and the surgeon must maintain a level of "controlled paranoia" even if others do not. The surgeon, even a recent residency graduate, is often the most clinically experienced physician on board who possesses the greatest capacity to identify a patient who is truly "sick." Additionally, as discussed in Chaps. 6, 7, and 23, planning, training, and drilling for a mass casualty incident (MCI) and activation of the walking blood bank (WBB) usually is in the purview of the surgeon.

Nearby Ships

Surgeons often receive consultations by telephone or email from neighboring ships in the Carrier Strike Group (CSG) or Amphibious Readiness Group (ARG) or mission. The logistics of transfer to evaluate the patient in person to make a diagnosis or provide treatment, knowing there is a risk for ADDITIONAL transfer to shore, adds extra layers of complexity to decision-making. Not only is it potentially difficult to virtually determine the urgency of a patient's medical status in any situation, but now a surgeon must take this potentially incomplete information to make a decision whether to direct transfer ashore or accept a patient knowing that they may require further transfer ashore.

Ancillary Studies (Laboratory and Radiology)

For all maritime platforms, there are limited ancillary studies available compared to shore-based facilities. Furthermore, capabilities vary by platform in both equipment and technician credentials, experience, and skill (see Chap. 8 for laboratory tests and radiographs commonly available on larger platforms where surgical teams will be).

The surgeon is likely to be considered the best "radiologist" on board. Fortunately, modern digital radiography technology allows for radiographs to be read ashore, albeit non-urgently. Having a point of contact at the local MTF (in radiology AND orthopedics) can be enormously helpful.

Importantly, point-of-care ultrasound (POCUS) is available on most ships with surgical capability, and surgeon practice with this modality is expanding. A deploying surgeon is well served to seek training and practice opportunities in POCUS (see Chap. 9 for an overview of common uses for POCUS). The surgeon should also be familiar with the ship's POCUS equipment prior to deployment. Perhaps the most important POCUS skill that SOMEONE aboard should possess is the ability to confidently identify or rule out an IUP.

It is critical to be reminded that false negatives with any laboratory test or radiographic study are possible; the chance of a false negative radiographic study is indirectly proportional to the experience and training of the individual interpreting the test. A negative POCUS and a normal white blood cell (WBC) count may be reassuring, but by no means do they entirely rule out serious disease.

History and physical exam are the hallmarks of diagnosis. Diagnostic laparoscopy should be used liberally as a DIAGNOSTIC study, especially if hemorrhage, tissue necrosis, or sepsis are of concern. On a ship, a negative laparoscopy is hardly a failure, but rather a victory. It can make the diagnosis and resulting plan much clearer, and it has the added bonus of allowing the surgeon to sleep at night.

Timing

Perhaps the most common diagnosis is non-specific abdominal pain. Because this is not necessarily emergent, it may also create the most significant dilemma regarding whether to operate, observe, or transfer. An additional challenge is that the shipboard surgeon is likely to encounter a patient after only a few hours or minutes of pain, unlike in a hospital where the patient has likely spent at least a few hours in an emergency department prior to surgical consultation. Fortunately, in the absence of peritonitis or hemodynamic instability, there are few conditions that require immediate intervention.

A Captive Audience for Observation

One of the greatest advantages of being on a ship is that a patient can be re-evaluated fairly readily since the ship is a small floating city with nowhere to hide. Additionally, the berthing in the medical department is likely better than the patient's current quarters, reducing the incentive to discharge to "home" to allow for ongoing observation within the department itself if necessary. Of course, this can present a different social challenge once the patient realizes HOW MUCH more pleasant it may be.

Regardless, a patient boarding on the ward or convalescing in their own berthing is easily followed up as regularly as desired. In the absence of the advanced laboratory testing and immediate advanced imaging results available in garrison utilized to arrive at a diagnosis, repeated exams, serial vital signs, and basic ancillary studies can provide invaluable data to guide treatment and the urgency thereof.

Prior to and throughout the period of observation, the surgeon must take into account the current available options and those that are to come, especially when considering MEDEVAC. How long will it take? Where will the patient go? Short of peritonitis on exam, other signs of serious disease must be continually evaluated, such as severe constant pain, especially localized pain, fever, tachycardia, and failure to respond to fluid and pain management.

General Surgery Emergencies

While trauma cases, especially orthopedic (and in particular hand) trauma, are common occurrences in any forward-deployed setting, these will be addressed elsewhere in this text (Chaps. 19, 22, 23, and 24). Similarly, obstetric, gynecologic, and urologic conditions are fairly common and addressed separately in Chap. 17, as is the conundrum of biliary disease at sea in Chap. 15, and the multiple conditions diagnosed and managed with endoscopy in Chap. 18. This section addresses other specific surgical conditions and makes recommendations for management for surgical conditions in the maritime deployed setting. Remember though, this is MUCH more of a set of guidelines than rules; there are almost always rational arguments for an alternative plan depending on specific circumstances.

While the term "acute abdomen" suggests a tremendously wide range of conditions, the patient population aboard United States (U.S.) Navy vessels narrows the field quite a bit. Non-specific abdominal pain remains the most likely diagnosis for a patient presenting with acute abdominal pain. Unsurprisingly, appendicitis typically follows in frequency. However, different from the civilian population, nephrolithiasis may take second position in frequency [2].

Nephrolithiasis

It is important for a surgeon to be prepared to manage kidney stones for several reasons. First, the definitive diagnostic study, CT, is not available. The surgeon may be best positioned to interpret plain film X-rays. The surgeon is also likely to be called for ANYONE aboard with abdominal pain or any other severe illness. Therefore, while a general surgeon is rarely consulted at a land-based hospital for kidney stones, this consult is far more likely on board a ship. While most cases are managed without MEDEVAC, the ability to identify a stone, particularly one larger than 7–8 mm, may be a significant factor in determining the course and LOCATION of care that ensues.

Appendicitis

While there are few conditions that should ALWAYS be managed on board, the surgical management of appendicitis should always be considered as the primary option. The situations in which MEDEVAC are most appropriate are as follows:

- When the diagnosis is in doubt (unless observation is chosen)
- When complicated appendicitis (with phlegmon or abscess) is suspected

Of course, MEDEVAC is not appropriate in either of these situations when the patient is ill and requires immediate diagnosis and definitive treatment (i.e., diffuse peritonitis). It is also not necessary in the absence of an emergent indication, as observation may be a reasonable option if the diagnosis is in doubt. On the other hand, transfer in both cases may be best, especially if imaging (i.e., CT) could change the management to avoid an operation AND the recovery is expected to be prolonged regardless of whether there is an operation. These situations also require that appropriate care is immediately available. One should also consider what follow-up care is required, including convalescence, and where all this will take place. For example, transferring a stable, afebrile, healthy young female with a normal WBC and RLQ pain, in hopes that a CT may help avoid an operation, MAY make sense during a 2-week exercise off the coast of the ship's home port. On the other hand, transferring the same patient to the United Arab Emirates while transiting the Suez Canal may lead to a CT or a laparotomy, and will result in a prolonged MEDEVAC process back to the U.S. regardless of management. In the second case, a trial of observation followed by diagnostic laparoscopy if no improvement or worsening clinical picture (or even laparoscopy immediately) can rule out serious disease, thereby saving the command, the mission, and the patient considerable inconvenience.

While most ships with surgical capability have laparoscopic equipment, it may not function properly, and troubleshooting efforts may fail [4]. Laparoscopic equipment that many surgeons have grown accustomed to routinely using may not be available, such as endoGIA™ staplers and/or energy devices like LigaSure™. Many surgeons use one or both to take the appendiceal mesentery and divide the base of the appendix. What to do if the ship's staplers are expired and there is no energy device? The expeditionary maritime environment is like any austere environment so surgeons and surgical teams must be prepared to perform procedures multiple ways. Most shipboard ORs have the ability to utilize hook cautery or a "hot" Maryland dissector. Just like in a pediatric surgery rotation in residency, the appendiceal mesentery can be taken with cautery close to the appendix. Then the base of the appendix and the remaining mesentery with the appendiceal artery can both be secured with an endoloop and the appendix divided and removed. The catch here is that endoloops are ALSO not typically found in a ship's AMAL; consider tactically acquiring them prior to joining the ship.

In the recent decade, open appendectomy may have become an "index" case for a resident [1]. However, U.S. Navy surgeons must be capable and prepared to take out the appendix through a single incision. In the case of uncomplicated appendicitis, a midline laparotomy with its inherent complications (hernia) should not be necessary, and MEDEVAC solely because laparoscopic capability is not available is unacceptable.

Nonoperative management of uncomplicated appendicitis, while becoming an accepted option for this disease, should have limited applicability (in the author's opinion—none) at sea, unless the patient is not able to be evaluated and treated by a surgeon. With few exceptions (perhaps short periods near homeport), uncomplicated appendicitis should be managed with appendectomy and recovery on board to avoid the unpredictability of failure of nonoperative management or recurrence.

Understanding the current MEDEVAC options is particularly important in the case of suspected complicated perforated appendicitis. A presentation after more than 4–5 days, high fever, significant WBC elevation, and/or mass on physical exam should make MEDEVAC the primary option. However, the surgeon must consider whether the patient will have immediate access to appropriate care, with the understanding that the treatment may not be exactly what the surgeon on the ship would have personally planned. If MEDEVAC options are not acceptable, one must always be prepared for an operation. This operation can be definitive (including ileocecectomy or right hemicolectomy) or temporizing (e.g., washout and drainage), considering the potential complications and continued treatment that may be required.

Clinical Vignette 14.3

One morning aboard a large deck amphibious assault ship while deployed with a Fleet Surgical Team (FST), I was asked to see a young officer who was being managed by the ship's medical officer as an inpatient on the ward for the last 5 days. His gastroenteritis was not improving. He had lower abdominal pain, tenderness, fever, and an elevated WBC. We planned a diagnostic laparoscopy, suspecting appendicitis.

Even before an incision was made, we encountered great difficulty intubating him, as he was stocky (endearing Navy term for obese) with a difficult airway. Fortunately, we could bag him safely in between attempts. Even more fortunately, the certified registered nurse anesthetist (CRNA) had the foresight to bring a bronchoscope aboard, even though it was not part of the Authorized Medical Allowance List (AMAL) at the time. At the time, I do not recall even considering any other options besides operating. It was literally the first operation I performed as a staff surgeon, let alone on a ship. Not only that, I BELIEVED he had a condition I could treat. I gave little, if any, consideration to anything else.

A diagnostic laparoscopy revealed perforated appendicitis, without abscess or significant phlegmon. This led to a difficult but successful open appendectomy (including a portion of cecum), which was followed by another week of inpatient care for his prolonged ileus. Fortunately, he recovered on board without further intervention.

What I discovered for the first time during his postoperative care is how a young surgeon can perseverate over a problem, especially when it is the ONLY problem. It also made me realize that we were not well suited to diagnose or manage any complications effectively.

Should this patient have been managed on board in the first place? Again, the answer is not as simple as only considering medical decision-making. What if this was the ship's only dentist or Command Master Chief? What if this was during an exercise off the coast of San Diego? What if I had never done an open appendectomy? What if the laparoscopic equipment was not working properly? What if he developed a postoperative abscess or early small bowel obstruction? These questions are by no means posed to suggest MEDEVAC as the first approach. All of these issues can be addressed after immediate surgical control of uncontrolled infection and can be safely addressed postoperatively. However, I encourage the maritime surgeon not to necessarily ACT on the worst-case scenario but to be actively prepared for it.

In this case, there was little choice but to operate. The Sailor was the Commodore's assistant, a "1 of 1" billet. The ship was transiting the Atlantic Ocean during bad weather. MEDEVAC was not practical or safe.

Hopefully, this vignette points out the importance for the surgeon to remain flexible, consider all options, and consider what is best for the patient, all while understanding this must be weighed against the aforementioned mission and logistical variables. For any particular clinical scenario, WHERE each aspect of treatment takes place can be as important as the treatment itself. Once the operation is over, the challenge can continue, including duty limitations and potential delayed complications, especially since computed tomography (CT), the most common postoperative diagnostic study, is not available.

Decision-making directed at the most likely scenario may not always be the best course. All possible outcomes must be considered, weighing risks (and their likelihoods), and a decision made based on communication between the medical department and line chains of command. However, a surgeon CANNOT shy away from doing what is necessary (stop hemorrhage, prevent tissue necrosis, and control sepsis) or “best” (keeping Sailors on the mission) simply because something bad MIGHT happen.

Diverticulitis

The vast majority of diverticulitis is uncomplicated and treated as an outpatient without surgical consultation. Most surgeons typically only see the worst 10–15% of cases in the shore hospital setting. However, on a ship it is likely the surgeon will see EVERY patient who has this diagnosis and have a telephone or email consultation from providers on nearby ships. Therefore, it can be a challenge to balance caution against paranoia. After all, presuming the worst-case scenario might lead one to suggest urgent MEDEVAC in all cases. This is impractical and unnecessary in the vast majority. Knowing the natural course of diverticulitis and the predominance of uncomplicated disease, outpatient observation with dietary modification and antibiotics is likely to be the best initial approach. A lack of response within 24 h should prompt inpatient observation and initial discussion for consideration of MEDEVAC. Another 24 h of failure will likely lead to MEDEVAC provided there is a suitable destination. Observation for longer periods, as the surgeon may be accustomed to doing in the hospital setting, is not advised, as the failure of medical management becomes more likely.

A particular dilemma is the case of suspected complicated diverticulitis. Most such cases are contained perforations, and present with only localized peritonitis. A patient with severe pain, unresponsive tachycardia, high fever, significant leukocytosis, or mass on physical exam should prompt immediate arrangement for MEDEVAC WITH immediate consideration to whether an operation is necessary for some form of sepsis control prior to transfer. Short-term complications probably render convalescence on board futile and risky. If an operation is required prior to MEDEVAC, a colectomy with an anastomosis may be too aggressive. SOME operation, however, may be necessary simply to diagnose the extent of the problem. If you do perform an anastomosis after sigmoid diverticulitis, consider performing a protective diverting ileostomy. In the absence of free perforation, laparoscopic washout and drain placement is a rational initial approach in the maritime environment. Free perforation will likely require resection or at least exclusion, as a "damage control" measure. While it may seem blasphemous, MEDEVAC without ANY incisions MAY be a consideration depending on patient stability, and time, distance, and type of definitive therapy available after transfer off the ship. Extreme caution must be taken, as transport time can vary frequently and expedience is necessary. A final consideration must be whether the patient may need to remain intubated, which adds an extraordinary level of complexity for transport.

Small Bowel Obstruction (SBO)

While small bowel obstruction (SBO) is a tremendously common admitting diagnosis in a shore-based hospital, it is quite unusual in the deployed population. However, one should always be prepared for the potential diagnosis. In this population, incarcerated hernia and prior surgery are uncommon but are clearly a critical part of the history and physical exam. After that history, an important part of the physical exam is a digital rectal exam to rule out impaction, a much more common condition in the deployed setting. While this may seem unlikely in young patients, it is much more common in the deployed setting. Sailors and Marines err on the side of dehydration, have low fiber diets, and "hydrate" with energy drinks.

Plain films are a tremendously useful adjunct to confirm air in the colon and raise or lower one's suspicion of SBO and its severity. Perhaps the most common confounding diagnosis is gastroenteritis. A reliable indicator is the onset of pain relative to nausea and vomiting. **If pain precedes nausea and vomiting, it is much more concerning.** Once a diagnosis of SBO is confidently made, provided there are no signs of ischemia, the decision must be made for the location of observation with all the factors previously discussed. Even with failure of nonoperative management, an operation can potentially lead to quick recovery and return to work, though the possibility of prolonged recovery must be considered. In patients with prior abdominal surgery and an SBO, most surgeons initiate resuscitation, nasogastric tube (NGT) decompression, and a "Gastrografin challenge." However, Gastrografin or any contrast is not in shipboard AMALs. Consider "tactically acquiring" contrast prior to deployment.

The use of Gastrografin is associated with lower rates of surgical exploration and shorter hospital stays. An example of a "Gastrografin challenge" would be mixing 100 mL of Gastrografin with 50 mL of water, pushing the solution down the NGT, then clamping the NGT for 6–8 h. Only attempt this after at least 2 initial hours of NGT decompression or patient clinical improvement. If the patient has a bowel movement or has contrast in the colon on plain X-ray within 24 h of Gastrografin administration, it is safe to advance their diet [5]. Gastrografin can cause pulmonary edema or a very severe aspiration pneumonitis that can result in death and should only be administered via an NGT after it has been confirmed to be in the stomach (not orally).

A patient with SBO in a virgin abdomen is probably best suited by MEDEVAC (though laparoscopy may be necessary to confirm the absence of ischemia prior to this). This may seem counterintuitive, as nearly all of these patients will require a definitive operation. However, most of these patients will have a prolonged ileus postoperatively. Also, in the case of neoplasm as a cause, there is a concern for the transfer of the pathology specimen and a high likelihood there will be further diagnostic studies and treatment required.

Peptic Ulcer Disease (PUD)

While peptic ulcer disease (PUD) is quite uncommon in today's society, it is not rare and can present a particular challenge underway. It is amazing how many young Sailors and Marines think 1600 mg of Motrin must surely work better than 800 mg. This chapter discusses the complications of the disease: perforation and bleeding.

As in garrison, a suspected acute duodenal perforation should be managed with urgent laparotomy or laparoscopy and is easily diagnosed intraoperatively if firm edematous omentum is mounded atop the duodenum in the appropriate clinical scenario. If in doubt, this can be taken down, though it is essentially nature's Graham patch. Even without identifying gross spillage, wide drainage of the area should be added in a ship because of the chance for complications and transfer delays. In the case of delayed perforation, exploration is still advised to rule out free perforation prior to MEDEVAC. Transferring the patient without doing so, or observing such a patient on board, is an invitation to catastrophe. Endoscopic leak test is discouraged, not only because it could worsen the problem, but it is technically difficult or impossible for the surgeon to perform both the endoscopy and surgical portions of the procedure simultaneously. The goal is prevention and control of contamination, followed by MEDEVAC.

Upper Gastrointestinal Bleeding (UGIB)

Upper gastrointestinal bleeding (UGIB) is uncommon in this patient population but is possible and can be a catastrophe leading to unnecessary morbidity and even mortality. If there is concern for UGIB, it must be confirmed or ruled out with prompt esophagogastroduodenoscopy (EGD). While surgeons are not typically responsible for the diagnosis or management of UGIB in garrison, they are the ones who manage this on a ship. EGD is not particularly difficult, and there are educational videos available as well as instructions and photos in Chap. 18. Even if intervention is not possible (for a variety of reasons), direct visualization at a minimum provides tremendously useful information regarding the rate of ongoing bleeding (or hopefully the absence of it), allowing better decision-making for timing of blood transfusion and/or MEDEVAC. Additionally, the importance of the WBB and the ability to safely and rapidly transfuse blood is addressed in Chap. 23 and cannot be overstated.

While surgeons rarely manage the bleeding complications of PUD in garrison, they are the ones who must manage this on board a ship. If an UGIB is expected, it must be confirmed or ruled out similar to garrison care. However, the surgeon's ability to treat an UGIB with EGD is limited by a likely lack of experience in these techniques as well as a lack of equipment to perform them. In the last few decades, most surgical residents have likely never performed or even witnessed these procedures. Despite that, it may be necessary, allowing better decision-making for timing of blood transfusion and/or MEDEVAC. Early transfusion should be considered, as persistence or recurrence of bleeding is common (especially without the ability to effectively treat), and MEDEVAC may be delayed. As for equipment, clips and even injecting needles are not part of the AMAL and may need to be "tactically acquired" (see Chap. 12). Additionally, any endoscopy equipment must be tested regularly to ensure it will function in an emergency. A common oversight and troubleshooting problem is the ability to use irrigation. See Chap. 18 for extensive insights about endoscopy underway.

Lower Gastrointestinal Bleeding (LGIB)

Lower gastrointestinal bleeding (LGIB) is even less common in this population, but the poor dietary habits of Sailors and Marines make anal bleeding MORE common. Perhaps the most useful instrument in the shipboard surgeon's armamentarium is an anoscope. Prior to getting underway, the surgeon should find the anoscope(s) (or "tactically acquire" some) on the ship. Lighted disposable anoscopes have only recently been recommended as an addition to some AMALs, and are the author's preference. Confirming if the source of a LGIB is located distally in the anus versus proximally is reassuring because it can be managed with direct pressure and precludes need for MEDEVAC. More proximal LGIB should always prompt a discussion for MEDEVAC at some point. The only remaining tool to evaluate for a source of LGIB is the colonoscope. See Chap. 18 for extensive insights about endoscopy underway.

The ship's equipment is probably not of the highest quality, diagnostic yield even in the hospital setting is low, therapeutic options are limited, and rebleeding is not infrequent. See Chap. 18 for more discussion. Again, the importance of the WBB and consideration of transfusion prior to MEDEVAC cannot be overstated.

Inflammatory Bowel Disease (IBD)

Among the list of diagnoses commonly discovered while deployed [2] is inflammatory bowel disease (IBD). This is typically a presumed diagnosis, and the management is as with other causes of the acute abdomen, potentially including colonoscopy and/or diagnostic laparoscopy for diagnosis and to rule out other etiologies. See Chap. 18 for a more in-depth discussion.

Foreign Bodies

Foreign bodies in orifices seem to occur more frequently in the deployed setting. In particular, esophageal food bolus is not uncommon. Sailors and Marines are in a hurry to eat, and poorly chew their food (often overcooked meat … no offense intended to the hard-working Navy culinary specialists). Meat-based food boluses will commonly pass spontaneously. However, observation in an inpatient setting is warranted, with the head of bed elevation and aspiration precautions. Any inability to tolerate secretions should prompt an EGD under general anesthesia for airway control. MEDEVAC without clearing the obstruction is ill-advised, as the transfer is rarely urgent and the aspiration risk cannot be mitigated as patient transfers typically occur with the patient flat. Many of these boluses can be easily pushed forward into the stomach (see Chap. 18).

It is also the author's observation, for whatever reason, that rectal foreign body impaction is not uncommon. A rectal foreign body can almost always be managed on board, using the same algorithm as in garrison.

Non-general Surgery Emergencies

There are a few other uncommon conditions that bear mentioning, not otherwise addressed in this text.

Vascular

While vascular trauma is addressed elsewhere, there are a few other conditions to be on the lookout for:

- Venous thromboembolism (VTE): While not common in the young, fit, healthy population, it has been known to occur. Unilateral leg edema, especially with pulmonary complaints, necessitates urgent MEDEVAC. There is no reliable way to confirm the diagnosis (although POCUS can be used to look for proximal lower extremity VTE as demonstrated in Chap. 9), the ability to treat is limited, and the worst-case scenario can be devastating. In the patient with a left lower extremity deep venous thrombosis consider the diagnosis of May–Thurner syndrome, where the left iliac vein is compressed by the right iliac artery. In the deployed environment, risk factors include dehydration and prolonged sitting. In addition to anticoagulation, vascular surgery consultation is required and MEDEVAC of the ship for further evaluation may be necessary.
- Acute limb ischemia: While exceedingly rare from thromboembolic disease in this population, limb ischemia threatening compartment syndrome from a differ-

ent cause is an entirely possible scenario in the deployed setting. Deployed Sailors and Marines are more dehydrated, consume products high in protein, and exercise with more vigor. As a result, acute rhabdomyolysis is a relatively frequent occurrence. One must be aware of the potential for the development of compartment syndrome in the affected limb (or even paraspinous muscle by one report). Incomplete fasciotomy (or none at all), either by inadequate incision length or missing a compartment is not uncommon and can have devastating consequences. Furthermore, while general surgeons are expected to know how to perform lower extremity fasciotomy, one must be prepared to do so in the upper extremity (or even the back).

Pneumothorax

Unlike the management of spontaneous pneumothorax in garrison, there is likely little role for simple observation of a pneumothorax aboard ship, with the possible exception of inpatient observation with an anticipated return to homeport within a few days. Even if MEDEVAC is planned, it is likely best done only after placing a tube of some kind and keeping it in place, to avoid tension pneumothorax while in transfer. It is prudent to inspect equipment prior to departure to know what options are available.

Ophthalmologic Emergencies

Other than traumatic globe injury, the main urgent concern for the eye is periorbital cellulitis. Additionally, pain with vision disturbances are hallmarks of dangerous conditions. While surgical intervention onboard is not likely, the guidelines of ophthalmologic emergency management aboard ship are simple: immediate patch of the affected eye, antibiotics, and arrangement for MEDEVAC in conjunction with DIRECT subspecialist communication.

Otolaryngology (ENT)

While many non-urgent conditions can occur, one urgent or emergent condition worth mentioning is peritonsillar abscess. Antibiotics with arrangement for MEDEVAC are warranted, but incision and drainage may be necessary to not only control sepsis prior to any delay in MEDEVAC but also avoid airway compromise en route. On some platforms, particularly aircraft carriers (CVNs), an oral maxillofacial surgeon (OMFS) is on board and can typically best manage this. If not, direct telephone expert consultation is warranted.

Testicular Mass

Different from a breast mass, any patient with a testicular mass (as opposed to a scrotal mass) should be rapidly evacuated for the presumed diagnosis of testicular cancer.

Elective/Non-urgent

There is wide variation of opinion regarding the performance of less urgent or even non-urgent elective procedures while deployed with rational arguments for and against them. The Joint Trauma System (JTS) Clinical Practice Guidelines (CPGs) [2] are most applicable to Role 2 land-based facilities, or other shipboard contingency operations intended to be limited to trauma management. On such platforms (e.g., Role 2 Light Maneuver (R2LM), Expeditionary Resuscitative Surgical System (ERSS), Forward Resuscitative Surgical System (FRSS)), the performance of elective cases is strongly discouraged. Surgeons in these units may be moved in a physical location, be required to do so with short notice, and equipment and supplies may be even more limited. If elective procedures are performed, they are likely most appropriate with an FST on a large deck amphibious assault ship or with the ship's surgeon on a CVN. The following opinions are heavily weighted by the author's own experience and bias, having performed many elective procedures on board. Some should be advocated for. Some should be avoided.

First, the surgeon must carefully consider the mission requirements of the patient, understanding that the expected outcome may only require a brief convalescent period but a prolonged convalescence in the setting of complications is also possible. The availability of equipment and supplies must also be considered, ensuring enough availability for true emergencies. No ship is generally supplied to support a great number of non-urgent procedures. Antibiotics, narcotics, and anesthesia medications are in short supply. Oxygen supplies must be monitored to ensure availability for an emergency. For these reasons, some propose that any elective surgery is inappropriate. However, others argue that any surgical team best prepares to function as a team when it is necessary by performing actual surgical procedures together. Finally, many elective procedures are performed for quality of life (and quality of work), which is also important on a deployment where every person's role matters.

The best answer is a balanced approach to consider performing elective procedures that will enhance the patient's quality of life and performance of their duties after an acceptable recovery period [6]. This probably becomes decreasingly advantageous toward the end of a deployment. However, some patients' duties (e.g., a Marine on an amphibious ship after the ground mission is complete) may have little mission impact after undergoing a procedure. A patient with symptoms, even one who may require weeks of recovery, who presents early in the deployment may best be served by early operation to recover on board. These decisions should be individualized after review with both the medical department and line leadership chains of command prior to proceeding [7]. Similar to paperwork used on shore, chits routed through the CoC preoperatively to discuss planned postoperative duty limitations and their potential extensions for complications is not an unreasonable way to ensure everyone has the same expectations of recovery prior to surgery (see Chap. 6).

Hernias

Elective hernia surgery should be considered if it is expected to improve the quality of life and work, despite a convalescent period. Repair of an asymptomatic hernia is strongly discouraged. While laparoscopic hernia aboard ship has been described (and happens to be many surgeons' personal preference in the hospital), its role on ships is limited [8]. Some particular equipment may not be available, and carbon dioxide and oxygen supplies that are not readily available for resupply can be used up quickly [4].

Biliary Disease

As mentioned elsewhere in this text (Chap. 15), elective cholecystectomy is highly discouraged. It consumes supplies as mentioned above, and it invites unnecessary potential complications. Biliary disease requiring emergent surgery is an uncommon occurrence.

Benign Anorectal Disease

Acute anal pain is another common occurrence while deployed. The critical distinction is to differentiate abscess from fissure or other non-urgent conditions. Obviously, there are few situations in which a delay in initial abscess management is appropriate. Abscesses require drainage (in both this region and in the rest of the body). However, postoperative wound care can be more challenging in a shipboard environment. Consider placement of a Malecot catheter or a vessel loop tied onto itself through an incision and a counter-incision to minimize frequency of painful dressing changes (also described in Chap. 34).

On the other hand, while anal pain without abscess is rarely urgent, it is also quite likely that management aboard ship is suboptimal, particularly if it is severe. Bowel habits are difficult to manage, medication options are limited, recovery can be prolonged, risks of long-term pain and thus likelihood of long-term inability to be full duty and perform are high. Non-urgent MEDEVAC for workup and treatment may be in the patient's and command's best interests. In these situations, communication is critical; recommendation for MEDEVAC for anal pain is not typically met with immediate understanding. While the medical management of anal fissure is beyond the scope of this chapter, the topical medications commonly used are not on shipboard pharmacy AMALs. Topical diltiazem and particularly topical nitroglycerin may not be appropriate for the shipboard environment. Consider discussing anal pain patients with a colorectal surgeon prior to MEDEVAC.

Pilonidal Disease

While elective definitive surgical management with wide local excision of pilonidal disease can be considered, the postoperative recovery is typically the limiting factor. On one hand, most patients can work with an open wound, and as stated previously there is a captive audience for frequent wound evaluation. However, the cleanliness on a ship in general and in many workspaces in particular (e.g., reactor Sailors working hours on end 6 days a week in a hot damp environment) coupled with the lack of wound care supplies commonly leads to suboptimal postoperative wound care. For this reason, the various definitive rotational flap procedures should not be performed in the shipboard environment. Preoperative frequency and severity of symptoms should guide treatment and be weighed against the mission impact, including the need for daily wound care. For symptomatic disease without a frank abscess, the minimally invasive "Gips" procedure may be an appropriate shipboard option. While the trephines used to perform this procedure are not available on ship, using a combination of an appropriately sized skin biopsy hole punch and curettes, pilonidal pits with underlying fistulous tracts and hair debris are extirpated. This allows treatment of symptoms and return to work and the deployed mission in most instances. Obviously, pilonidal abscess is treated urgently and subsequent postoperative wound care is dealt with on board. See benign anorectal disease above for discussion of abscess management.

Breast Disease

While abscess and mastitis are easily managed on board, a common presentation is a palpable breast mass. The vast majority of these could probably be observed. However, the clinical scenario may warrant a more urgent diagnosis (e.g., high-risk patient, rapid growth). While a biopsy may be technically simple and low risk, the potential delay of histopathologic diagnosis or even loss of the specimen must be considered. As discussed previously, dividing any specimen when the surgeon has concerns for malignancy (or any other reason the histology is critical) and retaining a portion on board in formalin until the diagnosis is complete should be considered. Additionally, it may be a consideration to routinely MEDEVAC a high-risk patient with a particularly concerning presentation for more urgent evaluation, expecting further diagnostic studies and treatment to follow anyway.

When considering elective breast surgery, while the author has performed gynecomastectomy while deployed in several different settings, it is generally discouraged as it is a completely elective procedure with a not infrequent rate of hematoma and seroma complications. Routine recovery typically requires duty limitations that preclude many Sailors and Marines from doing their jobs and any complications would only prolong those limitations.

Urologic Elective Procedures

Historically, a few elective urologic procedures have been performed frequently on board a ship, including by the author.

- Circumcision: Strongly discouraged except in the emergency management of paraphimosis, which cannot be otherwise reduced with penile manipulation alone. Recovery after circumcision is awkward (to put it mildly), and the required convalescent period is significant.
- Vasectomy: It can be reasonably performed on board, provided a surgeon has obtained the appropriate training ahead of time and other preoperative planning occurs. However, there must be a clear understanding not only of the expected recovery but also of the possibility of prolonged limitations in the event of scrotal hematoma or other complications. It is not a requirement for a man to have his spouse/partner be a part of his decision-making. Additionally, it is the surgeon's discretion whom to operate on—sometimes there can be an onslaught of men trying to have this procedure performed at sea or men that the surgeon does not feel comfortable performing the procedure on. This is completely elective and not performing it at sea does not preclude anyone from pursuing it on shore. Finally, the follow-up for this procedure to ensure the appropriate outcome has been attained is a bit more complex than most general surgery procedures and far more complex than if it is done at a shore facility. First, the segments of vas deferens should be sent to pathology as specimens to confirm the vas was removed. Next, two post-vasectomy semen analyses should be performed more than 30 days after the procedure to confirm azoospermia. At a shore MTF, the physician performing the procedure would typically order and follow up on these studies. Deployment pathology results often result long after the procedure was performed, and sometimes after the deployment has finished. Semen analysis is not available at all on board a ship and must be performed in port. Many Sailors and Marines return to completely different commands after deployment (e.g., embarked aviation units from across the country) with no available follow-up with the surgeon who performed the procedure. Therefore, patients should be educated and counseled appropriately preoperatively to get these tests and results confirmed with their primary care provider prior to having unprotected sex. If

vasectomy is performed on the ship, it may be best done toward the end of the deployment so the pathology specimens can be sent to the home-port MTF pathology department and appropriate follow-up can be arranged upon return.

Conclusion

Shipboard surgery presents a unique challenge, of which clinical decision-making is only a part. True surgical emergencies are unusual. However, any condition in which there is suspected ongoing hemorrhage, tissue necrosis, or uncontrolled infection requires immediate intervention. The decision to operate, observe, or transfer is complicated, multi-factorial, and heavily influenced by the ship's location and mission. Decision-making is even more nuanced in the setting of urgent or elective conditions. The maritime general surgeon should consider the worst-case scenario, be flexible, adapt to changing circumstances, and communicate early and often with the ship's medical and operational command to optimize clinical outcomes and support the ship's mission.

Declaration of Interest The views expressed in this chapter are those of the authors and do not necessarily reflect the official policy or position of the Department of the Navy, Department of Defense, nor the US Government.

Funding This research did not receive any specific grant from funding agencies in the public, commercial, or not-for-profit sectors.

Conflict of Interest Statement The authors declare no conflict of interest.

References

1. Nealeigh MD, et al. Surgery at sea: exploring the training gap for isolated military surgeons. J Surg Educ. 2019;76(4):1139–45.
2. Joint Trauma System. Emergency general surgery in deployed locations. Clinical Practice Guideline (CPG ID-71). 2018.
3. Lin H, et al. Surgery in expeditionary strike group. Mil Med. 2009;174:241–4.
4. Thoman DS. Laparoscopy at sea: overcoming unique challenges. Bull Am Coll Surg. 2004;89(8):12–7.
5. Zielinski MD, the EAST SBO Workgroup, et al. Multi-institutional, prospective, observational study comparing the Gastrografin challenge versus standard treatment in adhesive small bowel obstruction. J Trauma Acute Care Surg. 2017;83(1):47–54.
6. Fontana M, et al. Surgery aboard ship: is it safe? Mil Med. 1999;164:613–5.
7. Fisher RA, et al. Peacetime surgery in the aircraft carrier battle group. Mil Med. 1990;155:332–4.
8. Cubano MA, et al. First laparoscopic hernia repair onboard an aircraft carrier at sea. Mil Med. 1997;162:219–20.

Chapter 15
The Tyranny of Distance and the Difficult Gallbladder

Joseph A. Diaz, Laurier Tremblay, and Matthew D. Tadlock

In the history of warfare, a succession of bold ideas and weapons had promised to curb the tyranny of distance … The tyranny of distance still prevailed.

Geoffrey Blainey

Beware of the easy-looking gallbladder and the overconfident surgeon.

From Moshe Schein's A Companion to Aphorisms and Quotations for the Surgeon

Author deployment experience	
Joseph A. Diaz	Team Medic, Special Boat Team TWENTY-TWO, Joint Combined Exercise in Training, Thailand, 2004
	Team Medic, Special Boat Team TWENTY-TWO, Joint Combined Exercise in Training, Malaysia, 2004
	Boat Crew Leader, Special Boat Team TWENTY-TWO, Operation Iraqi Freedom, Iraq, 2006
	Team Leading Petty Officer, Special Boat Team TWENTY-TWO, Operation Iraqi Freedom, Iraq, 2009
	Team Chief Petty Officer, Special Boat Team TWENTY-TWO, Joint Combined Exercise in Training, Colombia, 2010
Laurier Tremblay	Ship's Surgeon, USS Constellation (CV-64), 1986–1987; Northern Pacific Cruise, INDOPACOM Area of Responsibility, 1986
	WESTPAC, INDOPACOM Area of Responsibility, 1987

J. A. Diaz · L. Tremblay
Navy Medicine Readiness and Training Command San Diego, San Diego, CA, USA

Department of Surgery, Naval Medical Center San Diego, San Diego, CA, USA
e-mail: joseph.a.diaz52.mil@health.mil

M. D. Tadlock (✉)
Department of Surgery, Naval Medical Center San Diego, San Diego, CA, USA
e-mail: matthewtadlockmd@gmail.com

M. D. Tadlock, A. A. Hernandez (eds.), *Expeditionary Surgery at Sea*,
https://doi.org/10.1007/978-3-031-21893-4_15

Author deployment experience	
Matthew D. Tadlock	Flight Surgeon, Carrier Air Wing Three (CVW-3), embarked on the USS Harry S. Truman (CVN-75) in support of Operation Iraqi Freedom, Fifth Fleet Area of Responsibility, 2004–2005; supporting Humanitarian Aid Disaster Relief (HADR) operations following Hurricane Katrina, 2005
	Resident Surgeon, USNS Mercy (T-AH-19), Pacific Partnership, Micronesia and Papua New Guinea, 2008
	Ship's Surgeon, USS Carl Vinson (CVN-70), WESTPAC, INDOPACOM Area of Responsibility, 2011–2012
	Officer in Charge, Forward Resuscitative Surgical System/Shock Trauma Platoon, Charlie Surgical Company, Native Fury, CENTCOM Area of Responsibility, 2016
	Chief of Trauma, NATO Role 3 Multinational Medical Unit, NATO Resolute Support and Operation Freedom's Sentinel, Kandahar Airfield, Afghanistan, 2017–2018
	Staff Surgeon, Expeditionary Resuscitative Surgical System Pacific, 2019–2020; Provided embarked Role 2 Surgical Support, INDOPACOM Area of Responsibility, 2020

BLUF (Bottom Line Up Front)

1. The deployed surgeon should be adept and comfortable with the use of point-of-care ultrasound (POCUS).
2. There is no role for elective cholecystectomy at sea. Surgical teams augmenting Role 1 shipboard medical departments without a formal operating room (OR) should also not perform cholecystectomy.
3. Check the OR equipment, instruments, and/or consumables before deployment, and "tactically acquire" what is needed to damage control the difficult gallbladder.
4. "Eat when you can, sleep when you can, and whatever you do, do not injure the common bile duct (CBD) during a cholecystectomy."
5. If the right upper quadrant (RUQ) looks "like a bomb went off," place a laparoscopic cholecystostomy tube and "get out of dodge."
6. When present, Rouviere's sulcus is an important landmark that serves as a reference point for the plane of the CBD. Always perform dissection above this plane, NEVER below.
7. Always obtain a "doublet" critical view of safety (CVS) prior to dividing the cystic duct and cystic artery.
8. Before needing to perform with an actual patient, train as an OR team and practice the steps required in performing a portable X-ray flat plate intraoperative cholangiogram (IOC).
9. Converting to open cholecystectomy does not magically make a challenging laparoscopic dissection easier or prevent a common bile duct injury (CBDI); consider performing a fenestrating subtotal cholecystectomy when converting to an open procedure.
10. Placement of a T-tube fashioned from a Red Rubber Robinson catheter may be necessary to temporize ascending cholangitis or to control a small CBDI in preparation for medical evacuation (MEDEVAC).

Introduction

Clinical Vignette 15.1

Two months into a 7-month Pacific deployment, a 40-year-old Sailor presented to the aircraft carrier's medical department with 8 h of unrelenting, constant, postprandial right upper quadrant (RUQ) pain. He had associated mild nausea and vomiting, but he had not experienced any fevers, jaundice, acholic stools, or choleuria. He has had intermittent epigastric and RUQ pain for years attributed to "indigestion."

His past medical history was pertinent for long-standing hypertension managed with appropriate medication and being treated 4 months prior to deployment as an outpatient with oral antibiotics for a clinical diagnosis of diverticulitis. However, he disclosed his pain and tenderness when he was given the diagnosis of diverticulitis was in his epigastrium, not his left lower quadrant.

He was afebrile and not tachycardic. Murphy's sign was present. His white blood cell (WBC) count was 13.8 × 10^9/L, and he had normal liver function tests (LFTs). Figure 15.1 *shows representative images of the point-of-care ultrasound (POCUS) performed by the ship's surgeon on board.*

While the diagnosis of routine acute calculous cholecystitis is likely based on this clinical vignette, the differential is broad, potentially involving the liver, biliary system, and upper gastrointestinal tract. In the expeditionary maritime environment, shipboard medical departments have limited resources to both diagnose and definitively treat acute calculous cholecystitis and other gallstone-related diseases.

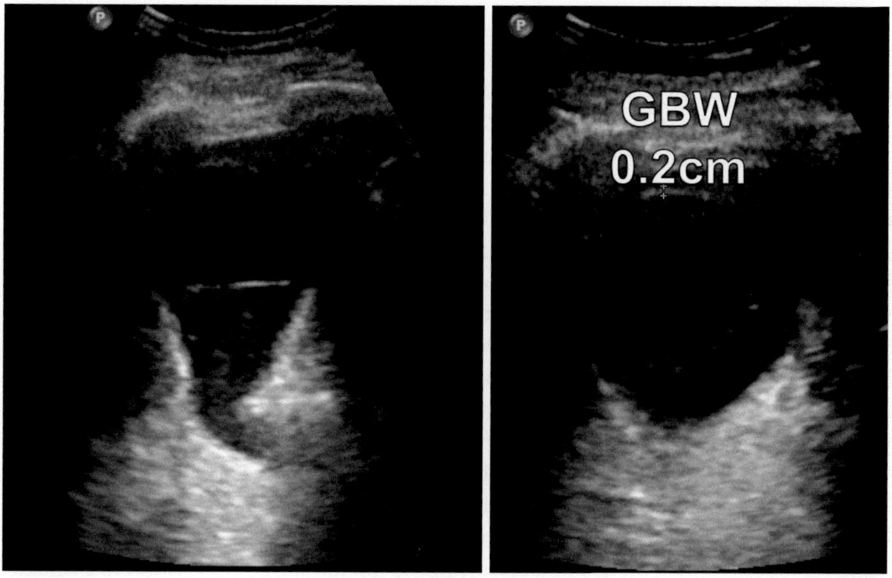

Fig. 15.1 Representative point-of-care ultrasound (POCUS) images of the patient in Clinical Vignette 15.1. Note the gallbladder is full of sludge, however there is an absence of large gallstones, gallbladder wall thickening, or pericholecystic fluid. *GBW* gallbladder wall. (Source: Photo courtesy of Matthew D. Tadlock, MD)

Approximately 10–20% of Americans have gallstones. Of these people, approximately 20% will experience symptoms as a result, and 1–2% will experience complications such as acute cholecystitis, cholangitis, and pancreatitis [1]. Between 2014 and 2018, the overall incidence of cholelithiasis in the active component across all services was estimated to be 1.2 per 1000 person years. During the same 5-year time period, 6470 cholecystectomies were performed in the active component with a cholecystectomy rate of 1.0 per 1000 person-years. Of these, 34.8% were performed in the inpatient setting [2].

A recent analysis of surgical cases performed on United States (U.S.) Navy warships included five aircraft carriers (CVNs) and eight large deck amphibious assault ships with an embarked fleet surgical team (FST) and examined over 200 months of deployment between 1995 and 2017. It found that four open cholecystectomies were performed (0.1–0.3 cases per 7-month deployment) and six laparoscopic cholecystectomies were performed in the 2000s (0.4 cases per 7-month deployment) [3]. However, in the author's (MDT) personal experience as the ship's surgeon during a 6-month deployment on a CVN, four patients with acute calculous cholecystitis were evaluated. One underwent medical evacuation (MEDEVAC) for definitive management because of a concern for choledocholithiasis on surgeon-performed POCUS, and three underwent laparoscopic cholecystectomy because of inability to MEDEVAC the patients during blue water operations.

Diagnosis

At sea, the diagnosis of acute calculous cholecystitis and gallstone-related diseases (Fig. 15.2) is largely clinical and confirmed by laboratory data and surgeon-performed POCUS. Common symptoms and physical exam findings consistent with biliary colic and acute cholecystitis include postprandial RUQ and/or epigastric pain, nausea, vomiting, fever, and RUQ tenderness. Before considering surgery, ensure there is no evidence of choledocholithiasis, pancreatitis, the less common Bouveret's syndrome or gallstone ileus. Rarely, a fistula develops between the gallbladder and the stomach or duodenum. Large stones then pass from the biliary system into the gastrointestinal tract and can cause gastric outlet obstruction (Bouveret's syndrome) or a small bowel obstruction (gallstone ileus) when the stone becomes lodged in the bowel. Patients with gallstone ileus will typically have symptoms of a distal small bowel obstruction with evidence of bowel obstruction on plain films, possibly a radio-opaque gallstone in the right lower quadrant, and/or pneumobilia.

Basic laboratory studies are available on most maritime surgical platforms that have surgical capability (see Chap. 8 for full discussion of laboratory capabilities). Patients with cholecystitis may have normal WBC count or a mild leukocytosis. A basic metabolic panel, LFTs, and serum lipase should all be performed to evaluate for appropriate renal function and evidence of biliary obstruction or pancreatitis.

While most surgeons are familiar with the Focused Assessment Sonography for Trauma (FAST) exam, surgeon-performed POCUS for the diagnosis of biliary

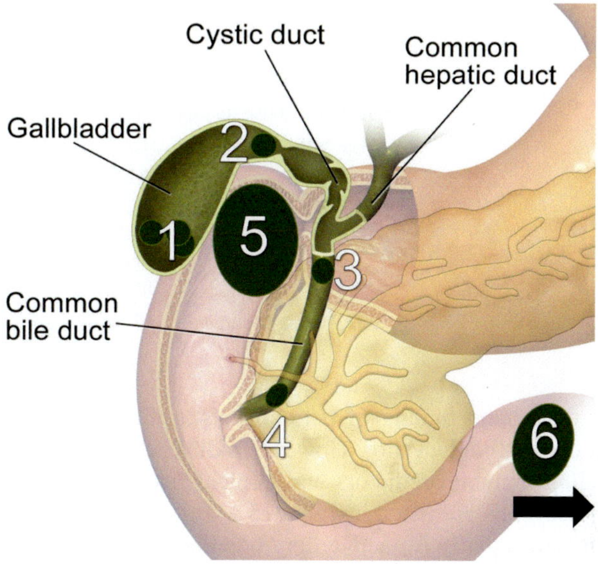

Fig. 15.2 Spectrum of Gallstone-related Diseases. 1-Cholelithiasis; 2-Calculous cholecystitis from cystic duct obstruction; 3-Choledocholithiasis; 4-Gallstone pancreatitis; 5-Bouveret's syndrome (acquired fistula to stomach where gallstone subsequently lodges in duodenum and causes gastric outlet obstruction); 6-Gallstone ileus (acquired fistula to small bowel where gallstone typically lodges at ileocecal valve and causes a distal small bowel obstruction); Mirizzi syndrome not pictured. (Source: Image adapted by the authors from "Gallbladder" by Bruce Blaus, available under a creative commons attribution share alike license from https://commons.wikimedia.org/wiki/File:Gallbladder_(organ).png)

disease is not a ubiquitous surgeon skill. Prior to deployment, the surgeon should spend time with experienced ultrasonographers to be able to identify gallstones, gallbladder wall thickening, pericholecystic fluid, common bile duct (CBD) diameter, and basic liver anatomy, thereby gaining the skills to use POCUS to help confirm a clinical diagnosis. Chapter 9 also discusses the use of POCUS in the diagnosis of biliary disease.

Prior to developing a management strategy and considering an operation, first try to predict which patients may be challenging at operation. While many younger active-duty members are relatively healthy, there will always be a deployed population with well-controlled medical problems such as hypertension or with potentially undiagnosed medical problems such as coronary artery disease. Furthermore, many sailors and marines, particularly males, are more likely to present with acute on chronic or gangrenous cholecystitis because they have either ignored their biliary colic symptoms for years or have been misdiagnosed with gastroesophageal reflux disease (GERD) due to atypical symptoms. Years of isometric contraction of gallbladder smooth muscle against a partial or temporary obstruction from gallstones or sludge causes a locoregional inflammatory response. After repeated episodes, a local ischemic response may result in irreversible organ injury. This prolonged ischemia can eventually result in complicated or gangrenous disease [4–6].

Table 15.1 Predictors of complicated or gangrenous cholecystitis [4–6]

Patient risk factors	Clinical risk factors
Male sex	Heart Rate >90 beats/min
Hypertension	Fever
Alcohol abuse history	WBC >13 × 10^9/L
Age >45 years	Total Bilirubin >1.2 mg/dL
	ALT >50 U/L
	Gallbladder wall thickening and/or absence of pericholecystic fluid on ultrasound

WBC white blood cell, *ALT* alanine aminotransferase

The classic ultrasound finding of pericholecystic fluid may not be present in complicated or chronic cholecystitis. However, gallbladder wall thickening remains a common finding. Patient predictors and clinical risk factors of complicated or gangrenous cholecystitis are listed in Table 15.1. Beware of relative tachycardia in the healthy, cardiovascularly fit, active-duty population. A heart rate of more than 90 beats/min may be an ominous sign, as is any degree of leukocytosis. Most patients with true acute cholecystitis have a normal to mild leukocytosis, therefore a WBC count greater than 13 × 10^9/L may be indicative of complicated disease.

The patient in Clinical Vignette 15.1 has several risk factors for gangrenous cholecystitis: male sex, hypertension, and WBC greater than 13 × 10^9/L. Figure 15.1 shows the patient's POCUS from the vignette. Despite typical symptoms of cholecystitis, note the absence of large gallstones, gallbladder wall thickening, or pericholecystic fluid; however, the gallbladder is full of sludge. Finally, he had a long history of likely biliary colic symptoms [4–7], which were previously misdiagnosed; he also likely had an episode of acute cholecystitis, misdiagnosed as diverticulitis.

Management

Patients with biliary colic should be managed with dietary modification alone, as there is no role for elective cholecystectomy in the deployed maritime environment given the potential risks and complications and limited resources, personnel, and access to tertiary care facilities.

Once the diagnosis of acute calculous cholecystitis or other acute gallstone-related diseases is made, several considerations must be made when determining the ideal management strategy when deployed at sea. Regardless, intravenous (IV) antibiotics that cover common biliary organisms should be started. Depending on what is available in the medical department, piperacillin/tazobactam (Zosyn), ampicillin/sulbactam (Unasyn), or ceftriaxone with metronidazole are all appropriate. Ertapenem is commonly available and can also be used; however, if one of the other listed antibiotic regimens are available (see Chap. 16 for discussion of antimicrobials), they should be preferentially utilized. Additionally, initiate IV hydration, appropriate pain control, and nil per os (NPO).

There are many factors to consider before performing a laparoscopic cholecystectomy at sea (Fig. 15.3). First, does the patient have evidence of sepsis or tissue ischemia? Next, are there appropriate diagnostic and surgical capabilities? For example, if the surgical team is augmenting a shipboard Role 1 medical department without a formal operating room (OR) (e.g., a destroyer or cruiser), then there is no role for cholecystectomy. Finally, as with all surgical decision-making, the ultimate decision to operate is not the surgeon's alone and instead involves both the medical and line chains of command (see Chaps. 6 and 14). Is MEDEVAC an available option? Is the patient stable for MEDEVAC? If so, does the receiving facility have the appropriate standards of care to manage the patient? If any answer is no, the patient will likely need an operation at sea.

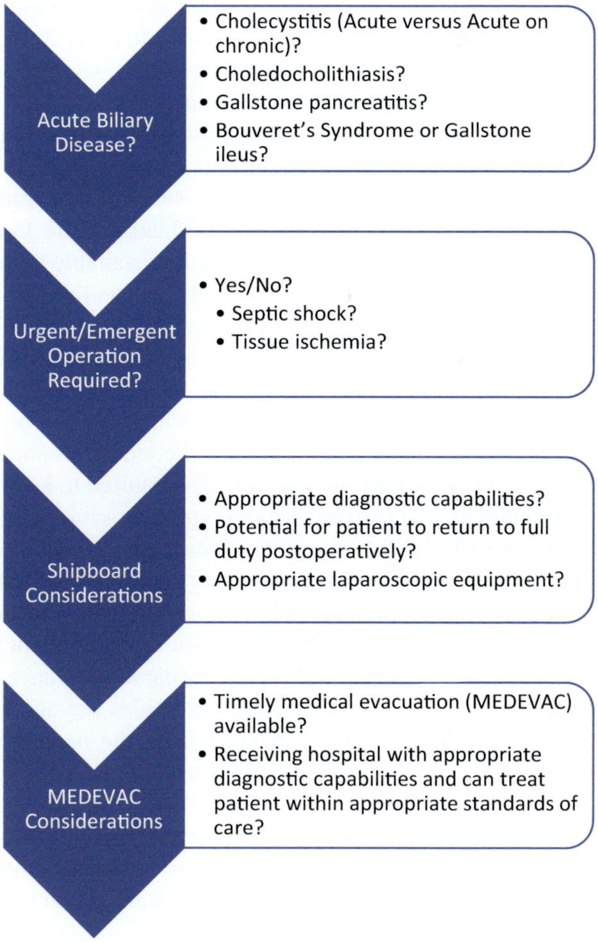

Fig. 15.3 Diagnosis and management considerations for acute gallstone-related diseases in the maritime surgical environment. (Source: created by authors)

Table 15.2 Damage control approaches to the difficult gallbladder

Placement of cholecystostomy tube (laparoscopic versus open)
Subtotal cholecystectomy (laparoscopic versus open)
• Fenestrating
– With closure of cystic duct orifice
– Without closure of cystic duct orifice
• Reconstituting
Conversion to open procedure

The primary goals should be to treat or temporize the acute process and do no harm. While there are many variations, a well-known surgical dictum is "eat when you can, sleep when you can, and don't mess with the pancreas." However, given how common surgical gallstone disease is, perhaps a more relevant dictum for the modern general surgeon, particularly in the expeditionary environment, is "eat when you can, sleep when you can, and whatever you do, don't injure the CBD during a cholecystectomy." A major common bile duct injury (CBDI) can be devasting for a patient. Long-term complications after CBDI include stricture (either from primary repair or post-hepaticojejunostomy), significant degradation in quality of life, potential ineligibility for continued military service, and overall increase in morbidity and mortality. At 1 year post-CBDI, the all-cause mortality in the general population is 7.2%, and it doubles to 14.5% at 5 years [8]. Therefore, before proceeding with surgery the surgeon and surgical team must be prepared for the "tyranny of distance and the difficult gallbladder." Be familiar with the various exit strategies and damage control approaches available in the event laparoscopic cholecystectomy cannot be performed safely at sea (Table 15.2).

If the RUQ looks like "a bomb went off" upon initial laparoscopic visualization, it may be best to temporize the situation and minimize risk to the patient by placing a cholecystostomy tube, which can be performed via an open or laparoscopic approach. Virtually any standard surgical drain can be used as a cholecystostomy tube including standard flat or round silicone drains and Red Rubber Robinson catheters. However, a purse-string suture is required to keep these types of drains in the gallbladder, which may be challenging laparoscopically with inflamed tissue. Foley catheters with the balloon partially inflated, Malecot catheters, and interventional radiology drains such as percutaneous pigtail or suprapubic catheters may be easier to employ as they may not require laparoscopic suturing to stay secure within the gallbladder (Fig. 15.4). Plan ahead prior to deployment for this contingency. Check the standard shipboard authorized medical allowance list (AMAL), verify what equipment, instruments, and/or consumables are actually present in the OR, and "tactically acquire" what is needed from the nearest military medical treatment facility (MTF) to be prepared to damage control the difficult gallbladder (as discussed in Chaps. 5 and 12).

If the plan is laparoscopic cholecystectomy, several things can be done to minimize the risk of CBDI. Even for the most seasoned surgeon, it is prudent to periodically review the steps of a safe laparoscopic cholecystectomy; for the waterborne

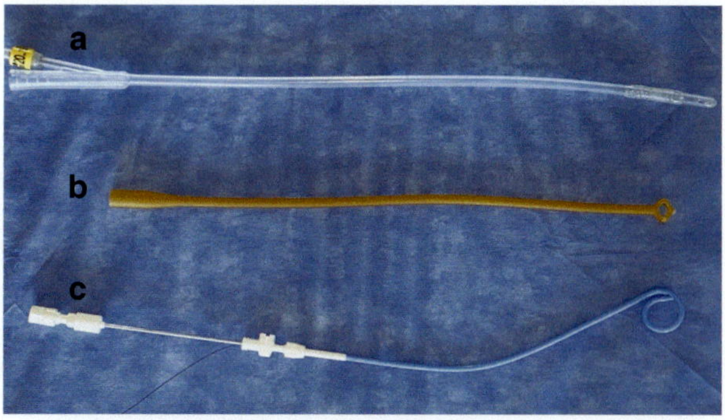

Fig. 15.4 Examples of potential cholecystostomy tubes. (**a**) 20 French Foley catheter; (**b**) 18 French Malecot catheter; (**c**) 10 Fr × 25 cm pigtail catheter. (Source: Photo courtesy of Matthew D. Tadlock, MD)

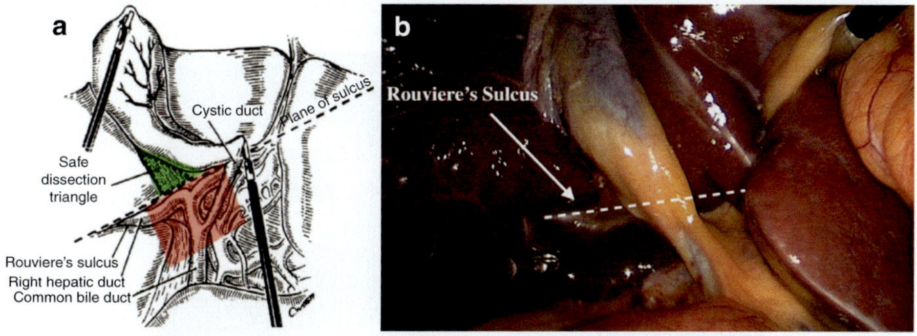

Fig. 15.5 (**a**) Diagram of Rouviere's sulcus demonstrating the safe triangle of dissection above the sulcus (**b**) Intraoperative photo demonstrating Rouviere's sulcus. (Source: Image adapted from O'Rourke TR. (2018) Operative Anatomy and Surgical Landmarks of the Biliary System. In: Cox M, Eslick G, Padbury R. (eds) The Management of Gallstone Disease. Springer, Cham. https://doi.org/10.1007/978-3-319-63884-3_1; Photo from Callahan ZM, Deal S, Alseidi A, Pucci MJ. (2020) Basic Principles of Safe Laparoscopic Cholecystectomy. In: Asbun H, Shah M, Ceppa E, Auyang E. (eds) The SAGES Manual of Biliary Surgery. Springer, Cham. https://doi.org/10.1007/978-3-030-13276-7_3)

surgeon, this may be even more true. Several points from the 2018 Tokyo guidelines [9] and the SAGES Safe Cholecystectomy Program [10] bear emphasizing:

1. Consider gallbladder decompression prior to dissection if markedly distended.
2. Use Rouviere's sulcus (Fig. 15.5) as a landmark, particularly in patients with marked hepatocystic triangle inflammation. Only dissect above the plane of the CBD, NEVER below. Rouviere's sulcus serves as a fairly reliable landmark and should be used, when present (approximately 80% of cases), as a reference point for the plane of the CBD [9, 11, 12].
3. Obtain a "doublet" critical view of safety (CVS). The standard CVS is obtained from the medial vantage point when the hepatocystic triangle is clear of fat and fibrous tissue, the lower one third of the gallbladder is separated from the liver

to expose the cystic plate, and only two structures are seen entering the gallbladder. The "doublet" view is the CVS from the standard medial view and the additional lateral view (Fig. 15.6).

4. Understand the potential of aberrant anatomy.
5. Consider a fundus-first dissection if the CVS cannot be obtained.
6. If the fundus-first approach is not feasible, convert to a subtotal cholecystectomy.
7. Make liberal use of intraoperative cholangiogram (IOC) – see next paragraph.
8. Conduct an intraoperative pause prior to clipping, cutting, or transecting ductal structures.
9. "5 mm ports are free" in laparoscopic surgery. However, their need may indicate that conversion to an open approach is prudent.
10. DO NO HARM! DO NOT injure the CBD!

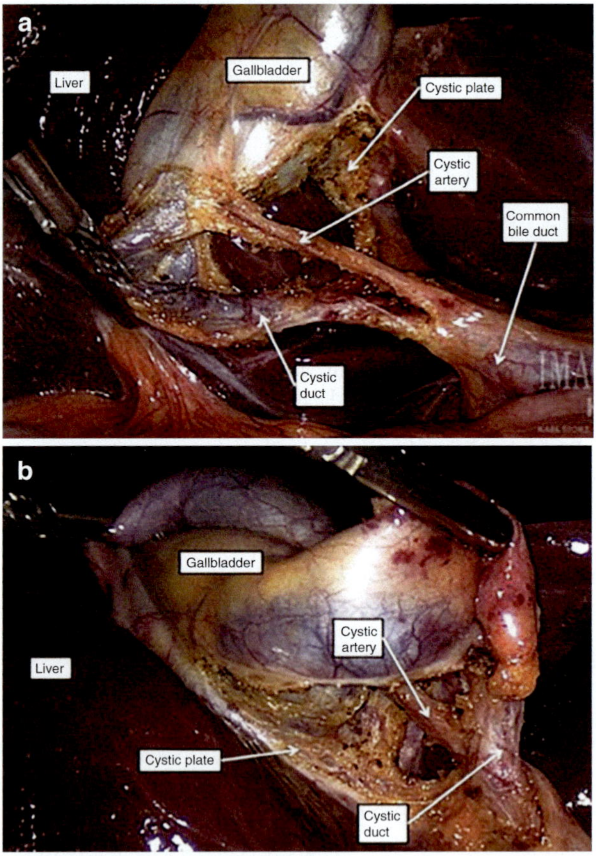

Fig. 15.6 "Doublet" critical view of safety (CVS) (**a**) Medial view (**b**) Lateral view. (Source: Images from Callahan ZM, Deal S, Alseidi A, Pucci MJ. (2020) Basic Principles of Safe Laparoscopic Cholecystectomy. In: Asbun H, Shah M, Ceppa E, Auyang E. (eds) The SAGES Manual of Biliary Surgery. Springer, Cham. https://doi.org/10.1007/978-3-030-13276-7_3)

Fluoroscopy is not available in the expeditionary maritime environment, but single-shot "flat plate" IOC can be performed since most ships with OR capabilities have portable X-ray capabilities as well. Whether the surgeon's shore-based practice is routine or selective IOC, it should be performed routinely at sea so the surgical team is ready and trained for a true surgical emergency. Remember, Omnipaque is not in the ship's AMAL, so acquire some prior to deployment. Furthermore, confirm the presence and type of laparoscopic cholangiogram clamp and cholangiogram catheter prior to deployment. Consider practicing on a surgery team member by taking abdominal X-rays on the OR table so the team is prepared for an actual operation. Finally, be cognizant of the type of portable X-ray machine on the platform (see Chap. 8). A computed radiography (CR) machine can only take one radiograph per plate and requires time for processing. Digital radiography (DR) machines can take multiple radiographs per plate with much faster and convenient processing. The following steps when performing an IOC are recommended:

1. Prior to injecting the contrast into the biliary system, take a scout shot in order to confirm adequate placement of the X-ray system (if using DR).
2. Prior to performing the IOC, inject sterile saline to wash out any small stones that may be present.
3. Use full strength Omnipaque 240 (not diluted) during the IOC to highlight the biliary tree to the maximal extent.
4. Approximately 5 s after injecting contrast, take the X-ray in order to allow adequate time for the ducts to fill with contrast.
5. If unable to visualize the entire biliary tree (from intrahepatic ducts to the normal taper at the duodenum), consider repeating Step 4 after adjusting the X-ray such that multiple shots will overlap, collectively incorporating all of the applicable anatomy.

What if there is so much inflammation in the hepatocystic triangle that it is not safe to do a complete cholecystectomy laparoscopically? One option is to perform a partial cholecystectomy. However, this is the least ideal of the damage control exit strategies because a significant portion of gallbladder remains, and there is a significant risk of recurrent cholecystitis. If forced to do this, first decompress the gallbladder and remove all gallstones.

If it can be done, a subtotal cholecystectomy is preferable to a partial cholecystectomy. Subtotal cholecystectomy is divided into two techniques, fenestrating and reconstituting. In the fenestrating type, the anterior wall of the gallbladder is removed, leaving the back wall connected to the cystic plate intact and may include suture ligating the cystic duct orifice from inside the infundibulum if possible. Some authors recommend leaving the entire back wall intact to minimize injury from dense fibrous adhesions to critical structures. It is important to leave approximately 1–2 cm (measured from the internal cystic duct orifice) of the anterior gallbladder wall left at the infundibulum to minimize the risk of CBDI and injury to other structures (Fig. 15.7). The steps are similar in a reconstituting subtotal cholecystectomy, except that the gallbladder is nearly completely removed and the remnant gallbladder wall is closed [9, 10, 13]. In the shipboard setting, if still laparoscopic, the authors prefer performing a fenestrating subtotal cholecystectomy without closure of the cystic duct orifice, leaving the entire back wall intact to minimize the risk of

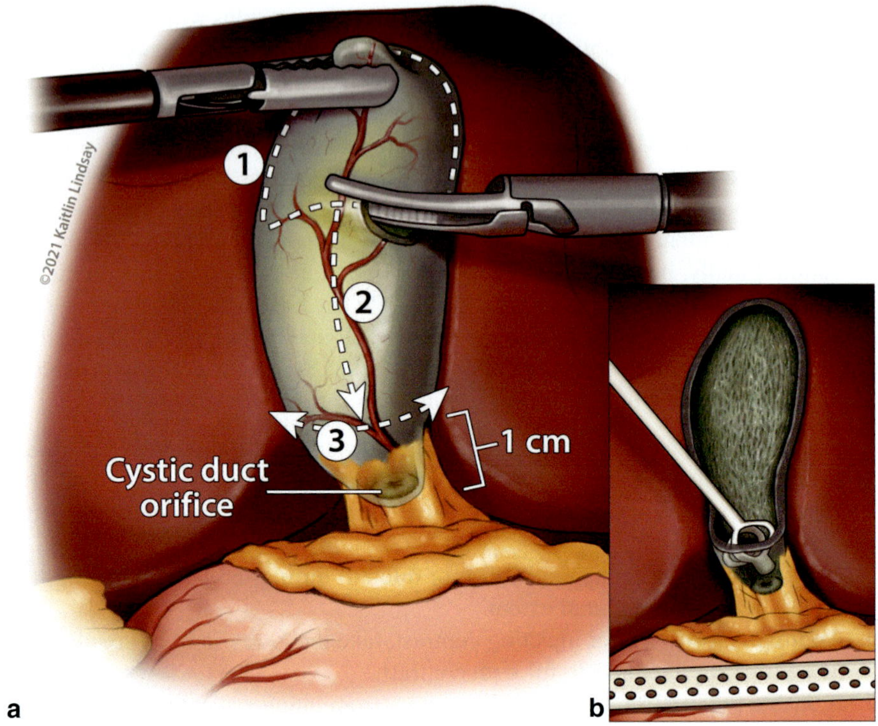

Fig. 15.7 Technique of fenestrating subtotal cholecystectomy (**a**) Essential steps of subtotal cholecystectomy. 1-divide gallbladder wall approximately 1 cm from liver; 2-guide incision down to infundibulum; 3-ensure 1–2 cm of anterior gallbladder wall remaining. (**b**) Fenestrating subtotal cholecystectomy, widely drained with a fluted drain in the gallbladder fossa and a drain in the remnant gallbladder infundibulum. Placing a drain in the remnant gallbladder is especially important to control a potential future bile leak when the cystic duct orifice is not closed. Note that 1 cm of anterior gallbladder wall is left at the infundibulum to minimize injury to the bile duct and surrounding structures. (Source: Image Copyright 2021 Kaitlin Lindsay, used with permission)

injury to critical structures and leaving drains. Closing the cystic duct orifice and suturing the remnant gallbladder closed laparoscopically may be more challenging at sea, particularly in the setting of inflammation and dense adhesions. Furthermore, the reconstituting technique has a higher incidence of recurrent cholecystitis. The fenestrating technique without cystic duct orifice closure has a higher likelihood of bile leak, as high as 18% in some studies, but the majority usually close on their own or after endoscopic retrograde cholangiopancreatography (ERCP) and sphincterotomy [13]. Figure 15.7 shows the basic steps in performing a fenestrating subtotal cholecystectomy.

The final damage control option is conversion to open cholecystectomy through a subcostal Kocher incision using a fundus-first approach [9]. Table 15.3 describes the key steps in performing an open cholecystectomy. However, converting to open cholecystectomy does not magically make a challenging laparoscopic dissection easier or prevent a CBDI. Therefore, if converting to open, particularly when the ship is 2–3 days or 2000–3000 miles away from the nearest land-based hospital, the most prudent thing to do may be to perform an open subtotal cholecystectomy and leave drains. Table 15.4 lists the key steps in performing an open subtotal cholecystectomy. Open or laparoscopic, the essential steps in performing a subtotal cholecystectomy are the same (Fig. 15.7).

Table 15.3 Key steps to the open cholecystectomy

Make right subcostal (Kocher) incision.
Take down gallbladder adhesions, look for possible fistula to duodenum or stomach.
Use rolled laparotomy pads to pack away small bowel and the hepatic flexure to improve exposure. Place laparotomy pads in between the liver edge anterior to the fundus (the edge of segments IV and V at Cantlie's line) and any hand-held or self-retaining retractors (ideal) to protect the liver and improve exposure.
Incise peritoneum over the gallbladder about 1 cm from liver edge with cautery.
Decompress the gallbladder; use cautery to open the fundus and remove any bile and stones.
Use a large clamp or ringed forceps to close the hole and aid in retraction during dissection.
Develop a plane between the gallbladder and liver with blunt dissection and electrocautery. The gallbladder will usually "shell out" if in correct plane (this will be bloody). Expeditious dissection will minimize blood loss.
Cauterize obvious bloody points. Primarily rely on a dry sponge and pressure until the gallbladder is removed.
Open peritoneum over the lateral hepatoduodenal ligament.
Bluntly dissect. Try to identify, ligate, and divide cystic artery early (it is shorter and not as elastic as the cystic duct, therefore more likely to be avulsed at likely origin from hepatic artery if stretched too vigorously).
Dissect, ligate, and divide cystic duct with or without cholangiogram.
Divide remaining peritoneal attachments. Remove the gallbladder.
Hemostasis is achieved using cautery, topical agents, and holding pressure for at least 10–15 min before looking at the area.
Place drains as indicated.
Close the wound in layers. It is ideal to close the fascia posterior to the rectus separately then the anterior fascia.

Table 15.4 Key steps to the open fenestrating subtotal cholecystectomy

Enlarge the opening at the fundus used to decompress gallbladder and insert a finger.
Using cautery, divide the gallbladder wall approximately 1 cm from the liver.
Use a finger to guide the incision from the fundus down to the infundibulum to unroof the entire gallbladder.
At the infundibulum, ensure there is 1–2 cm (measured from the internal cystic duct orifice) of anterior gallbladder wall left to minimize the risk of common bile duct injury (CBDI) and injury to other structures.
Suture ligate the cut end of the cystic artery in the wall of the gallbladder (this is usually quite apparent with pulsatile bleeding).
Obtain hemostasis along the gallbladder edge using cautery or a running locked suture (preferable).
Look for the cystic duct orifice in the base of the infundibulum. Consider a cholangiogram through the orifice.
If possible, suture ligate the cystic duct orifice from inside the gallbladder to avoid a potential postoperative bile leak.
Leave drains; be sure to place an additional drain in the remnant gallbladder if cystic duct orifice not closed.
Close in the usual fashion.

Complications

It is also worth considering how to handle the various challenges and complications that may arise during the difficult gallbladder. The following are some possible complications, along with reasonable bail out options.

Filling Defects on Intraoperative Cholangiogram (IOC)

Should the surgeon find that there are filling defects in the distal biliary system, there are a few simple interventions that should be attempted to clear the system. First, the anesthesia provider should administer IV glucagon (up to 2 mg), followed by copious saline flushes. Should the defects persist, it is reasonable to attempt clearance by introducing a biliary Fogarty balloon (3 or 4 Fr). If unsuccessful, it is recommended that the surgeon continue the cholecystectomy in the usual fashion, with the exception that the cystic duct stump should be closed using a polydioxanone synthetic absorbable laparoscopic endoloop suture. Postoperatively, the patient should have a MEDEVAC arranged for an ERCP as soon as is feasible. There is no role for laparoscopic or open CBD exploration at sea, as there is not the appropriate equipment to safely perform these procedures. However, in the rare unlikely scenario of a floridly septic patient with ascending cholangitis, most likely from choledocholithiasis, the maritime surgical team may need to perform a choledochotomy to place a T-tube (Fig. 15.8). While this scenario is unlikely, the basic steps required are listed in Table 15.5.

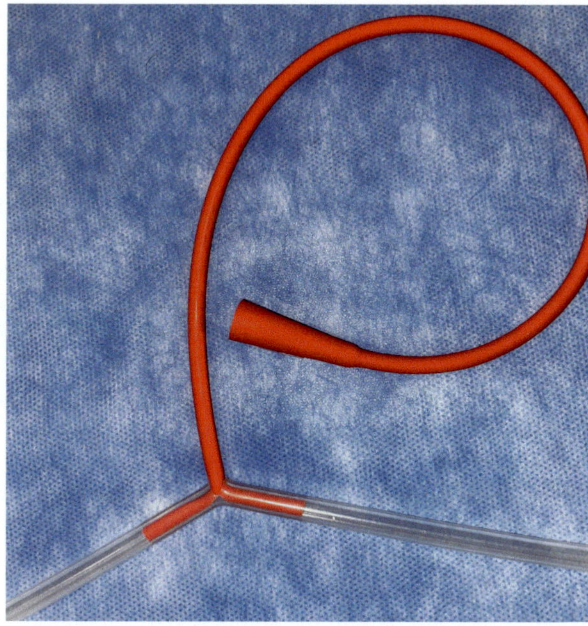

Fig. 15.8 Fourteen French Red Rubber Robinson catheter fashioned into a T-tube placed in a simulated common bile duct (CBD). Each portion of the "T" proximal and distal to the injury is approximately 1.5–2 cm. (Source: Photo courtesy of Matthew D. Tadlock, MD)

Table 15.5 Key steps to surgically decompress ascending cholangitis

After performing a Kocher maneuver, place stay sutures of 3-0 silk low on common bile duct (CBD).
Make a longitudinal incision on the CBD between stay sutures with #15 scalpel. Extend as necessary, but keep as small as possible.
LOOK inside for floating stones.
Irrigate CBD proximally and distally with Red Rubber Robinson catheter to float out stones.
Insert T-tube into CBD. Close CBD around tube with 3-0 or 4-0 absorbable suture.
Flush T-tube with saline to assure patency and absence of leak.
Perform a T-tube cholangiogram.
Exteriorize tube and connect bile drainage bag.
Leave a drain in a dependent position (Morrison's Pouch).
Close in the usual fashion.

Common Bile Duct injury (CBDI)

While not a common complication, CBDI can occur, with an incidence of 0.1–0.6%. Historically, the risk of CBDI was 2–3 times greater using the laparoscopic approach, however more contemporary data suggests that the incidence is similar between open and laparoscopic cholecystectomy [8]. This may be due to the fact that most modern surgeons are more comfortable with the laparoscopic approach, and open cholecystectomies are generally performed in patients with more complicated anatomy after inability to safely perform the procedure laparoscopically. If at any point during the operation a CBDI is suspected, it is imperative that the injury either be identified or ruled out. If the injury is not suspected until the postoperative period, it is equally imperative that the proper actions are taken as soon as possible.

If a CBDI is identified, the extent of the injury dictates the management. In this difficult situation the surgeon must remain focused on the ultimate goal, the safety of the patient. If a complete transection of the common duct has occurred or if the injury is greater than approximately 30%, do not proceed with hepaticojejunostomy. The best thing is to widely drain the area around the injury with closed suction drains to control the bile leak until the patient can be managed by an expert in hepatobiliary reconstruction. Small pinpoint injuries are also best managed with wide drainage to control the bile leak. Regardless of size, MEDEVAC off the ship should be arranged as soon as possible for ERCP.

If a small injury is identified (less than 20–30% circumference), do not primarily repair the injury as this is associated with a high rate of either CBD stricture or persistent bile leak. The best option is to repair the injury over a T-tube if MEDEVAC is not available in a timely fashion. Usually the T-portion of the tube is cut so it is 3–4 cm long and then cut longitudinally so 50% of the circumference remains. This "T" portion of the tube is then placed in the CBD with approximately 1.5–2 cm both proximal and distal to the injury. T-tubes are not commonly stocked in shore-based hospitals, nor are they in the ship's AMAL; therefore, it is unlikely that an actual T-tube will be available. Thankfully, almost any drain or catheter can be fashioned into a T-tube. Silicone catheters are not ideal as they can disintegrate over time. Polyvinyl chloride is inert and causes minimal tissue reaction, therefore a tract will not form. Latex is ideal, but a Red Rubber Robinson catheter can be used. To fashion a T-tube, take an appropriately sized Latex Malecot or a Red Rubber Robinson catheter and cut the tip off in an axial orientation. Then cut the end of the tube longitudinally so that the "T" portion is 2–4 cm long. After placing the T-tube through the injury, close around the tube with 3-0 or 4-0 absorbable suture and perform an IOC. Figure 15.8 shows an example of a Red Rubber Robinson catheter fashioned into a T-tube, placed in a simulated CBD. Alternate uses of common catheters are also discussed in Appendix A.

Intraoperative or Postoperative bleeding

As with any patient post-cholecystectomy, the patient must be closely monitored for signs of bleeding. The shipboard environment does not greatly influence how this is done. However, what is impacted are the resources available for management. If the surgeon suspects that there is poor intra-abdominal hemostasis, it is reasonable for initial investigation to be via a diagnostic laparoscopy. In most cases, postoperative bleeding can be addressed in a minimally invasive approach. If this is deemed inappropriate or hemostasis is not able to be achieved laparoscopically, it may be necessary to convert to an open approach through a right subcostal (Kocher) incision. Whatever the approach, the primary means of hemostasis should be via direct pressure or hemostatic agents, as electrocautery can lead to significant injury, making a bad situation worse.

Management of Other Acute Biliary Diseases

Gallstone Pancreatitis

Initial shipboard management of this disease is similar to that of hospital-based treatment. The patient should receive IV fluid resuscitation, pain control, and early enteral feeding. However, one should strongly consider a routine MEDEVAC for delayed cholecystectomy off the ship as soon as is feasible given the high rate of recurrence.

Mirizzi Syndrome

This process is a form of obstructing jaundice that is caused by impaction of a gallstone in the cystic duct or infundibulum leading to compression of the biliary tree. If expeditious MEDEVAC is not possible, it is recommended that the surgeon plans for a subtotal cholecystectomy with a low threshold for converting to an open approach.

Bouveret's Syndrome and Gallstone Ileus

Chronic inflammation within the gallbladder can cause fistula formation between the gallbladder and stomach. If a large enough stone passes from the stomach through the pylorus, gastric outlet obstruction can occur if the stone becomes lodged in the duodenum. On a ship, it is recommended that the stone be removed via a gastrotomy and the fistula left alone.

If a fistula instead is formed between the gallbladder and small bowel, usually the duodenum, that stone may become impacted anywhere in the small bowel. It most commonly occurs at the ileocecal valve in the terminal ileum, leading to a small bowel obstruction. This process is best managed by performing an enterotomy proximally in healthy, non-inflamed bowel, milking the stone proximally, and removing it through the enterotomy. As with Bouveret's syndrome, on a ship it is recommended that the enterotomy be closed and the fistula left alone.

Clinical Vignette 15.1 Conclusion

Upon laparoscopic visualization of RUQ, the patient had a significant amount of chronic inflammation. An attempt to dissect the medial peritoneum above Rouviere's sulcus was made, but a safe dissection could not be performed. While attempting a laparoscopic fundus-first dissection of the gallbladder, it was so gangrenous that the gallbladder wall was tissue paper thin and could not be grasped.

A laparoscopic fenestrating subtotal cholecystectomy was performed, and the back wall of the gallbladder could not be safely dissected off the liver bed so it was fulgurated with electrocautery. All bile was suctioned and stones removed. Closed suction drains were placed through the subcostal port sites. Postoperatively there was no bile leak after starting a regular diet, and the drains were removed on postoperative day 3.

Conclusion

As demonstrated in the clinical vignette for this chapter, the patient with complicated cholecystitis remained on ship for his recovery. However, in the setting of damage control cholecystectomy for complicated cholecystitis, routine MEDEVAC when able to is recommended. Many of the diagnostic modalities to identify complications should they occur (e.g., retained stone, bile leak, etc.) and their treatment (e.g., ERCP, Interventional Radiology procedures) are only available off ship.

In summary, while there is no role for elective cholecystectomy in the expeditionary maritime environment, the shipboard surgeon may have to manage patients with acute calculous cholecystitis and other gallstone-related pathology. If expeditious transfer off the ship to an appropriate level of care is possible, this may be the ideal management strategy. However, cholecystectomy has and can be safely performed at sea. The maritime surgeon must be comfortable with POCUS and familiar with various damage control exit strategies when managing complicated biliary disease to minimize CBDI and injury to other structures. In preparation, the surgical team may need to "tactically acquire" supplies prior to deployment, including Omnipaque, endoloops, cholangiogram clamps and catheters, and drains that can be used as cholecystostomy tubes and can be fashioned into T-tubes. It is imperative that the deployed maritime surgical team is as prepared as possible with regard to resources, personnel, and experience.

Declaration of Interest The views expressed in this chapter are those of the authors and do not necessarily reflect the official policy or position of the Department of the Navy, Department of Defense, nor the US Government.

Funding This research did not receive any specific grant from funding agencies in the public, commercial, or not-for-profit sectors.

Conflict of Interest Statement The authors declare no conflict of interest.

References

1. Stinton LM, Shaffer EA. Epidemiology of gallbladder disease: cholelithiasis and cancer. Gut Liver. 2012;6(2):172–87.
2. Lormand DK, Williams VF, Fedgo A, Stahlman S. Update: gallbladder disease and cholecystectomies, active component, U.S. Armed Forces, 2014–2018. MSMR. 2019;26(12):8–13.
3. Nealeigh MD, Kucera WB, Bradley MJ, et al. Surgery at sea: exploring the training gap for isolated military surgeons. J Surg Educ. 2019;76(4):1139–45.
4. Bourikian S, Anand RJ, Aboutanos M, Wolfe LG, Ferrada P. Risk factors for acute gangrenous cholecystitis in emergency general surgery patients. Am J Surg. 2015;210(4):730–3.
5. Ganapathi AM, Speicher PJ, Englum BR, Perez A, Tyler DS, Zani S. Gangrenous cholecystitis: a contemporary review. J Surg Res. 2015;197(1):18–24.
6. Wu B, Buddensick TJ, Ferdosi H, et al. Predicting gangrenous cholecystitis. HPB (Oxford). 2014;16(9):801–6.
7. Yokoe M, Hata J, Takada T, et al. Tokyo Guidelines 2018: diagnostic criteria and severity grading of acute cholecystitis (with videos). J Hepatobiliary Pancreat Sci. 2018;25(1):41–54.
8. Cohen JT, Charpentier KP, Beard RE. An update on iatrogenic biliary injuries: identification, classification, and management. Surg Clin North Am. 2019;99(2):283–99.
9. Wakabayashi G, Iwashita Y, Hibi T, et al. Tokyo Guidelines 2018: surgical management of acute cholecystitis: safe steps in laparoscopic cholecystectomy for acute cholecystitis (with videos). J Hepatobiliary Pancreat Sci. 2018;25(1):73–86.
10. Michael Brunt L, Deziel DJ, Telem DA, et al. Safe cholecystectomy multi-society practice guideline and state-of-the-art consensus conference on prevention of bile duct injury during cholecystectomy. Surg Endosc. 2020;34(7):2827–55.
11. Pere G, Benvegnu V, Merce C, Maulat C, Carrere N, Lopez R. The sulcus of the caudate process (Rouviere's sulcus): anatomy and clinical applications-a review of current literature. Surg Radiol Anat. 2020;42(12):1441–6.
12. Cheruiyot I, Nyaanga F, Kipkorir V, et al. The prevalence of the Rouviere's sulcus: a meta-analysis with implications for laparoscopic cholecystectomy. Clin Anat. 2021;34(4):556–64.
13. Dissanaike S. A step-by-step guide to laparoscopic subtotal fenestrating cholecystectomy: a damage control approach to the difficult gallbladder. J Am Coll Surg. 2016;223(2):e15–8.

Chapter 16
Infectious Disease Pearls for Maritime Surgical Teams

Matthew J. Carr and Ryan C. Maves

Humanity has but three great enemies: fever, famine, and war; of these by far the greatest, by far the most terrible, is fever.

Sir William Osler

Author deployment experience	
Matthew J. Carr	Flight Surgeon, Carrier Air Wing Seven (CVW-7), embarked on the USS Harry S. Truman (CVN-75), Operation Enduring Freedom, Fifth Fleet Area of Responsibility, 2015–2016
Ryan C. Maves	Flight Surgeon, Carrier Air Wing Seventeen (CVW-17), embarked on the USS George Washington (CVN-73), 2001–2003; Operation Noble Eagle, New York, NY, USA, 2001; Operation Southern Watch and Operation Enduring Freedom, Fifth Fleet Area of Responsibility, 2002
	Director for Medical Services and Infectious Diseases consultant, NATO Role 3 Multinational Medical Unit, Operation Enduring Freedom, Kandahar Airfield, Afghanistan, 2012

BLUF (Bottom Line Up Front)

1. The maritime surgical team should know the diagnostic capabilities and pharmacologic options on their deployed platform. They will be significantly less robust than on shore, so take inventory of options as a team early.
2. Surgical teams should utilize the Advanced Virtual Support for Operational Forces (ADVISOR) system, a 24/7 consultative service for deployed units,

M. J. Carr
Navy Medicine Readiness and Training Command San Diego, San Diego, CA, USA
e-mail: matthew.j.carr4.mil@health.mil

R. C. Maves (✉)
Wake Forest University School of Medicine, Winston-Salem, NC, USA
e-mail: rmaves@wakehealth.edu

M. D. Tadlock, A. A. Hernandez (eds.), *Expeditionary Surgery at Sea*,
https://doi.org/10.1007/978-3-031-21893-4_16

where the shipboard surgical team can seek advice from infectious disease (ID) specialists along with other specialties.

3. The expeditionary surgical team may be called to care for trauma, surgical, or non-surgical diseases in organ systems they may not be familiar with, and they need to be prepared for the basics of antimicrobial treatment, including the central nervous system (CNS), otolaryngology (ENT), pulmonary, ophthalmology, and gastrointestinal systems.
4. When necrotizing soft tissue infection (NSTI) is suspected on a maritime platform, treatment should first consist of either surgical debridement or the very least an operative exploration of the wound by the surgical team. Broad-spectrum antibiotics should also be initiated with coverage including agents that inhibit bacterial exotoxin synthesis.
5. Diseases such as malaria, tuberculosis (TB), and neglected tropical diseases are relatively rare in the United States (U.S.) but common in many developing countries. The deployed surgical team should maintain a high index of suspicion for such entities in endemic regions.

Introduction

Surgical teams are regularly deployed to austere settings where infection is an ever-present risk. The military surgeon is often one of the most experienced clinicians present and will be faced with infectious diseases that they do not frequently, or ever, encounter in their usual practice. Additionally, they will be equipped with fewer diagnostic capabilities than in a more familiar hospital setting. It is in the patients' best interests that the maritime surgical team is prepared to provide quality care despite unfamiliar diseases, reduced equipment, and limited pharmacologic agents. While this chapter is far from comprehensive, it provides a starting point to understand some of the more frequent infectious disease topics encountered in austere medical care.

Diagnostic Tools at Hand

The surgical team may not have the vast breadth of diagnostic capabilities they previously enjoyed in a tertiary referral center, but they will still have some familiar albeit basic capabilities. Laboratory testing, including point-of-care tests, brings to mind the medical school adage that tests should support a diagnosis rather than provide it.

At the time of publication, common tests available on most platforms are complete blood count (CBC), urinalysis, urine human chorionic gonadotropin (HCG), occult blood, rapid influenza antigen, and blood glucose. Tests that typically are only

Table 16.1 How to prepare various specimen slides

Dry Mount	Wet Mount	Smear Slide
1. Place specimen sample onto the liquid 2. Place a side of the cover slip against the slide at an angle, slowly laying it down over the specimen, avoiding air trap bubbles	1. Place a drop of fluid in the center of the slide 2. Place specimen sample onto the liquid 3. Place a side of the cover slip against the slide at an angle, slowly laying it down over the specimen, avoiding air trap bubbles	1. Place a liquid sample, such as blood, onto the slide 2. Using a second slide, slowly smear the sample to create an even thin coat 3. Place a side of the cover slip against the slide at an angle, slowly laying it down over the specimen, avoiding air trap bubbles

available on larger platforms with designated laboratory technicians are basic metabolic panel (BMP), comprehensive metabolic panel (CMP), liver function test (LFT), and prothrombin time/partial thromboplastin time (PT/PTT). See Chap. 8 for a discussion of the laboratory and radiology capabilities and limitations of maritime medicine. If available, a laboratory technician should be able to perform basic microscopy as well. However, the deployed clinician may take it upon themselves to prepare their own slides. A simple guide to basic slide preparation is listed in Table 16.1.

In terms of radiology capabilities, many larger platforms are able to perform standard radiography, such as a plain chest radiograph or abdominal film. Point-of-care ultrasound (POCUS) machines are usually available as well, although an ultrasound technician is not present and the results of any ultrasonographic studies are therefore dependent on the skill and experience of the operator.

The most useful tools of deployed surgeons and surgical teams in the management of infectious diseases are their hands, eyes, and ears. Although the clinical specialty of infectious disease (ID) medicine requires a detailed knowledge of microbiology, the care of the potentially infected patient depends principally on understanding the patient's history, their presenting syndrome, and their potential exposures to disease. A careful history, a thorough physical examination, and an appreciation for the patient's demographic risk factors for given pathogens, including multidrug-resistant organisms, will be the key features that determine initial therapy. The Advanced Virtual Support for Operational Forces (ADVISOR) system is a 24/7 consultative service for deployed units where the shipboard medical and surgical team can seek advice from ID specialists along with other specialties. See Chap. 5 for detailed information regarding both emergent (COMM 833-238-7756 or DSN 312-429-9089) and non-emergent consults.

The Maritime Pharmacy

A thorough inventory of the pharmacy should be one of the first tasks of any newly billeted surgeon. While the spectrum for the available medications is reasonably broad with relatively few gaps in coverage for a generally healthy and immunocompetent population when all medications are present, it is possible that specific items could be missing. While requesting additional medications is always possible, distance and supply chain limitations make this unreliable in terms of timeliness once deployed.

At the time of this publication, Table 16.2 shows the current antimicrobial drugs included in an authorized medical allowance list (AMAL) for a deployed pharmacy of the medical department of an aircraft carrier (CVN). Joint Trauma System (JTS) guidelines also cover prophylactic coverage for trauma exposures.

Table 16.2 Current antimicrobial drugs included in the Authorized Medical Allowance List (AMAL) for a deployed pharmacy of the medical department of an aircraft carrier (CVN)

Oral	Injectible	Ophthalmologic/otic	Topical
Albendazole 200 mg tab	Ampicillin 1 g	Ciprofloxacin 0.3% ophthalmic drops	Bacitracin Ointment
Amoxicillin 500 mg cap	Ampicillin-Sulbactam (Unasyn) 3 g	Erythromycin 0.5% ophthalmic ointment	Clindamycin 1% solution
Amoxicillin/clavulanate 875/125 mg tab 500/125 mg tab	Cefazolin 1 g	Moxifloxacin 0.5% ophthalmic solution	Clotrimazole 1% cream
Atovaquone/proguanil (malarone) 250/100 mg tab	Cefoxitin 2 g	Polymyxin B/ trimethoprim 10,000 U/1 mg ophthalmic solution	Ketoconazole 2% cream
Azithromycin 250 mg tab	Ceftriaxone 2 g 250 mg		Mupirocin 2% ointment
Cephalexin 500 mg cap	Ciprofloxacin 400 mg/200 mL	Ciprofloxacin/ dexamethasone 0.3%/0.1% otic drops	Nystatin-triamcinolone Cream
Ciprofloxacin 500 mg tab	Clindamycin 150 mg/mL		Silver sulfadiazene 1% topical
Clindamycin 150 mg cap	Doxycycline 100 mg		Terbinafine 1% cream
Dicloxacillin 500 mg tab	Gentamicin 40 mg/mL		
Doxycycline 100 mg tab	Levofloxacin 25 mg/mL		
Fluconazole 150 mg tab	Metronidazole 5 mg/mL (100 mg bag)		
Isoniazid 300 mg tab	Nafcillin 1 g		
Itraconazole 100 mg cap	Penicillin G 20 million U		
Levofloxacin 500 mg tab	Penicillin benzathine Suspension		

Table 16.2 (continued)

Oral	Injectible	Ophthalmologic/otic	Topical
Metronidazole 500 mg tab	Trimethoprim/ sulfamethoxazole 400/80 mg		
Nitrofurantoin 100 mg cap	Vancomycin 1 g		
Nystatin 100,000 U oral solution		Not included but can be ordered, mentioned in chapter	
Oseltamivir 75 mg cap		Artemether/ lumefantrine (Coartem) 20/120 mg tab	
Penicillin 500 mg tab		Linezolid 600 mg tab	
Praziquantel 600 mg tab		Moxifloxacin 400 mg tab	
Primaquine 26.3 mg tab		Artesunate 110 mg	
Rifampin 300 mg cap		Ertapenem 1 g	
Terbinafine 250 mg tab		Meropenem 1 g	
Trimethoprim/ sulfamethoxazole 800/160 mg tab		Piperacillin-tazobactam (Zosyn) 3.375 mg	
Valacyclovir 1 g tab 500 mg tab		Remdesivir 100 mg	

Neurological Infections

The non-deployed surgeon treats meningitis and encephalitis infrequently, with regular reliance upon consultants for definitive management. The deployed surgeon does not typically have that option and as such may be called upon to initiate treatment when the suspicion arises for one of these clinical presentations.

Penetrating Central Nervous System (CNS) Trauma

Traumatic central nervous system (CNS) wounds should be treated with prophylactic antibiotics. Penetrating brain injuries should be covered with intravenous (IV) cefazolin (2 g every 8 h) with the addition of IV metronidazole (500 mg every 8 h) coverage for gross organic debris. Alternatively, IV vancomycin (weight-based dosing), administered as a 15 mg/kg dose (maximum 2 g/dose) every 12 h in a typical adult patient and IV ciprofloxacin (400 mg every 12 h) may be used in rare cases of anaphylaxis to penicillin. Treatment should be for five days or until any leak has been closed. Penetrating wounds to the spinal cord may be treated in the same way, with IV metronidazole added for concurrent intraperitoneal injury. Burr holes should be treated as an open wound and treated with similar coverage. Obviously, the medical evacuation (MEDEVAC) process is indicated for these critically ill patients.

Meningitis

Meningitis involving the subarachnoid space can be differentiated clinically from encephalitis afflicting the deeper brain tissue. Nuchal rigidity, attempting to minimize irritation to the meninges, raises suspicion for meningitis, whereas alterations in behavior, seizures, focal neurologic deficits, and delirium are consistent with encephalitis. It is important to note that these entities may overlap ("meningoencephalitis") and that patients with a "pure" meningitis may present with delirium that is difficult to distinguish from an encephalitis that primarily affects the brain parenchyma.

When meningitis is suspected, immediate empiric antibiotics are indicated and should not be delayed in favor of a lumbar puncture (LP) or neuroimaging. The anesthesia provider on board the ship may be available to assist with an LP and is likely the most experienced operator with regards to this procedure. It is acceptable to give antibiotics before the LP if there is any chance of a delay. LP should not be performed in patients with focal neurologic findings or seizures unless neuroimaging is obtained first to exclude a mass-occupying lesion; as a practical matter, this precludes LP in such patients at sea as neuroimaging would require a MEDEVAC [1].

The major causes of bacterial meningitis in an immunocompetent military-aged individual are *Streptococcus pneumoniae* and *Neisseria meningitidis*. The disease course may be rapid, with progression from nausea, emesis, and photophobia to seizures and coma within hours. A MEDEVAC of the affected individual should be planned immediately. Empiric treatment should begin with IV ceftriaxone (2 g every 12 h) in combination with IV vancomycin. In pregnant women, patients over the age of 50 years, and patients with active alcohol abuse (all of which are infrequent but not unheard of in the deployed environment), IV ampicillin (2 g every 4 h) may be added for coverage of *Listeria*. If LP can be performed, the ship's laboratory technician may be able to perform a Gram stain. If the cerebrospinal fluid (CSF) is visibly purulent or if organisms are visible on microscopy, consideration should be made for empiric IV dexamethasone (0.15 mg/kg every 6 h) and given at the same time as the antibiotics. This will be an 8–16 mg dose of dexamethasone for a typical military member and is given for 2–4 days.

Meningitis due to *Neisseria meningitidis*, or meningococcus, is highly acute and fulminant. Septic shock and rash (purpura fulminans) are common findings that suggest meningococcal disease when present. In cases of suspected meningococcal meningitis, early involvement of public health authorities to determine the need for antibiotic prophylaxis of close contacts is mandatory. The majority of senior medical officers (SMOs) have formal public health and preventive medicine training and are valuable resources in this setting.

The majority of viral meningitis may be treated with supportive therapy alone, but differentiating bacterial versus viral within the prehospital deployed setting may not be possible, therefore empiric antibiotics remain indicated.

Encephalitis

Encephalitis in the immunocompetent military-aged individual is typically viral and often due to herpes simplex virus 1 (HSV-1). When suspected, empiric antivirals should be initiated without delay. IV acyclovir is the drug of choice but is not stocked onboard warships routinely. Oral valacyclovir (1 g three times per day) may achieve adequate therapeutic levels in the CSF based on limited data and is a reasonable short-term alternative until MEDEVAC is available for definitive care [2].

Infections of the Head and Neck

Clinically relevant infections of the head and neck for the deployed surgeon range from sinusitis to facial trauma resulting in open fractures. Most acute sinusitis may be treated as an outpatient, only occasionally requiring antibiotics and rarely requiring MEDEVAC.

Facial Trauma

Maxillofacial fractures, whether open or with foreign bodies to include fixation devices, should be covered for 24 h with IV cefazolin with IV clindamycin (900 mg every 8 h) as an alternative in the case of penicillin allergy. MEDEVAC to an appropriate level of care should be initiated during that time.

Peritonsillar Cellulitis and Abscess

An abscess forming within the peritonsillar region is typically a progression from acute tonsillitis and is common in the military-aged population. In early stages, it spreads as cellulitis, eventually developing into an abscess. A typical presentation is unilateral sore throat, fever, odynophagia, and otalgia. Additionally, muffled voice, drooling, trismus, deviation of the uvula toward the unaffected side, and edema or cellulitis can be appreciated on exam. Causative organisms reflect the flora of the oral cavity and include *Streptococcus pyogenes*, *Streptococcus anginosus*, or *Fusobacterium necrophorum*.

Once suspected, antibiotics such as IV ampicillin/sulbactam (Unasyn) (3 g every 6 h) should be administered, with eventual transition to oral amoxicillin/clavulanate (875/125 mg twice daily) once stable and tolerating oral medications. While an incision and drainage or a tonsillectomy may be performed, a needle aspiration may be the safest course, given the unfamiliar territory for a general surgeon. This can be aided with ultrasound guidance if the patient tolerates it. If deployed on a CVN, consultation with the onboard oral-maxillofacial surgeon (OMFS) is mandatory for assistance in treatment. Antibiotics should be continued for 14 days after drainage.

Submandibular Abscess and Ludwig's Angina

Submandibular abscesses present as bilateral infections within the submylohyoid and sublingual spaces, arising from the floor of the mouth. While this can be a progression from the second or third mandibular molar teeth, it can also present as an ongoing, untreated peritonsillar abscess. These infections are an aggressive form of cellulitis, usually without lymphadenopathy, which can rapidly spread to the parapharyngeal space, retropharyngeal space, and finally the superior mediastinum, posing danger to the airway as they spread.

On presentation, patients may present with a muffled voice or even an inability to speak. Dangerous late signs are difficulty breathing, stridor, and cyanosis. They will have bilateral erythema, induration, and tenderness in the submandibular region. Treatment is primarily in the form of broad-spectrum antibiotics, most often IV ampicillin/sulbactam (Unasyn). IV ceftriaxone (2 g every 24 h) and IV or oral metronidazole (500 mg every 8 h) is an acceptable alternative regimen, particularly for patients with reported anaphylaxis to penicillin. Airway compromise is a concern, and the patient must be monitored closely. Anesthesia providers should be made aware of the patient, as rapid sequence intubation may be necessary should the airway continue to worsen despite antibiotics. Due to the edematous nature of the airway, this may be a difficult airway requiring fiberoptic intubation (if available) or an emergency surgical airway. As the predominant effects arise from cellulitis rather than a distinct abscess, surgery may not be beneficial and drainage may be ineffectual.

Pulmonary Infections

Timely and adequate care of pulmonary infections is a common issue for surgeons both deployed and stateside. While some pulmonary disease is inherently surgical, such as thoracic trauma, there are also initially non-surgical infections that may progress to empyema and require operative intervention.

Penetrating Thoracic Trauma

Thoracic trauma resulting in a dirty wound, typically from penetrating trauma, warrants coverage with IV cefazolin with IV clindamycin as an alternative for allergy. If there is a concern for esophageal involvement, IV metronidazole should be added to cefazolin and continued until 24 h following closure of the injury.

Thoracic trauma resulting in hemothorax or pneumothorax and warranting a chest tube does not routinely warrant antibiotic prophylaxis when placed in a controlled environment. Prophylaxis should be considered in the event of a prehospital-placed chest tube by an advanced forward provider in a nonsterile environment. Chest tubes not placed in the operating room (OR), particularly while deployed at sea, should also be considered "nonsterile" even under "sterile" conditions in a treatment room. Therefore, prophylaxis with IV cefazolin is recommended by many experts.

Retained hemothorax, or hemothorax persisting despite adequate tube thoracostomy, predisposes the trauma patient to empyema. Complete radiographic resolution of the hemothorax following tube thoracostomy can result in an empyema in 2% of cases, though incomplete resolution of the hemothorax increases the risk of empyema up to 26.8% [3].

Empyema may further result from trauma to surrounding organs, such as an esophageal injury, or as an evolution from an infectious cause, such as a parapneumonic effusion. While effusions are common in pneumonia, fewer than 5% will eventually result in empyema [4]. Pneumococci and anaerobes are typical causes of empyema in the military population. Overall, empyema will frequently require treatment via video-assisted thoracoscopic surgery (VATS) following initiation of antibiotic treatment and initial tube thoracostomy. After initiating antibiotics and placing a chest tube, efforts should be made to obtain a MEDEVAC for the patient as soon as possible, as it is generally not appropriate to perform a VATS at sea. A thoracotomy could be performed but only in the rare situation when a MEDEVAC is not available. Consultation with a thoracic surgeon is recommended before considering thoracotomy.

Pneumonia

Not all pulmonary infections presenting to the surgeon will be surgical in nature nor warrant surgical intervention. In the austere environment, pneumonia is an ever-present concern. Community acquired pneumonia (CAP) may present as fevers, chills, productive or nonproductive cough, sweats, dyspnea, or pleuritic chest pain. The medical and surgical team typically has a complete blood count (CBC) to identify a leukocytosis and a chest X-ray to evaluate for airspace consolidation at their disposal on most larger platforms.

Viral pneumonia is common in military settings [5], but available diagnostics are not sufficient to withhold antibiotics for patients with established pneumonia even if a viral pathogen (such as influenza) is identified [6]. Typical bacterial causes of pneumonia in military personnel include *Streptococcus pneumoniae*, *Haemophilus influenzae*, *Mycoplasma pneumoniae*, and *Chlamydia pneumoniae*. Treatment for ambulatory patients without comorbidities should be oral amoxicillin (1 g three times daily) or oral doxycycline (100 mg twice daily). Ambulatory patients with comorbidities (such as asplenia or diabetes mellitus) should receive either combination therapy with oral amoxicillin/clavulanate plus oral azithromycin (500 mg daily) or monotherapy with oral levofloxacin (750 mg daily) or oral moxifloxacin (400 mg daily). Patients requiring admission to the ship's medical ward should receive IV ceftriaxone (2 g every 24 h) in combination with oral azithromycin or doxycycline at the doses listed above. All CAP therapy should last for 5–7 days, assuming clinical improvement.

Tuberculosis (TB)

Tuberculosis (TB) has been a scourge of military clinicians throughout the centuries. Today, it can be encountered in many theaters of operation. Latent TB is treated with rifampin, which is in the AMAL. Pulmonary TB may initially cause only mild symptoms including mild malaise and pleuritic chest pain, followed by progression to fevers, drenching night sweats, generalized malaise, or weakness. The focus for the maritime surgical team is recognition and diagnosis of TB, especially in patients with high suspicion (see Chap. 35 for discussion of the care of detainees). Oral treatment (multiple regimens with multiple weight-based agents) should be initiated promptly in probable cases. Since the typical military surgeon will have limited experience in the management of TB, consultation via ship's telephone (i.e., via ADVISOR) or electronic mail with ID specialists is advisable before initiating anti-TB therapy.

It is equally important to isolate the patient from others and to identify those with whom they have been in close contact. Instances of multi-drug resistant TB are increasing, though this will likely be identified by the receiving physicians once the patient has been evacuated. Consultation with preventive medicine on isolation and outbreak investigation at sea is also necessary; again, the ship's SMO is a resource in this setting. See Chap. 35.

Coronavirus Disease 2019 (COVID-19)

Recently, coronavirus disease 2019 (COVID-19) has become a great hindrance to military movement [7]. Treatment of the COVID-19 patient with acute respiratory distress syndrome (ARDS) is beyond the scope of this chapter, though the symptoms of COVID-19 are often mild in the typical military-aged individual. However, the patient must be placed in strict isolation, and quarantine must be considered for any other members who were in close proximity to the patient for two days prior to symptom onset. This will frequently include an entire crew of a ship or company in a field unit; a diagnosis of COVID-19 should be quickly routed through the chain of command (CoC).

Severe COVID-19, defined as evidence of pneumonia with hypoxemia (i.e., oxygen saturation (SaO2) of less than 94% on room air), may be treated with a combination of oral or IV dexamethasone (6 mg daily) and IV remdesivir. Dexamethasone is likely to be available in the deployed environment; some CVNs have now deployed with remdesivir onboard. It is acceptable to give dexamethasone without remdesivir in hypoxemic patients. However, most patients without hypoxemia do not benefit from steroids [8] or antivirals [9] (based on evidence at the time of this writing), and there is evidence of harm when steroids are administered to patients with normal peripheral saturation of hemoglobin (SpO2). Oral antiviral drugs, such as nirmatrelvir/ritonavir (Paxlovid) play a role in the treatment of mild-to-moderate COVID-19 for patients at high risk of progression, particularly unvaccinated patients and those with medical comorbidities. Monoclonal antibody treatments for ambulatory patients with COVID-19 have shown benefit, but the monoclonal landscape changes rapidly in light of emerging viral variants. Convalescent plasma preparations were widely used early in the pandemic but are not currently recommended.

Ultimately, the best therapy for COVID-19 is vaccination and prevention. The two mRNA vaccines (manufactured by Pfizer and Moderna) are highly effective and safe; additional vaccines, including adenovirus vector vaccines (manufactured by Johnson and Johnson and AstraZeneca) and protein subunit vaccines (manufactured by Novavax) are also likely to be effective. It is likely that all military members will be required to be vaccinated by the time of this publication. However, it is the duty of all medical officers to encourage immunization, both by word and by example.

Gastrointestinal Infections

Infections of the gastrointestinal tract and of the abdomen, in general, are an area of comfort for the deployed surgeon in regard to diagnosis and treatment. However, in the forward-deployed maritime setting, surgeons will find themselves without many of their usual diagnostic tools, such as computed tomography (CT) or ultrasonography performed by expert technicians. It is here where a clinician will need to rely upon their history and physical examination to arrive at the correct diagnosis.

Penetrating Abdominal Trauma

Abdominal trauma presents as an obvious source of infection for the deployed surgeon. Penetrating trauma violating the fascia will result in an exploratory laparotomy and a thorough evaluation of the abdominal cavity. Prophylactic antibiotics will be regularly utilized and tailored as the surgeon sees fit to the injuries they have cataloged.

Common Surgical Diagnoses

Common surgical diagnoses which the operational surgeon will encounter include appendicitis, cholecystitis, and diverticulitis. Acute appendicitis will undoubtedly be encountered by many deployed surgeons, though it may be at a time when surgery is impractical or impossible (see Chap. 14). The role of nonoperative appendicitis management has become a widely debated topic internationally and is best reserved for select patients. In the forward-deployed setting, appendicitis is ideally treated as a surgical emergency, and the patient should undergo an appendectomy or be transported to a location where operative intervention is possible. However, patients with appendicitis may not be on a submarine or ship with a surgeon present, or MEDEVAC to a surgeon may not be possible. In this situation, non-operative management of appendicitis is recommended, but the non-surgeon should do so in consultation with a surgeon.

While trials have shown the use of antibiotic-first appendectomy treatment in acute and uncomplicated appendicitis, a CT scanner would be required preoperatively to both make the diagnosis of uncomplicated appendicitis and select an appropriate patient [10]. Antibiotic choices vary between institutions. A typical intra-abdominal regimen includes IV ceftriaxone (2 g every 24 h) in combination with IV or oral metronidazole, with duration based upon clinical response. Also acceptable would be IV or oral fluoroquinolones like ciprofloxacin (400 mg every 12 h; 500–750 mg twice daily) plus IV or oral metronidazole. For broader coverage (if available), IV piperacillin-tazobactam (Zosyn) (3.375 g every 6 h) or IV ertapenem (1 g every 24 h) can be used as a first-line treatment. As surgery is the ideal treatment for appendicitis in the deployed setting for the young, healthy, active-duty service member, antibiotics should be seen as a bridge to surgical therapy and not a definitive treatment.

Often in the deployed environment, a patient with appendicitis presents with four days or more of pain and a history consistent with possible perforated appendicitis with a likely walled-off abscess. These patients typically have the standard periumbilical pain migrating to the right lower quadrant (RLQ) followed by a time interval of initial relief, then frank peritonitis followed by an improvement in symptoms as the small bowel or omentum walls off the abscess. Ileus and even symptoms of a small bowel obstruction (SBO) can occur from abdominal sepsis. Surgeon-performed POCUS may be helpful in diagnosing an intra-abdominal abscess. In the stable patient, IV fluid resuscitation and IV ceftriaxone and IV or oral metronidazole are appropriate with subsequent MEDEVAC of the ship when able. In general, in the expeditionary shipboard environment, only unstable patients with suspected perforated appendicitis should be operated on (see Chap. 14 for full discussion of the decision to observe, operate, or transfer). Finally, if non-operative management of appendicitis is performed for either complicated or uncomplicated appendicitis, interval appendectomy is recommended for active-duty sailors and Marines given the risk of recurrence during future deployments.

Cholecystitis may be frequently encountered, and its treatment as always will depend upon the severity of presentation. Simple biliary colic in-theater should respond to diet changes, with the plan for eventual surgical intervention post-deployment. Acute cholecystitis, concerns for emphysematous cholecystitis, or cholangitis will prompt initiation of antibiotics and possible surgery in-theater or emergent MEDEVAC (see Chap. 15 for an in-depth look at biliary disease for the maritime surgical team). Infections of the biliary tract should include anaerobic coverage. Cholangitis with evidence of shock may warrant IV meropenem if available (1–2 g every 8 h), though clearance of the common duct will be of the greatest priority. Regarding antibiotic choice, the following regimens could be considered:

- IV piperacillin-tazobactam (Zosyn)
- IV ampicillin-sulbactam (Unasyn)
- IV ceftriaxone plus IV or oral metronidazole
- IV or oral ciprofloxacin plus IV or oral metronidazole

Sigmoid diverticulitis in the acute setting is also a familiar diagnosis for most surgeons. Acute onset of left lower quadrant (LLQ) abdominal pain will prompt concerns for sigmoid diverticulitis, though, without the availability of a CT scan, this may become a clinical diagnosis. If the patient has a history of diverticulitis or a known history of diverticula on colonoscopy, the surgeon may be more reassured with the diagnosis. Empiric therapy with typical gastrointestinal antibiotics should result in clinical improvement within a few days. Worsening diverticulitis or non-responders may warrant MEDEVAC from the theater if stable for transfer. While sigmoid diverticulitis is most commonly encountered, remember that diverticula and diverticulitis can occur anywhere in the colon.

Diarrhea in the Returning Traveler

Service members on liberty, or otherwise interacting with the local environment, frequently present to the medical department with complaints of diarrhea. While distressing for the patient, these complaints are frequently short-lived and self-limited. Patients should be counseled that prevention is the best strategy: they should only eat well-cooked meals and consume bottled or boiled liquids.

Frequent causes of travelers' diarrhea include enterotoxigenic bacteria such as *Escherichia coli*, *Campylobacter jejuni*, *Shigella*, *Salmonella*, viruses such as norovirus, and amoebae such as *Entamoeba histolytica*, among others. The vast majority of these are self-limited and can be symptomatically treated with loperamide and rehydration. Moderate-to-severe diarrhea, including diarrhea that limits activities of daily living or is accompanied by fever or dysentery, may be treated empirically with oral azithromycin for three days; fluoroquinolones are no longer generally recommended due to high rates of resistance. It is generally acceptable to combine antibiotics with loperamide, even in cases of dysentery, and this combination has led to more rapid recovery time in deployed service members [11].

Ophthalmologic Injuries

Ophthalmologic injuries are infrequently encountered by trauma surgeons in the civilian environment and are another field where consultation with a subspecialist is appropriate. However, in the deployed setting, there will rarely be an available subspecialist. Non-penetrating injuries to the eye, including simple abrasions, may be covered with an erythromycin ophthalmic ointment (apply four times a day and as needed). Penetrating injuries are more significant, and the use of topical agents should be avoided until a discussion with an ophthalmologist. IV or oral levofloxacin (750 mg every 24 h), as well as IV vancomycin, will suffice until MEDEVAC and repair.

Skin Injuries and Infections

Burns

Burns are frequent concurrent injuries encountered in battlefield trauma. Loss of the protective epidermal layer will predispose these wounds to infection. Burn wounds and significant injury in the forward environment are unlikely to become infected at the initial point of presentation but are frequent during the MEDEVAC process to higher levels of care. Prophylactic care will ensure that these wounds are protected from eventual infection as these patients are transferred through the MEDEVAC system and undergo long-term rehabilitation.

Partial-thickness wounds can be dressed with topical antimicrobials such as silver sulfadiazine during daily dressing changes. If available, silver-impregnated dressings may be used and changed every 3–5 days, which may also help with patient comfort.

Deeper wounds, including deep partial-thickness burns and full-thickness burns, may be treated in the same fashion, though these will be best served with excision of tissue and skin grafting. As the forward-deployed shipboard environment is not ideal for skin grafting, MEDEVAC of these patients should be pursued for definitive care and the rehabilitation they will likely require. See Chap. 26 for an in-depth discussion of burn management.

Lacerations

Lacerations in the austere environment can rapidly progress from minimal issues to serious soft tissue infections which may necessitate MEDEVAC. Therefore, proper wound care is of the utmost importance in preventing infectious complications in war wounds. Thankfully, this is an area where most surgeons and surgical teams are comfortable.

Infection control begins with irrigation and debridement of the area. A bleach-based solution such as Dakin's solution is ideal, though potable water alone can be used if it is all that is available. Following thorough irrigation, the area should be debrided. The area should then be dressed and changed daily. Antibiotic coverage at the time of initial wound management may be IV cefazolin. If oral antibiotics are preferred, moxifloxacin or clindamycin (300 mg three times a day) are available [12].

For more broad coverage, IV ertapenem (if available) can be used as a first-line treatment, particularly in complex dirty wounds where the timing of MEDEVAC to definitive care is unknown. Given the broad spectrum of this agent, it is best to reserve it for more complex or severe infections.

In damp, aquatic, or humid jungle-like environments, or injuries occurring in fresh or saltwater, oral levofloxacin or oral doxycycline may cover aquatic pathogens such as *Vibrio* or *Aeromonas* species [13].

Necrotizing Soft Tissue Infections (NSTI)

A small inciting wound provoking overwhelming skin and soft tissue infections has been a feared and commonplace event throughout military medicine's history. What is labeled as "necrotizing fasciitis" can span a range of soft tissue infections, though true necrotizing fasciitis is a rare and quite deadly disease. These infections may be classified under the broader term of necrotizing soft tissue infections (NSTI). The cornerstone to the diagnosis of this lethal condition is a consistently high clinical suspicion. In some presentations, the affected skin may appear normal or slightly red, and an inciting wound may never actually be found. In other presentations, the skin may be grossly involved with overlying crepitus, bullae, and a grossly contaminated wound. The hallmark of presentation will be "pain out of proportion" upon examination of either of these presentations. Laboratory diagnostics which may help include serum sodium, serum creatinine, serum glucose, white blood cell (WBC) count, and C-reactive protein (i.e., the Laboratory Risk Indicator for Necrotizing Fasciitis (LRINEC) score) [14], though diagnostic studies should never create unnecessary delays to surgical debridement.

When suspected on a maritime platform, treatment should first consist of either surgical debridement or the very least an operative exploration of the wound by the surgical team with concomitant broad-spectrum antibiotic therapy and appropriate crystalloid resuscitation if indicated. On examination, there will be tissues easily broken-apart with finger sweeps, destruction of fascial planes, and turbid and likely foul-smelling "dishwasher fluid." When these findings are encountered, formal surgical debridement of all affected tissues is warranted with the frequent return to the OR for further debridement at regular intervals or sooner if clinical deterioration is noted. Broad-spectrum antibiotics are warranted; however, they do not take the place of wide surgical debridement to healthy tissue. Empiric antimicrobial therapy should cover staphylococci, streptococci, Gram-negative pathogens, and clostridia; it should also include a drug that inhibits bacterial exotoxin synthesis in group A streptococcal infection such as clindamycin or linezolid (only available orally and would likely need to be ordered separately from the AMAL at this time). Typical regimens available on board a warship to serve this purpose include:

- IV clindamycin plus IV vancomycin plus IV piperacillin-tazobactam (Zosyn)
- IV clindamycin plus IV ceftriaxone and IV metronidazole
- Oral linezolid plus IV piperacillin-tazobactam (Zosyn)
- Oral linezolid plus IV ceftriaxone and IV metronidazole

The deployed surgical team should do everything necessary to get urgent MEDEVAC for a patient with NSTI to an appropriate level of care. As continued debridement is likely necessary, temporary coverage should be performed. There is no clinical benefit to vacuum dressings, though they may be helpful for transport. Any dressing used must allow for monitoring of skin edges in case of progression of disease.

Vector-Borne Infections

Clinical Vignette 16.1

In 2003, a Marine Expeditionary Unit (MEU) was deployed to Liberia as additional security for the United States (U.S.) Embassy amid regional unrest. Upon returning to their ship, a significant number of Marines presented to the medical department with fever and diarrhea. Only through the diligence of the general surgeon attached to the embarked FST, who obtained and reviewed a peripheral blood smear, was the final diagnosis of Plasmodium falciparum *correctly established and the Marines evacuated to definitive care.*

The continued presence of U.S. forces in austere environments will always raise the concern for tropical infections, and the deployed surgeon must be vigilant in their workup and knowledgeable in their craft. Malaria is the most important parasitic disease for humans, with roughly 1 million deaths per year. *Plasmodium falciparum* remains the most common and deadly, with *Plasmodium vivax* being the next most common (and the dominant form of malaria in Afghanistan). The remaining species, *Plasmodium ovale*, *Plasmodium knowlesi*, *Plasmodium malariae*, and the recently described *Plasmodium simiae* make up the remaining cases.

Febrile patients with recent exposure to malaria-endemic regions have malaria until proven otherwise. Malaria may be difficult to diagnose initially, with nonspecific symptoms predominating the initial course, like in Clinical Vignette 16.1. Fatigue, myalgias, and headaches commonly precede fever. Severe disease may result in altered mental status, coma, anemia, renal failure, pulmonary edema and adult respiratory distress syndrome (ARDS), shock, convulsions, and bleeding with disseminated intravascular coagulation (DIC). Diagnosis may be via peripheral blood smear with identification of the parasite on a thin or thick smear or by use of whole blood rapid tests such as the BinaxNOW kits, which are widely available in deployed settings. Initially, negative smears should be repeated at 12-hour intervals for higher yield in the setting of continued clinical suspicion.

Given the high incidence of chloroquine resistance in *Plasmodium falciparum*, chloroquine is **not** the recommended empiric therapy for malaria in the absence of expert consultation. Mild to moderate cases of malaria in alert, ambulatory patients able to tolerate oral medications may be treated preferentially with oral artemether-lumefantrine (Coartem, 4 tablets initially in eight hours then twice daily on days 2 and 3); oral atovaquone-proguanil (Malarone, 4 tablets daily for three days) is an acceptable alternative if the preferred choice is unavailable [15].

Severe malaria is defined as malaria with signs of organ failure, including but not limited to delirium, hypotension, or acute kidney injury. The preferred therapy for severe malaria is IV artesunate with the duration of therapy depending on the severity of illness and parasitemia. If artesunate is not available, oral therapy as above should be started as a stop-gap measure. Immediate ID consultation is required upon diagnosis; the suspicion of malaria alone should prompt the maritime surgical team to seek the guidance of ID specialists. See Chap. 33 for an example of a mission anticipating severe malaria bringing and subsequently using IV artesunate during a humanitarian and disaster relief (HADR) mission.

The most effective treatment of malaria is prevention, and all units deploying to malaria-endemic regions should be provided with the recommended prophylactic medication, most often daily atovaquone/proguanil (Malarone) or doxycycline. In addition, vector avoidance, including the use of permethrin-treated clothing and the use of insect repellents on the skin, is necessary to reduce risk.

Other mosquito-borne infections, including dengue, Zika, and chikungunya, are similarly more common in the deployed environment or in the care of detainees or pirates (see Chap. 35). These viruses share overlapping clinical syndromes including fever, headache, rash, myalgia, arthralgia, and often subtle laboratory findings to include cytopenias and transaminase elevations. The primary preventive strategy for these infections is vector avoidance; there is a licensed dengue vaccine, but it is not currently recommended for military personnel due to limitations in its efficacy. Care is generally supportive and includes IV crystalloid resuscitation and acetaminophen. Corticosteroids are not effective, and nonsteroidal anti-inflammatory drugs (NSAIDs) should be avoided in suspected cases due to the risk of bleeding.

Severe disease due to dengue (and rarely Zika) often presents with hemorrhagic manifestations including petechiae and mucosal bleeding, along with signs of plasma leakage such as pleural effusions. Severe dengue is most often due to reinfection with a different dengue serotype following an earlier prior infection; as such, it is rare in US military personnel. Febrile disease with hemorrhagic manifestations should thus prompt immediate isolation and ID consultation due to concern for other viral hemorrhagic fevers, such as Lassa fever or Congo–Crimean hemorrhagic fever, the latter of which was responsible for at least one active-duty death in Operation Enduring Freedom.

Conclusion

This chapter serves as an introduction to the wide scope of infections that the surgical team may be asked to treat while underway. It is difficult to predict the entire range of infectious diseases that may be encountered at sea. Despite this, the goal remains the same: to recognize the severity of illness using limited tools, take the initial steps in stabilizing the patient using limited agents, and reach out for appropriate consultation when support is required to guide management. While the maritime surgical team is frequently alone, they are seldom far from advice if wise enough to seek it.

Declaration of Interest The views expressed in this chapter are those of the authors and do not necessarily reflect the official policy or position of the Department of the Navy, Department of Defense, nor the US Government.

Funding This research did not receive any specific grant from funding agencies in the public, commercial, or not-for-profit sectors.

Conflict of Interest Statement The authors declare no conflict of interest.

References

1. Tunkel AR, et al. Practice guidelines for the management of bacterial meningitis. Clin Infect Dis. 2004;39(9):1267–84.
2. Pouplin T, et al. Valacyclovir for herpes simplex encephalitis. Antimicrob Agents Chemother. 2011;55(7):3624–6.
3. DuBose J, et al. Development of posttraumatic empyema in patients with retained hemothorax: results of a prospective, observational AAST study. J Trauma Acute Care Surg. 2012;73(3):752–7.
4. Christie NA. Management of pleural space: effusions and empyema. Surg Clin N Am. 2010;90(5):919–34.
5. Sanchez JL, et al. Respiratory infections in the US military: recent experience and control. Clin Microbiol Rev. 2015;28(3):743–800.
6. Metlay JP, et al. Diagnosis and treatment of adults with community-acquired pneumonia. An official clinical practice guideline of the American Thoracic Society and Infectious Diseases Society of America. Am J Respir Crit Care Med. 2019;200(7):e45–67.
7. Vicente D, et al. US Navy's response to a shipboard coronavirus outbreak: considerations for a medical management plan at sea. Mil Med. 2021;186(1-2):23–6.
8. Horby P, Lim WS, et al. Dexamethasone in hospitalized patients with Covid-19. N Engl J Med. 2021;384(8):693–704. https://doi.org/10.1056/NEJMoa2021436.
9. Beigel JH, Tomashek KM, Dodd LE, et al. Remdesivir for the treatment of Covid-19 - final report. N Engl J Med. 2020;383(19):1813–26. https://doi.org/10.1056/NEJMoa2007764.
10. Salminen P, et al. Antibiotic therapy vs appendectomy for treatment of uncomplicated acute appendicitis: the APPAC randomized clinical trial. JAMA. 2015;313(23):2340–8.
11. Riddle MS, et al. Trial evaluating ambulatory therapy of travelers' diarrhea (TrEAT TD) study: a randomized controlled trial comparing 3 single-dose antibiotic regimens with loperamide. Clin Infect Dis. 2017;65(12):2008–17.

12. Barsoumian, Col Alice, et al. Infection prevention in combat-related injuries (CPG ID: 24).
13. Shackelford, Col Stacy. Acute traumatic wound management in the prolonged field care setting (CPG ID: 62).
14. Wong C, et al. The LRINEC (laboratory risk indicator for necrotizing fasciitis) score: a tool for distinguishing necrotizing fasciitis from other soft tissue infections. Crit Care Med. 2004;32(7):1535–41.
15. Taylor D, et al. Sepsis management in prolonged field care (CPG ID: 83). 2020.

Chapter 17
But…I'm a General Surgeon! Obstetric, Gynecologic, and Urologic Emergencies

Sheila Mulligan, Kristin M. DeSantis, Patrick L. Scarborough, and Amy A. Hernandez

Chance Favours the Prepared Mind
Louis Pasteur
We're surgeons. Sometimes wrong, but never unsure. Make a decision

CAPT (R) Rodd Benfield

Author deployment experience	
Sheila Mulligan	Battalion Surgeon, 9th Engineer Support Battalion, multiple operations, Okinawa, 2012–2013; Operation Guahan Shield, Guam; Cobra Gold and U.S. Humanitarian Mine Action Program, Thailand; Korea Military Exchange Program, South Korea
	Staff Obstetric and Gynecologic Surgeon, forward deployed Naval Hospital Yokosuka, 2017–2019
	Staff Obstetric and Gynecologic Surgeon, forward deployed Naval Hospital Rota, 2019–present
Kristin M. DeSantis	Staff Obstetric and Gynecologic Surgeon, Naval Hospital Camp Pendleton and 1st Marine Logistics Group, 2018–present
Patrick L. Scarborough	Human Intelligence Collector, 2nd Infantry Division, 8th U.S. Army and U.S. Army Special Operations Command, multiple deployments, Republic of Korea, 1997–2003
	Staff Urologic Surgeon, forward deployed Naval Hospital Guam, 2017–2019

S. Mulligan
Navy Medicine Readiness and Training Command Rota, Rota, Spain
e-mail: sheila.mulligan.mil@health.mil

K. M. DeSantis · P. L. Scarborough (✉)
Navy Medicine Readiness and Training Command Camp Pendleton, Camp Pendleton, CA, USA
e-mail: kristin.m.desantis.mil@health.mil; patrick.l.scarborough.mil@health.mil

A. A. Hernandez
Navy Medicine Readiness and Training Command San Diego, San Diego, CA, USA

M. D. Tadlock, A. A. Hernandez (eds.), *Expeditionary Surgery at Sea*,
https://doi.org/10.1007/978-3-031-21893-4_17

Author deployment experience	
Amy A. Hernandez	Battalion Surgeon, 7th Engineer Support Battalion, Operation Enduring Freedom, Camp Leatherneck, Afghanistan, 2011
	Ship's Surgeon, USS Carl Vinson (CVN-70), WESTPAC, INDOPACOM Area of Responsibility, 2017
	Department Head, Federal Emergency Management Agency (FEMA) and Defense Support of Civilian Authorities (DSCA), COVID-19 Community Vaccination Center mission, St. Louis, MO, USA, 2021

BLUF (Bottom Line Up Front)

1. Plan for pregnancy-related conditions prior to leaving port; despite rules against pregnancy at sea, it still occurs. A pregnancy test will shorten the differential.
2. There is typically personnel in many larger shipboard medical environments with labor management experience. Work together to optimize both maternal and fetal outcomes if a woman presents in labor.
3. If in breech and the baby needs to be rotated, grasp the baby by the hips, not the abdomen, to prevent fetal spleen laceration.
4. If in breech position and delivery is not imminent, do a cesarean. If a single hand or foot is presenting, do a cesarean.
5. Do not underestimate how much a laboring uterus can bleed; there is approximately 1 L of blood a minute being shunted to the uterus while the patient is in labor so she can bleed a lot and fast! Bimanual massage after delivery of the placenta is the first step in the prevention of postpartum hemorrhage (PPH).
6. In an emergent cesarean, making vertical lower midline skin, fascial, and uterine incisions provides quick access to the uterus. The surgeon should stand on the same side of the patient as their dominant hand (i.e., right-hand dominant surgeon stands on the patient's right side) so they can use their dominant hand to elevate and deliver the presenting part.
7. An ectopic pregnancy is a significant cause of maternal morbidity and mortality. Treatment at sea is surgical.
8. Physical exam and imaging can be inconclusive; do not let the skin get in the way if ovarian torsion is suspected. Do not excise an ischemic or necrotic ovary, as the majority of ovarian function will return.
9. Vaginal lacerations can result in vaginal hematomas, and vaginal hematomas can result in retroperitoneal bleeding. Take the patient with a vaginal laceration complaining of excessive pain and rectal pressure or becoming slightly unstable seriously.
10. Testicular torsion and testicular rupture are surgical emergencies. Do not wait for imaging to surgically explore if suspicion is high. Penetrating scrotal trauma requires exploration of both testicles.
11. Given the limited diagnostic abilities while deployed, if urethral injury is suspected given mechanism of injury and physical exam, place a suprapubic tube and plan a medical evacuation (MEDEVAC) for the patient.

Introduction

The gynecologic organs (uterus, ovaries, fallopian tubes, and vagina) are unique in that only a small percentage of service members have them. However, these organs come with their own set of pathologies that may require surgical treatment. While efforts are made to ensure pregnancy does not occur while underway, human factors are never completely controllable. Pregnancy needs to be considered in the differential for female service members presenting with pelvic pain with or without abnormal vaginal bleeding. Gynecologic case urgency ranges from the routine to emergent. It is important for the surgeon to maintain a broad differential to provide correct and competent care. While general surgeons can safely enter the abdominal cavity, there are nuances to laparoscopic port placements to optimize the approach to the pelvic anatomy. Most urologic surgical disease is not emergent, but a few emergencies require immediate intervention and familiarity. The goal of this chapter is to review obstetrical delivery and common gynecologic and urologic surgical diagnoses and treatments to prepare the expeditious maritime surgical team.

Female Reproductive Anatomy

While military general surgeons spend a lot of time in the abdomen, they do not typically spend a lot of time operating on the gynecologic organs. Here is a basic summary of female reproductive anatomy (see Fig. 17.1). Additionally, patient position is key for gynecologic exams.

- Uterus: Reproductive organ composed of a thick myometrium with a thin endometrial glandular layer. It is separated into the uterine corpus and cervix. The

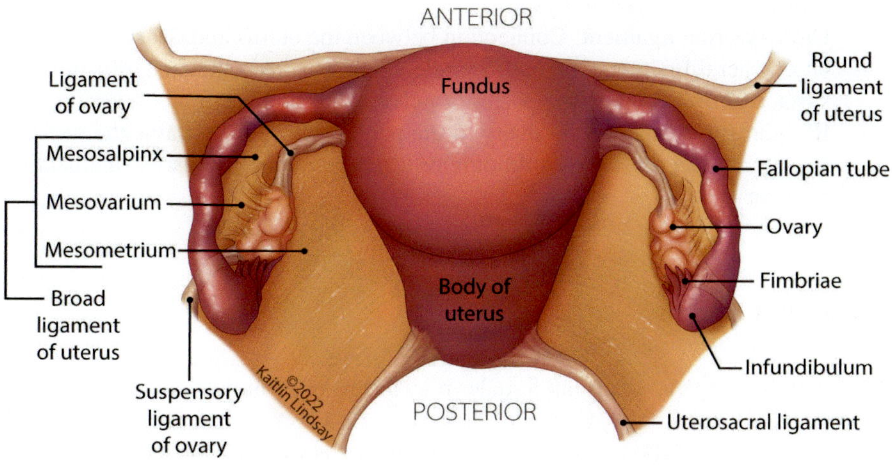

Fig. 17.1 Basic female reproductive anatomy (Source: Image Copyright 2022 Kaitlin Lindsay, used with permission)

uterine isthmus is the transition point between the corpus and cervix, as well as the endometrium and endocervix. The endometrium thickness changes throughout the menstrual cycle.

- Blood supply
  - Uterine artery: Primary blood supply to the uterus. It is a branch of the anterior internal iliac artery. It passes below the ureter before entering the uterus at the level of the cardinal ligaments at the uterine isthmus. The blood supply then separates into ascending and descending branches.
  - Ovarian artery: Supplementary blood supply to the uterus. It runs through the infundibulopelvic (IP) ligament.
  - Vaginal artery: Supplementary blood supply to the uterus.
- Ovary: Typically white in appearance with small follicles studding the surface. Ovarian cysts can be physiologic, benign, or malignant in nature. It is suspended by the utero-ovarian and IP ligaments. Only one ovary is needed to maintain fertility and hormonal physiologic support.
- Fallopian tube: Tubular structure extending from the uterine cornua to the ovary. It is composed of four components (proximal to distal): interstitial, isthmus, ampulla, and fimbriated end. Only one fallopian tube is needed to maintain fertility.
- Ligaments
  - Broad ligament: Double layer of peritoneum that extends from the lateral walls of the uterus to the pelvic walls.
  - Round ligament: Smooth muscle extension from the uterine cornua to the pelvic sidewall. It passes retroperitoneally through the inguinal canal to anchor on the labia majora. It may contain a small branch of the uterine or ovarian artery called the artery of Sampson.
  - Cardinal ligament: Perivascular connective tissue extending from the pelvic sidewall to the uterine isthmus to provide uterine support. It contains blood supply for the uterus and vagina.
  - Utero-ovarian ligament: Connection between the uterus and ovary.
  - Utero-sacral ligament: Smooth muscle extending from the posterior inferior surface of the cervix to the posterior pelvic walls and sacrum.
  - IP ligament: Suspends the ovary to the pelvic sidewall. Contains the ovarian vessels and nerves. Also commonly referred to as the suspensory ligament of the ovary.

Pregnancy at Sea

Prior to embarking underway, all females may have a urine human chorionic gonadotropin (HCG) test within 10 days of departure. However, not all pregnancies will be captured by this laboratory test if the pregnancy is early in conception. Once a patient is determined to be pregnant while underway, determine the gestational age of the pregnancy based on the approximate last menstrual period (LMP), timing of intercourse, and physical exam. Point-of-care ultrasound (POCUS) evaluation can then be used to determine location of the pregnancy (see Chap. 9 for a discussion of POCUS).

While sexual activity is not permitted underway, that in NO WAY means it is not happening, in particular during port/liberty when there are far more opportunities. A negative HCG test can be reassuring but does not rule out luteal phase pregnancy, so a good menstrual history can be helpful. While women often have a hunch that they are pregnant, the authors have also taken care of patients who may be hiding a possible pregnancy because they want to stay on deployment or to avoid perceived or potential disciplinary action depending on the circumstances.

Gestational week calculators are available to determine the estimated due date (EDD). On physical exam, the uterine height should be evaluated by palpating the abdomen. The uterus is a pelvic organ until approximately 12–14 weeks. A 20-week uterus will palpate approximately at the umbilicus. The fundal height can also be measured by calculating the distance from the pubic bone to the fundus in centimeters (i.e., 24 cm approximates 22–26 weeks pregnancy in a normally growing fetus).

Once an intrauterine pregnancy (IUP) is diagnosed, the patient is typically transferred off the ship at the next available opportunity. However, delivery at sea has occurred. A recent example in the media is of a Sailor reporting to the medical department with abdominal pain and no knowledge of her pregnancy and delivering a full-term baby hours later on the USS Dwight D. Eisenhower (CVN-69) in 2016 [1].

Once delivery is determined to be imminent, then the medical team should assemble a maternal team and a neonatal team. The maternal team is responsible for the delivery of the baby, delivery of the placenta, and monitoring postpartum bleeding; the maritime surgical team is most likely going to be a part of this team. The neonatal team is responsible for the resuscitation of the newborn. Blankets should be warmed in preparation for the infant. A clean sock can be used to cover the newborn's head and should also be warmed. Consultation with obstetrics and pediatrics is available via remote access (see Chaps. 5 and 14 for a discussion of resources like Advanced Virtual Support for Operational Forces (ADVISOR)) which should be engaged. On many platforms, there are family practice (FP) or emergency medicine (EM) physicians with more recent and thorough training in labor management than a general surgeon. Anesthesia providers, nurses, physician assistants, independent duty corpsmen (IDC), surgical technologists (STs), and general duty corpsmen all may also have prior labor deck experience. Everyone should work collaboratively to optimize the care of BOTH of the patients. Never forget to call for help!

Spontaneous Vaginal Delivery

The most likely situation is a patient that goes into labor with the fetus head down. When checking her cervix with a sterile glove, the hard, bony structures of the skull will be felt. If the amniotic sac is ruptured, hair may even be felt. In un-medicated labor, the patient will have uncontrollable shaking due to the hormone surges and will be relatively unable to not push during contractions. She may need to deliver in a squatting or kneeling position which is physiologically normal. When the head starts to separate the labia, gently place a gloved dominant hand over the perineum to protect it from tearing and a gloved non-dominant hand at the top of the fetal head by the urethra and clitoris.

As the head starts to deliver, gently protect the perineum anteriorly by the urethra and clitoris, as the fetal head can extend and tear the tissue. Once the head delivers, take a breath. Have the woman stop pushing for a moment. The head will restitute (rotate); feel for the umbilical cord at the neck. If there is a cord present, try to reduce it (i.e., gently pull it over the fetal head). If too tight and unable to reduce, deliver the remainder of the body through. Hold the baby by the head and apply downward traction until the anterior shoulder is visible, then guide the baby upward to deliver the posterior shoulder. Have the patient gently push to help deliver the remainder of the body, with care to protect the perineum so the arms and legs do not tear it. Place the baby onto the maternal abdomen and have the neonatal team stimulate, suction, and warm the baby.

In a hospital setting, the obstetric team usually waits 30–60 s before clamping the umbilical cord with two clamps, cutting in between them, and administering 10 units of intramuscular (IM) oxytocin (brand name: Pitocin). Oxytocin is currently on the aircraft carrier (CVN) Authorized Medical Allowance List (AMAL). The remaining umbilical cord can now act as a lever to help deliver the placenta. Place a towel over the pubic bone and provide suprapubic pressure over the abdomen with a gloved non-dominant hand while gently pulling on the cord to actively deliver the placenta. Cord lengthening and a gush of bright red blood indicate placental separation from the uterus. The entire placenta must be removed. Occasionally there are trailing membranes from the amniotic sac or a cotyledon that remains in the uterus. Facilitate delivery by using a ring forceps, twisting the membranes, or by placing a gloved dominant hand into the uterus and removing clots and remaining tissue.

Once the placenta is removed, provide uterine massage externally and bimanual massage internally to help regain uterine tone and decrease the chance of hemorrhage. Next, examine the perineum in a clockwise fashion looking for vaginal and perineal lacerations. Small, hemostatic lacerations near the urethra or on the labia minora do not need repair. If bleeding, use interrupted sutures to provide hemostasis with a delayed absorbable suture like polyglactin (i.e., Vicryl).

Perineal Laceration Repair

On the perineum, decide which type of laceration has occurred (Table 17.1) and repair as below. The first tenet of laceration repair is to stop the bleeding. Use pressure and interrupted or figure-of-8 sutures to stop pumping from exposed branches of the vaginal artery. Next, use the following recommendations to reapproximate the remaining tissues.

Table 17.1 Types of perineal lacerations

Degree of Laceration	Depth of Laceration
First degree	Vaginal mucosa
Second degree	Vaginal mucosa + vaginal muscles (STP + bulbous)
Third degree	Vaginal mucosa + vaginal muscles + EAS/IAS
Fourth degree	Vaginal mucosa + vaginal muscles + EAS/IAS + rectal mucosa

STP superficial transverse perineal, *EAS* external anal sphincter, *IAS* internal anal sphincter

- 1st degree lacerations
  - Suture: 3-0 or 4-0 absorbable synthetic like polyglactin suture on a CT-1 or SH. Chromic can also be used, but it has a slight increase in inflammation and irritation. These can also be closed with Dermabond if sutures are not readily available.
  - These lacerations only go through the vaginal mucosa, and if they are not bleeding and cosmetically look normal (remember, vaginal mucosa in a newly postpartum woman will be edematous), no intervention is required. If bleeding, repair with an interrupted figure-of-8 or running suture. While locking the suture for hemostasis is an option, use caution with this method at perineal skin as it can cause necrosis if the locking is excessive.
- 2nd degree lacerations
  - Suture: 2-0 or 3-0 absorbable synthetic like polyglactin suture on a CT-1.
  - As these lacerations tear through the bulbocavernosus and superficial transverse perineal (STP) muscles, there is a little bit more skill involved. The tear is typically in two planes thought of as two opposing triangles or as a diamond bent at a 90-degree angle, where the laceration changes planes with one triangle deep into the vagina and the other triangle on the perineal side. The authors will typically locate the apex in the vagina and place the anchoring suture 0.5 cm cephalad. Then re-approximate the vaginal mucosa and underlying tissue with a running, locked suture until the hymenal remnant is re-approximated (the blue-hued tissue close to the opening of the vagina). At this point, change planes and focus on re-approximating the bulbocavernosus and STP muscles with the crown-stitch; take the needle perpendicular to the plane of the body to ensure a good grasp on the muscle on each side. This will help re-approximate the muscles at the midline to decrease the chance of gaping introitus. Now, the perineal body can be re-approximated in a running manner, and the subcuticular skin can be closed with suture or Dermabond.
- 3rd degree lacerations
  - Suture: 2-0 or 3-0 delayed absorbable sutures like polyglactin or polydioxanone (i.e., PDS).
  - If it appears that the anal sphincter may be torn, a formal rectal exam may be needed to truly determine the degree of injury. If it is torn, the capsule of the

anal sphincter will have a ratty appearance to the fibers. If only a few fibers appear to be torn, reinforce the muscle with 0-Vicryl figure-of-8 sutures, placed in a horizontal manner to incorporate the tear. If there is a partial- or full-thickness tear, the authors prefer an end-to-end repair (as opposed to overlapping). Grasp the two ends with Allis clamps and use four separate sutures, which will be placed in a figure-of-8 fashion to re-approximate the muscles in the posterior-inferior-superior-anterior fashion. Do not tie down the sutures until the last suture is placed. After tying, perform a rectal exam to ensure rectal patency remains. Repair the remainder of the 2nd-degree laceration as described prior.

- 4th degree lacerations
  - Suture: 3-0 or 4-0 delayed absorbable polyglactin or chromic.
  - As with the discovery and repair of a 3rd-degree laceration, a rectal exam is necessary. If there is no identifying septum between the vaginal and rectum, there is a definite 4th-degree laceration. There will be a tear of the rectal mucosa, which is much smoother than the anal sphincters; use interrupted sutures to repair it and repair the remainder of the laceration as above.
- Note: Remember to replace the glove used for the DRE prior to finishing any repair or doing a vaginal exam. Consider 2 gm of intravenous (IV) cefoxitin for 3rd and 4th degree lacerations to decrease the risk of wound breakdown and infections.

Breech Presentations

If no fetal skull is felt when doing a cervical check and instead a squishy butt is felt or there is fecal matter on the glove, it is likely a breech presentation. The preferred and safest method is to bring the patient to the operating room (OR) for a cesarean (see section on cesarean delivery). If the fetus is either in complete breech or frank breech (legs crossed as if sitting on the ground or legs flexed at hips with both sets of ankles and toes near the head, respectively), then a vaginal delivery may be successful. **However, if a single foot or leg is hanging out of the vagina, this is an emergency! The fetus CANNOT deliver vaginally this way and an emergency cesarean delivery is necessary**.

The biggest risk with a breech delivery is fetal head entrapment. Take a breath and control the situation. Remember not to pull on the fetus. If the fetus needs to be rotated at any point, place hands at the bony prominences on the hips and rotate. The authors typically place their thumbs on the sacrum and forefingers on the iliac crests. **The fetal spleen can get lacerated if the abdomen is the point of rotation**.

The steps for vaginal delivery of a breech presentation are as follows:

1. Place mother in dorsal lithotomy position and bring her hips to the end of the bed or slightly over the end of the bed or table. This will provide the largest diameter

for hips and facilitate the easiest delivery to decrease body and head dystocia and to avoid delivering on the bed.

2. Determine that the baby is NOT in a jack-knife position (one leg presenting and the other leg either crossed or by the head), which requires cesarean delivery.
3. Have the patient push and deliver the fetal breech (the butt) in the sacrum anterior position, which is where the fetal spine is up toward the maternal urethra. If the baby is not in the sacrum anterior position, it can be gently rotated (*at the hips*) as described above.
4. If the hips and legs deliver spontaneously, then great. If they do not, follow up to the popliteal fossa, lightly grasp the femur, flex, and rotate away from midline to deliver the leg. To deliver the contralateral leg, rotate the fetus (*at the hips*) to facilitate easier palpation and delivery. This is called the Pinard maneuver.
5. Next, let the mom push until the bilateral scapula are present. Wrap a blue towel around the baby and support but DO NOT PULL ON THE BABY. It is hard to watch and wait during this time, but pulling will increase the risk of head entrapment.
6. If the arms do not deliver with maternal pushing efforts, rotate (*at the hips*) so that one shoulder is anterior and facing the urethra. Place fingers in and follow to the antecubital fossa, flex, swipe across the body, and deliver laterally. To deliver the other arm, rotate (at the hips) 180° and repeat the procedure. This is called the Loveset maneuver. It may be easiest to wrap the baby in a blue towel to help rotate.
7. For delivery of the fetal head, first, rest the body of the infant on the dominant forearm. Next, place index and middle fingers on the bilateral zygomatic processes (the cheeks) and flex the face down toward the fetal chest. Have an assistant place suprapubic pressure to flex the head forward. If the head does not easily deliver, give a uterine relaxant (i.e., IV nitroglycerin 100 mcg or IM terbutaline 0.25 mg) and try again. If this still does not work, use bandage scissors to cut the cervix via Duhrssen incisions (at 2, 6, and 10 o'clock). Remember that cervical branches come out at 3 and 9 o'clock on the cervix. These incisions can eventually be repaired once the baby is out with good visualization and 3-0 chromic in a running, locked fashion.
8. If the cervix was cut or if a uterine relaxant was given, prepare for postpartum hemorrhage (PPH).

Postpartum Hemorrhage (PPH)

One of the biggest risks after delivery is PPH; the most common etiology is lack of uterine tone. Other causes of PPH include trauma (inspect the perineum, vagina, and cervix), tissue (retained placenta), and coagulation defects (e.g., Von Willebrand's, disseminated intravascular coagulation (DIC)), described in Table 17.2. There is approximately 1 L of blood a minute being shunted to the uterus while the patient is in labor, so she can bleed a lot and fast! To combat

Table 17.2 4 Ts of postpartum hemorrhage (PPH)

Tone	Fundal massage, bimanual massage, uterotonic medications, uterine packing
Tissue	Remove entire placenta from uterus
Tear	Pack vagina or repair bleeding with sutures
Thrombin	Excessive bleeding can lead to disseminated intravascular coagulopathy (DIC)

Table 17.3 Uterotonic medications for use with postpartum hemorrhage (PPH)

Medication	Dose	Contraindications/considerations
Oxytocin (Pitocin)	10 U IM ×1 60-200 mU/min (10–40 U/1 L NS or LR)	Has ADH-like properties, so if rapid and undiluted IV use it can cause hyponatremia and hypotension
Misoprostol (Cytotec)	600 mcg buccal 800–1000 mcg rectal	Can cause fevers
Methergine	0.2 mg IM ×1 (can repeat ×1 in 30 min)	Contraindicated if cardiovascular disorder, hypertension, Raynaud's; not currently stocked on CVN AMAL
Hemabate	250 mcg IM every 15 min ×8	Contraindicated if reactive airway/asthma; can cause diarrhea; not currently stocked on CVN AMAL
Tranexamic acid (TXA)	1 g IV over 10 min (can re-dose in 30–60 min)	Not for atony, but will decrease blood loss

IM intramuscular, *NS* normal saline, *LR* lactated ringers, *ADH* antidiuretic hormone, *CVN* aircraft carrier, *AMAL* authorized medical allowance list, *IV* intravenous

hemorrhage, active management of the delivery of the placenta is recommended. After delivery of the placenta, infuse oxytocin (brand name: Pitocin) and the delivering provider should perform fundal massage with or without bimanual massage. Fundal massage is performed by covering the suprapubic area with a blue towel, cupping the top of the uterus (fundus), and rubbing aggressively. If bleeding continues, place a gloved dominant hand into the vagina and place a fist under the lower part of the uterus and cervix. Clamp the uterus between two hands and hold pressure. The majority of cases of PPH can be solved this way. Give available medications as described in Table 17.3. A common medication given in settings of PPH is IV tranexamic acid (TXA) 1 g over 10 min. This is an anti-fibrinolytic that will help decrease the amount of blood loss. However, it will not help regain uterine tone.

There are several ways to pack a uterus to help tamponade:

- Bakri balloon: Manufactured catheter with a balloon that can hold 500 mL of fluid. If available, it is placed into the uterus and filled with normal saline to tamponade. It can be left in place for 12–24 h, which is hopefully enough time to arrange for a medical evacuation (MEDEVAC). Unfortunately, it is not likely to be available in a maritime OR.
- Foley catheter with condom: "MacGyver" alternative to a Bakri. Inflate the bulb for the Foley catheter and then place a sterile condom over the end of the catheter.

Use silk or other suture to close the end of the condom over the catheter so that fluid does not leak out. The condom can be filled with up to 300 mL of normal saline (NS) or lactated ringers (LR), and this will ensure that it does not leak out. Place a hand into the uterus with the Foley and condom attached. Keep a hand inside the uterus while filling the condom through the urine drainage port with a Toomey syringe. Prepare for MEDEVAC as described with the Bakri balloon.

- Packing: Grab kerlix or lap pads and pack them as tight as possible into the uterus, making sure to count how many were placed. If anything is placed into the uterus for tamponade, place a black band (or any kind of identifying marking) on the patient's wrist to signify a foreign object is in place, and place a Foley catheter.
- **If bleeding from atony does not stop, go to the OR and consider a hysterectomy!**

If the uterus is firm but the patient is still bleeding, it can be a result of retained placental tissue. Look at the placenta and see if there are any missing pieces. Place the dominant hand through the dilated cervix into the uterus and remove tissue. This task is easier if the non-dominant hand directs the fundus externally. A sharp curettage can be performed, but this is typically done under POCUS guidance because the uterine muscle is thin at this point and the risk of perforation and damaging internal viscera is elevated.

As above in the delivery explanation, assess the perineum, vagina, and cervix for bleeding. Occasionally there are large pumping vessels. Remember that direct pressure can help in the interim. Get good visualization by disarticulating a speculum and using the bottom part for retraction or use Deavers, Sims, right-angle retractors, or half of a speculum. If she is still bleeding after any perineal bleeding is repaired, assess the cervix by using two ring forceps and walking around the cervix in a clockwise manner. Bleeding cervical lacerations are often repaired with 3-0 chromic in a running, locked fashion.

Lastly, consider bleeding disorders, most specifically DIC, which requires blood products quickly! On many platforms, this will require activation of the walking blood bank (WBB). O-negative is preferred if the blood type is unknown or if the patient is Rh-negative. See Chap. 23 for an in-depth discussion of the WBB.

Delayed Placental Removal or Avulsed Cord

If the placenta does not deliver by 30 min or if the umbilical cord avulsed from the placenta while attempting to actively deliver it, the surgeon must attempt manual removal of the placenta. Place the dominant gloved hand into the uterus and attempt to find a plane between the placenta and uterine tissue. Slide that hand in between that plane while stabilizing the uterus externally with the non-dominant hand; it should start to peel off like cellophane. Grab the placenta and twist to remove. Try to deliver the placenta intact, as there will be less bleeding and the entire placenta will deliver more easily. If it comes out in pieces, keep sweeping and trying to remove it. If a POCUS is available, that can help guide the sweeping motions or guide careful curettage as discussed prior. If all the tissue cannot be removed and she continues to bleed, place a Bakri balloon or another form of uterine packing in order to tamponade and MEDEVAC to a higher level of care.

Cesarean Delivery

There are specific reasons to proceed with cesarean delivery. Emergency situations include umbilical cord prolapse, placental abruption, placenta previa (placenta is covering the cervical os), and incomplete breech as described previously. If complete or frank breech and not imminently delivering, perform a cesarean to avoid the risks associated with head entrapment. Another indication includes arrest of dilation where the cervix has not changed or the patient has pushed for greater than 3–4 h.

If the situation is emergent due to maternal hemodynamic instability, active hemorrhage due to placental abruption, placenta previa, or uterine rupture, the book answer is to prep the abdomen quickly with betadine (dump the bottles over the abdomen in the place of the planned incision) and move forward with a low vertical midline incision on the abdomen. Not only is this a familiar incision for the average general surgeon and surgical team, but with this approach, the rectus muscles can be separated at the midline, the peritoneal cavity can be bluntly entered with a finger, and the rectus muscles can be spread laterally, providing good and quick access to the uterus. If the surgeon is right-hand dominant, then they should stand on the maternal right (vice versa for left-hand dominant). This may be different from the normal operating position, but it is important to use the dominant hand to elevate and deliver the fetal presenting part.

If the situation is urgent or routine, prep the abdomen with an alcohol-based skin cleanser like chlorhexidine. Current recommendations are to give IV cefazolin 2 g within 30 min of skin incision (for penicillin/cephalosporin allergy, alternate regimen is IV clindamycin 900 mg and IV gentamicin 5 mg/kg). If she has been laboring, add IV azithromycin 500 mg given over 1 h. All medications are currently available on the CVN AMAL except the IV azithromycin (see Chap. 16). Add sequential compression devices (SCDs) for venous thromboembolism (VTE) prophylaxis. Neuraxial anesthesia is typically preferred over general endotracheal anesthesia if possible, due to maternal and fetal risks with intubation and inhaled anesthetics. Place a Foley into her bladder once she is numb.

If the surgeon feels comfortable, perform a Pfannenstiel skin incision, enter the peritoneal cavity, and visualize the uterus. Expose the uterus by using a self-retaining retractor like an Alexis (medium size typically works well if available) or a Richardson placed cephalad and a bladder blade placed caudad. The surgeon should place the dominant hand inside the abdomen to feel the presenting part (usually the head), get a general idea of how big the baby is to help ensure that the sizes of the skin and fascial incisions are adequate to deliver the baby, and rock the body to see the movement needed for delivery.

A midline vertical uterine incision will be the easiest to deliver from for a surgeon with less experience with cesareans, as it gives the most exposure. The muscle is thicker closer to the fundus, so it will take longer to get through and to repair (typically performed in two layers). Obstetricians will typically make a low transverse incision at term, which gives the patient the opportunity to labor for her next pregnancy and is a quicker incision to close; however, it does take more skill and comfort to deliver the baby. To do this technique, make a semi-lunar horizontal incision of approximately 2–3 cm length and *take care* to avoid extending it through the uterine arteries at the lateral aspects of the uterine isthmus. Be cognizant that if a patient has had a prior cesarean delivery, her bladder serosa may be very adherent to the lower uterine segment and there is also danger in cutting or tearing through this!

When making the uterine incision, be careful to avoid cutting the baby. Use the back of the scalpel or the Yankauer suction to bluntly enter the uterus after thinning it out in order to avoid this. Then place two fingers into the hysterotomy and extend cephalad to caudad. As stated prior, the surgeon should place their dominant hand into the uterus, elevate the presenting part (without flexing the wrist), and bring it to the hysterotomy. The assistant surgeon should push on the fundus of the uterus with a CONSTANT pressure. This is NOT the time to mimic contractions with multiple small pushes; constant pressure is needed to facilitate delivery.

Head down: Once the head is delivered, gently place pressure in a downward motion to deliver the anterior shoulder, then move upward to deliver the posterior shoulder. Following this, deliver the baby onto the surgical field.

Breech: Refer to the vaginal breech section for the basic tenets of breech delivery. In brief, keep the sacrum anterior and deliver each leg by flexing at the popliteal fossa and hip, and sweep out. Place a thumb and forefinger *on each boney hip* to help guide the body out while the assistant surgeon is providing fundal pressure. The body may need to be rotated once at the scapula to deliver the arm (flex at the antecubital fossa, bring down and sweep laterally across the body). Rotate the body 180° (at the hips) and perform a similar procedure to deliver the contralateral arm. For the fetal head, the surgeon should place index and middle fingers on the zygomatic processes to flex the head while the assistant surgeon is helping flex with external pressure on the uterus at its occiput. Deliver the baby onto the surgical field.

If the baby has good tone and is making a crying effort, delay clamping the umbilical cord for 30–60 s. Stimulate and suction nose and mouth. Once ready, clamp the cord twice then cut across with bandage scissors. Pass the baby off of the surgical field to the neonatal team.

Once the baby is out, the next step is delivering the placenta. Place the nondominant hand onto the fundus of the uterus and place gentle traction onto the clamped umbilical cord. It should separate easily. If not, place the dominant hand into the uterus, find the plane, and separate the placenta off of the uterine wall. Check to ensure the placenta has been removed in its entirety then pass it off the field. Grab one moist and one dry lap, both completely opened. Exteriorize the uterus, wrap the uterus in the moist lap (laparotomy sponge) and use the dry lap to cover the fingers of the surgeon's dominant hand. Place the lap-wrapped hand into the uterus and into the cervix to wipe/remove the remaining placenta or placental fragments. This process can also be facilitated with a ringed forceps.

Once the placenta is completely removed, turn all efforts to quickly closing the hysterotomy. Replace the bladder blade. Use a 0-Vicryl on CTX (Circle Taper Extra Large) in a running, locked suture. Take care to ensure the lateral edges are closed because, again, the uterine arteries can continue to bleed. Once the first layer is complete, imbricate in a horizontal or vertical manner with another 0-Vicryl or 0-Monocryl for hemostasis and sturdiness or help hemostasis with multiple figure-of-8 sutures. Now feel behind the uterus and take a Poole-tipped suction to remove excess fluid. Place the uterus back into the abdomen. Re-examine and ensure the hysterotomy and bladder serosa are not bleeding. Wipe or suction the bilateral gutters. Turn attention to the rectus and ensure hemostasis. Most obstetricians will not re-approximate the rectus abdominal muscles, and only some will re-approximate the peritoneum. Close the fascia with a running, non-locked fashion with a delayed absorbable suture like 0-Vicryl or #1 PDS. If the subcutaneous tissue of the abdominal wall is greater than or equal to 2 cm in depth, re-approximate with 3-0 Vicryl. Close the subcutaneous tissue and then place either pressure dressing or Dermabond.

Gynecologic Emergencies

Ectopic Pregnancy

Clinical Vignette 17.1

A 28-year-old woman presented to an CVN medical department with abdominal pain and vaginal bleeding. She was hemodynamically unstable on presentation. Her HCG test was positive. The surgeon performed a Focused Assessment with Sonography in Trauma (FAST) exam with POCUS which was positive and consistent with blood throughout the abdomen. The WBB was activated, and she received four units of fresh whole blood (FWB).

Exploratory laparotomy was performed and upon opening of the peritoneum, she became unstable initially requiring blood resuscitation and intermittent vasopressor support. After packing off the abdomen and evacuation of hemoperitoneum, findings consistent with a ruptured right tubal ectopic pregnancy were identified. Open salpingectomy was performed. She made a full recovery and returned to full duty six weeks after the incident.

Approximately 2% of all known pregnancies are ectopic pregnancies. Ruptured ectopic pregnancies continue to be a significant cause of pregnancy-related morbidity and mortality. 90% of ectopic pregnancies occur in the fallopian tube. Alternate sites include the abdomen (1%), cervix (1%), ovary (1–3%), and cesarean scar (1–3%). An ectopic pregnancy can occur simultaneously with an IUP, with an incidence of 1 in 4000 to 1 in 30,000 in spontaneously occurring pregnancies.

Ectopic pregnancies are suspected by history and physical exam. Definitive diagnosis is made with surgery and pathologic diagnosis of products of conception outside the uterus. Symptoms of an ectopic pregnancy include vaginal spotting or bleeding, abdominal pain that is typically unilateral in nature, and/or signs of peritonitis/surgical abdomen if rupture has occurred. Hemodynamic instability can also be found with profound rupture and hemorrhage. If an ectopic pregnancy is considered after confirming pregnancy with a positive HCG test, an abdominal POCUS can be performed to attempt to locate the pregnancy. The uterus and adnexa should be evaluated for a gestational sac, yolk sac, fetal pole, and possible cardiac activity; see Chap. 9 for more details on how to use POCUS for this indication. **If these structures are identified outside the uterus, then surgical treatment should be pursued as medical management is not typically available while remote from a medical treatment facility (MTF)**. If time permits and it is available, consultation with an obstetrician is recommended. Obviously the patient presented in the clinical vignette, was a surgical emergency, and emergent laparotomy was warranted.

Surgery can be performed with laparoscopy or laparotomy; the route should be chosen by the surgeon with consideration to the patient's hemodynamic status, available resources, and surgical team experience. The minimally invasive approach is preferred unless hemodynamic instability is encountered, as seen in Clinical Vignette 17.1. Salpingostomy and salpingectomy have similar fertility outcomes, however, salpingectomy is preferred with complete removal of the fallopian tube if the contralateral fallopian tube is normal in appearance. If the contralateral tube is not normal in appearance, salpingostomy may be attempted to preserve fertility, but it does have a risk of scarring and future ectopic pregnancy that a salpingectomy would not incur.

Once the abdomen has been entered, explore the abdomen and pelvis. Place the patient into the Trendelenburg position and sweep the bowel. Blood may need to be suctioned. The uterus, fallopian tubes, and ovaries should be identified. Typically, the ectopic pregnancy is visible as a violaceous bulge in the fallopian tube. The tube may be ruptured or have bleeding from the distal end. The pregnancy may be expelled from the fallopian tube, and it is typically then found in the posterior cul-de-sac.

Laparoscopic salpingectomy: Port placement for gynecologic surgery typically consists of a 5 or 10 mm umbilical port with 5 mm ports in bilateral lower quadrants approximately 2 cm anterior and medial to the anterior superior iliac spine (ASIS). Place the lateral ports with care to avoid the inferior epigastric artery. Once the ectopic pregnancy and fallopian tube are identified, place the affected tube on tension by grasping the fimbriated end. Use a bipolar device (e.g., LigaSure) to clamp the mesosalpinx while attempting to hug the fallopian tube. After activation and transection, repeat the same process of clamp, burn, cut. The proximal end of the fallopian tube is typically coagulated twice before transection. Inspect the mesosalpinx for hemostasis. The specimen can be removed in a bag-removal device through a 10 mm port and sent to pathology. If no bipolar energy device is available and the mesosalpinx does not look very vascular, then one option is to cauterize along the fallopian tube using traditional Bovie electrocautery (the technique similar to doing a pediatric appendectomy) and place a PDS endoloop on the proximal fallopian tube, however, if any doubt or lacking appropriate tools, the safest option is laparotomy and salpingectomy.

Laparotomy with salpingectomy: Once the ectopic pregnancy and fallopian tube are identified, elevate the affected tube with distal and proximal Babcock clamps to place the mesosalpinx on tension. Beginning at the fimbriated end of the tube, place one Kelly clamp or hemostat across a 2 cm section of the mesosalpinx hugging the fallopian tube. Place a second clamp similarly across the mesosalpinx near the ovary. Transect the mesosalpinx with scissors. Tie the ovarian pedicle with 2-0 or 3-0 delayed-absorbable suture, and remove the clamp. The clamp on the fallopian tube side remains. Repeat the process of clamp, cut, tie to the cornua. Place the final clamp across the proximal mesosalpinx and fallopian tube, cut, and similarly tie. Inspect the adnexa for hemostasis and send the specimen to pathology.

If salpingostomy is attempted, grasp the fallopian and put on tension. Make a 1–2 cm incision lengthwise across the ectopic pregnancy. Gently grasp and remove the products and send as a specimen. Achieve hemostasis with electrocautery. Leave the tube to heal by secondary intention.

Ovarian Torsion and Ruptured Hemorrhagic Cysts

Clinical Vignette 17.2

A 24-year-old nulliparous female with an LMP of 25 days prior presented with acute right lower quadrant (RLQ) pain. She was not using contraception and denied recent sexual intercourse. Her pain began acutely 3 h ago, colicky in nature with a severity of 10/10 at peak pain. She had intermittent nausea and vomiting associated with the severe pain. She had no significant medical or surgical history. Abdominal exam was notable for normoactive bowel sounds, tenderness to palpation in bilateral lower quadrants, and positive guarding and peritonitis.

HCG test was negative. POCUS was negative for intra-peritoneal fluid, however a 6 cm mass with mixed echogenicity was noted in the RLQ.

Concern was high for ovarian torsion so the patient underwent diagnostic laparoscopy. On examination of the pelvis, the right ovary was torsed and dusky in appearance. An ovarian cyst was found; cystectomy was performed. Intraoperative rupture was notable for yellow-green mucus and hair, confirming the diagnosis of dermoid cyst (mature teratoma).

Symptomatic ovarian cysts can arise causing abdominal pain, discomfort, and pressure; however, these are typically not surgical emergencies. If a hemodynamically stable woman presents with acute onset abdominal pain, negative HCG, and free fluid in the pelvis with an adnexal mass on POCUS, then a ruptured hemorrhagic cyst may be suspected. Most hemorrhagic cysts can be treated with nonsteroidal anti-inflammatory drugs (NSAIDs), acetaminophen, and narcotics as needed. However, if the patient experiences hemodynamic instability, then surgical intervention should be considered to achieve hemostasis.

The need for a more urgent/emergent ovarian cystectomy may also arise in the case of ovarian torsion. When ovarian cystectomy is pursued, the goal is to remove the cyst with the preservation of as much normal ovarian tissue as possible. Most cystectomies can be performed safely with laparoscopy, however larger ovarian cysts (>10 cm) may need laparotomy.

If a woman presents with acute abdominal or pelvic pain, associated nausea and vomiting, and negative HCG with an adnexal mass typically >5 cm, then ovarian torsion should be considered as part of the differential. Physical exam and adjuncts like POCUS cannot definitively rule out the diagnosis. Ovarian torsion is a surgical emergency, and diagnostic laparoscopy is warranted if it is suspected. A common cause of ovarian torsion are dermoid ovarian cysts given the inherent differences in tissue density that increase the propensity to torse, similar to the patient in Clinical Vignette 17.2. Cysts >5 cm increase the risk for torsion, regardless of the cyst appearance. Other adnexal masses can also present with torsion, such as large paratubal cysts. The goal of surgery is to detorse the ovary, restore normal anatomy, and remove any cause of torsion like a cyst. **The ovary should not be removed, even in the setting of ischemia or necrosis, as ovarian function is preserved in 90% of cases at 3 months after surgery**.

As with ectopic pregnancy, minimally invasive or open surgery can be performed, taking into consideration the patient's hemodynamic status, available resources, and surgical team experience. The minimally invasive approach is preferred, unless hemodynamic instability is encountered. Port placement is similar to described above with a 5 or 10 mm umbilical port and 5 mm ports in bilateral lower quadrants. Once the abdomen has been entered, explore the abdomen and pelvis and identify anatomy. Place the patient into the Trendelenburg position and sweep the bowel. Blood may need to be suctioned.

Once the ovarian cyst is identified, normal anatomy should be returned in the case of ovarian torsion. Make an incision along the antimesenteric side of the affected ovary with either a scalpel or electrocautery. The placement of the incision here is to minimize dissection into the vessels at the ovarian hilum. The incision should be deep enough to encounter the cyst wall without rupture. Use sharp and blunt dissection to remove the overlying ovarian stroma from the cyst next. Place Allis clamps along the ovarian stroma to gently pull the stroma from the cyst wall. Use of the principles of traction and countertraction will assist with dissection. Once the hilum is reached, increased bleeding should be expected. If an intraoperative rupture is encountered, the pelvis should be thoroughly irrigated. After the cyst wall is removed, trim excess ovarian stroma to assist to return normal anatomy. If the ovarian hilum is hemostatic, suture may not be needed. If ongoing bleeding persists, then close the hilum in layers using 3-0 or 4-0 delayed-absorbable suture. Care should be taken to avoid sutures on the exterior of the ovarian stroma, as it promotes adhesions. Once hemostasis is achieved, place the adnexal structures into their anatomic positions. There is no need to perform an oophoropexy procedure to affix the ovary to the sidewall to prevent future torsion.

Straddle Injuries/Vaginal Lacerations

The most common mechanism of injury for a straddle injury on a ship is falling and hitting the perineum with excessive force, which can occur in a variety of locations from one of the many ladderwells or from the top rack in a three-person stacked berthing. Like injuries to the face, this area can bleed a lot because it is so well vascularized.

Small areas on the vulva can be re-approximated with Dermabond, but larger lacerations with muscle involvement or extensive bleeding will require formal suture repair.

First, determine where the injury is. Most commonly, it will be the labia which can be infiltrated with local anesthetic, cleansed, and closed using a series of interrupted or running locked sutures (the authors prefer 2-0 or 3-0 polyglactin suture). If it is on the posterior fourchette, this area will likely be bruised and painful, but the same suture can be used to repair it. If a laceration is close to the urethra, place a Foley catheter into the urethra during the repair to ensure the lumen is not compromised during the repair. If the laceration is close to the clitoris, try to use as little suture as possible and only repair areas for hemostasis. Scar tissue, structuring, and chronic pain can occur from laceration repairs in this area. As described in the Obstetrics section, a vulvar laceration is fairly self-limited. Swelling and hematoma can occur, but this can be treated with ice and direct pressure. It does not need to be opened and explored.

If there is a perineal laceration, see the obstetrics section for details on repair.

If there is a vaginal laceration (think about falls and sexual assault, e.g.), make sure that there is adequate visualization. The speculum can be taken apart and used as a speculum if needed. If the laceration can be visualized, repair it with local anesthetic. Cleanse the vagina with betadine. Heaney needle drivers are useful in deep areas of the vagina. Repair with interrupted figure-of-8 or running locked sutures. If the laceration cannot be visualized and/or the bleeding is extensive, pack the vagina with kerlix (can place Premarin or lubrication) and bring the patient to the OR. Use Deavers, Sims, right-angle retractors, or half of a speculum to assist in visualization.

Watch patients with vaginal lacerations carefully, as vaginal lacerations can result in vaginal hematomas, and vaginal hematomas can result in retroperitoneal bleeding. If the laceration seems superficial and the patient is hemodynamically stable, vaginal packing is not necessary. If there is concern about a hematoma, pack the vagina as stated above. **These patients can bleed large volumes into the retroperitoneum before they become unstable, so if they are complaining of excessive pain, rectal pressure, or are becoming slightly unstable, take this seriously**. Feel the vagina for fullness, do serial exams and vitals, and have a low threshold for formal exploration. If there is a concern for a retroperitoneal bleed that is not controlled, the gynecologist would call the general surgeon, so the maritime surgical team should feel comfortable proceeding without further discussion in this chapter.

Bartholin's Cyst and Abscess

A Bartholin's cyst is a common female genital "bump" that causes patients to present for medical care. The glands are located at the 4 o'clock and 8 o'clock positions of the vaginal opening, and their function is to lubricate the vulva and vagina and secrete mucus. To identify a Bartholin's cyst, place one digit into the opening of the vagina to palpate a discrete, well-circumscribed mass in the appropriate location. If there is no evidence of infection and it is not too painful, a cyst can often be treated expectantly with Sitz baths and warm compresses. However, this is quite difficult to accomplish in the not-so-private heads (bathrooms) of a ship.

While a cyst is not an emergency, it can develop into an abscess. If it looks infected or if the patient has significant pain and it continues to grow despite expectant management, there are a few available operative options (Table 17.4).

First is the classic incision and drainage, start by placing the patient in the low lithotomy position. Cleanse the area with betadine, pull the Bartholin's gland into view with one hand (place index finger into vagina and grasp between index finger and thumb). Take an 11-blade scalpel and make a stab incision through the vaginal mucosa and cyst wall immediately inside the hymenal ring. Drain area, break up loculations and irrigate with normal saline (the 10 mL pre-packaged syringes work well for this). Incision and drainage are easy and can be done with minimal local anesthetic, however, the recurrence rate is much higher than with other methods.

Another option with a lower recurrence rate is doing an incision and drainage then leaving a drain. The best drain for this is a Word's catheter (not usually in the AMAL) if the patient does not have a latex allergy. Fill a Word's catheter with 3–5 mL of saline via a 25-gauge needle placed into the catheter. Place the balloon portion into the stab incision after irrigation (do not make the incision too big or the catheter will fall out immediately), and introduce saline through the needle, remove the needle, and tuck the end of the Word's catheter into the vagina. The concept behind a Word's catheter is that a tract epithelializes and eventually pushes the catheter out. If it does not fall out on its own by 4 weeks, remove it once the tract has epithelialized.

Another option is marsupialization. Classically, these are done in the OR under general anesthesia but can certainly be done in a non-OR setting with good local anesthesia and proper patient selection. Plan for the incision to be 2–3 cm directly inside the hymenal ring in the vagina to hide the incision. Infiltrate local anesthetic then pull the gland to the surface with thumb and forefinger. Make an elliptical incision with a 15-blade scalpel through the vaginal mucosa and then the cyst wall.

Table 17.4 Treatment of Bartholin's cyst and abscess

Expectant (warm compresses, Sitz baths, ± antibiotics)
Incision and drainage
Incision and drainage with Word's catheter placement
Marsupialization
Excision *NOT TO BE DONE ON SHIP*

Drain area, break up loculations and irrigate as stated previously. Use a series of interrupted 2-0 delayed absorbable sutures (like polyglactin) to suture vaginal mucosa to cyst wall, leaving cyst open to re-epithelialize.

Lastly, Bartholin's gland excisions are only performed if marsupialization fails a few times; do NOT try this on a ship. Branches of the pudendal artery sit behind the cyst and can bleed enormously. Leave this for board-certified gynecologists in an OR at an MTF.

Aftercare includes 2 weeks of vaginal rest: no tampons, no intercourse, no baths. They are usually polymicrobial (so cultures are not helpful) but consider a Methicillin-resistant *Staphylococcus aureus* (MRSA) swab and gonorrhea/chlamydia polymerase chain reaction (PCR), as the population is at high risk for both.

Lastly, Bartholin's cysts are rarely cancerous. If the patient is a woman who is over 40 years or if suspicious for malignancy (fixed, solid mass, or palpable mass within the cyst), biopsy the back wall of the cyst. The average age of Bartholin's malignancy is about 57 and is typically adenocarcinoma.

Male Genital Emergencies

Testicular Torsion

Clinical Vignette 17.3

A 22-year-old male presented to sick call on a CVN with complaints of acute onset of right-sided testicular pain approximately 2 h prior. He states that the pain began without warning and was the most severe pain he has ever experienced in his life. It stopped him in his tracks and he had to sit down for about 10 min. He then attempted to walk the pain off. However, it continued to worsen. Vital signs were normal except for an elevated heart rate to 110. On physical exam, the patient's right testicle was swollen, lying in a somewhat horizontal fashion, and seemed to be somewhat higher than the left. It was exquisitely tender, and he cursed constantly during the examination. A POCUS confirmed ongoing but relatively decreased blood flow to the right testicle as compared to the left.

He went to the OR for immediate surgical exploration, detorsion of the right testicle, and right orchiopexy. Postoperatively his pain was completely resolved. He recovered uneventfully and went on to finish the deployment.

Testicular torsion is one of the few true urologic emergencies and occurs in approximately 1 in 4000 males younger than the age of 25. Signs and symptoms are classically described as a sudden onset of intense, one-sided testicular and scrotal pain, severe enough at times to cause the patient to be unable to stand or move, although this is not always the case. This is often accompanied by nausea and emesis. The scrotum is generally significantly swollen and edematous on the affected side, with obvious erythema noted. A "high-riding" testicle is usually seen, as demonstrated in Clinical Vignette 17.3. The cremasteric reflex is sometimes absent, although the presence or absence of this reflex should not be considered diagnostic.

Diagnosis is based on the history and physical exam. If a POCUS is readily available, it may be performed; however, treatment should never be delayed in order to obtain imaging in cases with a high suspicion of torsion. POCUS will show decreased or absent blood flow to the affected testicle when compared to the contralateral side. See Chap. 9 for a discussion of technique and sample images of normal and torsed testicles on POCUS.

Testicular torsion can masquerade as orchitis, epididymitis, torsion of a testicular or epididymal appendage, or even as a varicocele. If increased blood flow to the affected testicle is seen, the diagnosis is orchitis. For orchitis, no surgical intervention is necessary, and antibiotics should be initiated. A reactive hydrocele may also be present.

However, the surgeon should always bear the old adage that "time is testicle" in the forefront of their mind. A general rule followed by the majority of urologists is that a torsed testicle can be salvaged if scrotal exploration and detorsion is performed within 6 h of pain onset. Orchiectomy is usually required if more than 12 h have passed since the patient first experienced symptoms. In short, if there is any possibility of torsion and a POCUS is not available, easily performed, or conclusive, the patient should immediately be taken to the OR for scrotal exploration.

Treatment consists of immediate surgical exploration, detorsion, and possible orchiectomy if the torsed testicle is no longer viable. If the affected testicle is able to be saved, it is sutured into place in the ipsilateral scrotum. Orchiopexy of the contralateral testicle may also be performed to prevent future occurrences if the surgeon feels comfortable. In the patient in the vignette, the decision was made not to do contralateral orchiopexy after discussion with local MTF. If planning to operate on both sides of the scrotum, a midline scrotal incision is generally preferred (Fig. 17.2), although bilateral horizontal incisions are also acceptable (Fig. 17.3).

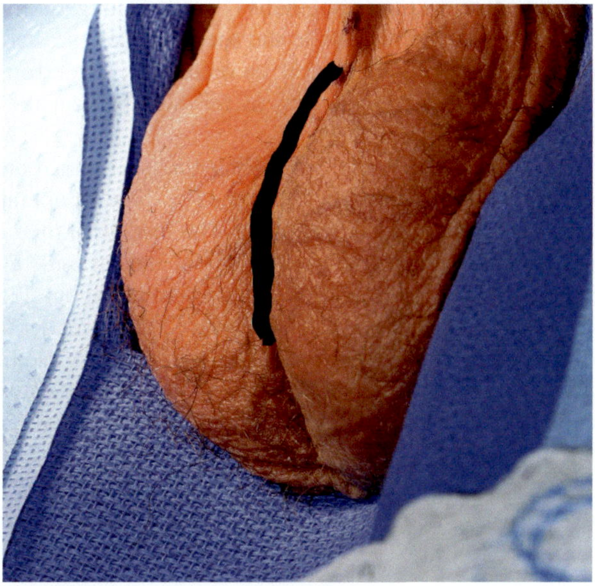

Fig. 17.2 Planned midline scrotal incision (Source: Photo courtesy of Patrick L. Scarborough, MD)

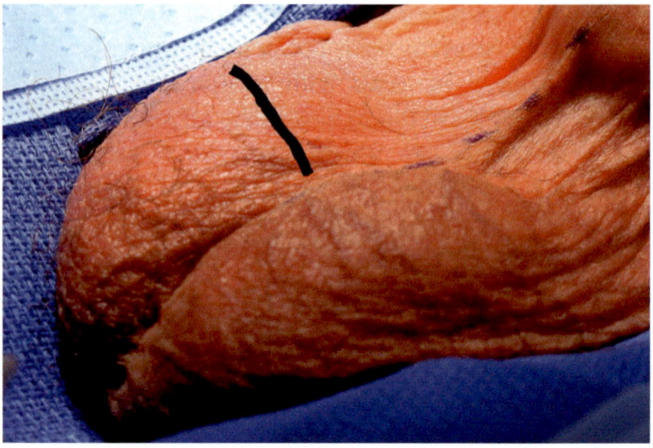

Fig. 17.3 Planned horizontal scrotal incision (Source: Photo courtesy of Patrick L. Scarborough, MD)

Carry out dissection down to the overlying tunica vaginalis using gloved fingers and electrocautery. Deliver the testicle into the operative field. The surrounding cremasteric muscle fibers are either bluntly freed from the testicle or divided with electrocautery. Divide the gubernaculum at this point, as the testicle will be either sutured into place or removed. This is generally accomplished with electrocautery. However, there are occasionally prominent gubernacular veins that must be ligated using 2-0 silk sutures. The spermatic cord should also be freed of surrounding attachments and dissected proximally as far as possible, preferably to the level of the ipsilateral external inguinal ring. This will provide adequate length for either the planned orchiopexy or the possible orchiectomy.

Once the testicle is completely freed from its scrotal attachments, open the tunica vaginalis with Metzenbaum scissors. Evacuate any fluid surrounding the testicle. The presence of a hematocele generally confers a poor prognosis for testicular salvage. Ensure the tunica vaginalis is opened along the entire length of the testicle and reflected back on the testicle and spermatic cord so there is no subsequent compression of the spermatic cord if an orchiopexy is performed. Remove excess tunica vaginalis with electrocautery, as this will prevent the subsequent formation of a hydrocele.

Perform inspection of the testicle and spermatic cord with notation made of the degree and direction of the twist; see Fig. 17.4 for operative findings of a patient like the one in Clinical Vignette 17.3. The testicle is then detorsed, wrapped in gauze soaked in warm normal saline solution, and set aside to allow time for reperfusion. If appropriate, turn attention to the contralateral unaffected testicle at this time. If a midline scrotal incision was used, it is a simple matter to bring the other testicle out of the same incision in the same manner that was used for the affected testicle. If a horizontal scrotal incision was used, a matching incision should be made on the contralateral scrotum with a similar approach to deliver the testicle into the operative field.

Access to the contralateral testicle is performed in the same manner. Once exposed and evaluated, create a subdartos pouch in the hemi-scrotum using a Kelley

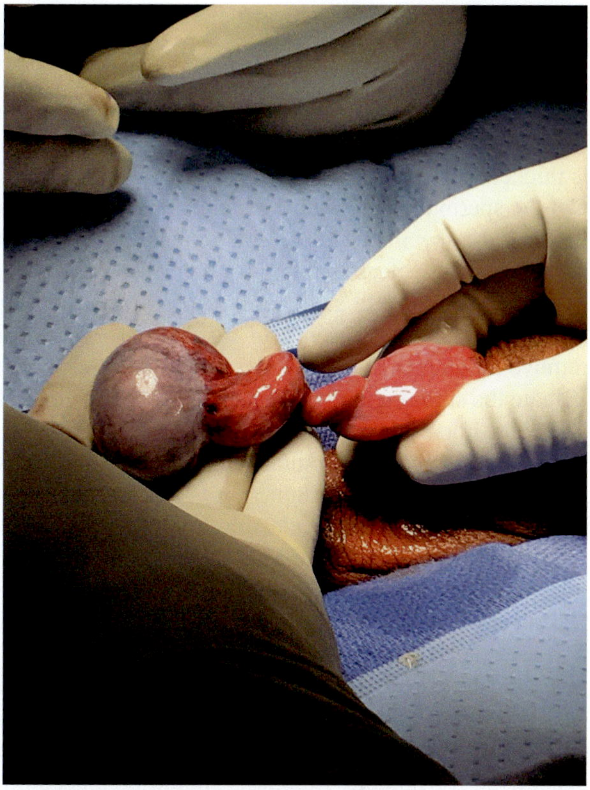

Fig. 17.4 Testicular torsion with a 360-degree clockwise twist (Source: Photo courtesy of Patrick L. Scarborough, MD)

hemostat. Suture the testicle into place in the scrotum in three dimensions using a permanent suture (the author prefers 4-0 polypropylene (i.e., Prolene)) with one suture placed in the scrotal skin inferiorly, one medially, and one laterally. On the scrotal side, take care to ensure that the sutures placed do not penetrate through the scrotum. On the testicular side, place the sutures through the tunica albuginea to ensure that the testicle is unable to twist once healing occurs.

After addressing the contralateral testicle, the previously torsed testicle is unwrapped and re-inspected for viability. The decision as to whether a testicle is viable is not always clear. However, if there is significant doubt, make a small incision in the inferior portion of the testicle with observation for bleeding. If bright red blood is observed, the testicle is adequately perfused. If deoxygenated blood is observed or no bleeding is seen, the testicle is not salvageable and should be removed. Care must be taken to make this incision in the tunica albuginea, avoiding the epididymis, as scarring in the epididymis will inevitably lead to infertility of the affected testicle. If the testicle is salvageable, close the incision in the tunica albuginea with a small absorbable suture.

If the testicle is viable, proceed with orchiopexy as previously described. If the testicle is not viable, perform an orchiectomy. Clamp the spermatic cord with a

Peon hemostat distal to the ipsilateral external inguinal ring, allowing adequate room for the placement of sutures. Perform a stick tie with a large permanent suture, either 0 polyester or silk, proximal to the previously placed clamp. Place a hemostat on this tie for later inspection of the spermatic cord stump for hemostasis. Place a second free tie using the same suture proximal to the stick tie. If the spermatic cord is thickened, it may be separated into two halves, which can then each be stick-tied. Cut the spermatic cord with Metzenbaum scissors between the clamp and the stick tie. Pass the specimen off the field for submission to pathology. Burn the spermatic cord stump with electrocautery for hemostasis.

Inspect the testicle and spermatic cord to ensure hemostasis and proper placement, as well as an absence of inadvertent torsion. Once hemostasis is ensured, remove all clamps and allow the spermatic cord to retract into the inguinal canal. Irrigate the scrotum with normal saline solution. Scrotal drains are not necessary. If a separate horizontal incision was performed, closure of the scrotum is completed in two layers: an absorbable suture, generally a running 3-0 chromic gut, at the Dartos fascia followed by 3-0 chromic gut in a horizontal mattress fashion at the skin. If a midline incision was used, closure is performed after completion of the orchiopexy or orchiectomy of the torsed testicle and in a manner similar to closing a horizontal incision. Take additional care to include the scrotal septum in the closure of the Dartos fascia. Bacitracin is placed on the incision and fluffed gauze and scrotal support are placed as a dressing.

Postoperative care consists generally of adequate pain control and rest. On board during a ship deployment, the patient should be given at least 7 days on a Sick-In-Quarters (SIQ) status, followed by at least 3 weeks of light-duty. Jockstrap can be considered if available. Emphasis should be placed on no significant exercise and activity during the recovery period, as a painful postoperative scrotal hematoma commonly occurs if the patient becomes active too soon following surgery. Fertility and hormonal function following orchiectomy are generally unaffected as long as the contralateral testicle was normal but this can be followed once the patient returns from deployment.

Testicular Injury

Injury to the testicles generally occurs as the result of either blunt force or penetrating trauma, with blunt force trauma being the most commonly encountered. Given the nature of the mission during deployments, the maritime surgeon may encounter both and be required to quickly diagnose and intervene in order to preserve hormonal function and fertility. Relatively innocuous activities may lead to severe testicular damage, sometimes resulting in a delay in diagnosis. Signs and symptoms consist of scrotal swelling and edema, generally in combination with obvious ecchymosis, as well as moderate-to-severe testicular pain. Depending on the mechanism of injury, there may be significant visible damage to the scrotal skin with the possibility of a testicle or other scrotal contents being visible during the initial physical exam.

Diagnosis is similar to the approach for testicular torsion and is based on the history, physical exam, and mechanism of injury. Again, if a POCUS is readily available it may be performed, although surgical exploration should not be delayed in the absence of imaging, particularly if significant swelling and ecchymosis are observed. Penetrating injuries generally require bilateral scrotal exploration, while blunt force trauma may or may not require surgery. If a non-expanding scrotal hematoma is observed on ultrasound without underlying disruption of the testicular tunica albuginea and the patient's pain is well controlled, then observation is reasonable. However, if the hematoma is expanding, there is disruption of the tunica albuginea with extrusion of seminiferous tubules on ultrasound or the patient's pain is not well controlled, then exploration of the affected hemi-scrotum is required.

The approach to surgical exploration is similar to the approach for testicular torsion, with a midline scrotal incision preferred for bilateral exploration and a horizontal scrotal exploration acceptable if only one side is to be addressed. Assess for any devascularized tissue with removal if necessary. Evacuate any hematomas and obtain hemostasis. Remove any foreign bodies with care to ensure hemostasis. Fully assess the testicle after opening the tunica vaginalis, particularly if imaging was concerning for testicular rupture.

In the event of a visible testicular rupture with extrusion of seminiferous tubules, the overall viability of the testicle is assessed. If it is not viable with the absence of blood flow or more than 50% of the testicular contents have been pushed outside of the testicle, perform orchiectomy as previously discussed. If the testicle is viable and there is enough remaining testicle for salvage, debride all seminiferous tubules outside of the testicular tunica albuginea with electrocautery and the tunica albuginea is reapproximated with an absorbable suture [2] and orchiopexy is performed.

Verify hemostasis, irrigate with normal saline solution, and place a 1/2-inch Penrose drain in the dependent portion of the scrotum. Secure the Penrose to the skin with a 2-0 silk suture. Closure of the wound is then accomplished as previously described.

It is worth noting that there may be instances where a significant portion of the scrotal skin has been damaged or lost during a traumatic event. If the skin is not viable, it is of course removed. Generally, up to 50% of scrotal skin may be removed without difficulty and with excellent cosmetic results.

Post-operative care mirrors that described for testicular torsion. The Penrose drain should be removed 3–5 days postoperatively. Adequate rest and recovery are again critical following surgery. Hormonal function and fertility are generally adequate as long as one normal testicle is present and can be monitored upon return from deployment.

Urethral Injury

Fortunately, urethral injury is uncommon. However, it remains a possible complication of severe pelvic injury and should be in the forefront of the mind of the deployed surgeon if a trauma patient presents with blood at the urethral meatus. Given the limitations of available diagnostic equipment and supplies while deployed, it is reasonable to treat any patient with blood at the urethral meatus following trauma as if there is a significant urethral injury.

Diagnosis of urethral injury is usually confirmed with either direct visualization via cystoscopy or after the performance of a retrograde urethrogram. While a retrograde urethrogram could be performed while on ship using flat-plate pelvic X-ray, the contrast required is not part of any ship's AMAL. Consider "tactically" acquiring contrast for this contingency. Given these limitations, the treatment for suspected urethral injury becomes relatively straightforward. If blood is noted at the urethral meatus during a trauma evaluation, particularly if there is a pelvic injury, then urethral injury is assumed. An attempt may be made to place a Foley catheter, but if any resistance or difficulty is encountered with placement of the catheter, the surgeon should proceed with the placement of a suprapubic catheter.

Placement of a suprapubic catheter is relatively straightforward. There are percutaneous kits and catheters that are not typically found on the AMAL, so if they are not available a Foley catheter can be placed suprapubically using open technique. After appropriate shaving and sterile preparation, make a 2–3 cm incision in the skin approximately two finger breadths superior to the pubic symphysis. Carry down dissection to the underlying bladder using electrocautery. Place stay sutures in the bladder muscle and elevate the bladder. Enter with electrocautery. Verify hemostasis at this time. The Foley catheter, generally 14–16 French in size, is then placed directly into the bladder and the balloon inflated with 10 mL of sterile water. Close the incision around the Foley catheter with an absorbable suture, and secure the catheter to the skin with 2-0 silk suture. If available, POCUS can be used intraoperatively to guide placement of the suprapubic incision but is not strictly necessary as the procedure is performed under direct visualization.

Postoperatively the catheter should remain in place for at least 3–4 weeks to allow for the proper epithelialization of the suprapubic tract. The patient should be MEDEVAC to a higher level of care at the earliest opportunity for a full evaluation of the urinary tract by a subspecialist.

Conclusion

In a woman presenting with acute lower abdominal pain and/or bleeding, asking the patient for her potential for pregnancy and getting an HCG test will help rapidly narrow the differential diagnosis and determine the fastest, safest approach for management. In the case of a woman presenting in labor, use the people with more recent training in labor management to work collaboratively to care for the mother, deliver the baby, repair lacerations, and prevent or treat PPH. Be prepared for the management of breech deliveries and cesarean sections. While most gynecologic conditions can be managed medically and electively, a handful are true emergencies requiring surgical intervention at sea. The maritime surgical team needs to prepare, drill, and be familiar with the diagnosis and surgical treatment of ectopic pregnancy, ovarian torsion, and vaginal laceration. While the majority of testicular complaints do not require an immediate journey to the OR, it is important to always remember and rule out emergencies like testicular torsion and rupture. If there is any question in the deployed surgeon's mind and imaging has not shed any additional light on the diagnosis, the answer is to surgically explore.

Finally, this chapter is an overview of multiple surgical subspecialty topics that an expeditionary surgical team may have to care for at sea. As stated in several other chapters, help is usually only a phone call or email away. Never hesitate to communicate with on-call subspecialists to use the resources available in the middle of the ocean to best care for the patient (or both patients)!

Declaration of Interest The views expressed in this chapter are those of the authors and do not necessarily reflect the official policy or position of the Department of the Navy, Department of Defense, nor the US Government.

Funding This research did not receive any specific grant from funding agencies in the public, commercial, or not-for-profit sectors.

Conflict of Interest Statement The authors declare no conflict of interest.

References

1. Larter, David B., "A U.S. sailor delivered a baby at sea – in the middle of the ISIS war." The Navy Times. September 12, 2016. Available at: https://www.navytimes.com/news/your-navy/2016/09/12/a-u-s-sailor-delivered-a-baby-at-sea-in-the-middle-of-the-isis-war/.
2. Urotrauma: American Urological Association Guideline, Genital Trauma, Pg 16, 2014

Further Reading

Comprehensive Handbook Obstetrics and Gynecology by Thomas Zheng
Pocket Obstetrics and Gynecology by K. Joseph Hart
Penn Clinical Manual of Urology by Philip Hanno, Thomas Guzzo, S. Bruce Malkowicz, and Alan Wein

Chapter 18
Haze, Gray, and Endoscopy Underway

Thomas Mellor, Diego A. Vicente, and R. Daniel Lawson

Non nova, sed nove. (Not new things, but in a new way.)

Latin proverb

Author deployment experience	
Thomas Mellor	Staff Physician, Battalion Aid Station Papa Ocho, Operation Allies Refuge, Sigonella, Italy, 2021
	Staff Gastroenterologist and Division Officer, Navy Medicine Readiness and Training Command Bremerton, Bremerton, WA, USA, 2021–present
Diego A. Vicente	Ship's Surgeon, USS Harry S. Truman (CVN-75), Operation Inherent Resolve, AFRICOM Area of Responsibility, 2015–2016
	Officer in Charge, Role 2 Light Maneuver team, embarked on the USS Hershel "Woody" Williams (ESB-4), 2020; Provided embarked Role 2 Surgical Support, AFRICOM Area of Responsibility, 2020
R. Daniel Lawson	Staff Gastroenterologist, USNS Mercy (T-AH-19), Pacific Partnership, INDOPACOM Area of Responsibility, 2010
	Staff Gastroenterologist, USNS Mercy (T-AH-19), Pacific Partnership, INDOPACOM Area of Responsibility, 2012
	Staff Gastroenterologist/Interventional Endoscopist, Navy Medicine Readiness and Training Command San Diego, San Diego, CA, USA, 2013–2021

T. Mellor
Navy Medicine Readiness and Training Command Bremerton, Bremerton, WA, USA

D. A. Vicente
Navy Medicine Readiness and Training Command San Diego, San Diego, CA, USA
e-mail: diego.a.vicente.mil@health.mil

R. D. Lawson (✉)
MultiCare Rockwood Clinic, Spokane, WA, USA

M. D. Tadlock, A. A. Hernandez (eds.), *Expeditionary Surgery at Sea*,
https://doi.org/10.1007/978-3-031-21893-4_18

BLUF (Bottom Line Up Front)

1. Endoscopy is an effective and potentially lifesaving diagnostic and therapeutic modality employed by the deployed surgical team in austere environments.
2. Understanding the endoscopic equipment, tools, and personnel capabilities available at sea are critical for successful execution of endoscopy.
3. The risks of endoscopy are low and include cardiopulmonary events, aspiration, abdominal pain, bloating, bleeding, perforation, splenic injury, and rarely death. It is crucial to know the patient, endoscopist, and procedural factors that augment these risks.
4. Endoscopy ergonomics include appropriate endoscopist, patient, and equipment positioning and should be optimized prior to beginning any endoscopic procedure.
5. Endoscopic procedures are often challenging; there are multiple troubleshooting options available that should be approached in a systematic fashion when faced with a difficult procedure or malfunctioning equipment.
6. Resistance during endoscopy indicates tension on the gastrointestinal (GI) tract and attempts should always be made to reduce resistance if encountered. **Never push against fixed resistance as this can result in perforation.**
7. Patients with esophageal foreign body impactions should be assessed for complications and intubated prior to endoscopy, which should be performed on an urgent basis.
8. There are many presentations and etiologies for dysphagia. Some can be managed on board and some need higher levels of care.
9. Treatment of GI bleeding is variable and based on etiology. On the ship, it may include injection of vasoconstricting agents (epinephrine), use of electrocoagulation, hemostatic clips (through the scope), and Argon Plasma Coagulation (APC), depending on what is stocked. The combination of two treatment modalities often further reduces the risk of recurrent bleeding.
10. If in doubt, and not a risk to the patient, abort the procedure and defer management until return from sea or medical evacuation (MEDEVAC) if necessary.
11. There are multiple incidental findings that can be encountered during endoscopy, which should not be addressed while at sea unless an immediate threat to the patient.

Introduction

Clinical Vignette 18.1

A 20-year-old male presented with repeated presentations to the medical department for 1 year of intermittent reflux refractory to anti-acid therapy, unintended 10-pound weight loss, persistent cough, and a taste of regurgitated contents when supine. Symptoms also included progressive dysphagia, first with solids and then with liquids. Work up included barium swallow with static X-rays demonstrating a dilated esophagus with distal tapering (Bird's beak appearance). A likely diagnosis of achalasia was made, and the patient was transferred to a continental United States (CONUS) medical treatment facility (MTF) where manometry, dynamic esophagram, and esophagogastroduodenoscopy (EGD) supported this diagnosis. He ultimately underwent laparoscopic Heller myotomy with a Dor fundoplication (Table 18.1) [1].

Table 18.1 Combined endoscopy experience of two surgeons for combined total of 14 months during different deployments on aircraft carriers (CVNs)

Patient presentation	Endoscopy performed	Findings on endoscopy	Final diagnosis and disposition
Substernal chest pain with difficulty swallowing	EGD	Distal esophagitis	Pill esophagitis
BRBPR, progressive abdominal pain	EGD Colonoscopy	Normal EGD; Inflammation of TI on colonoscopy	TI biopsies consistent with CD, medical management initiated with asynchronous GI consult
Nausea, vomiting, epigastric pain following uncomplicated cholecystectomy	EGD	Normal EGD	All laboratory data performed during port call normal, including LFTs, CT abdomen, and MRCP
BRBPR, melena, early satiety	EGD Colonoscopy	Normal EGD; 1.5 cm ascending colon polyp requiring snare biopsy	No snare biopsy capability, sent off ship for colonoscopy and biopsy
BRBPR	Colonoscopy	Normal colonoscopy, internal hemorrhoids only	Medical management
BRBPR	Colonoscopy	Inflammation of TI on colonoscopy	TI biopsies consistent with CD, medical management initiated with asynchronous GI consult

(continued)

Table 18.1 (continued)

Patient presentation	Endoscopy performed	Findings on endoscopy	Final diagnosis and disposition
BRBPR, progressive abdominal pain	Colonoscopy	Inflammation of cecum on colonoscopy	Cecal biopsies consistent with CD, MEDEVAC initiated given progression of symptoms
Family history of colon cancer; age > 50 years	Colonoscopy	Normal colonoscopy	Repeat screening colonoscopy in 5–7 years
Retching and sialorrhea 1 h after eating	EGD	Complete obstruction at GEJ (grilled chicken)	Endoscopic disimpaction with biopsy forceps, piecemeal reduction in food bolus then push technique successfully performed. See Fig. 18.1
Retching and sialorrhea 1 h after eating	EGD	Complete obstruction at GEJ	Food bolus dislodged using push technique
History of lupus without dysphagia presented with retching and sialorrhea 2 h after eating	EGD	Complete obstruction at thoracic inlet (steak)	Food bolus was easily dislodged from the impaction at the thoracic inlet. However, subsequent impaction at the GEJ required extensive piecemeal reduction in food bolus then push technique successfully performed
Three symptomatic esophageal impactions with retching and sialorrhea after eating	EGDs	Complete obstruction at thoracic inlet	First presentation was diagnosed clinically with MEDEVAC to a civilian medical facility ashore for endoscopic management. During second and third presentations, MEDEVAC not possible so both times food bolus dislodged using push technique
12 months of intermittent reflux symptoms and 10-pound weight loss that progressed to solid food dysphagia	Modified timed barium swallows only	Dilated esophagus with distal tapering and delayed emptying of the esophagus	No EGD performed. MEDEVAC to CONUS MTF where EGD and dynamic esophagram confirmed achalasia diagnosis. Subsequent laparoscopic Heller myotomy with Dor fundoplication was performed

EGD esophagogastroduodenoscopy, *CD* Crohn's disease, *BRBPR* bright red blood per rectum, *TI* terminal ileum, *GI* gastroenterology, *LFTs* liver function tests, *CT* computed tomography, *MRCP* magnetic resonance cholangiopancreatography, *GEJ* gastroesophageal junction, *MEDEVAC* medical evacuation, *CONUS* continental United States, *MTF* medical treatment facility

Clinical Vignette 18.2

A 38-year-old previously healthy male aviator presented to the medical department with 1 h of postprandial retching and sialorrhea. Vital signs and physical examination were unremarkable. Work up included barium swallow study with static X-rays demonstrating complete esophageal obstruction proximal to gastroesophageal junction (GEJ) (Fig. 18.1). *He was diagnosed with esophageal food impaction. EGD was performed. Biopsy forceps were utilized for piecemeal reduction of food*

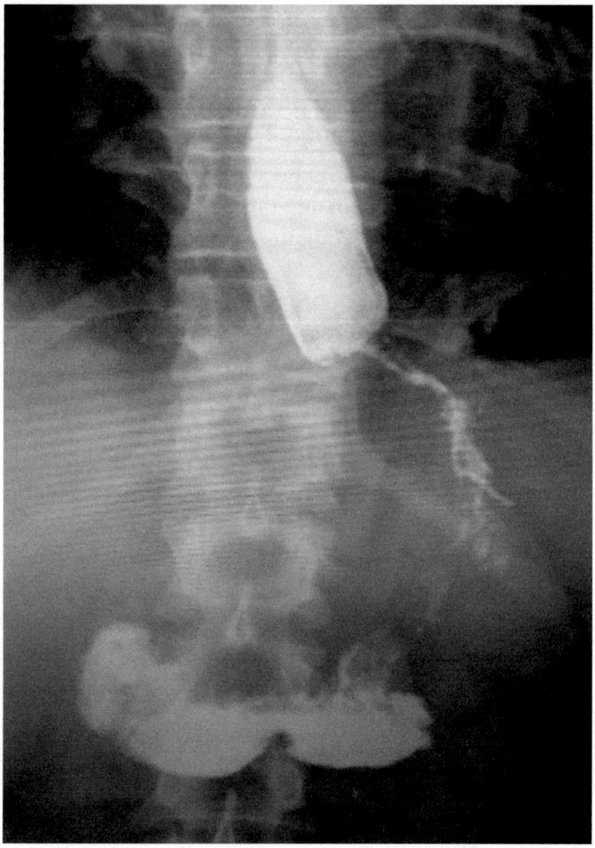

Fig. 18.1 Shipboard barium swallow study showing complete esophageal obstruction proximal to the gastroesophageal junction (GEJ). (Source: Image courtesy of Diego A. Vicente, MD)

bolus (grilled chicken) followed by push technique to advance food bolus into the stomach (Table 18.1) [1].

Endoscopy has become a critical skill set for civilian and military surgeons. General surgery Accreditation Council for Graduate Medical Education (ACGME) requirements mandate a minimum of 35 upper endoscopic procedures and 50 colonoscopies for graduation. However, graduating military general surgeons are expected to perform not only diagnostic endoscopy, but also lifesaving endoscopic therapeutic procedures in austere environments. This chapter has been developed based on feedback from junior surgeons who found themselves at sea managing a complexity of acute gastrointestinal (GI) pathology while out of immediate medical evacuation (MEDEVAC) range.

For context, Table 18.1 demonstrates the combined endoscopy experience of two surgeons for combined total of 14 months during different deployments on aircraft carriers (CVNs). For example, during one of the author's (DAV) first deployment as a new general surgery residency graduate, he and his team diagnosed one patient with Crohn's disease (CD) and one patient with achalasia, endoscopically managed six food bolus esophageal impactions, and surgically treated one gastric volvulus over the course of an 8-month CVN deployment [1]. Endoscopy was a critical tool in the evaluation and management of these patients as well as a useful adjunct during surgical intervention.

In addition to a good endoscopic background to manage acute GI pathology at sea, preparation to evaluate and manage these patients begins before deployment. Surgeons should contact their pharmacy department to ensure that there is oral contrast available on-board prior to deployment. While cross-sectional computed tomography (CT) and fluoroscopic imaging capabilities are not currently available at sea, well-timed oral contrast static X-ray images can aid in the diagnosis of upper and lower GI pathology prior to invasive intervention, demonstrated in both clinical vignettes. Surgical technologists (STs) should ensure they are familiar with the equipment, consumables, and setup as well as with high level disinfection, especially if they have not been responsible for this process previously during their careers (see Chap. 12). Furthermore, given the risk of aspiration with any GI pathology, early close communication and planning between the surgeon, anesthesia provider, and medical team is vital to successful mitigation strategies and to minimize the risks of intubation when indicated. Finally, early objective assessment of capabilities at sea and indications as well as plans for MEDEVAC and long-term management of these patients should be considered prior to deployment. This chapter will discuss the equipment, technical considerations, GI pathologies, and most importantly pitfalls that all deploying surgeons should prepare to manage at sea.

Endoscopy Equipment

GI endoscopy equipment, both brand/model of processor and model of scopes, is not standardized throughout the United States (U.S.) Navy. Though Olympus is the most common brand, military physicians may be required to use equipment manufactured by Pentax or Fujifilm. Despite subtle differences in appearance, connectors, and button layout (among others), the basic components and approach to set-up are similar between brand and models to allow for certain generalizations. It is also important to note that all the equipment has required maintenance that needs to be performed regularly and consumables that need to be ordered regularly, see Chap. 12.

The "Equipment Tower"

The Equipment Tower is comprised of five critical (and one optional) integrated components to which the endoscope attaches (Figs. 18.2, 18.3, and 18.4).

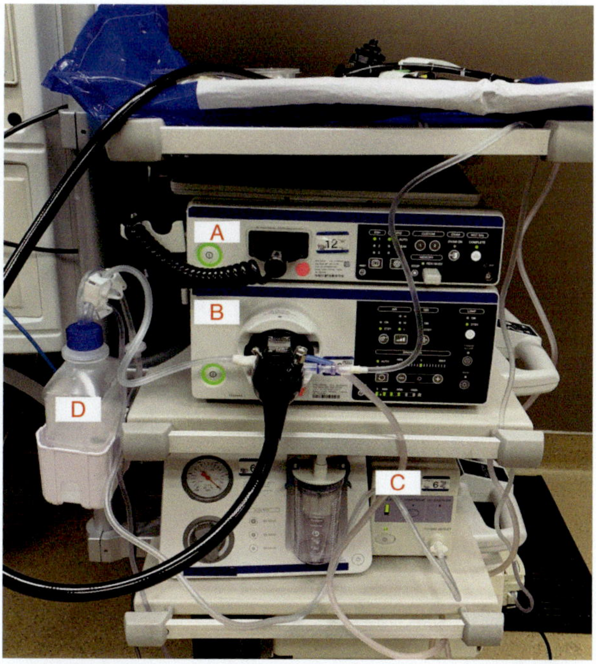

Fig. 18.2 Endoscopy tower. *A*—Video processor; *B*—Light source; *C*—Carbon dioxide pump; *D*—Canister attached to tubing for carbon dioxide insufflation. (Source: Photo courtesy of R. Daniel Lawson, MD)

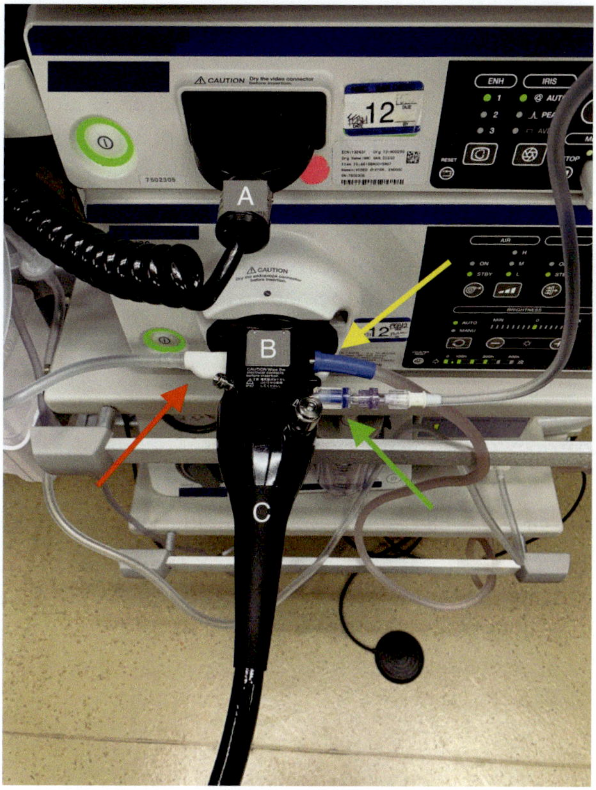

Fig. 18.3 Endoscopy tower. *A*—Coiled cable of video processor; *B*—Light source connector; *C*—Umbilical (universal) cord; Yellow arrow-tubing attached to suction port; Green arrow-irrigation port with anti-reflux valve attached; Red arrow-Two-prong attachment for carbon dioxide insufflation and scope lens cleaner. (Source: Photo courtesy of R. Daniel Lawson, MD)

Fig. 18.4 Water irrigation pump with arrow indicating direction of water flow. (Source: Photo courtesy of R. Daniel Lawson, MD)

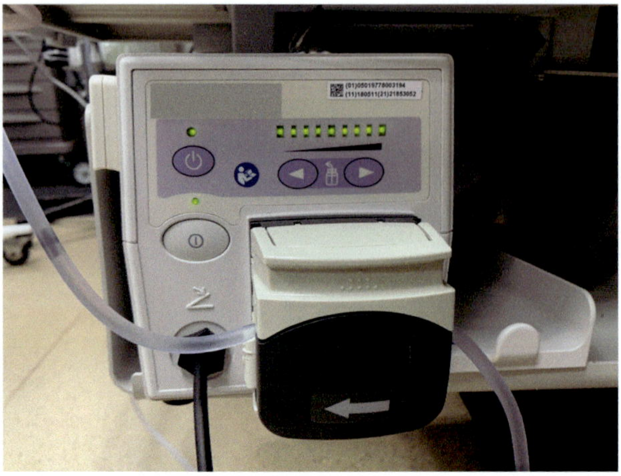

- Video processor
- Light source
- Monitor(s)
- Water irrigation pump
- Suction pump
- Carbon dioxide pump (optional, but considered standard of care)

The video processor and light source produced by a given manufacturer are uniquely compatible with endoscopes of the same brand and vary slightly in configuration. Olympus and Fujifilm house the video processor and light source into separate boxes, whereas Pentax combines these two components into a single box. Monitors, water irrigation pumps, suction pumps, and/or carbon dioxide pumps need to be compatible but not necessarily the same brand as the video processor/light source.

The umbilical (or universal) connector and cord attach the handle into the Equipment Tower. Water irrigation, suction, and combined insufflation/lens irrigator are all attached to the connector. Some models also have a plug to connect a cable that links the endoscope to the video processor.

Endoscopes

All endoscopes have similar configurations. An endoscope consists of the parts shown in Figs. 18.5 and 18.6.

1. **Insertion tube:** the longest section of the endoscope that is inserted into the patient's body and is held in the endoscopist's right hand.
2. **Flexible (bending) tip:** distal 10–15 cm of the scope that can be deflected along all axes, controlled by dials on the handle.

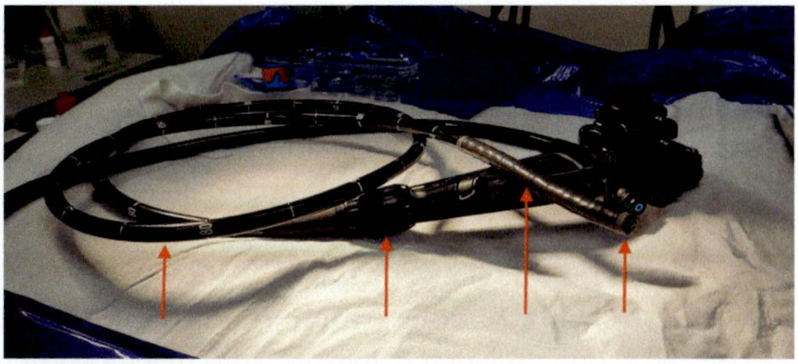

Fig. 18.5 Colonoscope with arrows from left to right indicating: Insertion tube; Variable stiffness knob; Flexible (bending) tip; Distal tip. (Source: Photo courtesy of R. Daniel Lawson, MD)

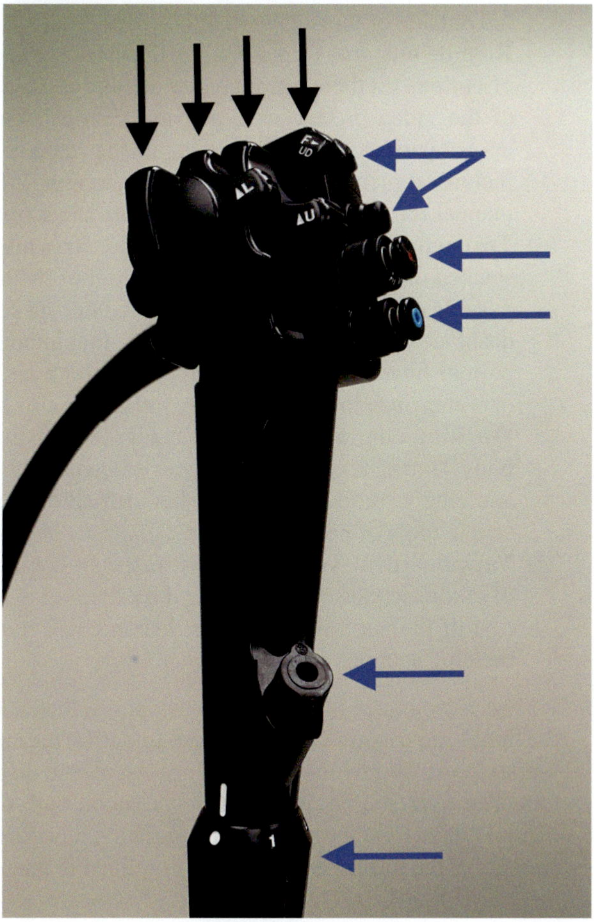

Fig. 18.6 Control body of endoscope. Black arrows from left to right indicating: Small control dial locking knob; Small control dial; Large control dial; Large control dial locking knob. Blue arrows from top to bottom indicating: Remote buttons; Suction valve; Air/Water valve; Working channel; Variable stiffness knob. (Source: Photo courtesy of R. Daniel Lawson, MD)

3. **Distal tip:** flat end of the bending section containing the light guide lens, objective lens, air/water nozzle, instrument channel outlet, and suction port.
4. **Handle (control body):** held in the endoscopist's left hand and houses multiple controls used to operate the endoscope (Fig. 18.6).

(a) **Two control dials (small and large):** These dials are rotated to deflect the bending section of the scope along two axes that are perpendicular to each other. Turning the larger dial, especially in the counterclockwise direction, generates the most deflection. Turning both dials in the counterclockwise direction will produce maximal deflection, referred to as "candy caning" of the scope, which is useful when performing retroflexion maneuvers (such as rectal retroflexion).
(b) **Two locking knobs (small and large):** The desired angle of deflection of the scope tip can be "locked" into place by either pushing forward the locking knob adjacent to the big wheel or rotating clockwise the locking knob on the outside of the small wheel.
(c) **Remote buttons**: Depending on the model of endoscope, there are a number of buttons on the control head that can be programmed within the software of the video processor to activate various processor functions depending upon operator preference (e.g., image capture, image freeze, near focus, picture-in-picture, and narrow band imaging). See the manufacturer's user manual for details on how to configure the scope remote buttons.
(d) **Two cylinder openings (suction and air/water):** These are two openings stacked on top of each other at the front of the handle into which either disposable or reusable valves are inserted during scope set-up. The top valve is designed for suction and is typically manipulated by the endoscopist's left pointer finger. The bottom valve is for both air insufflation (light pressure) or water rinse to clean the lens (full depression).
(e) **Working channel:** Is located below the valves on the front of the control body. During scope set-up a cap is placed on this working channel so that air and enteric fluids do not leak but still allow the endoscopist to pass endoscopic tools or perform flushes.
(f) **Variable stiffness knob:** The stiffness of the insertion tube of some models of colonoscopes can be adjusted by rotating a dial located at the distal portion of the control body. This does not affect stiffness or flexibility of the bending section.

The video image is obtained by the lens of the endoscope with assistance from the light source, converted to a digital image by the camera head (within the endoscope), processed within the video processor, and displayed on one or more monitors. The light source typically uses a xenon bulb due to its similarity to clear, natural, white light. For successful operation it is imperative that the various components of the tower be connected as outlined in the model-specific user manuals.

Electrocautery Unit and Argon Plasma Coagulation (APC)

Though not a critical component of the Equipment Tower, an electrocautery unit is required to perform many common endoscopic procedures such as removal of large polyps and hemostasis. Argon plasma coagulation (APC) is used less frequently, but the generator is incorporated within the electrocautery unit or is attached. APC is a useful modality to treat arteriovenous malformations (AVMs), residual polyp tissue following polypectomy, and gastric antral vascular ectasias (GAVE); however, it requires specialized training for safe use.

Preparing Equipment for a Case

Maritime surgical teams should have appropriately trained STs, proficient in gastrointestinal endoscopy equipment set-up, endoscopist support during procedures, and high-level disinfection. However, it is helpful for all members of the maritime surgical team to have a general awareness of how the equipment is prepared for each case.

Ancillary consumables are required for equipment operation and must be compatible. After completion of cases these consumables should be exchanged, including:

- Air/water channel adaptor connected to water bottle
- Tubing for water irrigation
- Tubing for gas insufflation
- Tubing for suction and suction canister (changed between procedures)
- Suction valve and air/water valve (changed between procedures)
- Instrument channel cap (changed between procedures)

To help pass the endoscope and perform procedures, the following should be readily available:

- Lubricant
- 4 × 4 gauze
- Specimen cups with formalin (specimens should be labeled, sent to the laboratory, processed, and followed up like any other specimen, see Chap. 12 for details)

Equipment Set-Up

Please review the model-specific user manuals and team ST knowledge for specific instructions on setting up the particular brand and model of endoscopy equipment on board the ship. The following is intended to provide the maritime surgical team (outside of the ST) a broad overview of the process of setting up the equipment. Refer to Figs. 18.2, 18.3, 18.4, 18.5, and 18.6.

1. Make sure that all components of the tower (except for monitors) are turned OFF.
2. Attach the endoscope to the endoscopy tower by sliding the umbilical connector into the light source until it locks into place, being sure to carefully align the light tube into the appropriate channel. Some brands (such as older generation

Olympus models) require attachment of the umbilical connector to the video processor via a coiled cable.
3. Place a cap onto the working channel of the endoscope handle.
4. Firmly insert the two valves into the cylinder openings (suction and air/water) of the handle (larger valve inserts into the lower opening).
5. Attach the anti-reflux valve to the irrigation port (water auxiliary inlet) located on the umbilical connector. Some endoscopes, such as older models or pediatric endoscopes, will not have a water irrigation channel.
6. Connection of the appropriate tubing. There are three tubes: water irrigation, suction, and air insufflation.

   (a) Water irrigation:

      - Attach the anti-reflux valve (previously connected to the umbilical connector) to one end of the long water irrigation tube.
      - Attach the other end of the irrigation tube to a 1 L bottle of sterile water (usually this has a special connector).
      - Snake the water irrigation tubing through the head of the irrigator pump so that the direction of pumped water flow is toward the scope. Usually, the head of the irrigator pump will have an arrow indicating pump flow direction that makes this step straightforward. The head of the pump usually has a clamp arrangement that when fully depressed firmly approximates the tubing with the rotating pumping mechanism.

   (b) Suction tubing:

      - Attach one end of suction tubing to the large suction port on the umbilical connector.
      - Attach the other end of the suction tubing to the suction canister fitted with disposable/sealable canister.

   (c) Air insufflation and lens cleaner:

      - There is a two-prong attachment on the umbilical connector into which one end of the special tubing attaches by first inserting onto the larger prong then slightly rotating the tubing until it securely sits on the smaller prong.
      - There are two loose ends at the other end of this tubing. One attaches to a bottle with a tight seal and special connectors, and the other end is attached to the carbon dioxide supply connector.
      - Though carbon dioxide insufflation is the preferred gas for insufflation this requires both an insufflator pump and source of carbon dioxide. Alternatively, room air can be used and is controlled through buttons located on the light source. When carbon dioxide is used, the room air insufflator is switched to "off" or "standby."

Once the equipment is attached, turn on the power to all of the equipment on the endoscopy tower: turn on the lamp to the endoscope, turn on source of suction, and turn on gas flow for insufflation of either air (located on the light source) or carbon dioxide (located on the carbon dioxide insufflation pump). At this point, the quiet whistling sound of suction should be heard through the endoscope. Appropriate setup is indicated by all buttons and valves functioning and successful video displaying on the monitor.

1. Suction (top valve):
   (a) Insert the tip of the endoscope into a basin of water on the field and firmly depress the top valve while examining the suction tubing and canister for water movement.
   (b) If suction is absent or weak, check to make sure the valve is firmly seated, the connections are tight, the suction canister is sealed, and the suction source is turned on.
      - If the valve is removed but suction is still felt in the channel with a finger over the channel, then the valve should be cleaned or replaced.
      - If the suction channel stops working during the case, the channel may be clogged. It can be cleared by flushing irrigation fluid through the working channel and/or passing a brush through the suction channel toward the scope tip and then through the channel in the umbilical cord to the connector.
2. Gas insufflation and lens cleaner (bottom valve):
   (a) With the scope tip in the basin of water, cover the hole in the middle of the bottom valve but do not depress. A gentle continuous stream of gas should be felt on the fingertip and a stream of steady bubbles should be seen in the basin of water emitting from the tip of the scope.
   (b) If there are no bubbles, check to make sure the valve is firmly seated, all connections are tight, the water bottle is filled approximately to the halfway mark, the lid is tight, and the source of gas is turned on.
      - If the valve is removed and air flow is still felt in the channel with a finger over the channel, then the valve should be cleaned or replaced.
      - If there is no air flow during the case, then the insufflation circuit will need to be thoroughly evaluated for leaks.
   (c) Remove the scope tip out of the basin of water and firmly depress the bottom valve. The image should blur on the monitor, indicating water trickling over the lens.
      - If the lens cleaner is not working despite operational air insufflation, check to make sure the water bottle is at least filled halfway with water and the lid is sealed.
3. If video images are not displayed on the monitor(s) then
   (a) Make sure the monitor is turned on.
   (b) Check to make sure that the cable connecting the processor to the monitor is connected to one of the "video out" ports on the back of the processor and to the "video in" port on the back of the monitor.

(c) Ensure that the appropriate input is selected on the monitor. This is done by activating the menu on the monitor and navigating to an option along the lines of "Image Input." The choice selected should match the port to which the cable is connected on the monitor.
(d) If everything is properly connected and monitor is appropriately configured as above and image still not displaying, the cable may need to be replaced and/or a different "video in" port on the monitor should be tried (which will then require the port to be changed in the menu settings on the monitor).

Once the procedure is completed, cleaning of the endoscope must immediately begin in the procedure room before the endoscope is transported to the scope-wash room/area for high-level disinfection. The STs should have good knowledge of this process. The following should be readily available:

- Scope cleaning sponge
- Two containers with 500 mL capacity
- Enzymatic detergent
- Two containers of 1 L sterile water
- Air/water channel adaptor
- Cleaning brush
- Either an impermeable bag (there are a variety of manufactures of scope transport bags) or clean hard plastic bin with appropriate biohazard labels that are used to transport used endoscopes to the scope-wash room

Endoscopic Instruments

The maritime surgical team should have a variety of basic endoscopic tools that can be passed through the instrument channel to allow the endoscopist to perform important diagnostic or therapeutic inventions while at sea [2, 3]. The basic list might include the following, but it cannot be emphasized enough that the surgical team should perform a thorough inventory of all endoscopy gear, to include equipment, consumables, and injectables (i.e., oral contrast, epinephrine, India ink), prior to deployment as outlined in Chaps. 5 and 12.

- **Biopsy Forceps:** small grasping tools used for tissue sampling and removal of small (<3 mm) polyps.
- **Snares:** loops of monofilament or braided wire within a plastic catheter that is used to remove polyps or other types of tissue, different types of snares can be used with or without cauterization and come in a variety of shapes and sizes.
- **Grasping Forceps**: forceps with larger opening size used to remove foreign bodies or impacted food boluses, come in a variety of shapes and sizes.
- **Roth Nets:** retractable nets attached to a loop of wire used to remove foreign bodies, impacted food boluses, large polyps following polypectomy, etc.

- **Injection Needles:** through the scope needles that are used to inject medications, tattoo into the submucosa, or lift the mucosa.
- **Bipolar Hemostasis Catheters:** catheters that are connected to electrocautery unit and used to treat bleeding.
- **APC Probes:** used in conjunction with APC generator/Argon gas to focally transmit targeted electrical energy to treat bleeding or devitalized tissue.
- **Hemostasis Clips:** through the scope metal clips used to treat bleeding, close mucosal defects, or provide landmark for future radiographic studies or interventions.

Risks of Esophagogastroduodenoscopy (EGD) and Colonoscopy

EGD and colonoscopy are generally safe procedures with low rates of complications. Both procedures have risks related to sedation as well as risks unique to each procedure. The most common adverse events are reviewed below and should be discussed with patients as part of informed consent.

Moderate Sedation/Monitored Anesthesia Care (MAC)

Cardiopulmonary adverse events related to sedation include aspiration, hypoxemia, cardiac arrhythmias, and hypotension, accounting for 60% of all adverse events. Rates are variable across studies ranging from 1 per 170 to 1 per 10,000 procedures. Patients at high risk are those with underlying cardiopulmonary disease, advanced age, and American Society of Anesthesiologists (ASA) Class III or higher, all of which are unlikely but always possible on the forward deployed maritime platform.

Factors associated with increased rates of **aspiration** include patient factors of advanced age, altered mental status, gastric outlet obstruction, those with nothing by mouth (NPO) for less than 2 h prior to sedation, and procedural factors such as prolonged procedures, prone position, and procedures where intubation of the esophagus is difficult [4]. Rates of airway management issues are higher with anesthesiologist delivered sedation (0.14%) vs non-anesthesiologist delivered sedation (0.02%) [5, 6]. For colonoscopy, aspiration requiring hospitalization is rare, occurring in 0.004–0.16% [7].

Systemic sedation is typically utilized for endoscopy, but is not absolutely necessary if contraindicated. The goal of sedation is to facilitate completion of a safe and effective procedure, and it is generally well tolerated. The most commonly used medications for minimal to moderate sedation are midazolam, fentanyl, and meperidine given in small intravenous (IV) bolus doses separated by short intervals until the target level of sedation is achieved. IV diphenhydramine can also be utilized as an adjunct to sedation and best when given 3–5 min before the procedure. Reversal agents should always be immediately available in the procedure room if needed. Topical sedation with benzocaine is associated with methemoglobinemia and should be avoided.

EGD: **Bleeding** is uncommon with EGD in the absence of coagulopathy or thrombocytopenia. There is a 4% risk of bleeding with tissue biopsies in patients with <50,000 platelets/microliter. **Perforation** is also rare ranging from 1 in 2500 to 1 in 11,000 EGDs. Factors increasing risk of perforation include the presence of anterior cervical osteophytes, Zenker's diverticulum, esophageal stricture, malignancy, and duodenal diverticula [4, 6, 8].

Colonoscopy: The most common adverse events are **abdominal pain** (5–10%) and **bloating** (25%), typically related to air insufflation required for mucosal examination. Symptoms are reduced with minimizing air insufflation, use of carbon dioxide, use of water immersion technique, and avoidance of looping. **Bleeding** occurs in 2.4 per 1000 colonoscopies, but occurs almost exclusively with polypectomy (9.8/1000) compared with 0.6/1000 without polypectomy. Risk factors for bleeding include patients with cardiovascular disease, size and number of polyps removed, recent anticoagulation, and polyps removed from the right colon. Prophylactic clipping of non-pedunculated polyps >2 cm in size in the proximal colon reduces the risk of bleeding. The rate of **splenic injury** is 1–4.5 per 10,000 colonoscopies with increased rates in patients with splenocolic adhesions, splenomegaly, and prior abdominal surgery. Procedure-related risks include difficult colonoscopies, deep sedation, maneuvers such as "hooking" the splenic flexure to straighten the colon, and application of abdominal pressure in the left hypochondrium. **Perforation** risk is 5.8 per 10,000 colonoscopies. Patient factors increasing risk include inflammatory bowel disease (IBD) (with an eightfold greater risk), diverticulosis, and corticosteroid use. Endoscopists performing low volumes of endoscopy (defined as <141 colonoscopies per year) also have higher rates of perforation. **Mortality** secondary to colonoscopy is exceedingly rare occurring in 3 per 100,000 procedures [5, 7, 8].

Techniques for Performing Esophagogastroduodenoscopy (EGD) and Colonoscopy

There are general principles that can be applied to both EGD and colonoscopy to reduce the procedural-related risks and maximize likelihood of success.

- Always position the monitors and equipment and height of the patient in such a way that maximizes ergonomics for the endoscopist.
- The monitor should be directly in front of and 20 cm lower than the height of the endoscopist resulting in the top edge of the monitor at eye level or below.

Assuming a 14-in. monitor, the optimal distance away from the endoscopist is between 52 and 182 cm [9].

- For both left- and right-handed endoscopists, the handle of the scope is held in the left hand and the insertion tube is held in the right.
- When patients become uncomfortable, try repositioning the scope, reducing scope loops, or removing excess gas before giving additional sedation.
- **When resistance is encountered while inserting the scope, STOP and try to determine the cause.** If resistance is the result of scope looping then loop reduction, subtle tip control to navigate around overlapping folds, and use of water immersion technique in the sigmoid colon with patient in the slightly head-down position should be considered. If it is a stricture that is offering resistance, options include switching to a smaller caliber scope or taking biopsies and aborting. In neither case should the endoscopist simply push harder as this may result in perforation.
- There should be no resistance during withdrawal of the scope. If there is resistance, then immediately stop and reposition the scope and loosen the knobs before reattempted scope withdrawal. Pulling harder is not a safe strategy.
- Avoid doing anything that may make it more difficult for performing follow-up endoscopic procedures. Do not biopsy polyps that can potentially be removed. Do not inject tattoo directly into an identified abnormality.
- If there is any doubt during the procedure and doing nothing poses no threat to the patient, then do nothing.
- When the scope tip is against the wall of the lumen and there is blanching of the mucosal vasculature then the scope should be repositioned to get off of the wall to reduce risk of perforation.
- Always consider complications of the procedure during and after the endoscopic exam if there are unexpected events.
- The goal of the endoscopic exam is to examine as close to 100% of the mucosal surface as possible.

Esophagogastroduodenoscopy (EGD)

Patient positioning: The patient should be placed in the left lateral decubitus position, but the procedure can be completed supine if necessary. Supine positioning may make it more difficult to pass the scope beyond the pylorus. The patient's mouth should be at a height that is comfortable for the endoscopist.

Scope handling/endoscopist position: Hold the insertion tube at approximately 15–20 cm from the tip with the right hand such that the major deflection of the scope is aligned with the pointer finger. This technique provides optimum scope control and avoids the need for repositioning of the hand during esophageal intubation. The umbilical connector should be in front of the endoscopist.

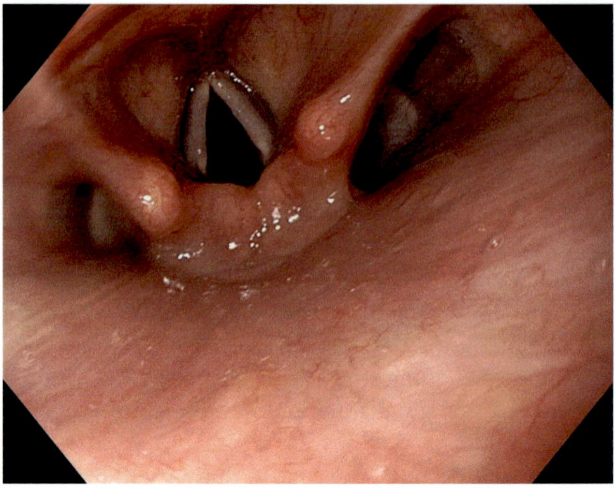

Fig. 18.7 Normal hypopharynx with vocal cords (top) and cricoarytenoid cartilage (bottom). (Source: Photo courtesy of R. Daniel Lawson, MD)

Scope advancement: Once the target level of sedation has been achieved, place the tip of the instrument on the tongue. Guide the scope through the mouth toward the soft palate with the tongue at the 12 o'clock and the uvula at 6 o'clock while slightly deflecting the tip of the scope with big wheel to maintain visualization. After passing the epiglottis, the cricoarytenoid cartilage and vocal cords will appear (Fig. 18.7). Deflect the tip of the instrument behind the cricoarytenoid cartilage and apply gentle pressure. Eventually with this gentle pressure, or with swallowing, the upper esophageal sphincter (UES) will relax enough to allow the scope to easily pass into the esophagus. Gentle side-to-side movement and torquing of the scope tip to maneuver out of the piriform sinuses may be required to traverse the UES. Never push hard as this can result in perforation.

Procedure: If there is no resistance to the scope, immediately and gently advance the endoscope to the stomach and immediately remove any residual liquid to help reduce risk of aspiration. Then either start the examination in the stomach and finish with the esophagus or withdraw the scope and start in the esophagus. Strategy will depend on endoscopist preferences and the indications for the procedure.

In the esophagus, examine the appearance of the GEJ and esophageal mucosa (Fig. 18.8). Patiently wait for any peristaltic waves to pass and the esophagus to relax to allow for complete inspection. In the left lateral position, fluid will accumulate along the left wall of the esophagus, which is the 6 o'clock position of the endoscopic view. Normal esophageal mucosa is shiny, pale, and white with superficial blood vessels running longitudinally. In the mid-esophagus there is extrinsic compression with indentation of the anterior wall from the aortic arch and left main bronchus. Left atrial pulsation can occasionally be seen. The GEJ is the transition zone from the esophagus to the stomach and identified by the proximal edge of the gastric folds (Fig. 18.9). The squamocolumnar junction is the transition zone from stratified squamous mucosa of the esophagus, characterized by the end of the

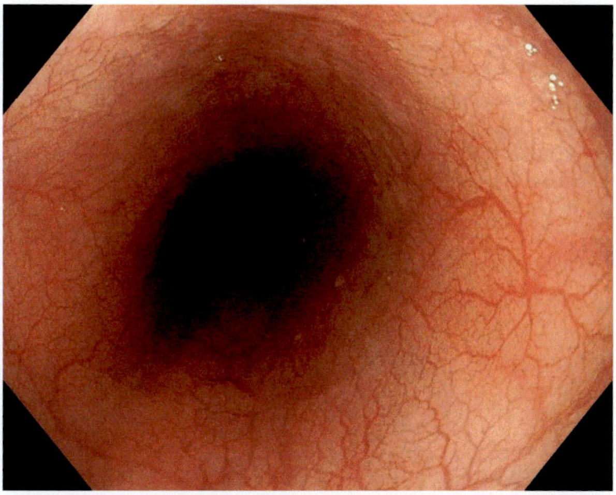

Fig. 18.8 Normal esophagus with shiny, pale, white mucosa. (Source: Photo courtesy of R. Daniel Lawson, MD)

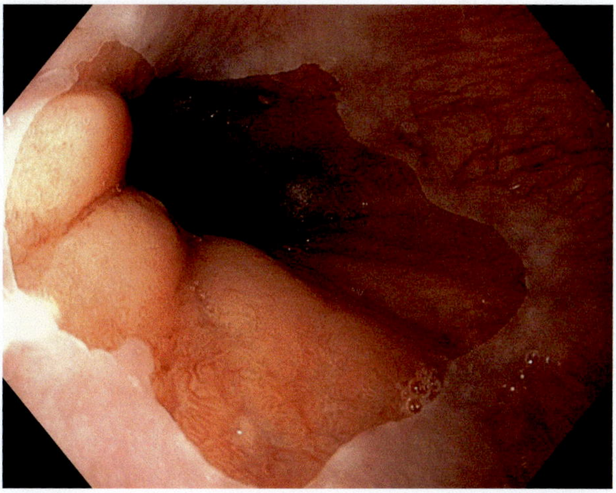

Fig. 18.9 Normal gastroesophageal junction (GEJ) with transition from longitudinal palisading vessels of the esophagus to the thick, red gastric mucosa. (Source: Photo courtesy of R. Daniel Lawson, MD)

longitudinal palisading vessels, and beginning of the thick, red mucosa of the stomach. The final important landmark in this region is identification of the diaphragmatic hiatus, which endoscopically appears as circumferential extrinsic compression often described as a "pinch." It normally occurs at the level of the GEJ, but can be below it in the setting of a hiatal hernia (Fig. 18.10) [10].

Once the endoscope has entered the stomach when the patient is in the left lateral decubitus position, the greater curvature will be at the 6 o'clock position, lesser curvature at 12 o'clock, anterior wall at 9 o'clock, and posterior wall at 3 o'clock [10]. Again, any retained fluid should be immediately suctioned. The stomach should be maximally insufflated with flattening of the rugal folds for adequate mucosal visualization. Incomplete insufflation should alert the endoscopist to the possibility of an underlying diffuse benign or malignant infiltrative disease (e.g., linitis plastica,

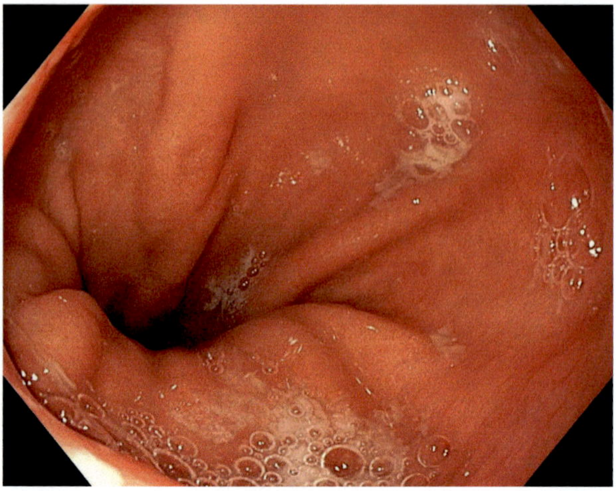

Fig. 18.10 Hiatal hernia with diaphragmatic hernia or "pinch" seen distal to the gastroesophageal junction (GEJ). (Source: Photo courtesy of R. Daniel Lawson, MD)

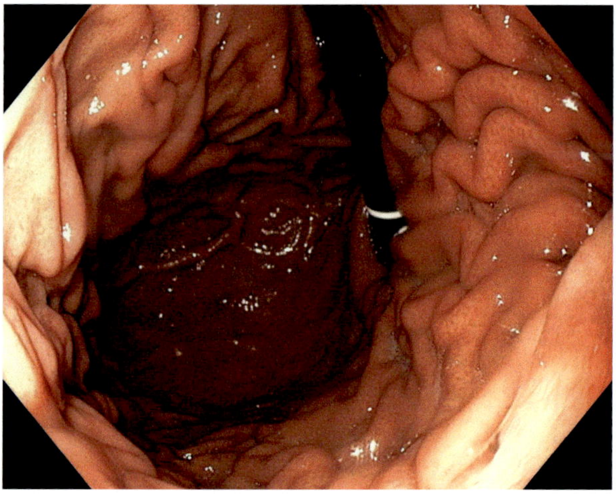

Fig. 18.11 Normal gastric mucosa with lesser curvature (foreground) and fundus (background) on retroflexion. (Source: Photo courtesy of R. Daniel Lawson, MD)

lymphoma, Ménétrier disease, scleroderma, sarcoidosis, CD). Visualization of the cardia, fundus, and the lesser curvature of the body is best accomplished through retroflexion (Fig. 18.11). This is performed by advancing the endoscope toward the antrum with maximal deflection of the tip up and to the left (big wheel and little wheel all the way down), creating the "candy cane" appearance of the scope tip. Torque of the scope to the left (counterclockwise) is often necessary to avoid the incisura. The endoscope should be advanced to the antrum, demarcated from the body at the angularis with transition from rugal folds to flat mucosa and ending in the pyloric ring [10]. The scope is advanced to and through the pylorus, which generally requires introduction of a loop into the J shaped stomach and will increase pressure in the patient's oropharynx resulting in some discomfort. If the patient is in the supine position and the endoscopist is unable to pass the scope into the duodenum because of looping then reposition the patient in the left lateral position.

Beyond the pylorus is the first portion of the duodenum, or duodenal bulb, identified by the transition from flat mucosa to the finger-like projections called villi that line the small intestinal mucosa. While patient is in the left lateral position, the anterior wall will be at the 9 o'clock position and the posterior wall at 3 o'clock. Adequate visualization of the posterior wall is important prior to advancing the endoscope as superficial scope trauma can occur when passing the duodenal sweep. Traversing the duodenal or "C" sweep involves reduction of the previously placed internal loop and shortening of the endoscope. This is accomplished by advancing the scope to the proximal edge of the sweep, right (clockwise) torque, and upward deflection of the tip of the scope (big wheel down). This is followed by internally rotating the left arm, turning the endoscopist's body to the right, and finally withdrawing the endoscope with the right hand which should result in the scope propelling forward. Ideally, the luminal tract should be kept in view throughout this entire maneuver, but with edema or anatomical variance, can be carefully performed with blind passage. If resistance is encountered this should be aborted immediately. At this point the scope is in the second portion of the duodenum and can be confirmed by visualization of the major and/or minor papillae (Fig. 18.12), although this is not always possible with a forward viewing endoscope.

Upon withdrawal, the mucosa of the duodenum should be examined in a 360° pattern ensuring that the mucosa on the proximal side of each fold is adequately seen. The posterior wall of the duodenum is notoriously challenging to visualize as the scope has a tendency to slingshot backward around this turn now that the gastric loop has been reduced. Ways to increase visualization of this wall are by utilizing the outside wheel or with the addition of a plastic cap attachment to the distal tip of the scope. The stomach can be examined again during withdrawal with retroflexion repeated if necessary. Before removing the scope from the patient's body, the stomach should be completely decompressed of gasses and fluids.

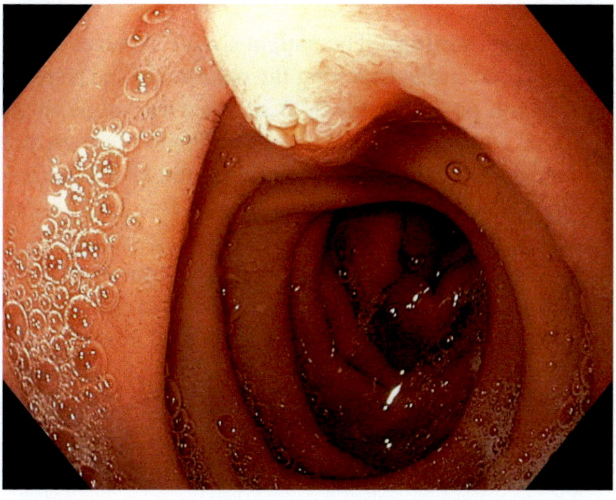

Fig. 18.12 Normal second portion of the duodenum indicated by villi and opening of the major papilla at 12 o'clock. (Source: Photo courtesy of R. Daniel Lawson, MD)

Regardless of whether the esophagus was examined earlier in the procedure, it is good practice to always carefully examine the entire length of the esophagus as outlined above during final withdrawal of the scope. It is not uncommon for novice endoscopists to simply pull the scope out of the body once the examination of the stomach and duodenum is completed even though little attention may have been given to the esophagus during scope insertion. After passing the UES, the oropharynx should be suctioned during removal of the scope to reduce aspiration risk.

Pitfalls: A common reason for failure of EGD is inability to intubate the esophagus. This can occur in the setting of an inadequately sedated patient, in which case gagging and patient discomfort prohibit esophageal intubation. If it is unsafe to give additional systemic sedation, topical pharyngeal anesthetic with viscous lidocaine can improve patient tolerability. If adequate sedation cannot be achieved, performing upper endoscopy transnasally with a neonatal endoscope is an option, as this is more tolerable for patients (when available, not likely to be on a non-T-AH maritime platform). Cervical osteophytes can also make intubation difficult as these deflect the tip of the scope anteriorly toward the vocal cords. In this case, approaching the esophageal opening from either piriform sinus and torquing the endoscope midline once beyond the cricoarytenoid cartilage can result in successful intubation. Additionally, anterior jaw thrust performed by an assistant can also facilitate easier intubation. In the difficult to intubate esophagus, consideration should also be given to an underlying Zenker's diverticulum or a proximal esophageal stricture, as there is increased risk for esophageal perforation. In this situation, using a neonatal scope with standard technique can be performed and is often successful (again, when available).

Colonoscopy

Patient positioning: The patient should be placed in the left lateral decubitus position. In some cases, changing the position of the patient to the supine, prone, or even right lateral position may help advance the scope to the cecum. Proper positioning is crucial for a successful examination and maintenance of proper ergonomics. The patient should be placed at approximately elbow height to 10 cm below elbow height so that the endoscopist's head, neck, back, shoulder, and elbow postures are neutral. Vector force is also important to consider. The angle of the patient should be such that the trajectory of the left colon is parallel to the vector of the pushing force. This reduces bowing of the colonoscope in the rectum and results in better one-to-one transmission of shaft movement to tip motion.

Scope handling/endoscopist position: The insertion tube should be held approximately 30 cm from the tip. The arms should be in a comfortable, neutral position. The umbilical connector should be behind the endoscopist.

Digital rectal exam (DRE): If maneuvers to assess anorectal function are indicated, the anorectal digital rectal exam (DRE) should be performed PRIOR TO initiation of sedation. Otherwise, once the target level of sedation is achieved, a DRE should be performed beginning with an external exam to assess for rashes, lesions, excoriations, fissures, fistulae, skin tags, hemorrhoids, and rectal prolapse. Next, a lubricated and gloved finger is slowly advanced into the rectum to assess for any masses or strictures. In men, the prostate should be palpated for any nodules or masses. Additionally, tenderness should be assessed to determine if additional sedation should be given prior to inserting the endoscope.

Scope advancement: The tip of the endoscope should then be advanced slowly through the anus into the rectum. If double-gloved for the DRE, then the top lubricated glove should be removed to improve scope grip. Immediately upon insertion there will be a red-out appearance while the rectum is insufflated and the scope rotated until the lumen is identified. The scope is advanced through the rectum, which is characterized by prominent vasculature and large, semi-crescent folds of mucosa referred to as the valves of Houston (Fig. 18.13). These alternate in a left-to-right orientation and are typically three in total (lower, middle, upper) and are useful landmarks when describing location of mucosal abnormalities. The rectum is approximately 15 cm in length and a retroperitoneal structure; thus, it is relatively fixed [11]. The endoscope should be advanced through this section with relative ease with mainly right and left torque to navigate the valves of Houston through the rectosigmoid junction and into the sigmoid colon.

Procedure: The sigmoid colon is an intraperitoneal structure that is usually freely mobile but can be fixed in the setting of prior lower abdominal surgery or inflammatory processes. The sigmoid forms a loop approximately 40 cm in length, which can

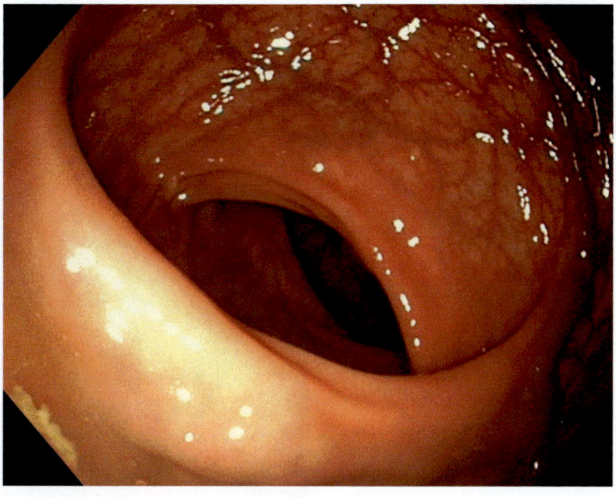

Fig. 18.13 Normal rectal mucosa with the semi-crescent valves of Houston. (Source: Photo courtesy of R. Daniel Lawson, MD)

be lengthened up to 70 cm from stretching during colonoscope insertion. Additionally, there are multiple curves with deep haustra and acute angulations, making this one of the most challenging portions of the insertion. The lumen is often collapsed and narrow and can be identified by the convergence of folds [11, 12]. Additional clues for the appropriate direction of the lumen are areas of shadow and the concave area of the arcs formed by folds. Experts recommend that up to two thirds of the total insertion time should be spent navigating the sigmoid colon, ensuring that the scope is as short as possible with all loops fully reduced prior to advancing beyond the splenic flexure [13]. It is in the sigmoid colon that using water immersion rather than gas insufflation with patient in slightly head-down position may be the most useful since the water weighs down and straightens the sigmoid [14].

The splenic flexure can occasionally be identified by a bluish hue indicating the luminal impression of the spleen. The transverse colon is traditionally marked by triangular shaped haustra (Fig. 18.14). This portion of the colon can be straightforward and allow for easy scope advancement but in some patients can be tortuous and difficult to traverse. The hepatic flexure is also often identified by a blue area from the impression of the liver (Fig. 18.15) and typically indicates the last turn into the ascending colon. The approach to this turn is similar to that of the duodenal sweep and involves advancing the tip of the scope to the proximal edge of the ascending colon, right (clockwise) torque of the scope, maximal deflection of the scope tip (big wheel down). This is followed by internally rotating the left arm, turning the endoscopist's body to the right, and finally withdrawing the endoscope with the right hand which should result in reduction of the colonoscope and advancement of the tip forward into the proximal ascending colon.

The colonoscope is then advanced into the cecum; often this requires slight luminal decompression and possibly external pressure applied in the transverse colon or right upper quadrant by an assistant. The cecum is identified by three major

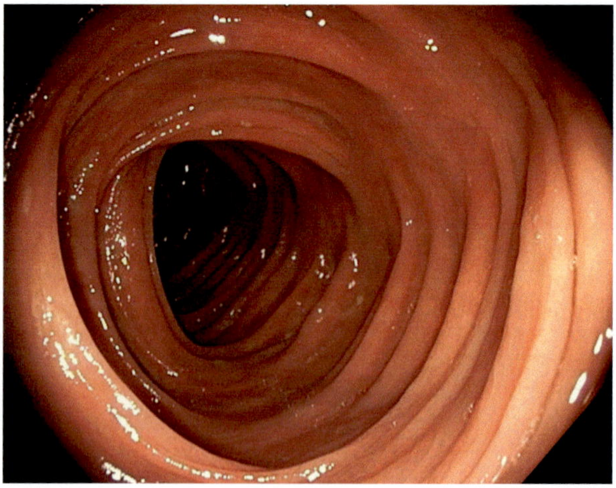

Fig. 18.14 Normal transverse colon with the triangular haustral folds. (Source: Photo courtesy of R. Daniel Lawson, MD)

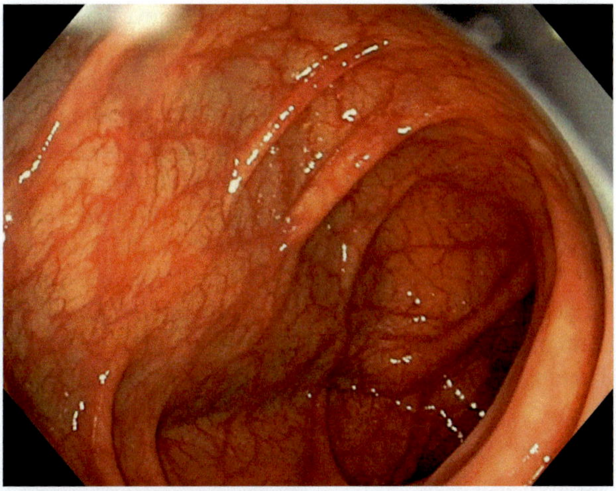

Fig. 18.15 Normal hepatic flexure indicated by blue area from impression of the liver. (Source: Photo courtesy of R. Daniel Lawson, MD)

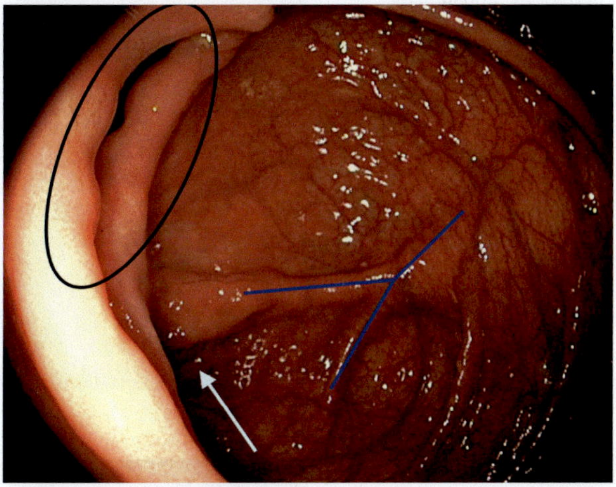

Fig. 18.16 Normal cecum with appendiceal orifice (AO) (arrow); ileocecal valve (ICV) (oval); taenia coli forming appearance of crow's feet (y-shaped lines). (Source: Photo courtesy of R. Daniel Lawson, MD)

landmarks: the appendiceal orifice (AO), ileocecal valve (ICV), and terminal ileum (TI), which should all be photo-documented and included in the procedure report for quality metrics. The cecum is the proximal end of the colon, which takes the appearance of a crow's foot formed by three bands of longitudinal taenia coli converging on the AO (Fig. 18.16). The AO is typically round or semilunar in shape [11]. It is important to identify all three landmarks to confirm cecal intubation since the hepatic flexure can mimic the appearance of the crow's foot in the cecum. Approximately 5 cm distal to the AO is the ICV that appears as an elongated, wide-mouthed opening along the ileocecal fold. In order to identify the ICV, the colonoscope should be withdrawn approximately 8–10 cm from the AO to bring the ileocecal fold into view, which appears as a thickened area on the first haustral fold from the cecal pole. Depending on the position of the ICV, it can be difficult to visualize the opening. Techniques to achieve ICV visualization include rotating the scope to reorient position as well as suctioning air from the lumen to reduce colonic distention and allowing the ICV orifice to fall into view. If this is unsuccessful, the bow and arrow sign can help identify the opening. This method includes using the curve of the AO as the bow and drawing an imaginary line perpendicular to the apex of the bow that points toward the opening of the ICV (Fig. 18.17) [15]. Finally, performing retroflexion of the colonoscope in the cecum can also bring the ICV into view and provide a retroflexed view of the ascending colon. Cecal retroflexion (Fig. 18.18) is accomplished by insufflating the cecum, then advancing the endoscope toward the AO while maximally deflecting the scope tip into the "candy cane" configuration by rotating both the big and little wheel toward the endoscopist and torquing the insertion tube clockwise or counterclockwise, depending on position.

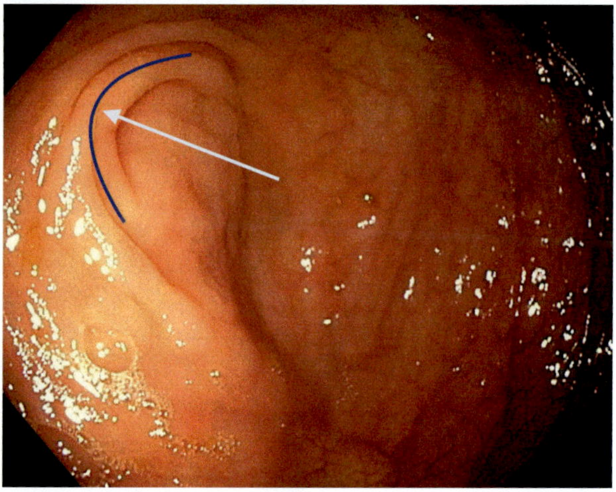

Fig. 18.17 Normal bow and arrow sign in the cecum, bow formed by the curve of the appendiceal orifice (AO) (curved line) and arrow pointing to the opening of the ileocecal valve (ICV). (Source: Photo courtesy of R. Daniel Lawson, MD)

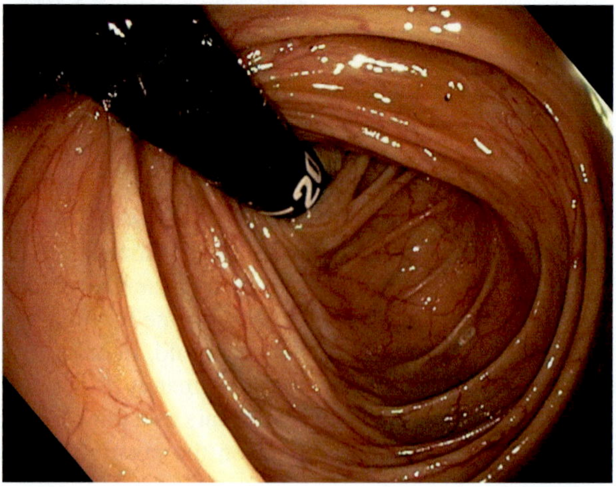

Fig. 18.18 Normal ascending colon visualized in cecal retroflexion. (Source: Photo courtesy of R. Daniel Lawson, MD)

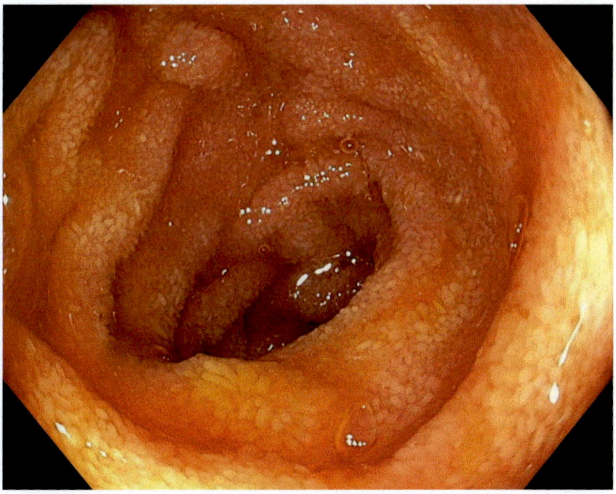

Fig. 18.19 Normal terminal ileum (TI) mucosa with villi. (Source: Photo courtesy of R. Daniel Lawson, MD)

Once the ICV has been identified, the TI should be intubated if possible. Ideally, this is accomplished by bringing the opening to the ICV in direct view and advancing the tip of the scope through the opening. This is not always possible and blind intubation of the TI can be accomplished by starting with the tip of the scope in the cecum and withdrawing slowly while deflecting the tip of the scope toward the opening of the ICV. Once villi of the ileal mucosa are visualized, slow movements with gentle puffs of air insufflation or water irrigation encourage opening of the valve and visualization of the TI lumen (Fig. 18.19). Ideally, this maneuver is performed with the ICV at the 9–12 o'clock position allowing for maximal radius of tip deflection. Prior to attempting blind intubation, reducing colonic tension by suctioning air from the colon can increase the likelihood of successful TI intubation. Finally, if all of the above are unsuccessful, the TI can be intubated in retroflexion. This is accomplished by retroflexion in the cecum (described above). Once the ICV is visualized, withdraw the scope until the tip of the scope is within the distal TI. The dials are then released while continuing to withdraw the scope slowly, which should result in propulsion of the scope tip deeper into the TI.

The TI indicates the most proximal and final location in standard colonoscopy. At this point scope withdrawal is initiated, during which detailed mucosal evaluation is performed. Appropriate withdrawal technique includes slowly removing the colonoscope while rotating in a 360° pattern ensuring all areas of the lumen are examined. If the indication for examination is colorectal cancer (CRC) screening, a second look in the right colon should be performed either en face or in retroflexion, which can facilitate better visualization of difficult to see areas. The most difficult areas to visualize are typically the cecal side of mucosal folds, particularly in the right colon. These folds can be pulled back and flattened out for inspection by using the tip of the scope or examined with the scope in retroflexed position.

Once the scope has reached the dentate line, the final step of the examination is retroflexion within the rectum (Fig. 18.20). This is accomplished using a technique

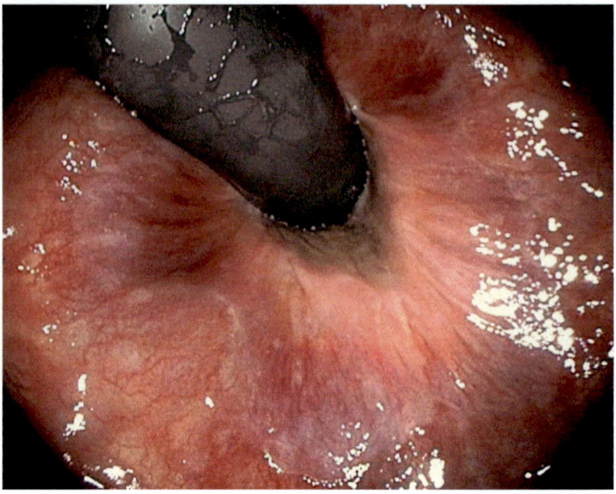

Fig. 18.20 Normal dentate line and distal rectum visualized in retroflexion. (Source: Photo courtesy of R. Daniel Lawson, MD)

similar to retroflexion in the cecum and stomach. This view should also be photo-documented for completion. All dials should then be relaxed and unlocked and the scope is then removed from the patient. Minimum withdrawal time for a complete exam during screening colonoscopy is 6 min; however, longer periods of time may be required to assure complete visualization of the colonic mucosa.

1. **Pitfalls**:

   - **Sigmoid Colon:** Given its tortuosity and mobility, the sigmoid colon is often the most challenging region to traverse during colonoscopy, especially in the presence of severe diverticulosis. Air insufflation should be minimized as this lengthens the colon and sharpens angulations at the flexures [14]. Sigmoid alpha and omega loops are commonly formed while advancing the endoscope through this section of the colon [16]. Loss of one-to-one transmission or paradoxical motion is indicative of loop introduction and should be reduced prior to moving forward. Loop reduction is typically performed by rightward (clockwise) torque, maintaining the luminal view with right-left controls, and withdrawing the scope until the shaft is straightened and one-to-one transmission is again obtained. Another common challenge in the sigmoid colon is navigating acute angulations. Keeping the arc of the folds at the 6 and 12 o'clock positions can be helpful in navigating these turns as tip deflection is maximal with the up-down control. Water immersion can help straighten the sigmoid segment and reduce loop formation, and placing the patient in the supine position can also open angulations [17]. If these techniques are not successful, the adult colonoscope can be exchanged for a pediatric colonoscope or gastroscope to navigate tight, fixed angulations [18]. **Importantly, pushing against fixed resistance should never be performed as this can result in perforation or other complications.**

- **Transverse Colon:** In the redundant colon and in patients with a large mesenteric fat pad, the formation of "U" loops and gamma loops (a circle formed within the coronal plane) can occur in the transverse colon. In these situations, stiffening the colonoscope via the variable stiffness knob or by applying gentle rightward (clockwise) torque while advancing can assist with creating a more linear push force. Insertion of a stiffening wire or biopsy forceps into the working channel can also provide increased scope stiffness in significantly redundant colons [18]. Additionally, transverse colonic abdominal pressure prior to advancing the scope can prevent the formation of these types of loops and keep the colonoscope straight [18]. This is performed by the assistant applying manual pressure posteriorly in the periumbilical region and then gently pulling cephalad.
- **Ascending Colon:** Right-sided colonic looping is common, making intubation of the cecum and/or TI challenging. Maintaining a straightened scope with frequent loop reduction while passing the scope through the distal colon is critical for success. In patients with a challenging ascending colon, the scope may need to be withdrawn, to the rectum if necessary, followed by meticulous attention to loop reduction at each turn during scope reinsertion to achieve one-to-one motion at the hepatic flexure. In some cases, this can be made difficult by large abdominal wall hernias in which case manual reduction of these hernias throughout the procedure can help with successful completion. Abdominal pressure can minimize loop formation in the right colon typically over the right lateral abdomen or via upward pressure under the cecum [19]. If the assistant is able to palpate the scope during loop formation, direct abdominal pressure over this area prior to scope advancement should be attempted. On occasion "sandwiching" is necessary in which two assistants apply pressure on both sides of the abdomen [18]. Changes in patient position either to the supine, prone, or right lateral position can also prove helpful in this situation.

Common Pathologies: Dysphagia and Odynophagia

Esophageal Foreign Body

Presentation: Classically presents as acute onset of dysphagia with or without odynophagia. In the setting of complete esophageal obstruction, there will also be inability to tolerate secretions (sialorrhea). Most patients will be able to identify the ingested foreign body or food bolus as well as the timing of ingestion. A classic presentation was shown in Clinical Vignette 18.2. Localization is non-specific, but sensation of retrosternal discomfort is suggestive of obstruction in the distal esophagus. The most common locations of impaction occur at the three sites of physiologic narrowing: the UES, aortic arch, and diaphragmatic hiatus (typically at the GEJ) [20]. Patients should be evaluated for signs and symptoms of airway compromise (i.e., stridor, choking), esophageal perforation (i.e., fever, persistent tachycardia >120 beats per minute, retrosternal chest pain, crepitus), and bowel obstruction [21]. In the setting of a food bolus, administration of IV glucagon 1 mg can be given in attempts to facilitate passage via smooth muscle and lower esophageal sphincter (LES) relaxation. Endoscopic removal should be performed within 24 h for most esophageal foreign bodies as delays beyond this increase risk for perforation. Emergent indications for immediate removal include complete esophageal obstruction due to risk of aspiration and ingestion of sharp objects or disk batteries due to risk of perforation [21]. Labs and imaging are not routinely required unless indicated clinically. Barium swallows with serial static X-rays (as seen in Clinical Vignettes 18.1 and 18.2 and Fig. 18.1) can help diagnose a number of upper gastrointestinal disorders and obstruction. Barium sulfate is an inert material, but it can rarely cause complications. Symptoms are rare after small volume aspirations, however aspiration pneumonitis, hypoxia, and/or acute respiratory distress syndrome have been reported in severe cases.

Pre-procedural intubation is recommended for airway control in all cases at sea.

Endoscopy: Intubation of the esophagus should be performed cautiously in the event of impaction of the foreign body in the proximal esophagus. The endoscope should be advanced slowly until the foreign body is identified (Fig. 18.21). Various retrieval devices are available for use and depend on availability, foreign body characteristics, positioning, and endoscopist preference. Ideally, a sharp object should be removed with the sharp edge directed distally. If available, overtubes or distal hood attachments can be utilized to protect the mucosa during removal of sharp objects. Impacted food is the most common esophageal foreign body in adults and usually indicative of underlying esophageal pathology (i.e., eosinophilic esophagi-

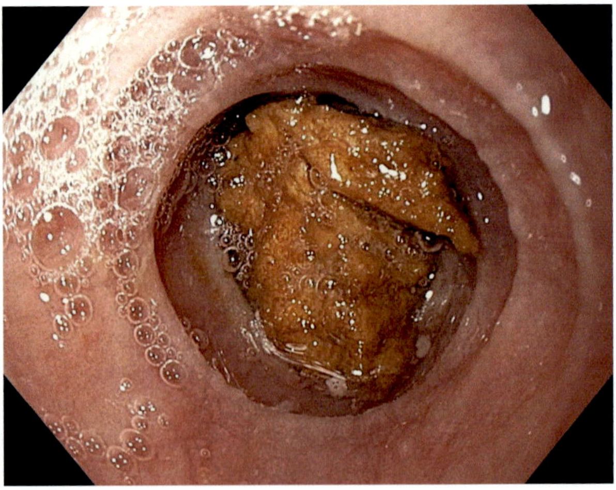

Fig. 18.21 Esophageal foreign body consisting of food bolus impaction with concentric rings or "trachealization" of the esophagus, suggestive of eosinophilic esophagitis (EoE). (Source: Photo courtesy of R. Daniel Lawson, MD)

tis (EoE)). In the absence of bones or other sharp components, attempt at advancing an impacted food bolus into the stomach with gentle scope pressure and air pressure can be performed. Excessive force indicated by bowing of the endoscope should be avoided as this can result in perforation. If the food bolus cannot be advanced, piecemeal removal can be performed with snare forceps, raptor forceps, or Roth nets. Once the foreign body has been cleared, the esophagus should be evaluated for underlying pathology, but biopsies and dilation should be deferred.

Post procedural management: Diet can be advanced as tolerated unless there is evidence of complications. If anatomical obstruction is identified, the patient should maintain nutrition with a pureed or liquid diet until return from sea and evaluation with repeat endoscopy. Given association with underlying pathology, these patients should be referred for formal evaluation with gastroenterology (GI) subspecialists at the end of deployment. Earlier evaluation via routine MEDEVAC may be required if a patient develops a second episode of esophageal impaction during deployment.

Eosinophilic Esophagitis (EoE)

Presentation: Symptoms are variable and range in severity. Subtle clinical manifestations include chronic reflux symptoms and gradual accommodation in eating behavior such as eating slowly, cutting food into small pieces, and drinking liquid to dilute food. Intermittent dysphagia to solids, liquids, and pills is common. Some patients will present with an esophageal food impaction as their index presentation. Common comorbidities include other atopic disorders such as asthma, eczema, allergic rhinitis, and anaphylactic food allergy [22].

Endoscopy: The most common findings are mucosal edema, eosinophilic exudates, linear furrows, esophageal rings, and strictures (Fig. 18.22). Multiple stacked concentric rings can form and appear as "trachealization" of the esophagus. An endoscopic scoring system has been developed and validated to standardize assessment of EoE known as the EREFS (edema, rings, exudates, furrows, strictures) score [23]. Four quadrant biopsies should be obtained from the distal esophagus, 3–5 cm above the GEJ, and the mid-esophagus at 10–15 cm above the GEJ to maximize the likelihood of detecting esophageal eosinophilia. Biopsies are best obtained by advancing the biopsy forceps beyond the distal tip of the endoscope. The forceps should then be opened and pulled back until hubbed against the endoscope. The tip should then be deflected toward the desired area of biopsy while suctioning air from the lumen. Once the lumen has collapsed, the forceps should be closed and biopsies taken. A firm sensation when taking biopsies can also be appreciated in the fibrostenotic form of EoE and referred to as the "tug sign."

Post-procedural management: Patients should be instructed to chew all food thoroughly and to avoid foods that trigger symptoms. If there is significant luminal

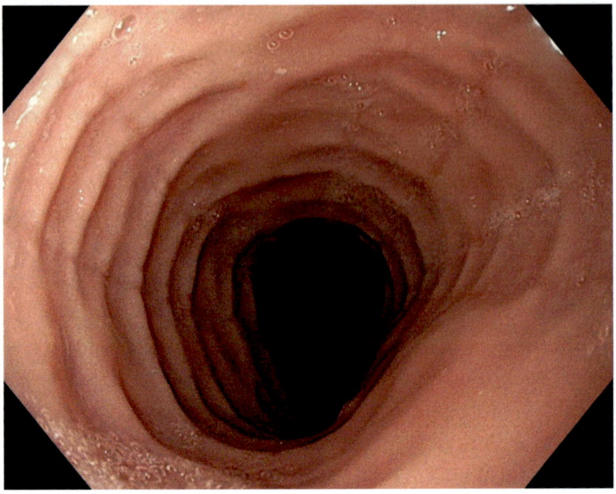

Fig. 18.22 Eosinophilic esophagitis (EoE) characterized by esophageal edema, furrows, and multiple concentric rings or "trachealization." (Source: Photo courtesy of R. Daniel Lawson, MD)

narrowing or strictures identified, the patient should maintain a pureed or liquid diet until returning from sea and evaluated by GI subspecialists. First-line medical treatment is with oral proton pump inhibitors (PPI), typically taken twice daily 30–60 min before a meal and titrated to lowest effective dose. Approximately 30–50% of patients will have histologic response to PPI therapy. In those that do not respond to PPI or those with significant inflammation and esophageal narrowing, topical steroids can be initiated. One option is via a fluticasone 220 μg aerosol inhaler with instructions for two puffs into the mouth and swallowed twice daily [24]. If available, a budesonide slurry can also be utilized but often requires special compounding by the pharmacy that is unlikely to be in the maritime pharmacy.

Drug-Induced Esophagitis

Presentation: Patients typically present with acute onset of retrosternal chest pain, odynophagia, dysphagia, and/or hematemesis. History is critical and should reveal recent initiation of a culprit medication. Medications known to cause esophageal mucosal injury include those with low pH such as doxycycline, ferrous sulfate, and ascorbic acid, those with hyperosmolar properties such as potassium chloride, those disrupting the cytoprotective mucosal barrier such as aspirin and nonsteroidal anti-inflammatory drugs (NSAIDs), and those with direct chemical injury such as oral bisphosphonates. Antibiotics account for approximately 50% of reported cases [20, 25]. Patients at increased risk are those with risk factors that delay esophageal transit such as altered esophageal anatomy, esophageal dysmotility, and conditions affecting saliva production and/or taking pills without adequate liquid and lying supine soon after ingesting medications [20].

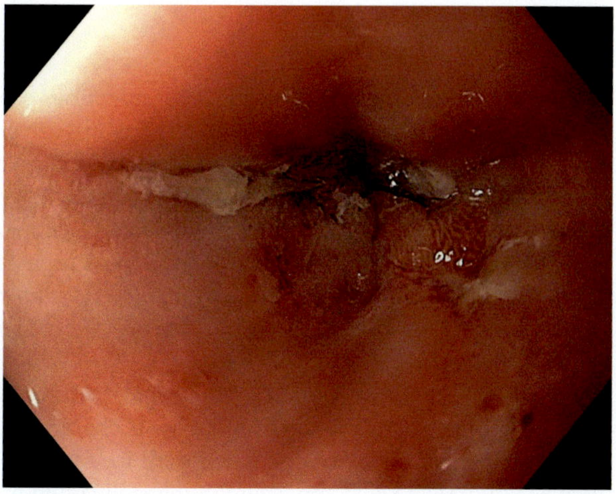

Fig. 18.23 Drug-induced esophagitis with classic "kissing ulcers." (Source: Photo courtesy of R. Daniel Lawson, MD)

Endoscopy: The most common anatomic locations where pills can become lodged in the esophagus are the mid-esophagus (at the aortic arch) and the GEJ [20]. Endoscopic appearance is variable and can be non-specific with erythema, edema, friability, erosions, and superficial ulcerations in typical locations. Remnant drug fragments and coating of the esophageal mucosa with drug material can be seen. A classic finding is the "kissing ulcer," which appears as two ulcerations on opposing walls of the esophagus representing two areas of contact injury from the previously trapped pill (Fig. 18.23) [26]. Chronic or severe drug-induced esophagitis can result in luminal narrowing and stricture, although this is uncommon. Infectious esophagitis with Herpes simplex virus (HSV) or cytomegalovirus (CMV) can mimic drug-induced esophagitis warranting superficial biopsies from the edge and center of any ulcers present. While bleeding ulcers are rare, if present or if high-risk features for recurrent bleeding are present, they should be treated similar to peptic ulcers.

Post-procedure Management: Drug-induced esophagitis is usually a self-limiting condition after discontinuing the offending agent, which is the primary treatment modality. A short trial (2–4 weeks) of PPI can reduce further mucosal injury from acid reflux. Oral sucralfate provides a local barrier and can help with symptoms and healing. Topical lidocaine can also be used to alleviate odynophagia. If difficulty swallowing is severe then patients can maintain nutrition with a liquid diet. To prevent drug-induced esophagitis, patients should also be educated to take all medications while upright with eight ounces of water and avoid lying supine or prone for at least 30 min after ingestion.

Infectious Esophagitis

Presentation: Patients at highest risk for infectious esophagitis are those who have immunosuppression either from an underlying disease process such as human immunodeficiency virus (HIV) or by treatment with an immunosuppressive therapy; however, this process can occur in the immunocompetent patient. The hallmark symptom of infectious esophagitis is acute or subacute odynophagia occasionally with concomitant dysphagia. The most common causal organism is *Candida* followed by HSV and CMV. Less common culprits include HIV, tuberculosis (TB), varicella zoster virus, among other viral, bacterial, fungal, and parasitic etiologies [27].

Endoscopy: There are classic endoscopic features depending on the causative infectious organism. Candidal esophagitis is characterized by thick, white, adherent plaques that are not easily dislodged with irrigation (Fig. 18.24). Biopsy of these plaques will reveal yeast and pseudohyphae invading mucosal cells [27]. The vesicular lesions seen in oropharyngeal and genital HSV infection are rarely seen in the esophagus. HSV esophagitis appears as multiple small, well-demarcated, shallow ulcers with normal intervening mucosa (Fig. 18.25). Biopsies should be obtained from the edge of the ulcer for highest diagnostic yield. This contrasts with CMV esophagitis that classically presents with linear, serpiginous, deep ulcerations affecting submucosal fibroblasts and vascular endothelium. Thus, biopsies should be taken from the base of the ulcer bed to make the diagnosis [28]. Other forms of infectious esophagitis are variable in appearance. If there is suspicion for bacterial or tuberculosis infection, separate biopsies should be taken, placed in sterile water, and sent to microbiology for culture and possibly polymerase chain reaction (PCR) testing.

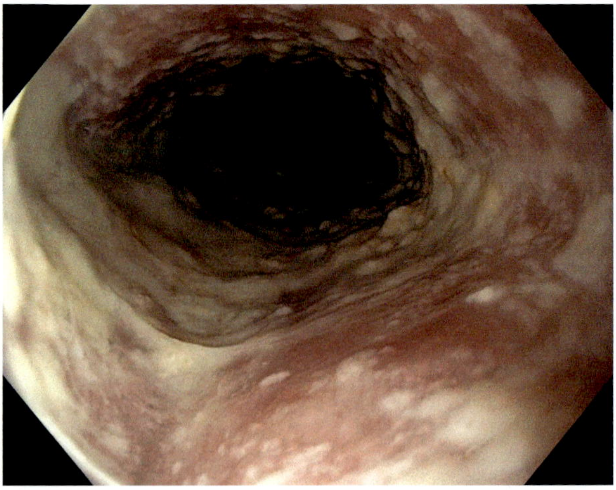

Fig. 18.24 Candidal esophagitis with classic thick, white plaques adherent to the esophageal mucosa. (Source: Photo courtesy of R. Daniel Lawson, MD)

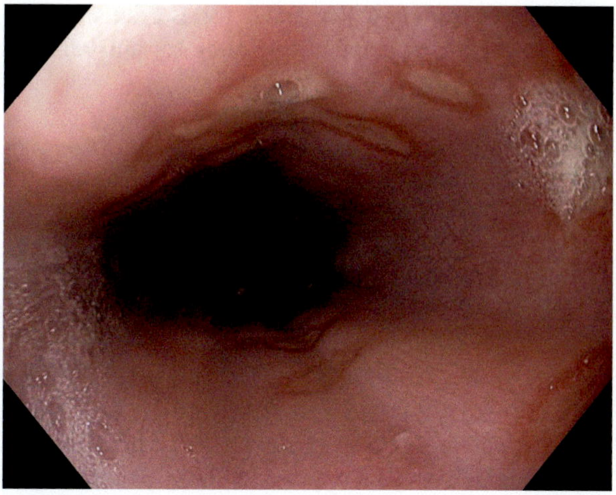

Fig. 18.25 Herpes simplex virus (HSV) esophagitis with small, well-demarcated, shallow ulcers and normal intervening mucosa. (Source: Photo courtesy of R. Daniel Lawson, MD)

Post-procedure management: Empiric antimicrobials are reasonable to initiate based on classic endoscopic appearance while awaiting histologic confirmation in symptomatic patients or those with evidence of systemic infection. First-line treatment of candidal esophagitis is systemic antifungal therapy with oral fluconazole 200–400 mg daily for 14–21 days [29]. HSV esophagitis is typically managed with oral acyclovir for 14–21 days in the immunocompromised. Immunocompetent patients will often resolve spontaneously, but a 7–10-day course can hasten symptomatic resolution. CMV esophagitis is treated with oral valganciclovir 900 mg twice daily for at least 14 days until clinical resolution and eradication of viremia (if present). IV ganciclovir is reserved for life-threatening infections [30]. While the other oral agents are available on the current CVN AMAL (see Chap. 16), ganciclovir is not typically present on forward deployed maritime platforms. There are additional options in patients with contraindications or resistance. Patients with gastrointestinal CMV infection warrant MEDEVAC given the side effects and close monitoring necessary while on therapy, if that therapy is even available on the ship at all.

Erosive Esophagitis

Presentation: Erosive esophagitis presents similar to non-erosive disease with the cardinal symptoms of heartburn and regurgitation. Response to PPI is suggestive of gastroesophageal reflux disease (GERD), but is not completely reliable as a diagnostic modality. Dysphagia can also occur but is considered an alarm symptom for possible underlying complications of GERD such as a ring or stricture or other sinister pathology and warrants early endoscopy [31]. Other indications for endoscopy in the setting of GERD symptoms include symptoms refractory to high dose anti-secretory therapy, screening for Barrett's esophagus in the appropriate risk demographic, pre-procedure planning for anti-reflux surgery, or any suspicion for complications.

Endoscopy: The Los Angeles (LA) Classification is used to describe and grade the severity of erosive esophagitis at the GEJ (Table 18.2) [32]. See Fig. 18.26 for an example of LA Grade B erosive esophagitis.

Post-procedure management: Patients with erosive esophagitis should be started on an oral PPI administered 30–60 min prior to meals twice daily. After 8 weeks of therapy with good clinical response, PPI can be titrated to the lowest effective dose. For patients with LA grade B esophagitis and above, maintenance therapy with once daily PPI is typically necessary as nearly 100% of patients will have recurrence of symptoms at 6 months [33]. Additionally, patients with LA grade C and D esophagitis should have repeat upper endoscopy performed after 8 weeks of PPI therapy to evaluate for healing and underlying Barrett's esophagus [31].

Table 18.2 The Los Angeles (LA) classification of erosive esophagitis at the gastroesophageal junction (GEJ)

Grade	Endoscopic appearance
A	One or more mucosal breaks no longer than 5 mm, does not extend between the tops of two mucosal folds
B	One or more mucosal breaks more than 5 mm, does not extend between the tops of two mucosal folds
C	One or more mucosal breaks that are continuous between the tops of two or more mucosal folds but which involve less than 75% of the esophageal circumference
D	One or more mucosal breaks which involve at least 75% of the esophageal circumference

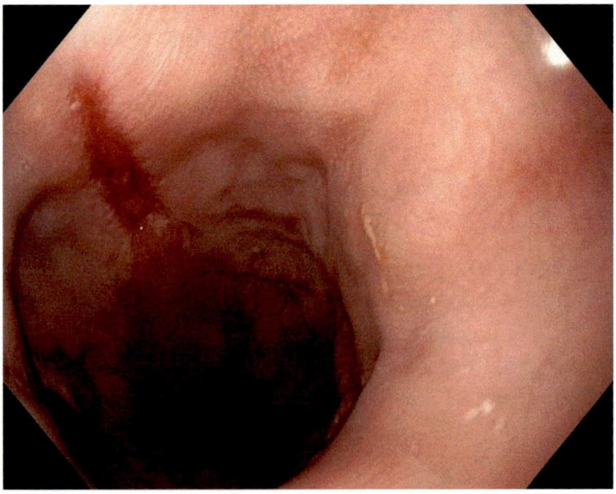

Fig. 18.26 Erosive esophagitis–Los Angeles (LA) Grade B. (Source: Photo courtesy of R. Daniel Lawson, MD)

Common Pathologies: Gastrointestinal (GI) Bleeding

Peptic Ulcer Disease (PUD)

Presentation: Peptic ulcer disease (PUD) is the most common cause of upper GI bleeding in adults and classically presents with melena, although hematochezia can occur with brisk upper GI bleeding. The most common symptomatic presentation of PUD is epigastric abdominal pain, followed by heartburn and GI bleeding [34]. The most common risk factors are *Helicobacter pylori* infection and NSAID use. In the setting of bleeding, EGD should be performed within 24 h of presentation. Prior to endoscopy, patients must be adequately resuscitated with a goal hemoglobin >7 g/dL. IV PPI should be initiated to reduce need for endoscopic therapy. IV erythromycin 250 mg given 20–90 min prior to endoscopy can improve diagnostic yield [35]. Oral azithromycin can be used if erythromycin is not available.

Endoscopy: The most common locations for peptic ulcers are the gastric antrum and proximal duodenum. Ulcers are characterized by the Forrest classification (Table 18.3), which indicates risk of rebleeding and guides need for endoscopic intervention [36]. Figures 18.27, 18.28, 18.29 demonstrate Forrest class IIA, IIC, and III, respectively. Treatment is indicated for active arterial bleeding (IA), active oozing (IB), and nonbleeding visible vessel (IIA). If an adherent clot (IIB) is encountered, vigorous irrigation is recommended to dislodge the clot and examine the ulcer bed for stigmata [35]. Before irrigation, injection of epinephrine is recommended before dislodging the clot in the event an active arterial bleed is provoked. If the clot cannot be removed or if in an unstable scope position that would make treatment difficult after removing the clot, endoscopic intervention is recommended. Endoscopic options for treatment include epinephrine injection, bipolar electrocoagulation, hemostasis clip placement (through the scope and over the scope), and APC. Epinephrine injection should always be combined with a second treatment modality. Hemostatic powder spray TC-325 is reserved for active ulcer bleeding

Table 18.3 Forrest classification of peptic ulcers with corresponding risks of rebleeding

Forrest class	Stigma	Frequency (%)	Risk of rebleeding (%)	Risk of rebleeding after endoscopic treatment (%)
IA	Active arterial bleeding	12	90	15–30
IB	Active oozing	14	10–14	0–5
IIA	Nonbleeding visible vessel	22	50	15–30
IIB	Adherent clot	10	33	0–5
IIC	Flat spot	10	10–25	0
III	Clean base	32	3	–

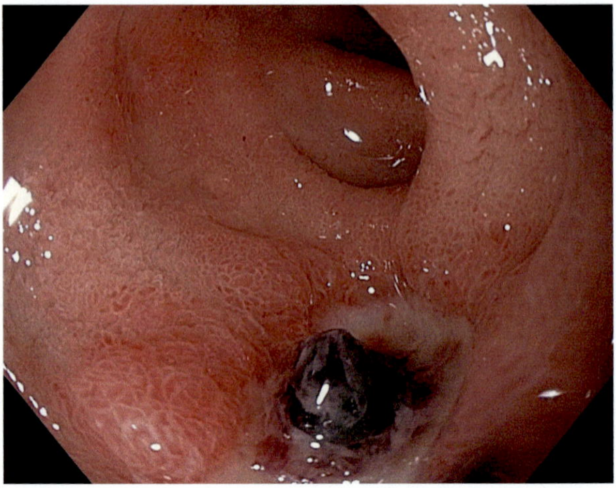

Fig. 18.27 Forrest class IIA: Duodenal ulcer with nonbleeding visible vessel. (Source: Photo courtesy of R. Daniel Lawson, MD)

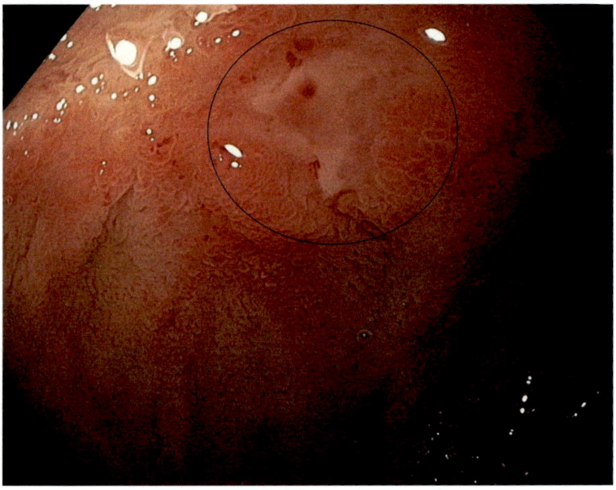

Fig. 18.28 Forrest class IIC: Ulcer with flat pigmented spot (oval). (Source: Photo courtesy of R. Daniel Lawson, MD)

only given its mechanism of action, and data is limited regarding use as definitive monotherapy. Over the scope clip placement is reserved for recurrent bleeding ulcers [35].

Treatment is not recommended for clean based ulcers (III) or those with flat pigmented spots (IIC). Biopsies are generally taken from the edge of gastric ulcers or suspicious duodenal ulcers to rule out malignancy. Gastric biopsies should also be taken from the antrum, greater and lesser curvatures 3–5 cm from the pylorus, incisura, as well as greater and lesser curvatures of the body, per the Sydney protocol to evaluate for *Helicobacter pylori*.

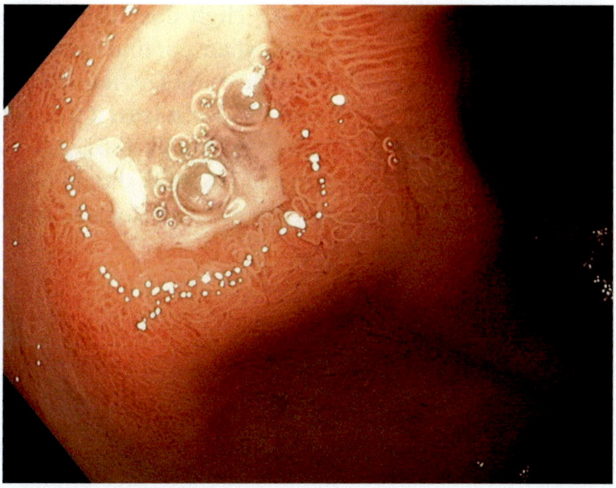

Fig. 18.29 Forrest class III: Clean-based ulcer. (Source: Photo courtesy of R. Daniel Lawson, MD)

Techniques:

- **Epinephrine injection:** Most commonly used in a 1:10,000 dilution, injected in 0.5–2 mL aliquots in a four-quadrant fashion. Circumferential blanching around the ulcer bed indicates successful injection into the submucosa. At least 10 mL of fluid should be injected to provide an additional tamponade effect.
- **Bipolar electrocoagulation:** Contact thermal therapy best used when in a stable scope position as prolonged contact is necessary for adequate coagulation. The heater probe should be applied with moderate pressure against the vessel or bleeding site. Power should be applied for 8–10 s and continued until the probe has been completely removed from the treatment site to avoid unroofing the newly formed eschar. Caution should be used in the small intestine and cecum as the luminal wall is thin and risk of perforation higher. Additionally, this modality is less effective in patients with coagulopathy.
- **APC:** Monopolar, non-contact thermal treatment less commonly used for ulcer bleeding. The tip of the monopolar probe should be positioned just above the desired area of treatment and power-delivered until coagulation has occurred.
- **Through the scope hemostasis clips:** Clips should be placed directly over the vessel of interest or bleeding site then mechanical pressure applied at the point of clip closure. Multiple successive clips can be placed until hemostasis is achieved. Clips can be difficult to place in fibrotic or broad-based ulcers as adequate purchase of normal adjacent mucosa is difficult.
- **Hemostatic powder spray:** Inorganic powder that clots upon contact with liquid and creates a mechanical barrier. This can only be used for actively bleeding sites and caution must be used to not allow the catheter tip to contact liquid as this will result in clot formation that will block further deployment of powder. Visualization is extremely limited after deployment of hemostatic powder and thus is typically reserved after failure of alternative therapies. Not currently available on maritime platforms.
- **Over the scope hemostasis clips:** Highly effective therapy indicated for recurrent ulcer bleeding. However, they are not currently available on platforms at sea.

Post-procedure management: High dose PPI, defined as at least 80 mg daily, should be given IV for 3 days either continuously or intermittently if endoscopic therapy is performed, as this reduces rebleeding and mortality. Patients should then be continued on high dose oral PPI for at least 2 weeks after endoscopy followed by an additional 2 weeks of once daily PPI [35]. All patients should be tested for *Helicobacter pylori* infection and NSAIDs should be avoided. In patients with gastric ulcers, repeat endoscopy should be performed after 8 weeks to confirm healing and rule out gastric cancer.

Dieulafoy Lesion

Presentation: A Dieulafoy lesion is a large submucosal artery protruding through a small mucosal defect without associated ulceration. As this is a high-pressure vessel, the presentation is often intermittent, massive bleeding. Melena is the most common presentation followed by hematemesis, hematochezia, and symptoms related to blood loss [36].

Endoscopy: The most common location is in the gastric fundus within 6 cm from the GEJ, but can occur anywhere along the GI tract. Dieulafoy lesions appear endoscopically as a pulsatile vessel through a mucosal defect <3 mm in size with normal surrounding mucosa (Fig. 18.30) [37]. These are notoriously difficult to find unless there is active bleeding due to the absence of mucosal ulceration. Endoscopic treatment should be performed with hemostasis clips, bipolar electrocoagulation, or injection therapy. Combination therapy may result in lower rebleeding rates [37]. Tattooing with India ink adjacent to the area should also be performed for ease of localization in the event of rebleeding.

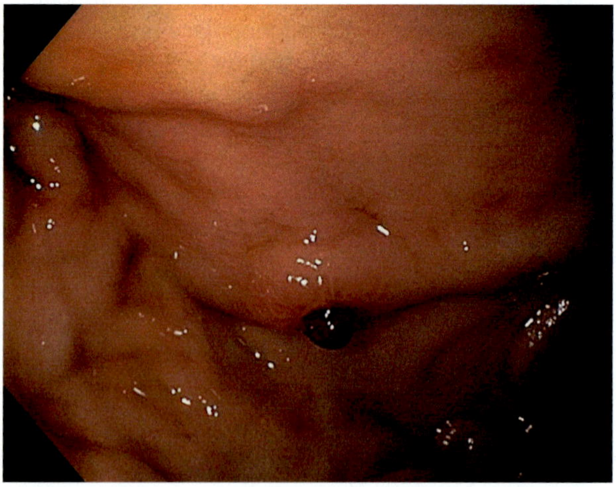

Fig. 18.30 Gastric Dieulafoy lesion characterized by a visible vessel protruding through a small mucosal defect with normal surrounding mucosa. (Source: Photo courtesy of R. Daniel Lawson, MD)

Post-procedure management: Endoscopic intervention is usually definitive. A short course of PPI can be utilized to enhance mucosal healing. NSAIDs and smoking should be avoided because they are risk factors.

Angiodysplasia (AD)

Presentation: Angiodysplasia (AD) is characterized by the focal accumulation of aberrant, dilated, tortuous blood vessels within the mucosa and submucosa. AD includes angioectasias and telangiectasias, which are considered acquired venous lesions. AD differs from AVMs, which are congenital arterial lesions [38]. AD is the most common cause of small bowel bleeding but can occur anywhere in the GI tract. Clinical presentation is variable and ranges from iron deficiency anemia to overt GI hemorrhage. Most AD occurs in patients older than 60 years of age [36].

Endoscopy: The lesions appear endoscopically as arborizing ectatic blood vessels that emanate from a central vessel (Fig. 18.31) and will blanch with gentle pressure, although this is not necessary to confirm the diagnosis [36]. Incidentally-found AD do not require treatment; however, treatment is indicated for bleeding and is typically performed with bipolar electrocoagulation or APC. Injection with epinephrine can also be performed and/or hemostasis clips placed [39].

Post-procedure management: Primary management includes iron repletion, blood transfusion if needed, and discontinuing anticoagulation if able as rates of rebleeding are as high as 45% [39]. Correction of any present underlying comorbidities, such as severe aortic stenosis, is indicated to reduce risk of recurrent bleed-

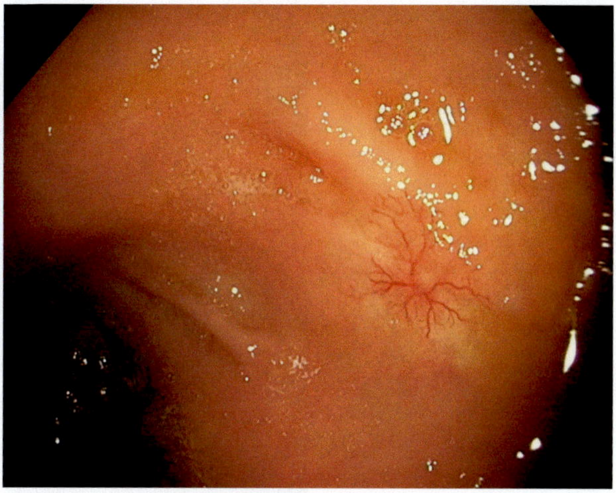

Fig. 18.31 Classic appearance of angiodysplasia (AD) characterized by arborizing ectatic vessels. (Source: Photo courtesy of R. Daniel Lawson, MD)

ing. Medical treatment options are limited and include somatostatin analogues and thalidomide among others but can be considered for patients with multiple recurrent episodes [38], which would not be available on a ship.

Colonic Ischemia

Presentation: The classic clinical presentation is cramping lower quadrant abdominal pain followed by bloody diarrhea in a patient with risk factors. Generally, patients at risk are the elderly with vascular disease. In the young, risk factors for development include medications such as NSAIDs or vasoconstricting medications [40]. Additionally, colonic ischemic can occur in the setting of intensive exercise. Patients with right-sided colonic ischemia should be further evaluated with cross-sectional CT with IV contrast to rule out a mesenteric thrombus (not available at sea).

Endoscopy: The most common locations for colonic ischemia are the watershed regions which occur in the splenic flexure (Griffith's point) and sigmoid colon (Sudeck's point). Aside from location, findings are relatively non-specific and include erythema, edema, and superficial ulceration. The linear stripe sign is a single inflammatory band of erythema with erosion and/or ulceration along the longitudinal axis of the colon and is more specific for ischemia (Fig. 18.32) [40]. Blue-black nodules with dusky appearing mucosa are suggestive of gangrene. Biopsies should be obtained from non-necrotic areas of inflammation to evaluate for infectious mimickers such as CMV.

Post-procedure management: The mainstay of treatment is supportive therapy and withdrawal of offending agents. Patients should be kept normotensive and

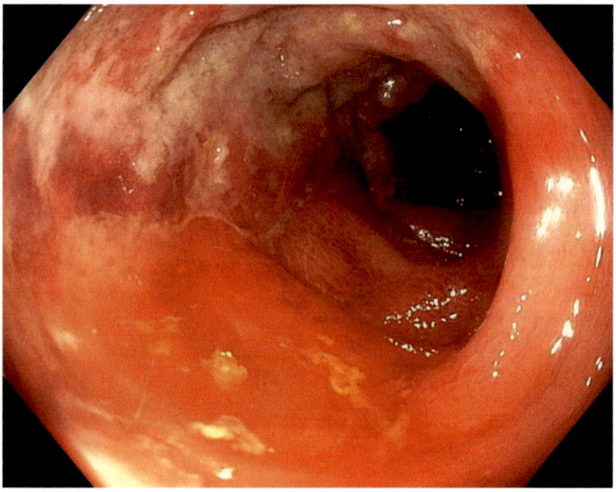

Fig. 18.32 Stripe sign: single inflammatory band of erythema with ulceration along the longitudinal axis of the colon seen in colonic ischemia. (Source: Photo courtesy of R. Daniel Lawson, MD)

encouraged to hydrate well. Antibiotics covering typical GI microbes (see Chap. 16 for regimens on maritime platforms) can be considered in moderate-to-severe disease for a course no longer than 7 days [40]. Patients should have a repeat colonoscopy after 6 weeks to rule out underlying CRC if they have not had a recent high-quality screening examination.

Diverticulosis

Presentation: Diverticular bleeding is an arterial hemorrhage that presents as large-volume painless hematochezia, though if bleeding originates in the proximal colon the patient may have crampy abdominal pain as a result of peristalsis. Right-sided lesions can present with melena or maroon-colored stool, although this is not typical. Patients often present with symptoms of acute blood loss, including hemorrhagic shock.

Endoscopy: Diverticuli appear as small- or wide-mouthed false lumens (Fig. 18.33) and can result in a tortuous and angulated colon with luminal narrowing. Left-sided diverticulosis is most common, but it can occur anywhere along the colon. Active bleeding, non-bleeding visible vessel, and adherent clot are all indications for endoscopic therapy [41]. Through the scope hemostasis clips are the preferred modality of treatment as this may be safer than bipolar electrocautery therapy and are more readily available than band ligation. Epinephrine injection can be utilized to control bleeding prior to definitive therapy.

Post-procedure management: Treatment is primarily supportive, including holding of anticoagulation until hemostasis is achieved.

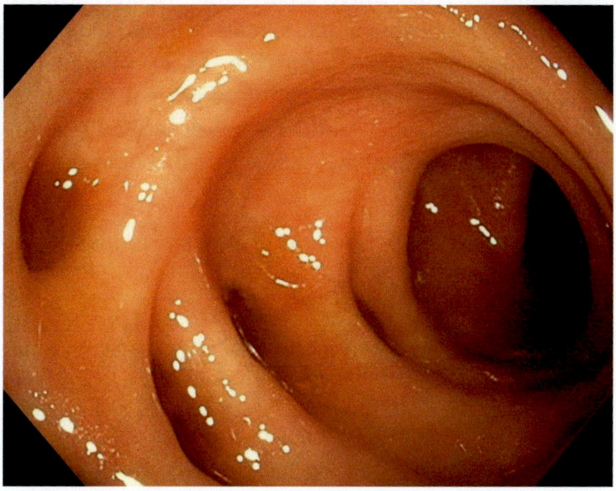

Fig. 18.33 Colonic diverticulosis. (Source: Photo courtesy of R. Daniel Lawson, MD)

Inflammatory Bowel Disease (IBD)

Presentation: Clinical manifestations are variable for IBD. Ulcerative colitis (UC) typically presents with bloody diarrhea, abdominal cramping, urgency, tenesmus with or without fevers [42]. CD is usually more subacute with hallmark symptoms of abdominal pain, watery diarrhea, and fatigue. Some patients present with complications of CD such as bowel obstruction from stricture, intra-abdominal abscess, or perianal fistula and/or abscess [43]. While CD can involve any portion of the GI tract, upper GI involvement in adults is rare. Extraintestinal manifestations of IBD include anterior uveitis, episcleritis, scleritis, erythema nodosum, pyoderma gangrenosum, axial and peripheral inflammatory arthritis, and primary sclerosing cholangitis. Malnutrition indicated by weight loss, iron deficiency anemia, and other nutrient deficiencies also raise suspicion for underlying IBD. Patients with diarrhea and suspected or confirmed IBD should be evaluated for infection, specifically *Clostridioides difficile*.

Endoscopy: A thorough rectal exam should be conducted prior to endoscope insertion to evaluate for evidence of perianal fistula, abscess, or atypical fissures. If IBD is suspected based on endoscopic findings, biopsies should be taken in a segmental fashion throughout the colon, regardless of macroscopic appearance, from the cecum, ascending colon, transverse colon, descending colon, sigmoid colon, and rectum and placed into separate specimen jars to stage the disease extent. Biopsies of normal-appearing TI generally are not recommended although controversy exists as to the clinical importance of microscopic ileitis and prognosis of developing clinical CD in the future.

- **Ulcerative Colitis (UC):**
  Typical mucosal findings of UC are erythema, edema, loss of vascular pattern, exudates, friability, spontaneous oozing, erosions, and ulcerations with severity classified by the Mayo Endoscopic Score shown in Table 18.4 [42]. Luminal involvement begins at the dentate line and extends proximally in a circumferential and contiguous manner (Fig. 18.34) with involvement of the entire colon or marked by an abrupt transition to normal mucosa at the proximal extent of disease involvement. Another well-described phenotype is the "cecal or peri-appendiceal red patch," defined as discontinuous involvement of the cecum in

Table 18.4 Mayo endoscopic score of ulcerative colitis (UC) severity

Mayo score	Endoscopic appearance	Disease activity
0	Normal	Inactive
1	Erythema, decreased vascular pattern, mild friability	Mild
2	Marked erythema, lack of vascular pattern, friability, erosions	Moderate
3	Spontaneous bleeding, ulcerations	Severe

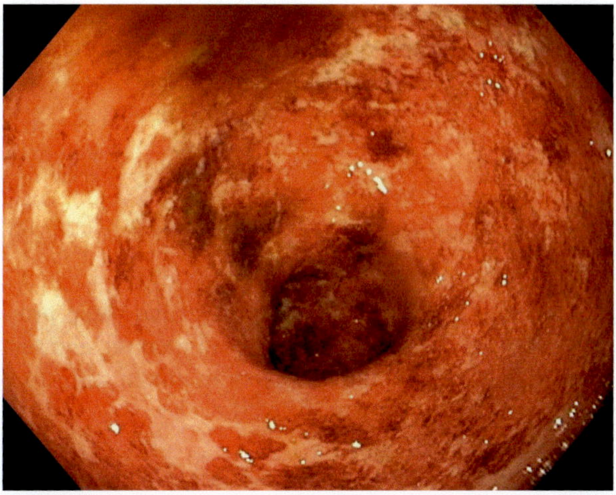

Fig. 18.34 Severe Mayo Class 3 ulcerative colitis (UC) with contiguous and circumferential erythema, friability, ulceration, and spontaneous bleeding. (Source: Photo courtesy of R. Daniel Lawson, MD)

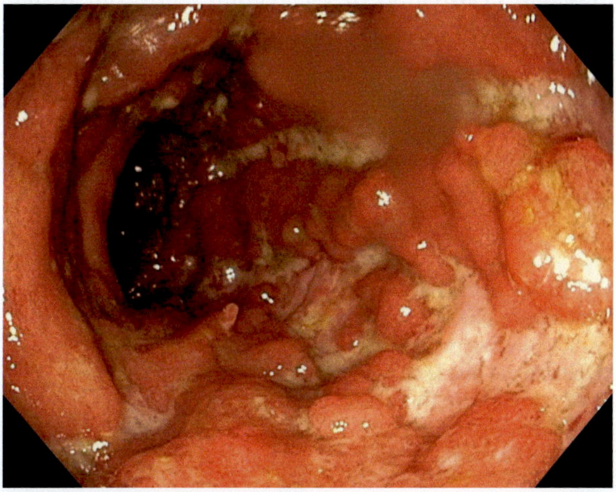

Fig. 18.35 Crohn's colitis with cobblestone appearance of the colonic mucosa and deep ulcerations. (Source: Photo courtesy of R. Daniel Lawson, MD)

patients with left-sided UC [44]. In the setting of ulcerative pancolitis, involvement of the distal ileum is sometimes referred to as "backwash ileitis" due to a dysfunctional ICV, but there is ongoing debate as to whether this represents UC or CD.

- **Crohn's Disease (CD):**

  CD can occur in any portion of the GI tract, most commonly in the TI. Segmental involvement called "skip lesions" is classic; however, the entire colon can be involved and mimics ulcerative pancolitis. Typical endoscopic findings include mucosal nodularity that can create a cobblestone appearance, edema, ulcerations, friability, stenosis, and fistulae (Fig. 18.35). Deep ulcerations are seen in CD and rarely occur in UC. Multiple scoring systems have been devised to standardize endoscopic findings; however, consensus is lacking [43].

Post-procedure management: Medical management of IBD is complex and outside the scope of this chapter. Generally speaking, mild disease can likely be managed symptomatically until return from sea; however, moderate or severe disease warrants MEDEVAC for appropriate care.

Internal Hemorrhoids

Presentation: Common symptoms include anal pruritus, painless hematochezia, anorectal pain, palpation of prolapsed mucosa, and sensation of sitting on a foreign body. Blood can coat the outside of or mix in with stool, drip into the toilet bowl, or be seen on tissue after wiping [45].

Endoscopy: Internal hemorrhoids are best viewed in rectal retroflexion (Fig. 18.36) and appear as deep purple, dilated, submucosal veins proximal to the dentate line. Maximal insufflation of the rectum can result in flattening of the hemorrhoidal plexus reducing diagnostic yield [36].

Post-procedure management: Management is primarily medical with fiber supplementation, stool softeners, and sitz baths. Symptomatic hemorrhoids can also be treated with topical glucocorticoids or rubber band ligation performed during anoscopy [45].

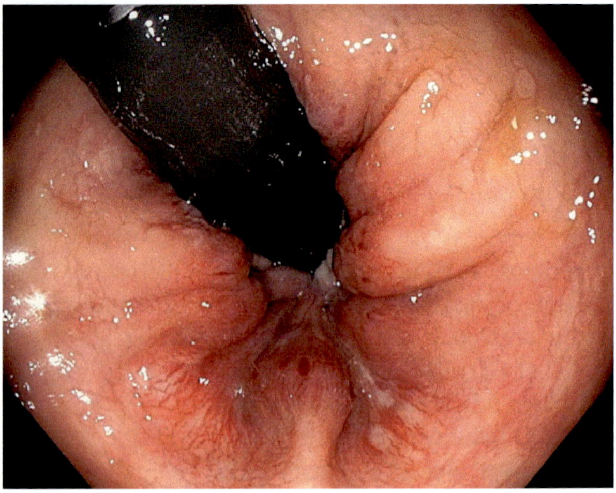

Fig. 18.36 Internal hemorrhoids characterized by dilated veins proximal to the dentate line seen in rectal retroflexion. (Source: Photo courtesy of R. Daniel Lawson, MD)

Incidental Findings

The following findings are commonly encountered during routine endoscopy and are non-emergent pathologies. If seen during the maritime endoscopic examination, it is recommended that these findings are photo-documented and the patients routinely referred to GI subspecialists upon completion of the time at sea.

Gastric Inlet Patch

A gastric inlet patch is an area of heterotopic gastric tissue found in the cervical esophagus. Endoscopically it appears as an island of salmon-colored mucosa (Fig. 18.37), which is lined by columnar epithelium and is rarely symptomatic (globus sensation) [46].

Barrett's Esophagus

Barrett's esophagus is the replacement of normal esophageal squamous epithelium with columnar lined epithelium with goblet cells, referred to as intestinal metaplasia. Endoscopically it appears as salmon-colored mucosa extending into the esophagus ≥1 cm proximal to the GEJ (Fig. 18.38), which is identified by the junction of the top of the gastric folds with the palisading vessels of the esophagus [47].

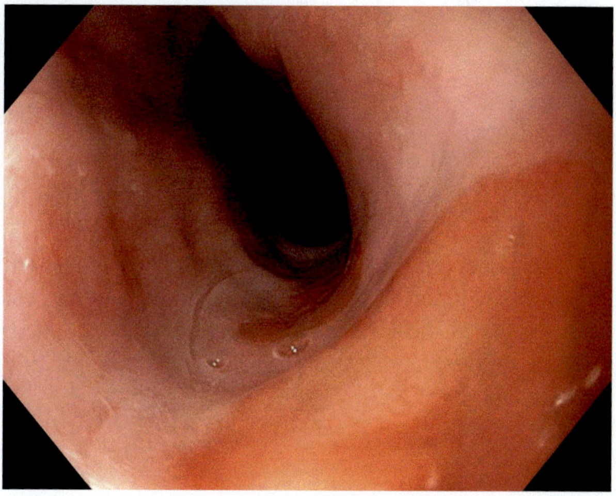

Fig. 18.37 Gastric inlet patch with islands of salmon-colored mucosa in the proximal esophagus. (Source: Photo courtesy of R. Daniel Lawson, MD)

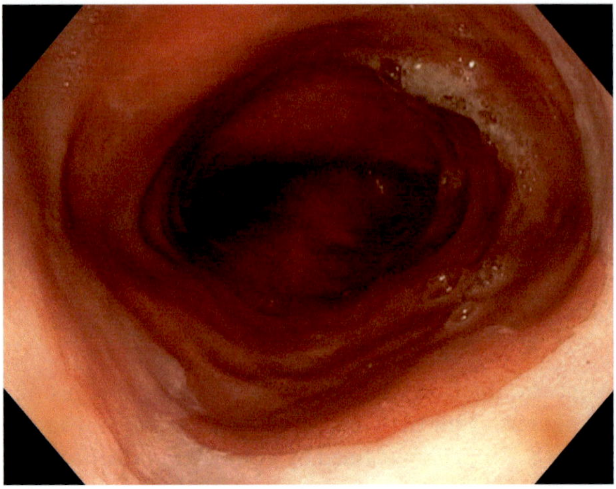

Fig. 18.38 Barrett's esophagus with salmon-colored mucosa extending from the top of the gastric folds proximally into the esophagus. (Source: Photo courtesy of R. Daniel Lawson, MD)

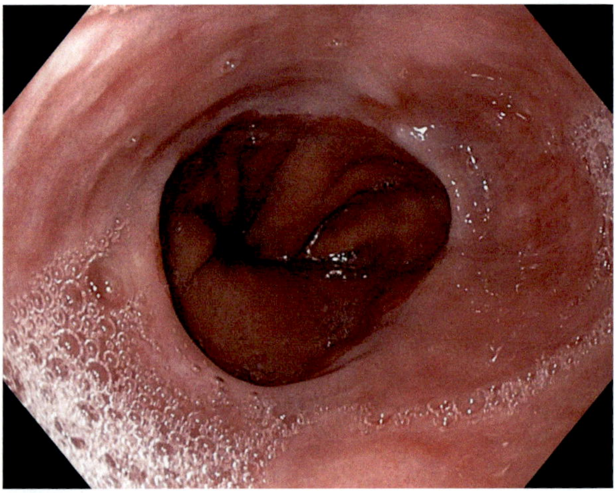

Fig. 18.39 Schatzki ring with a thin, fibrous, circumferential band at the gastroesophageal junction (GEJ). (Source: Photo courtesy of R. Daniel Lawson, MD)

Schatzki Ring

Schatzki rings are rings composed of mucosa and submucosa that form at the squamocolumnar junction [48]. Endoscopically they appear as thin, fibrous, circumferential bands at the GEJ (Fig. 18.39), often associated with a hiatal hernia. In the absence of dysphagia, they are not clinically meaningful; otherwise, dilation is indicated.

Pancreatic Rest

A pancreatic rest is an area of ectopic pancreatic tissue most commonly found in the antrum that endoscopically appears as a broad-based subepithelial lesion with central umbilication (Fig. 18.40) [48].

Polyp

A polyp is a raised protrusion of mucosa characterized by abnormal cellular proliferation (Fig. 18.41). Polyps can be benign, pre-malignant, or malignant and can be classified according to surface pattern characteristics or by morphology [46].

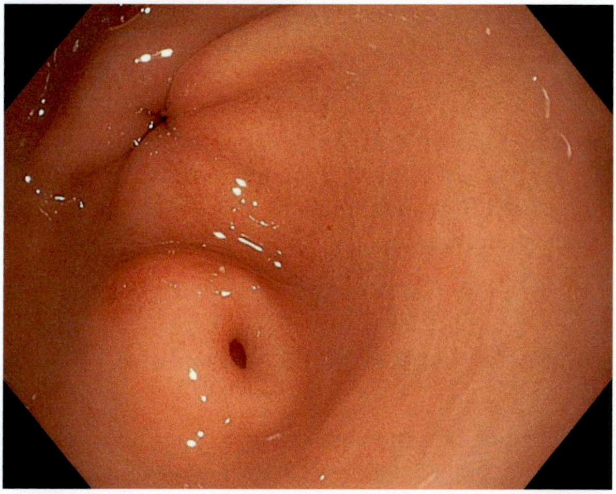

Fig. 18.40 Classic pancreatic rest characterized by a broad-based subepithelial lesion with central umbilication in the gastric antrum. (Source: Photo courtesy of R. Daniel Lawson, MD)

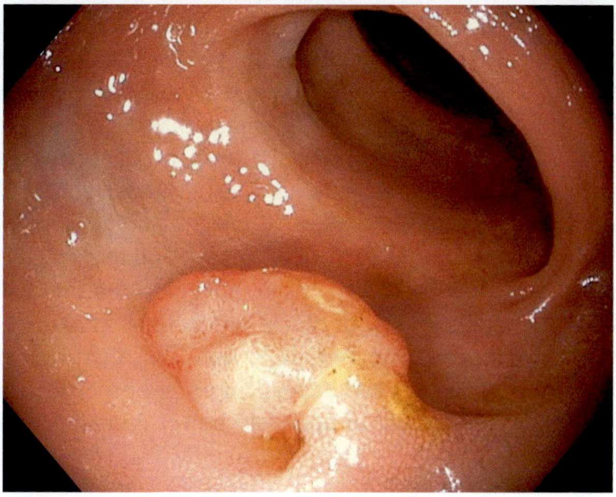

Fig. 18.41 Colonic polyp—tubular adenoma. (Source: Photo courtesy of R. Daniel Lawson, MD)

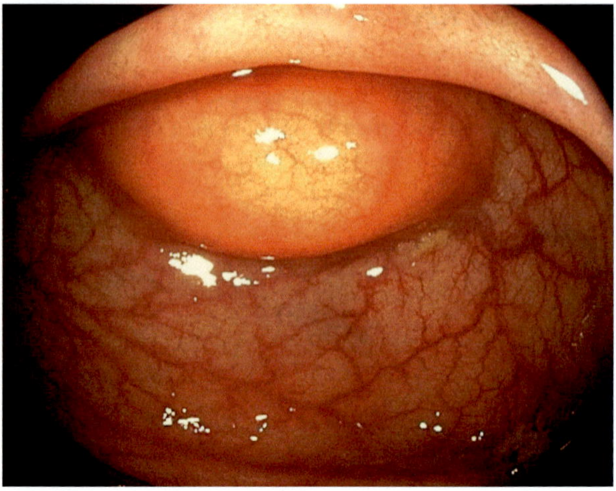

Fig. 18.42 Colonic lipoma characterized by a discrete, smooth, soft, subepithelial lesion with a yellow hue. (Source: Photo courtesy of R. Daniel Lawson, MD)

Lipoma

Lipomas in the GI tract are benign tumors that can occur anywhere. Endoscopically they appear as discrete, smooth, soft, subepithelial lesions with a yellow hue (Fig. 18.42). Lipomas are easily indented when probed with closed biopsy forceps, which is referred to as the "pillow sign" [46].

Colorectal Cancer (CRC) Screening

Recent guidelines from the United States Preventive Services Task Force (USPSTF) include recommendations for CRC screening in average-risk adults between the ages of 45 and 75 years old [49]. The American College of Gastroenterology recommends colonoscopy or annual fecal immunochemical testing (FIT) as the primary screening modalities [50]. Patients at increased risk for CRC should be screened according to individual guidelines. These patients include those with a prior diagnosis of CRC, adenomatous polyps, IBD, and those with a personal diagnosis or family history of known genetic disorders that increase their lifetime risk of developing CRC [49]. Depending on the ship's operational tempo, direction of leadership, and comfort of the maritime surgical team, offering CRC screening at sea may be an opportunity for the embarked sailors and marines to perform during their downtime.

If colonoscopy is performed for the intent of CRC screening, multiple quality indicators must be met to ensure adequate and optimal CRC screening. Complete colonoscopy consists of cecal intubation, proximal to the ICV, with photo-documentation of the AO, ICV, and TI. Adequate visualization of the colonic mucosa is necessary and dependent on pre-procedure bowel preparation. The most important component of adequate bowel preparation is the time interval between completion of bowel prep and start of procedure. Patients should be instructed to complete a split bowel prep, half the night before and the remaining half the day of the procedure. Patients should begin the second half 4–5 h before their scheduled procedure start time [50]. The quality of bowel cleansing should be documented by the endoscopist and must be adequate to detect polyps >5 mm in size. The Boston Bowel Preparation Scale is a validated preparation score that can assist with assessment of adequacy of bowel preparation. Withdrawal time must also be measured with a minimum withdrawal time of 6 min, although longer duration may be needed for a complete examination. Due to the lower rates of CRC prevention against right-sided colon cancer, a second look should be performed in the right colon. This can be accomplished in forward view or in retroflexion, performed in the cecum [51]. Finally, retroflexion must also be performed and photo-documented in the rectum.

Conclusion

The prior experiences of all the members of the maritime surgical team may not include much endoscopy. Preparing prior to deployment to understand and troubleshoot the endoscopic equipment and tools is critical for successful execution of endoscopy in the diagnosis and treatment of dysphagia, GI bleeding, or other etiologies. Having a working basic knowledge of potential endoscopic findings is also helpful. While there can be many challenges, endoscopy underway is a valuable tool for the maritime surgical team.

Declaration of Interest The views expressed in this chapter are those of the authors and do not necessarily reflect the official policy or position of the Department of the Navy, Department of Defense, nor the US Government.

Funding This research did not receive any specific grant from funding agencies in the public, commercial, or not-for-profit sectors.

Conflict of Interest Statement The authors declare no conflict of interest.

References

1. Carr M, Oxner C, Elster E, Ritter E, Vicente D. Management of acute upper gastrointestinal disease while at sea. Mil Med. 2018;183(9–10):e658–62.
2. Barkun A, Liu J, Carpenter S, et al. Update on endoscopic tissue sampling devices. Gastrointest Endosc. 2006;63(6):741–5.
3. Carpenter S, Petersen B, Chuttani R, et al. Polypectomy devices. Gastrointest Endosc. 2007;65(6):741–9.
4. ASGE Standards of Practice Committee. Adverse events of upper GI endoscopy. Gastrointest Endosc. 2012;76(4):707–18. https://doi.org/10.1016/j.gie.2012.03.252.

5. Vargo J, Niklewski P, Williams J, Martin J, Faigel D. Patient safety during sedation by anesthesia professionals during routine upper endoscopy and colonoscopy: an analysis of 1.38 million procedures. Gastrointest Endosc. 2017;85(1):101–8. https://doi.org/10.1016/j.gie.2016.02.007.
6. Sharma V, Nguyen C, Crowell M, et al. A national study of cardiopulmonary unplanned events after GI endoscopy. Gastrointest Endosc. 2007;66(1):27–34.
7. Kothari S, Huang R, Shaukat A, Agrawal D, Buxbaum J, Abbas Fehmi S, et al. ASGE review of adverse events in colonoscopy. Gastrointest Endosc. 2019;90(6):863–876.e33. https://doi.org/10.1016/j.gie.2019.07.033.
8. Levy I, Gralnek I. Complications of diagnostic colonoscopy, upper endoscopy, and enteroscopy. Best Pract Res Clin Gastroenterol. 2016;30(5):705–18. https://doi.org/10.1016/j.bpg.2016.09.005.
9. Singla M, Kwok R, Deriban G, Young P. Training the endo-athlete: an update in ergonomics in endoscopy. Clin Gastroenterol Hepatol. 2018;16(7):1003–6.
10. Kim KO. Normal upper GI findings and normal variants. In: Chun H, Yang S, Choi M, editors. Clinical gastrointestinal endoscopy: a comprehensive atlas. Heidelberg: Springer; 2014. p. 1–10.
11. Cha M, Jae. Normal colonoscopy findings. In: Chun H, Yang S, Choi M, editors. Clinical gastrointestinal endoscopy: a comprehensive atlas. Heidelberg: Springer; 2014. p. 318–43.
12. Canard JM, Letard JC, Penman I. Diagnostic colonoscopy. In: Houston M, Scott J, Garraway P, editors. Gastrointestinal endoscopy in practice. Edinburgh: Elsevier/Churchill Livingstone; 2011. p. 101–19.
13. Berzin T. Colonoscopic tips and tricks--advice from 3 master endoscopists. Gastrointest Endosc. 2009 Aug;70(2):370–1.
14. Rodrigues-Pinto E, Ferreira-Silva J, Macedo G, Rex D. (Technically) difficult colonoscope insertion – tips and tricks. Dig Endosc. 2019;31(5):583–7. https://doi.org/10.1111/den.13465.
15. Akere A, Tejan EA. How frequent does bow and arrow sign locate ileocecal valve during colonoscopy? J Dig Endosc. 2018;9:10–3.
16. Bruce M, Choi J. Detection of endoscopic looping during colonoscopy procedure by using embedded bending sensors. Med Devices (Auckl). 2018;18(11):171–91.
17. Waye J, Thomas-Gibson S. How I do colonoscopy. Gastrointest Endosc. 2018;87(3):621–4.
18. Rex D. Achieving cecal intubation in the very difficult colon. Gastrointest Endosc. 2008;67(6):938–44.
19. Prechel J, Young C, Hucke R, Young-Fadok T, Fleischer D. The importance of abdominal pressure during colonoscopy. Gastroenterol Nurs. 2005;28(3):232–6, quiz 237–8.
20. Saleem F, Sharma A. Drug induced esophagitis. [Updated 2020 Jun 23]. In: StatPearls [Internet]. Treasure Island: StatPearls Publishing; 2021. https://www.ncbi.nlm.nih.gov/books/NBK549818/.
21. Ikenberry S, Lue T, Anderson M, et al. Management of ingested foreign bodies and food impactions. Gastrointest Endosc. 2011;73(6):1085–91.
22. Furuta G, Katzka D. Eosinophilic esophagitis. N Engl J Med. 2015;373(17):1640–8.
23. Dellon E, Cotton C, Gebhart J, et al. Accuracy of the eosinophilic esophagitis endoscopic reference score in diagnosis and determining response to treatment. Clin Gastroenterol Hepatol. 2016;14(1):31–9.
24. Hirano I, Chan E, Rank M, et al. AGA Institute and the Joint Task Force on allergy-immunology practice parameters clinical guidelines for the management of eosinophilic esophagitis. Gastroenterology. 2020;158(6):1776–86.
25. Zografos GN, Georgiadou D, Thomas D, Kaltsas G, Digalakis M. Drug-induced esophagitis. Dis Esophagus. 2009;22(8):633–7.
26. Abid S, Mumtaz JW, Abbas Z, Shah H, Khan A. Pill-induced esophageal injury: endoscopic features and clinical outcomes. Endoscopy. 2005;37(8):740–4.
27. Hoversten P, Kamboj A, Katzka D. Infections of the esophagus: an update on risk factors, diagnosis, and management. Dis Esophagus. 2018;31(12) https://doi.org/10.1093/dote/doy094.

28. Park KS. Infectious and noninfectious esophagitis. In: Chun H, Yang S, Choi M, editors. Clinical gastrointestinal endoscopy: a comprehensive atlas. Heidelberg: Springer; 2014. p. 17–30.
29. Pappas P, Kauffman C, Andes D, et al. Clinical practice guideline for the management of candidiasis: 2016 update by the Infectious Diseases Society of America. Clin Infect Dis. 2016;62(4):e1–50.
30. Mulhall B, Wong R. Infectious esophagitis. Curr Treat Options Gastroenterol. 2003;6(1):55–70.
31. Katz P, Gerson L, Vela M. Guidelines for the diagnosis and management of gastroesophageal reflux disease. Am J Gastroenterol. 2013;108(3):308–28. https://doi.org/10.1038/ajg.2012.444.
32. Lundell LR, Dent J, Bennett JR, et al. Endoscopic assessment of oesophagitis: clinical and functional correlates and further validation of the Los Angeles classification. Gut. 1999;45:172–80.
33. Vigneri S, Termini R, Leandro G, Badalamenti S, Pantalena M, Savarino V, Di Mario F, Battaglia G, Mela GS, Pilotto A, et al. A comparison of five maintenance therapies for reflux esophagitis. N Engl J Med. 1995;333(17):1106–10.
34. Barkun A, Leontiadis G. Systematic review of the symptom burden, quality of life impairment and costs associated with peptic ulcer disease. Am J Med. 2010;123(4):358–66.e2.
35. Laine L, Barkun A, Saltzman J, et al. ACG clinical guideline: upper gastrointestinal and ulcer bleeding. Am J Gastroenterol. 2021;116(5):899–917.
36. Savides T, Jensen D. Gastrointestinal bleeding. In: Feldman M, Friedman L, Brandt L, editors. Sleisenger and Fordtran's gastrointestinal and liver disease, vol. 20. 11th ed. Philadelphia: Elsevier; 2021. p. 276–312.e8.
37. Malik T, Anjum F. Dieulafoys lesion causing gastrointestinal bleeding. In: StatPearls [internet]. Treasure Island: StatPearls Publishing; 2021.
38. Sakai E, Ohata K, Nakajima A, Matsuhashi N. Diagnosis and therapeutic strategies for small bowel vascular lesions. World J Gastroenterol. 2019;25(22):2720–33.
39. Jackson C, Strong R. Gastrointestinal angiodysplasia: diagnosis and management. Gastrointest Endosc Clin N Am. 2017;27(1):51–62.
40. Brandt L, Feuerstadt P, Longstreth G, Boley S, et al. ACG clinical guideline: epidemiology, risk factors, patterns of presentation, diagnosis, and management of colon ischemia (CI). Am J Gastroenterol. 2015;110(1):18–44.
41. Strate L, Gralnek I. ACG clinical guideline: management of patients with acute lower gastrointestinal bleeding. Am J Gastroenterol. 2016;111(4):459–74.
42. Rubin D, Ananthakrishnan A, Siegel C, et al. ACG clinical guideline: ulcerative colitis in adults. Am J Gastroenterol. 2019;114(3):384–413.
43. Lichtenstein G, Loftus G, Isaacs K, et al. ACG clinical guideline: management of Crohn's disease in adults. Am J Gastroenterol. 2018;113(4):481–517.
44. Nevin D, Genta R, Saboorian HM. The cecal patch is associated with a greater prevalence of symptoms in patients with ulcerative colitis. Am J Gastroenterol. 2012;107:S654.
45. Fontem RF, Eyvazzadeh D. Internal hemorrhoid. [Updated 2020 Aug 8]. In: StatPearls [Internet]. Treasure Island: StatPearls Publishing; 2021. https://www.ncbi.nlm.nih.gov/books/NBK537182/.
46. Qayed E, Shahnavaz N, editors. Sleisenger and Fordtran's gastrointestinal and liver disease. 11th ed. Philadelphia: Elsevier; 2021.
47. Shaheen N, Falk G, Iyer P, Gerson L, et al. ACG clinical guideline: diagnosis and management of Barrett's esophagus. Am J Gastroenterol. 2016;111(1):30–50.
48. Chun HJ, Yang S-K, Cho M-G, editors. Clinical gastrointestinal endoscopy: a comprehensive atlas. Heidelberg: Springer; 2014.
49. Davidson K, Barry M, Mangione C, et al. Screening for colorectal cancer: US preventive services task force recommendation statement. JAMA. 2021;325(19):1965–77.
50. Rex D, Schoenfeld P, Cohen J, et al. Quality indicators for colonoscopy. Gastrointest Endosc. 2015;81(1):31–53.
51. Desai M, Bilal M, Hamade N, et al. Increasing adenoma detection rates in the right side of the colon comparing retroflexion with a second forward view: a systematic review. Gastrointest Endosc. 2019;89(3):453–459.e3.

Chapter 19
Of Hatches and Hands: Management of Hand Injuries

Shian L. Peterson, John P. Waggoner, and Dominic T. Gomezleonardelli

The hand, more than any other organ except the brain itself, is symbolic of the mind and soul of a person. It represents his life, his work, his strength, and his love. One touch of a hand may mean more than a thousand words … it is a seal of the oneness of the sick person and the healer.

Dr. Paul Brand, 1992 Journal of Hand Surgery

Author deployment experience	
Shian L. Peterson	Resident Orthopedic Surgeon, Naval Medical Center San Diego, 2018–Present
John P. Waggoner	Platoon/Task Unit Officer in Charge, SEAL Delivery Vehicle Team TWO and SEAL Team ONE, multiple land and sea deployments supporting Joint Operations; service aboard aircraft carriers, large-deck amphibious ships, submarines, and patrol craft, 2001–2011
	Executive Officer, SEAL Team 17 Naval Reserve Unit, 2011–2014
	Acting Commanding Officer, SEAL Team 17 Naval Reserve Unit, 2013
	Resident Orthopedic Surgeon, Naval Medical Center San Diego, 2018–Present
Dominic T. Gomez-Leonardelli	Surface Warfare Officer, USS Pearl Harbor (LSD-52), 1998–2000; Western Pacific Bon Homme Richard Amphibious Readiness Group, WESTPAC, Operation Southern Watch, Eager Mace Exercise, Eastern Maverick Exercise, Sea Soldier Exercise, INDOPACOM Area of Responsibility, 2000
	Surface Warfare Officer, USS Chosin (CG-65), 2000–2002; WESTPAC, INDOPACOM Area of Responsibility, 2001
	Hand Surgeon, Naval Hospital Okinawa, sole hand surgeon supporting Western Pacific Area of Operations, 2014–2016
	Hand and Orthopedic Surgeon, Expeditionary Resuscitative Surgical System Pacific, 2019–2020; Provided embarked Role 2 Surgical Support, INDOPACOM Area of Responsibility, 2019–2020

S. L. Peterson · J. P. Waggoner · D. T. Gomezleonardelli (✉)
Navy Medicine Readiness and Training Command San Diego, San Diego, CA, USA
e-mail: shian.l.peterson.mil@health.mil; john.p.waggoner2.mil@health.mil; dominic.t.gomezleonardelli.mil@health.mil

M. D. Tadlock, A. A. Hernandez (eds.), *Expeditionary Surgery at Sea*,
https://doi.org/10.1007/978-3-031-21893-4_19

BLUF (Bottom Line Up Front)

1. More than half of all sick-call visits are musculoskeletal complaints, with hand and wrist injuries accounting for most of these visits. Historically, hand surgery accounts for <6% of all procedures performed on a deployment, and many hand-related sick-call complaints and diagnoses are appropriately treated by conservative, non-surgical treatment.
2. Underlying the diagnosis of most hand pathology is an understanding of hand anatomy and a sense of what normal looks like. Basic understanding of hand anatomy and familiarity with the orthopedic musculoskeletal exam are critical for managing hand injuries and communicating with specialists if required.
3. Evaluation and documentation of a thorough physical exam, to include neurovascular status, prior to administration of any local or general anesthesia is essential.
4. Orthopedic hand urgencies well documented on maritime deployments include open and/or unstable fractures and tendon or nerve lacerations, including combinations of these injuries such as in "hatch hand" situations.
5. Orthopedic hand emergencies include upper extremity amputations, dysvascular limbs, and high-pressure injections, which have not been documented on maritime deployments in the literature or surgical logs.
6. Lower acuity orthopedic hand injuries include fractures and/or dislocations of carpals, metacarpals, and phalanges.
7. Be creative with the supply locker and treatment options.
8. Prevention is just as important as treatment.

Introduction

Musculoskeletal complaints and injuries account for more than half of all visits to sick call in the shipboard environment, with hand and upper extremity problems accounting for the leading chief complaints [1, 2]. In a retrospective analysis of two separate carrier strike group (CSG) deployments, hand and wrist injuries alone accounted for 40.4% of all orthopedic injuries and the majority of lacerations (88%) and fractures (59%) [1]. Hand and wrist injuries appear to disproportionately affect the men and women serving in the deployed shipboard setting, almost five times more than the civilian population [2]. However, surgical management of hand and wrist injuries is less common, accounting for fewer than 7% of all procedures performed on deployed ships [3, 4]. While this chapter touches on surgical management, the vast majority of hand and wrist injuries encountered in the shipboard setting can be managed nonoperatively. The challenges include diagnosis, triage, management, and decision-making with limited resources.

Case 19.1

A 37-year-old Tactical Action Officer (TAO) was leaving his workspace after his night shift ended and let his fingers linger a little too long in a door opening. A heavy hatch slammed onto the fingers of his non-dominant hand with injuries to multiple digits. His co-worker wrapped his hand in a shirt and immediately escorted him to the medical department just as morning sick call was getting started.

"Hatch hand" refers to patients who sustain crush injuries to their hands from the "hatches" or doors aboard maritime vessels, often leading to multiple phalangeal and metacarpal fractures that may require surgical intervention, including closed reduction and percutaneous pinning or open reduction and internal fixation (ORIF) (Figs. 19.1 and 19.2). While hatches and doors may inflict injury both pier-side and on deployment, sharp lacerations and fractures are more common due to crew members using knives, working with sheet metal, opening cans, and participating in air operations [5]. As such, this chapter includes both hatch hands and related orthopedic hand injuries that a shipboard surgeon may encounter, including hypothetical case presentations.

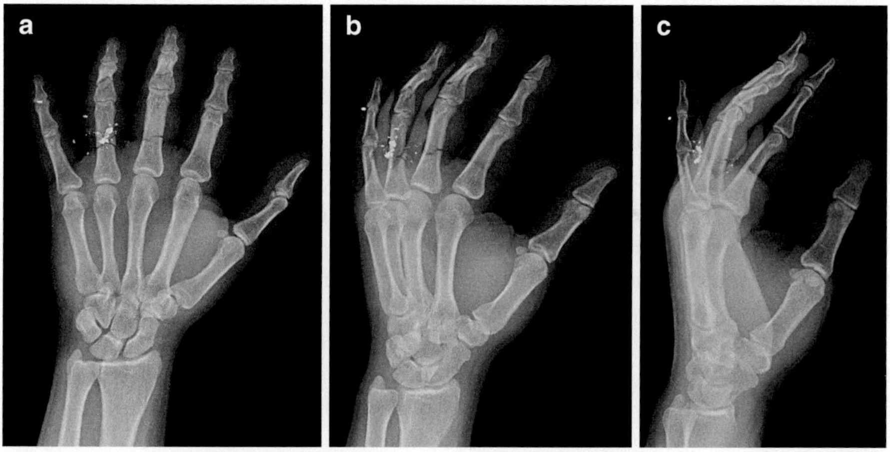

Fig. 19.1 (**a**) Anteroposterior (AP), (**b**) oblique, and (**c**) lateral X-rays of the left hand showing a 37-year-old right-hand-dominant male with a hatch hand injury, sustaining a left open ring finger proximal phalanx fracture, left ring finger middle phalanx fracture, left long finger proximal phalanx fracture, left long finger middle phalanx fracture, and a left ring finger partial extensor tendon laceration in extensor zone 4. (Source: Images courtesy of Navy Medicine Readiness and Training Command San Diego Radiology Department, used with permission)

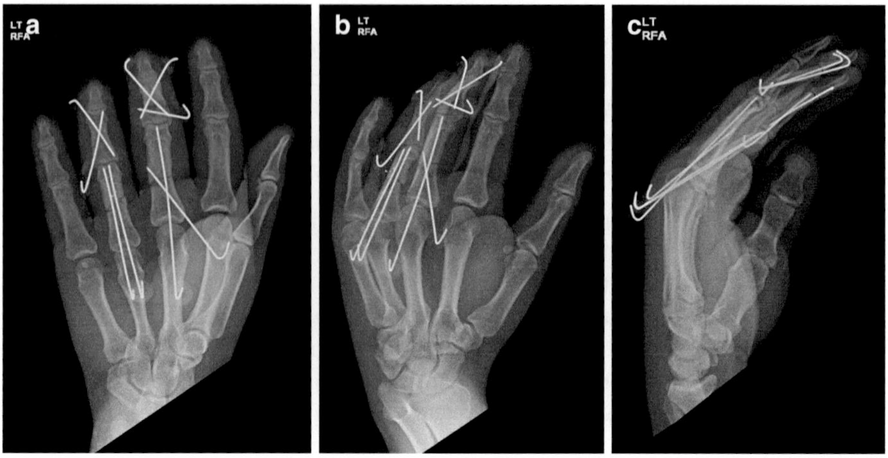

Fig. 19.2 (**a**) Brewerton anteroposterior (AP), (**b**) oblique, and (**c**) lateral X-rays of a 37-year-old right-hand-dominant male with a hatch hand injury after irrigation and debridement of his open wound, partial extensor tendon repair, and closed reduction and percutaneous pinning of his long and ring finger phalangeal fractures. This surgery would not be expected of a general surgeon; however, irrigation and debridement, loose closure, and splint with a medical evacuation (MEDEVAC) on an urgent basis would be appropriate. (Source: Images courtesy of Navy Medicine Readiness and Training Command San Diego Radiology Department, used with permission)

Basic Anatomy and Terminology

The hand is an intricately designed and highly functional living work of art. It exists in a wonderful balance between flexor and extensor tendons, with extrinsic components in the forearm and intrinsic muscles in the hand executing orders from the arborized nerves in the upper extremity. This intelligently woven fabric of soft tissue surrounds the bone and cartilage which provide a living scaffold for tendons and ligaments to assert their carefully allocated force. A network of blood vessels brings in nutrients and oxygen and brings out waste in a fairly predictable and frequently redundant system. At the level of the wrist, the nerves frame the vessels so that the vessels live relatively on the inside and the nerves live relatively on the outside [6]. **Underlying the diagnosis of most hand pathology is an understanding of hand anatomy and a sense of what normal looks like.**

Twenty-seven bones provide skeletal support for hand function, divided into eight carpal bones, five metacarpal bones, and 14 phalanges (Fig. 19.3). These bones space out the joints of the hand, starting with the radiocarpal joint, midcarpal joint, carpometacarpal joints (CMCJ), metacarpophalangeal joints (MCPJ), proximal interphalangeal joints (PIPJ), and distal interphalangeal joints (DIPJ) (Fig. 19.3). The thumb only has an interphalangeal joint due to its unique anatomy. Each joint has a synovial capsule and is stabilized with a volar plate and collateral ligaments on either side.

Orthopedic terminology utilizes the adjective "proximal" to describe being situated toward the center of the body and "distal" to describe being situated toward the

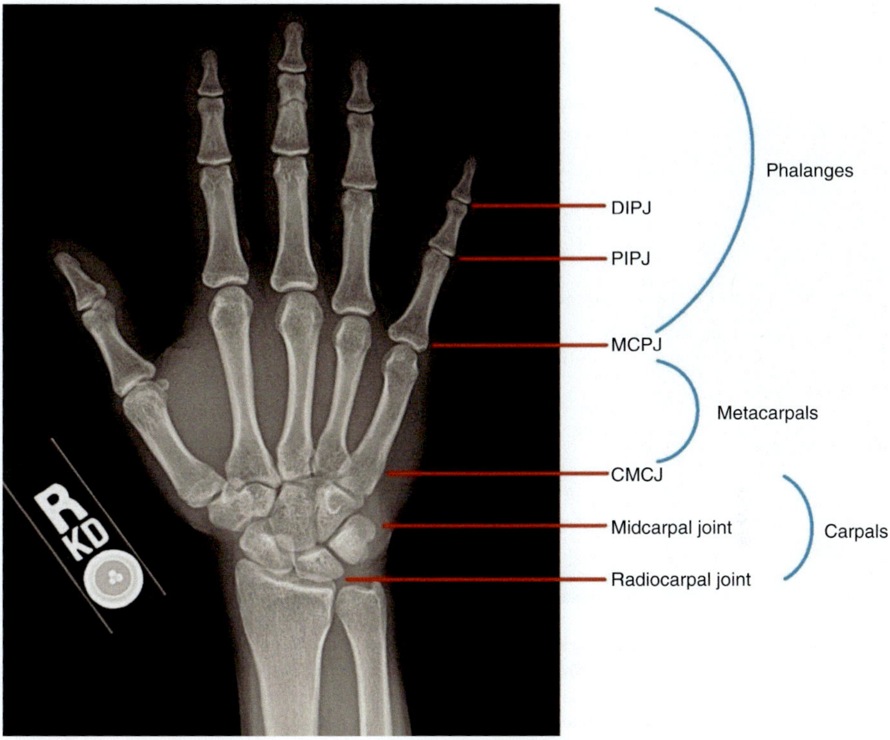

Fig. 19.3 Anteroposterior (AP) X-ray of the right hand. The hand contains eight carpal bones, five metacarpals, and 14 phalanges, spaced out with their respective joints. Note the transverse fracture across the long finger middle phalanx. The remainder of the X-ray appears normal. *DIPJ* distal interphalangeal joint, *PIPJ* proximal interphalangeal joint, *MCPJ* metacarpophalangeal joint, *CMCJ* carpometacarpal joint. (Source: Image courtesy of Navy Medicine Readiness and Training Command San Diego Radiology Department, used with permission)

periphery. Hand terminology also utilizes the descriptors of "radial" to describe direction toward the thumb, "ulnar" to describe direction toward the small finger, "volar" to describe the palm, and "dorsal" to describe the back of the hand. Rather than using numerical designators for phalanges, hand surgeons typically use thumb, index finger, long finger, ring finger, and small finger to describe a particular ray of the hand. In the absence of sharing X-rays by email or video with an orthopedic consultant, the appropriate verbiage can help immensely to paint a mental picture of what is happening with a patient.

The carpus breaks down into a proximal row, made up of the scaphoid, lunate, triquetrum and pisiform, and a distal row, made up of the trapezium, trapezoid, capitate, and hamate (Fig. 19.4a). While motion between carpal rows and bones is required for normal activity, abnormal dissociation can generate pain. Each carpal bone has unique anatomy. The scaphoid has a retrograde blood supply and is particularly vulnerable to trauma. The hamate can often be fractured in cases of a

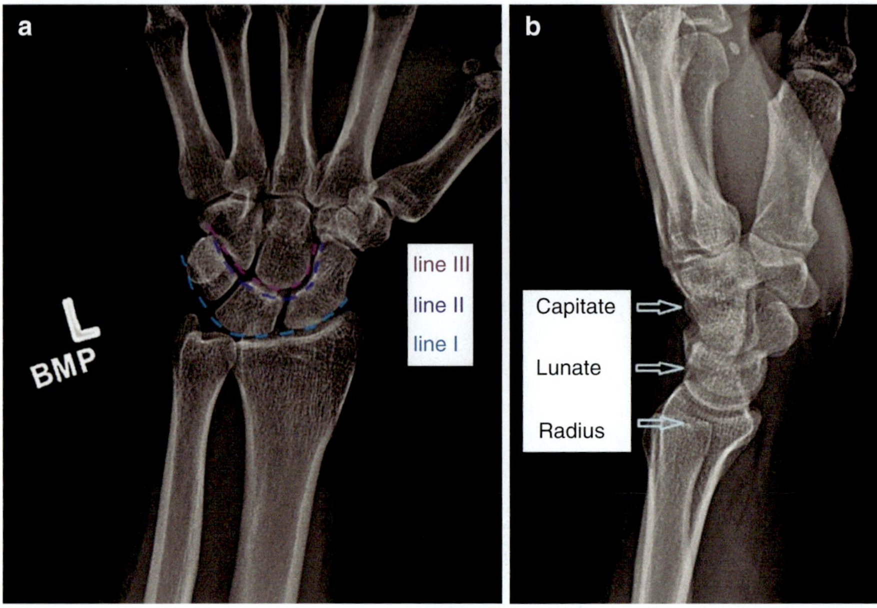

Fig. 19.4 (**a**) Normal anteroposterior (AP) X-ray of the left wrist demonstrating Gilula's lines. Carpal bones in the proximal row from radial to ulnar: scaphoid, lunate, triquetrum, and pisiform. Carpal bones in the distal row from radial to ulnar: trapezium, trapezoid, capitate, hamate. (**b**) Normal lateral X-ray of the left wrist demonstrating the colinear relationship of the capitate, lunate, and distal radius. (Source: Images courtesy of Navy Medicine Readiness and Training Command San Diego Radiology Department, used with permission)

fourth/fifth metacarpal base fracture-dislocation since it forms part of the CMCJ. The lunate can be a source of dorsal wrist pain while appearing completely normal in early stages of Kienbock's disease.

Perhaps the most critical anatomic relationship for a ship's surgeon to recognize in the carpus is the normal alignment of the carpal bones in the anteroposterior (AP) and lateral planes. Dr. Gilula, a late professor of radiology at Washington University in St. Louis and prior United States (U.S.) Army Captain described three critical lines in the AP X-ray of the wrist that align with the proximal aspect of the proximal carpal row (line I), the distal aspect of the proximal carpal row (line II), and the proximal aspect of the distal carpal row (line III), all of which should appear as smooth arcs (Fig. 19.4a) [7]. On the lateral X-ray, the capitate, lunate, and distal radius should create a collinear column (Fig. 19.4b). Deviations from these relationships on well-aligned X-rays should raise concern for dislocation or instability.

The metacarpals are numbered 1 through 5, with 1 referencing the most radial metacarpal at the base of the thumb and 5 referencing the most ulnar metacarpal. Alternatively, some orthopedic surgeons may also refer to the metacarpals as thumb, index, long, ring, and small finger metacarpals, corresponding to the respective distal phalanges. Each metacarpal has a head, neck, shaft, and base (Fig. 19.5). The head is part of the articulation between the proximal phalanx and the metacarpal,

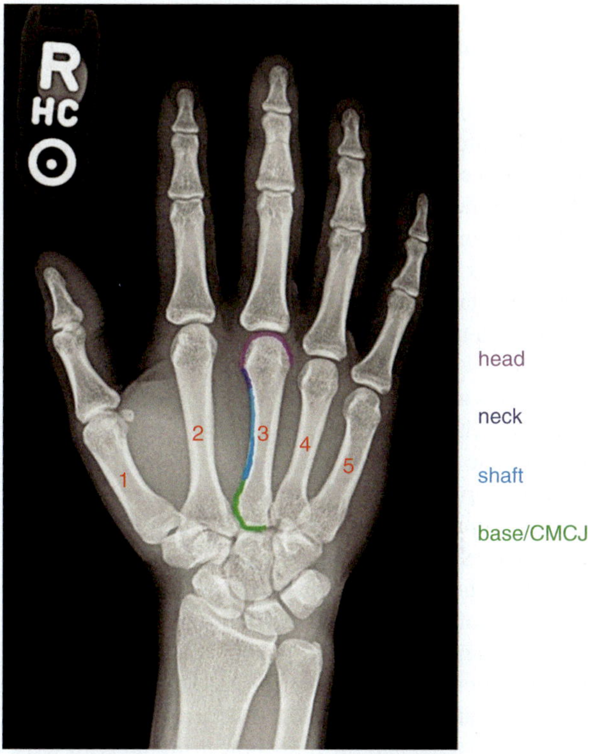

Fig. 19.5 Normal anteroposterior (AP) X-ray of the right hand with metacarpals 1–5 labeled. The metacarpal can further be described by its head, neck, shaft, and base, which extends into the carpometacarpal joint (CMCJ). (Source: Image courtesy of Navy Medicine Readiness and Training Command San Diego Radiology Department, used with permission)

also known as the MCPJ, and is covered in articular cartilage. The neck is the metaphyseal region connecting the head to the shaft, which serves as the hollow diaphyseal strut between the neck and the metacarpal base.

It is important to appreciate where one portion begins and the other ends, as displacement tolerances can vary depending on the region of the metacarpal. For example, an incomplete but 2.5 mm displaced fracture at the fifth metacarpal head, where the joint relies on congruency of the cartilage, can be much more problematic than a completely displaced and angulated fracture at the neck, where tolerances are much more forgiving since the functional costs of having an angulated fifth metacarpal neck are small.

As above, hand surgeons describe phalanges based on their respective finger, thumb, index finger, long finger, ring finger, and small finger, and further subdivide them into proximal, middle, and distal phalanges. For example, proper use of the nomenclature could be "proximal phalanx of the thumb" or "middle phalanx of the small finger." Note that the thumb only has a proximal and distal phalanx, while the index, long, ring, and small fingers each have proximal, middle, and distal phalanges.

The volar aspect of the distal phalanx serves as the insertion site for the flexor digitorum profundus (FDP), the tendon which bends the DIPJ. The volar aspect of the proximal phalanx serves as the insertion site of the flexor digitorum superficialis (FDS), which bends the PIPJ. The dorsum of the distal phalanx serves as the insertion site for the terminal portion of the extensor tendon, while the dorsum of the proximal phalanx serves as the insertion site for the central slip of the extensor tendon.

The flexor tendons run through the carpal tunnel along with the median nerve. Smooth fibro-osseous sheaths and pulleys hold the flexor tendons flush to the bone so that finger flexion and grip can occur without flexor tendon bowstringing. The FDP starts deep to the FDS in the carpal tunnel; however, it tunnels through the FDS to become more superficial at Camper's Chiasm, where the FDS splits into two slips as it inserts at the level of the proximal phalanx. Slender tendinous bands called vinculae attach the FDS and FDP to bone, providing blood to the tendons.

The extensor tendons that extend the wrist and fingers originate in the forearm and lateral epicondyle of the elbow. In general, the extensor digitorum communis (EDC) acts as the main powerhouse for MCPJ extension via the sagittal bands, PIPJ extension via the central slip, and DIPJ extension via the terminal extensor tendon and oblique retinacular ligament. The small finger and index finger usually each have additional extensor tendons, the extensor digiti quinti (EDQ), and extensor indicis proprius (EIP), respectively. The thumb has a separate tendon altogether called the extensor pollicis longus (EPL).

Within the dorsum of the hand, usually, more distally, juncturae tendinae are narrow bands of connective tissue that attach between the extensor tendons, often fooling examiners into thinking that an extensor tendon is intact when clinically testing patient function after lacerations. At the wrist level, the extensor retinaculum, a transverse and superficial band of connective tissue, holds the extensor tendons close to the wrist and prevents bowstringing with wrist extension.

Three main nerves and their terminal branches supply sensory and motor function to the hand: urgent/emergent hand injuries – the radial, ulnar, and median nerves. In broad strokes, the radial nerve provides dorsoradial hand sensation via the sensory branch of the radial nerve (SBRN). It also provides wrist and hand extension to the extensors via the posterior interosseous nerve (PIN). The SBRN emerges superficially about 6–8 cm proximal to the radial styloid [8].

The median nerve provides sensation to the palmar aspect of the thumb, index, long, and radial half of the ring finger, up to the dorsal distal phalanges via the palmar cutaneous branch and palmar digital branches. It also provides motor function to the thumb and radial finger flexors via the anterior interosseous nerve (AIN) and the recurrent branch of the median nerve. The palmar cutaneous branch of the median nerve branches off of the median nerve about 5 cm proximal to the transverse volar wrist crease [9].

The ulnar nerve provides sensation to the palmar and dorsal aspect of the small finger and ulnar half of the ring finger via palmar and dorsal cutaneous branches. It also provides motor function with flexion of the ulnar finger flexors and intrinsic hand musculature. The dorsal sensory branch of the ulnar nerve becomes subcutaneous about 5 cm from the proximal edge of the ulnar styloid [10]. The sensory branches of the median and ulnar nerve terminate as palmar digital nerves on both sides of the fingers and are volar to the digital arteries in the fingers.

The hand has a robust blood supply, with contributions from the ulnar and radial arteries which usually communicate through palmar arches in the hand. The superficial palmar arch is more distal in the hand with most of its blood supply coming from the ulnar artery, though there are usually contributions from the radial artery as well. The deep palmar arch is more proximal in the hand and receives most of its blood supply from the radial artery, with smaller contributions from the ulnar artery. Branches from the arches form the common digital arteries and the proper digital arteries which supply the fingers.

Anatomic variations of the arches exist in terms of vessel contributions and branches. Rich and redundant anastomoses also exist, as around 80% of individuals have complete palmar arches and 90% have functionally intact collaterals [11–13]. Furthermore, the proximal dorsal hand receives blood supply from the dorsal metacarpal arch, with variable contributions from the radial and ulnar arteries, and the distal dorsal hand receives blood from perforators coming from the deep palmar arch [14].

While this section certainly does not cover all of hand anatomy in an exhaustive sense, a basic review of hand anatomy will help surgeons to make the best decisions for injured sailors and marines. The authors highly encourage surgeons going on shipboard deployments to take opportunities to read and interpret normal X-rays of the hand, as this practice will help develop an understanding of hand anatomy and form a foundation upon which to judge pathology. Also, if opportunities arise to participate in cadaveric hand dissections or assist in hand surgical cases, those opportunities will only further the appreciation for the intricacies of hand anatomy.

Management of Urgent/Emergent Hand Injuries

Hatch Hand: Urgent/Emergent Hand Injuries: Likely Medical Evacuation (MEDEVAC)

The patient who presented in Case 19.1 is a typical presentation of a hatch hand injury. What to do to work it up? What to expect? Can this be managed on board or should the team start the process of initiating a medical evacuation (MEDEVAC)? This chapter should provide guidance to begin answering these questions.

Every acute hand injury, especially a hatch hand one, requires three-view X-rays of the hand and a detailed physical exam. Starting with X-rays, scrutinize boney anatomy for fractures and alignment. Any fractured finger may also warrant its own set of dedicated films.

The physical exam involves inspection, palpation, and a careful neurovascular exam. Starting with inspection, carefully assess the skin: If skin is compromised, it is important to note the depth and location. A deep laceration on the volar side of the index finger should make the surgeon think about ruling out a flexor tendon injury. A poke-hole laceration oozing deep dark blood is concerning for an open fracture.

Palpation should be done thoughtfully and ideally after having initially reviewed X-rays. Overt fractures do not require aggressive palpation; however, focused palpation of the hand may reveal additional tenderness that helps with clinical correlation or determining whether or not X-rays are necessary.

The neurovascular exam is critical, especially if there is a deep laceration which may involve a digital artery or nerve. Grossly, the motor exam consists of having the patient make a thumbs up to test the radial nerve, an "okay" sign to test the motor branch of the median nerve, and crossed fingers to test the motor branch of the ulnar nerve. More detailed testing of individual tendons will be covered later, but, in general, motion at all joints distal to a laceration should be tested. The sensory exam should test the radial, ulnar, and median nerve distributions: the examiner can test sensation over the dorsum of the thumb for the radial nerve, the volar aspect of the index finger for the median nerve, and the ulnar aspect of the small finger for the ulnar nerve. Finally, vascular status should be checked via capillary refill to the fingers, which should be less than 3 s.

Regarding hatch hand injuries or finger lacerations, two-point discrimination should be performed on all five fingers to better assess sensation. A tool to test two-point discrimination can be easily made with a paperclip, folded over so that the ends act as two separate points (Fig. 19.6). Each finger has radial and ulnar digital sensory nerves, and both should be tested if a nerve laceration might have occurred. The examiner asks patients if they feel one point or two points as patients look away, measuring the distance to which patients can distinguish two separate points. In the paperclip example, the measured distance means the distance between the

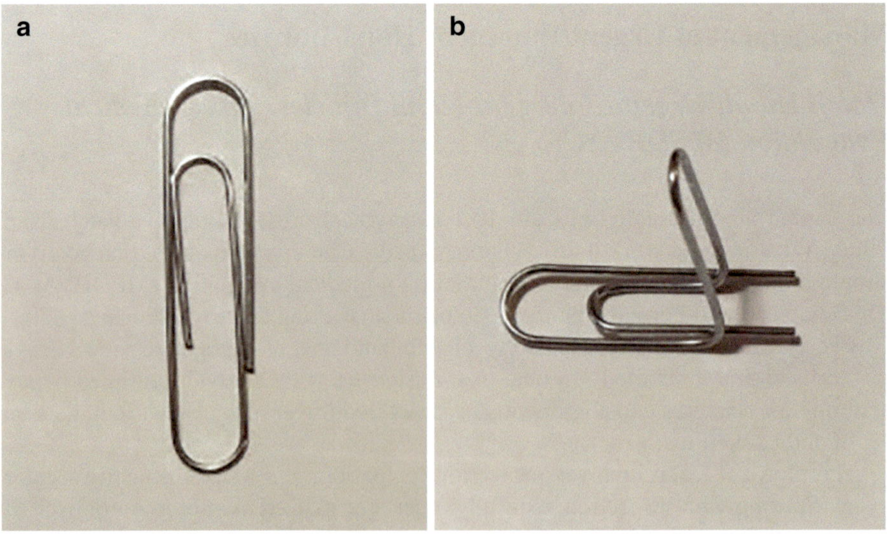

Fig. 19.6 (**a**) Paperclip. (**b**) Paperclip fashioned to test two-point discrimination. Width can be adjusted as needed for a smaller distance or a larger distance. (Source: Photos courtesy of Shian L. Peterson, MD)

two prongs of the bent paperclip. Normal sensation is 4–5 mm in the fingertips [15, 16]. Nerve injuries are most ideally repaired in an inpatient, hospital setting by a hand surgeon, thus any patient with a suspected nerve injury should get a MEDEVAC to a tertiary care center within 2–3 days after injury with a well-documented, thorough, neurovascular exam.

In general, a hatch hand injury may consist of multiple phalangeal fractures, nerve contusions from local swelling, tendon disruptions, and skin lacerations from the impact. After X-rays and a detailed examination, if there are any open fractures then broad-spectrum antibiotics should be administered and tetanus immunization should be verified/updated. Grossly contaminated wounds should be washed out with normal saline and significantly angulated fractures should be reduced to best reapproximate anatomic alignment; both can be done under local anesthesia only. During wound irrigation and debridement, the wound should also be explored and any damaged soft tissue structures that might require further intervention should be noted.

Once open wounds are cleaned, they should be loosely approximated with 4-0 nylon, dressed, and splinted appropriately. Kirschner wire (K-wire) placement to maintain fracture alignment is not routinely expected of a shipboard surgeon, nor should it be attempted without appropriate equipment, specifically fluoroscopy, power, and K-wires (none of which is available in the forward-deployed maritime environment outside of hospital ships).

If the skin is intact and fractures are nondisplaced, repeat X-rays in a week and splinting for 3–4 weeks is appropriate treatment for most phalangeal fractures, with subsequent gradual occupational therapy (OT) after the fracture is nontender to prevent stiffness. If fractures are severely angulated, highly unstable, or not otherwise amenable to shipboard care, routine MEDEVAC is recommended, as phalangeal fractures become increasingly difficult to fix in a closed manner if more than 2 weeks elapse from the time of injury.

When trying to make the decision as to whether a hatch hand injury needs routine care or urgent MEDEVAC or requires an orthopedic consultation, the minimum information needed includes a thorough physical exam and appropriate X-rays. For example, for the patient in Case 19.1 whose injuries are visualized in Fig. 19.1, the following statement helps clearly paint a picture in the mind of an orthopedic consultant being consulted via telephone:

> *I have a 37-year-old right-hand-dominant male with a left hatch hand injury that happened today, including a left open ring finger proximal phalanx fracture, left ring finger middle phalanx fracture, left long finger proximal phalanx fracture, left long finger middle phalanx fracture, and a left ring finger partial extensor tendon laceration in extensor zone 4 (discussed later in this chapter). He cannot extend his left ring finger at the PIPJ, but he has protective sensation and is perfusing all digits. We administered intravenous (IV) Ancef 2 gram, updated his tetanus status, performed an initial irrigation and debridement of his open wound, found a complete extensor tendon laceration, loosely closed his skin laceration, and placed him in a plaster volar resting splint.*

In this case, urgent MEDEVAC should be arranged, with the goal of getting the patient to tertiary care within 72–96 h. This would likely be the most severe hatch hand scenario that a ship's surgeon might face. The remainder of the chapter focuses on variations and specific shipboard injuries that also occur with hatches and hands.

Lacerations and Tendon Injuries: Likely Medical Evacuation (MEDEVAC)

Case 19.2

A 37-year-old male Boatswain's Mate (BM) lacerated the volar aspect of his dominant index finger while demonstrating how to cut sheet metal in the hangar bay. He presented to the medical department during the workday holding pressure over his finger complaining predominantly of extreme pain and was unable to flex his index finger.

How do the work-up and management differ between the patients in Cases 19.1 and 19.2? **The most important parts of evaluation still involve inspecting the wound to describe its location AND documenting a good neurological exam <u>prior to</u> anesthetizing the finger or exploring the wound.** When describing tendon lacerations, it is highly recommended to review the section on hand anatomy and terminology, as the location of the laceration and completeness of the injury makes the difference between a simple washout and skin closure versus consideration for a MEDEVAC. The correct decision might save the patient from a 6-month limited duty period for flexor tendon reconstruction to treat a chronic FDP laceration and/or permanent functional morbidity.

Hand surgeons divide the flexor and extensor tendons into different zones along the volar and dorsal aspect of the hand and wrist. The flexor tendon is broken up into five zones (Fig. 19.7) [17, 18].

- Zone I is distal to the insertion of the FDS, typically includes the area near the distal interphalangeal joint, and includes only the FDP tendon.
- Zone II encompasses the area from the distal palmar crease to the insertion of the FDS (typically at the middle aspect of the middle phalanx) and likely involves both the FDS and FDP tendons.
- Zone III extends from the distal edge of the transverse carpal ligament to the distal palmar crease.
- Zone IV lies deep to the transverse carpal ligament, essentially the carpal tunnel.
- Zone V is proximal to the carpal tunnel, including the forearm.

The extensor tendon zones are divided into eight zones (Fig. 19.7) [19, 20]. An easy way to remember these is to start at the DIPJ (Zone 1). The joints moving proximally are odd-numbered whereas even numbers occur over the shafts of the hand bones.

- Zone 1 corresponds to the DIPJ.
- Zone 2 overlies the middle phalanx.
- Zone 3 corresponds to the central slip and PIPJ.

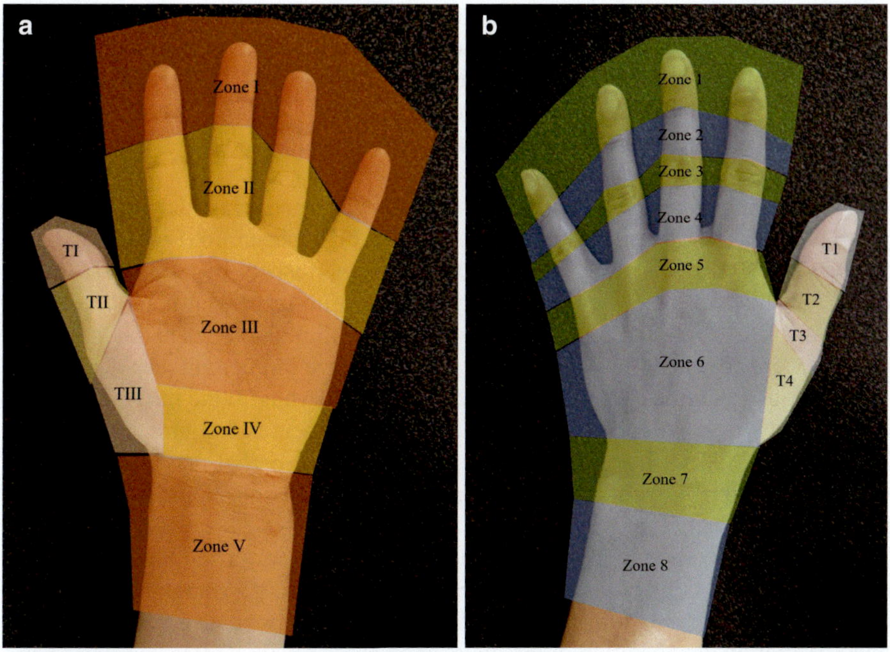

Fig. 19.7 (**a**) Flexor Tendon Zones. (**b**) Extensor Tendon Zones. Note that the thumb has its own designations for both flexor and extensor zone injuries. (Source: Photos courtesy of Shian L. Peterson, MD)

- Zone 4 encompasses the proximal phalanx.
- Zone 5 encompasses the MCPJs.
- Zone 6 corresponds to the dorsum of the hand.
- Zone 7 overlies the wrist.
- Zone 8 encompasses the distal forearm.

The thumb has its own classification (Fig. 19.7).
There are three flexor zones.

- Zone TI distal to the IPJ
- Zone TII encompassing the A1 pulley to the IPJ
- Zone TIII involving the thenar eminence

On the extensor side, the thumb has four zones.

- Zone T1 extending distally from the IPJ
- Zone T2 overlying the proximal phalanx
- Zone T3 involving the MCPJ
- Zone T4 encompassing the CMCJ

For the patient in Case 19.2, the evaluation initially includes inspection of the wound as previously described. If the laceration is overlying extensor Zone 1, it may be amenable to irrigation, debridement, and closure via tenodermodesis, where the skin and tendon are sutured in conjunction with the closure [19]. If it is deep and appears to be overlying flexor tendon Zone II then this injury would likely benefit from a formal wound exploration to determine the extent of the laceration. If it is complete, it would need MEDEVAC to a hand surgeon for operative repair, ideally within one week. The inspection portion of the exam alone gives a fairly good idea of the possible severity of the injury.

The next step is obtaining and documenting a good neurovascular exam. A good place to start is with two-point discrimination. Using a paperclip (Fig. 19.6), assess for two-point discrimination on the radial and ulnar aspect of the affected digit, distal to the laceration. This is especially important in flexor tendon injuries as the radial and ulnar digital nerves are more volar to the digital arteries in the finger and can be lacerated with a flexor tendon laceration. Nerve injury with an extensor tendon laceration is unlikely unless the laceration passes volar to the mid-axial line of the finger. Normal two-point discrimination in the fingers is 4–5 mm. Greater than 7 mm lack of discrimination should be concerning for partial nerve laceration or neuropraxia, while greater than 15 mm lack of discrimination should be highly suspicious for digital nerve laceration [15].

The digital nerves provide sensation along the borders of the hand, the radial digital nerve to the index finger, the ulnar digital nerve to the thumb, and the ulnar digital nerve to the small finger, which together provide protective sensation to the hand. Wallerian degeneration of the distal axon starts 48–96 h after transection and is complete by 1–4 weeks [16]. **Nerve repair is best done by a hand surgeon within 3–7 days of injury.**

After checking two-point discrimination in all the fingers, a digital nerve block can be provided to the patient for pain relief and to finish the exam. Prep the skin around the base of the proximal phalanx with iodine and alcohol. Infiltrate 4 mL of a 50/50 mixture of 0.25% Marcaine plain and 1% Lidocaine plain with a 23–25-gauge needle at the base of the proximal phalanx on both the radial and ulnar sides. If multiple digits need to be evaluated, do not exceed a single dose of 40 mL and calibrate according to the extent of the injury. After 5–10 min, assess the patient for the appropriate analgesia. While the patient may still feel pressure, they should no longer feel sharp pain. Other techniques also exist, such as an intrathecal block within the flexor tendon sheath [21, 22].

Capillaries should be tested next, by pressing on the distal tips of the finger and watching for the blush to return. Thankfully, the fingers have a robust blood supply from both digital arteries and collateral circulation from the dorsum of the hand [14].

Next, test for motor function and tendon integrity. As discussed previously, test radial, ulnar, and median nerves. If concerned for laceration, the most important step is to see if the tendon still functions. For example, if there is a concern for a flexor tendon injury to the index finger, it is helpful to know if the patient can flex at the DIPJ and PIPJ. If the patient cannot, this finding can help hand surgeons determine whether the injury is to FDP or FDS or both. It is especially important for the examiner to isolate each joint on the patient's hand separately using their own fingers (Fig. 19.8). If there is a concern for an extensor tendon injury, again assess

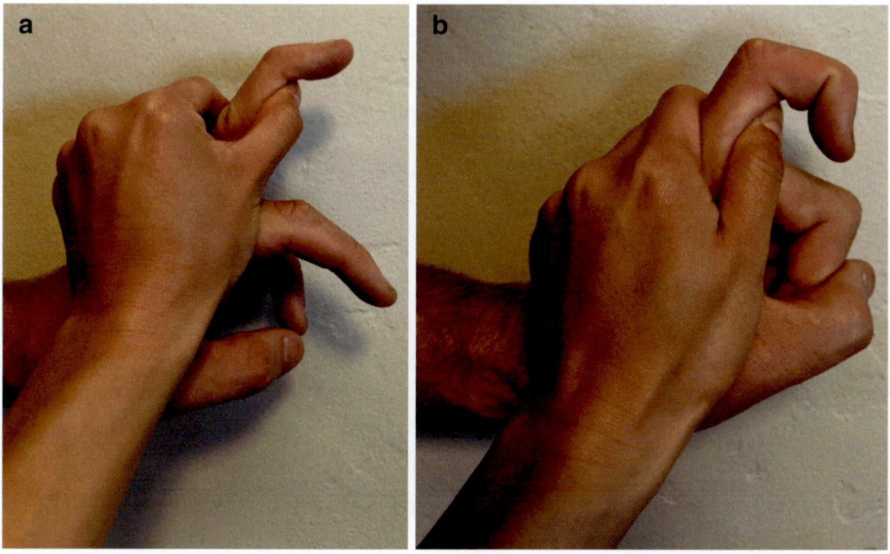

Fig. 19.8 Distal interphalangeal joint (DIPJ) and proximal interphalangeal joint (PIPJ) are isolated separately for examination purposes to examine the integrity of the flexor digitorum profundus (FDP) and the flexor digitorum superficialis (FDS), respectively. (**a**) The DIPJ of the long finger is tested. The FDP flexes the DIPJ. (**b**) The PIPJ of the index finger is tested. The FDS flexes the PIPJ. (Source: Photos courtesy of Shian L. Peterson, MD)

extension distal to the laceration, at the MCPJ, PIPJ, and DIPJ. This technique helps to tease out differences between a complete or partial tendon laceration.

The next step involves irrigating and further exploring the wound. Sometimes simply examining gross tendon integrity can give an idea of whether the laceration is complete or partial. Prepare a sterile field, ensure the hand has appropriate local anesthesia, and proceed to gently irrigate the wounds with 1–3 L of normal saline. While doing the irrigation, if the tendon is visible and it is completely intact, then simply close the skin laceration and manage the wound until healed.

However, if a partially or completely lacerated flexor tendon is visualized, finish irrigating, loosely close the skin with 4-0 nylon, place the hand in a splint, and arrange for MEDEVAC. Flexor tendon lacerations, particularly those that result in the inability to actively flex the DIPJ or PIPJ, are most appropriately addressed with surgical exploration and primary repair by a hand surgeon. **Expedited MEDEVAC (within 1–2 weeks of injury) is especially important in flexor tendon lacerations, as delayed treatment is associated with poor outcomes** [19].

Extensor tendon lacerations can be repaired, with differing techniques depending on the zone (Table 19.1) [20]. While an attempt at repairing extensor tendon injuries is reasonable while underway, formal OT is still highly recommended to ensure a good outcome. Therefore, transfer of complete tendon lacerations to a tertiary care center with a certified hand OT in a timely fashion, even in the setting of a successful repair of the tendon laceration, is recommended.

Table 19.1 Doyle's proposed techniques for extensor tendon repair

Zone 1 (DIPJ)	Running suture of the skin and tendon as a single unit, non-absorbable 4-0 suture, also known as tenodermodesis
Zone 2 (P2)	Running 5-0 stitch near cut edge of the tendon, oversewn with an epitendinous 5-0 cross stitch
Zone 3–5 (in fingers) and Zones 2–3 (thumb)	Modified Kessler suture of 4-0 synthetic material in the thickest portion of the tendon, oversewn with an epitendinous 5-0 cross stitch

DIPJ: distal interphalangeal joint; P2: middle phalanx

All finger injuries should be appropriately splinted for soft tissue rest and safety while healing or during transport. If the laceration involves the flexor tendons then splinting should occur in slight flexion with a dorsal blocking splint. If the laceration is on the extensor side, the finger should be splinted in extension with a volar-based splint.

Digital Nerve Injury: Likely Medical Evacuation (MEDEVAC)

If a patient presents with a sharp laceration that is deep and more volar, it is incumbent on the evaluating surgeon to maintain a high suspicion for a digital nerve injury until the nerve is proven to be intact. As described above, two-point discrimination can be tested with a paperclip folded in half (Fig. 19.6), which acts as a readily available substitute over the traditional Dellon-McKinnon Disk-Criminator used in a most hand clinics. If a nerve injury is suspected, two-point discrimination should be tested on all fingers, on both sides of the digits, to assess for the radial and ulnar digital nerve sensation to each finger. Traditionally, normal two-point discrimination in the digits is estimated to be around 4–5 mm; however, there is about 2 mm of interobserver difference. Therefore, compare the injured digits to the uninjured digits, document these findings, and send documented findings with the patient so that any changes over time will be noted by the receiving physician [16, 23, 24]. As stated previously, this evaluation is especially important to complete prior to providing local analgesia for pain relief and subsequent irrigation and debridement.

After a detailed neurovascular exam is performed, local analgesia via a digital block can be performed (see description previously described in this chapter), along with thorough irrigation with 1–3 L of normal saline.

The wound should be loosely closed with non-absorbable suture and dressed. If there are any associated fractures, those should be reduced and splinted. The patient should then get an urgent MEDEVAC, as definitive nerve repair or reconstruction is best performed in a tertiary care center with a hand surgeon. The ideal timing from a hand surgery perspective is digital nerve repair within three days of injury. Nerve lacerations that present to a tertiary center more than seven days from the time of injury may have too much tension at the laceration site to allow for a repair, and may require reconstruction with nerve allograft; thus, time is of the essence.

Amputations: Likely Medical Evacuation (MEDEVAC)

Case 19.3

A 37-year-old male Sailor was working night flight operations on the flight deck and attempted to blindly release a latch with a high-pressure spring-loading mechanism. The equipment malfunctioned and amputated the index finger of his dominant hand. He was immediately escorted to the medical department, holding the amputated finger he retrieved from the flight deck.

If a hatch, sheet metal, nautical line/cordage, or other shipboard hazard causes a finger or limb amputation or dysvascular limb, this situation requires an emergent MEDEVAC.

With regards to amputation of a digit like in Case 19.3, certain conditions must be met for replantation to even be a consideration. Some indications include a thumb, multiple digits, amputation at the level of the palm, wrist, or forearm, or a single digit distal to the FDS insertion. Sharp or guillotine injuries have better outcomes than crush or avulsion injuries, given the wider zone of injury. The time for viability for a digit from traumatic amputation to replantation or revascularization is 12 h of warm ischemia time (room or ambient temperature) or 24 h of cold ischemia time (iced cooler). Ischemia time basically means the time that the severed limb can survive and still possibly undergo replantation. These times are halved if the amputation is proximal; there is less time to work with when treating a more proximal amputation.

If it is not feasible to get an emergent MEDEVAC to a replant center in these time frames, the digit is unlikely to survive. If there is any chance of proximity to a replant center, wrap the tissue in saline-soaked gauze, place it in a plastic bag, and place this on a bed of ice with the goal of keeping the tissue cool without freezing it [25]. Be careful to avoid direct contact with ice, as this practice can damage the soft tissues. Irrigate the amputated stump if there is gross contamination, place a pressure dressing, elevate the affected limb, administer antibiotics, and update tetanus status. In the setting of a digit amputation, tourniquets and vessel ligation should be avoided.

Dysvascular or Crushed Limbs: Likely Medical Evacuation (MEDEVAC)

For a dysvascular limb where either the radial and/or ulnar artery are compromised from a direct laceration, operative repair is a surgical emergency if the hand is not perfused. A dysvascular limb often occurs in the context of a mangled extremity but can also occur as a sharp, deep laceration along the volar wrist [16]. If there exists any suspicion that the radial or ulnar artery is lacerated, assessment of vascular status is critical. This can best be done first by controlling the bleeding with direct pressure then inspecting the affected tissues and comparing them to adjacent or similar well-vascularized tissues. Most traumatic upper extremity vascular injuries can be controlled with direct pressure. Hemostasis is best achieved with 5–15 min of uninterrupted, digital, manual pressure and a compressive dressing [26]. Tourniquet use would only be recommended in an operative setting to explore the area of injury or in extreme cases of hypovolemic shock and circulatory collapse from blood loss and should be avoided for more than 2 h. Tourniquet use increases the risk of reperfusion injury, compartment syndrome, and ultimately the loss of a limb.

Assessment of the digital perfusion about the dorsal paronychia is more reliable than nailbed capillary refill, and return of pink color 1–2 s after application and release of pressure indicates healthy tissue [27]. Pale color indicates arterial insufficiency and dusky discoloration can indicate venous congestion. Assessment of overall hand perfusion can be checked with an Allen's test, though this may not be feasible depending on where the laceration is. Shipboard point-of-care ultrasound (POCUS), if available, can also be a useful tool to assess vascular status. Again, keep in mind that 80% of individuals have complete palmar arches and 90% have functionally intact collaterals [11–13], so an isolated, complete laceration of a radial artery does not automatically infer an ischemic, compromised limb. However, given the close proximity of the radial artery to the other volar tendons and nerves, the chance of concomitant damage is quite high and should not be ignored. In the absence of ischemia, thorough repair of the damaged structures is best performed within 24 h of injury [6]. If the limb is dysvascular and the distal tissues are ischemic, then shipboard surgeons have to decide whether to immediately explore and repair the vessels on their own or to send the patient on an emergent MEDEVAC.

Dysvascular limbs also result from shipboard crush injuries or otherwise mangled upper extremities. Any significant crush of the hand or upper extremity should raise clinical suspicion for compartment syndrome, and serial examinations to make sure that compartment syndrome does not develop is recommended. A severe hatch hand is one type of crush injury, but a sailor or marine's hand could also get caught in engine room machinery or run over by an onboard vehicle or aircraft. In these serious injuries, the crushing of various layers of tissue results in rapid myonecrosis, vascular and neurologic compromise, and likely fracture of multiple underlying bones [27]. The resultant direct injury to major vessels or branching perforators or the indirect crushing of endothelial or muscle cells can lead to varying degrees of macro- or micro-circulatory compromise and increasing pressures within the myofascial compartments [27]. While a full discussion of compartment syndrome is beyond the scope of this chapter, shipboard surgeons should be aware of crush injuries placing sailors and marines at high risk for compartment syndrome, and they should arrange for such injured personnel to get an emergent MEDEVAC.

If patients demonstrate extreme pain with passive stretch of their digits, have tense, swollen hand compartments, and increasing analgesic requirements in the context of a trauma that is consistent with a clinical picture of acute compartment syndrome, a shipboard surgeon may need to perform a hand compartment release prior to placing the patient in a splint and arranging an urgent/emergent MEDEVAC to a tertiary care center. If this scenario presents itself, contact with a hand surgeon using the references cited in this chapter (and in Chaps. 5 and 14) is recommended to discuss the situation and get step-by-step guidance; however, the basic sequence to release the hand compartments is outlined here.

1. If there is a compartment-pressure testing kit onboard or access to an arterial line setup, place the needle into the muscle compartment of concern. If the compartment pressure measures within 30 mmHg of the patient's non-anesthetized diastolic blood pressure, this diagnostic test can help to confirm the diagnosis of compartment syndrome. However, if clinical suspicion is high for compartment syndrome, no additional diagnostics are required for the diagnosis.
2. If required, keep in mind multiple incisions may be required to release all compartments in the hand, which is fraught with potential for harm. It is extraordinarily important to understand exactly where the incisions should be and to be familiar ahead of time with the neurovascular anatomy of the hand.
3. The following landmarks should be physically and/or mentally noted as they guide safe treatment:

   (a) The palmaris longus (stay ulnar to this, if too radial then could cause injury to the palmar cutaneous branch of the median nerve)
   (b) Hook of the hamate
   (c) Kaplan's cardinal line, which is drawn from the ulnar thumb crease to the hook of the hamate. The intersection with the line extended from the radial border of the ring finger line helps identify the location of the superficial palmar arch.
   (d) Note where the long finger bends down to touch the thenar eminence, which is commonly where the recurrent motor branch of the median nerve will pop out of the thenar eminence

4. Start with the extended carpal tunnel release along the volar wrist and hand. The landmarks help find the incision site, which is a 2–3 cm incision parallel and 6 mm ulnar to the thenar crease, made in line with the radial border of the ring finger, ulnar to the palmaris longus, with a Bruner incision approach across the wrist crease to avoid the palmar cutaneous branch of the median nerve, and then continued proximally 2–3 cm over the volar forearm (Fig. 19.9).
5. After the skin incision, spread through the deep dermal layer, getting down to the transverse carpal ligament. There may be a layer of muscle overlying it called the palmaris brevis, which can be feathered off with a knife, to visualize the fascia of the transverse carpal ligament. Find a spot over the fascia, pick it up, and either cut through it with a knife or incise it with tenotomies to pop into the carpal tunnel. The median nerve should be superficial and radial in the carpal tunnel. Use hemostats to spread underneath the fascia and lift it off the nerve, so the fascia can be safely cut with the knife, staying ulnar within the canal and in line with the radial border of the ring finger. Be aware that Guyon's canal, which houses the ulnar nerve, is just ulnar to the carpal tunnel. Advance distally until the palmar fat pad is visualized, which is the landmark that delineates where the superficial palmar arch is. In the distal portion of the incision, the volar fascia of the adductor pollicis can be released. Confirm the full release with a freer. Now

turning attention proximally, it can help to flex the wrist over a small towel bump, to allow the median nerve to fall away. Identify the proximal forearm fascia and free it up with tenotomies above and below it to brush away any extra tissue (this is in preparation to release it). As an added check, run a freer deep and superficial to the forearm fascia. Next, using just the tips of the scissors, aim dorsally and ulnarly and extend the release proximal up the forearm. Check with a freer that the antebrachial fascia is fully released.

6. Next, on the volar hand, make two additional longitudinal incisions along the radial aspect of the first/thumb metacarpal and the ulnar aspect of the fifth metacarpal to decompress the thenar and hypothenar compartments, respectively (Fig. 19.9).
7. Decompress the dorsal aspect of the hand with two longitudinal dorsal incisions between the second and third metacarpals and fourth and fifth metacarpals to allow access to the interosseous and adductor muscle compartments (Fig. 19.9). Additionally, the first dorsal interossei and dorsal aspect of the adductor pollicis can be released through an incision over the first dorsal web space.
8. Any grossly necrotic tissue should be debrided; anything questionable should be left. All incisions should be left open and the wounds appropriately dressed with a moist gauze dressing, which should be changed in the operating room in 24–48 h if immediate MEDEVAC is unavailable. The hand should be splinted in a neutral position to ensure the support of all of the digits prior to transporting the patient off of the ship.

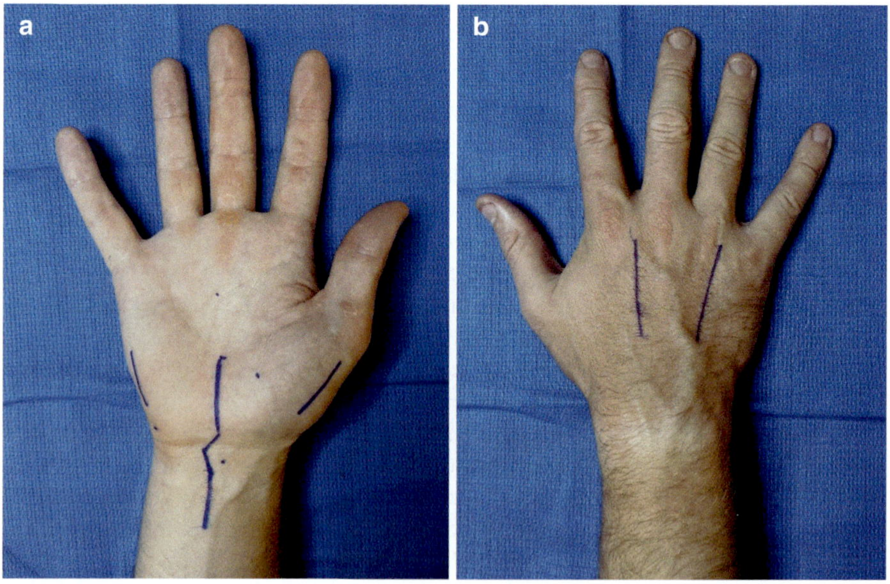

Fig. 19.9 (**a**) Extended carpal tunnel release incisions. (**b**) Volar and dorsal hand compartment release incisions. Note the dots made for the key landmarks as described prior to drawing incisions. (Source: Photos courtesy of Shian L. Peterson, MD)

Thankfully, no reported cases of shipboard upper extremity amputation or dysvascular limbs have been noted in the current military or medical literature; however, shipboard surgeons should be aware of the appropriate treatment protocols for this significant injury and worst-case scenario.

High-Pressure Injection, Burns, and Degloving Injuries: Likely Medical Evacuation (MEDEVAC)

Case 19.4

A 37-year-old male aviation mechanic sustained a high-pressure injection site injury on the ulnar aspect of his right hand, his non-dominant hand. Even though the wound was not that severe looking, he presented to the medical department for evaluation at the request of his immediate supervisor.

Sailors and Marines exposed to machinery and moving components aboard the ship and vehicles have higher risks of high-pressure injection, deep burns, skin degloving, and other severe soft-tissue injuries relative to the rest of the crew. Regardless of if high-pressure injections, burns, and skin degloving appear benign or extremely severe, they all likely require emergent MEDEVAC and formal operative intervention.

High-pressure injection injuries to the hands or fingers often appear benign as described in Case 19.4 and demonstrated in Fig. 19.10 [28], but they can cause significant soft-tissue damage and can result in amputation if not quickly diagnosed and surgically treated [29]. While these injuries are relatively rare in the civilian population, they are most common among those using pressurized tools, paints, greases, oils, and solvents [29], typical findings aboard any naval vessel across its various departments. Typically, the nondominant index finger or thumb is involved, with organic solvents thought to be most harmful to the underlying tissue

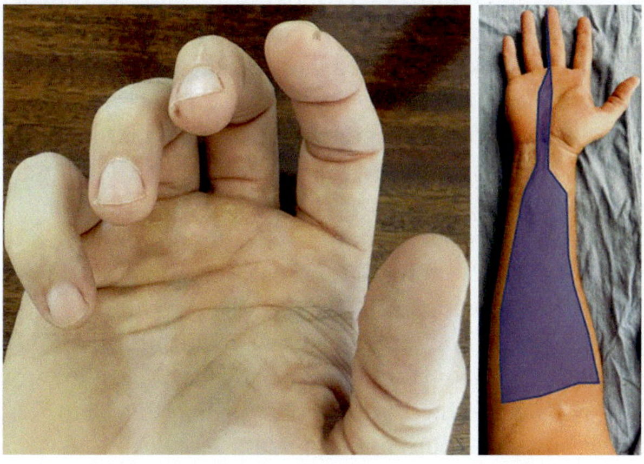

Fig. 19.10 Left: Representative image of small, benign-appearing, high-pressure injection site on ulnar aspect of long fingertip. Right: Likely dissection field required to achieve thorough debridement of this injury. (Source: Photos courtesy of John P. Waggoner, MD)

due to cytotoxicity [29]. Recent studies demonstrate that even water injections have significant morbidity and long-term sequelae, despite water being relatively biologically inert [30].

Because the high-pressure liquid travels along a path of least resistance, the injected substance usually travels along the same corridors as the nerves and vessels, shearing through the fascial planes and muscular compartments. Damage to tissue arises from the force of the initial injection, chemical irritation of the tissues, secondary inflammation, and secondary infection [29].

Given the severity of these injuries and the need for urgent/emergent surgical care, administer broad-spectrum antibiotics and update tetanus status while arranging for emergent MEDEVAC. If there will be a significant delay (>24 h) in MEDEVAC due to poor weather, transportation unavailability, or other unforeseen operational requirements, this injury would be indicated for shipboard irrigation and debridement to decompress neurovascular structures, clean tissues, clear flexor tendon sheaths to remove the irritating chemical, and provide prophylaxis against compartment syndrome and secondary inflammatory or infectious concerns.

If required, this procedure involves fully exposing the digit or limb, inspecting all neurovascular and connective tissue structures for damage, debriding away necrotic tissue, and removing the offending agents. Postoperatively, the wound should be dressed and inspected frequently, and the extremity should be splinted and elevated for soft tissue rest and to minimize swelling. Thankfully, no documented cases of high-pressure injection injuries requiring shipboard surgery appear in the military literature; however, understanding the severity of these injuries and the need for timely MEDEVAC remains paramount.

Similarly, severe burns and degloving injuries require urgent/emergent MEDEVAC so that soft tissue coverage can be rapidly restored, the patient's digits or limbs can be salvaged, and risks of severe negative sequelae minimized. Assessment of burns typically involves clinical judgment based on the mechanism of injury and physical exam. The American Society for Surgery of the Hand classifies burns as first through fourth degree, corresponding first degree burns having skin redness without blistering; second-degree burns including blisters; third degree including "white and leathery" skin; and fourth degree looking the same as third degree burns but also including visible damage to underlying connective tissue or bones [31].

First and second-degree burns of the hand should be treated conservatively with appropriate analgesia, topical creams, and soft protective wraps as required, third-degree burns, fourth-degree burns, and any burns resulting from high-energy mechanisms or with unknown penetration depth should get a MEDEVAC on an urgent/emergent basis for subsequent surgical exploration and soft-tissue coverage. Current literature describes minimal roles for prophylactic antibiotic administration for most burns [32]; however, these observations may not apply to maritime and other military environments. Consequently, the authors recommend broad-spectrum antibiotics for maritime military burns requiring MEDEVAC, given their likelihood for significant concomitant skin loss or laceration, environmental contamination, and low risks associated with prophylaxis. See Chap. 26 for an in-depth discussion about burns and burn management.

Degloving injuries are so-named because they result in a significant detachment of skin and underlying subcutaneous tissue from their deep muscular or boney scaffolds [33], and they can have quite a dramatic appearance. Degloving injuries may also have concomitant fractures underlying the soft-tissue defects, so it is important not to forget X-rays as part of the diagnostic workup once the patient is stabilized. By definition, these injuries are open injuries and should be treated similar to hatch hands and other high-morbidity injuries in this chapter. Rapid administration of broad-spectrum antibiotics and a tetanus status update are critical. Appropriate resources for soft tissue coverage are unlikely to be available on board any ship, so advanced reconstructive or skin-grafting options are not discussed in this chapter.

If an upper extremity or digital degloving injury occurs, the traumatized limb should be inspected and any life-threatening or severe vascular injuries addressed with direct pressure. Hemostasis for upper extremity vascular injuries can almost always be obtained with direct pressure alone, so tourniquet use is a last, life-saving resort. As previously stated, X-rays and physical examination to evaluate neurovascular status should follow, then appropriate analgesia should be administered promptly to keep the patient as comfortable as possible during the following steps and eventual MEDEVAC.

Analgesia can include IV or oral medications augmented by local tissue field or digital blocks with short- or long-acting agents. For local anesthesia, the authors prefer a 50/50 mixture of 0.25% Marcaine plain and 1% Lidocaine plain, typically not exceeding a single dose of 40 mL and calibrated according to the extent of the injury. Injured limbs should then be irrigated with 3 L of normal saline to remove gross contamination and moisten the tissues.

Use available skin to cover the underlying tissues and dress with petrolatum gauze or other moist, nonadherent dressing, such as wet-to-dry gauze, silver-impregnated dressings, or other commercial products designed for such purposes. Once all deep tissues are covered, the extremity should be splinted for protection and soft tissue rest and elevated to decrease swelling, if possible. If there is a delay in MEDEVAC, the wounds must be examined and moist dressings should be changed at least daily.

A Word on Damage Control Orthopedics (DCO)

It is highly unlikely that a maritime surgeon will be faced with one of these upper extremity orthopedic emergencies such as an amputation, dysvascular limb, or compartment syndrome as an isolated injury. Such an injury likely occurs in the context of polytrauma, so following the advanced trauma life support (ATLS) protocol is of the utmost importance. In a multiple-injury patient with chest injuries, head injuries, and mangled extremities, DCO emphasizes temporizing and controlling the injury rather than definitively repairing the extremity to minimize any additional physiologic insult from a prolonged and complex surgery [34]. See Chap. 24 for further discussion. For the ship's surgeon with a general surgery background, DCO would likely involve ATLS management followed by appropriate work-up and stabilization of fractures via X-rays, reduction and splinting, broad-spectrum antibiotics, tetanus prophylaxis, and irrigation and debridement as appropriate while awaiting a MEDEVAC.

Management of Lower Acuity Hand Injuries

Given the high rates of hand and wrist injuries among crewmembers [1, 35], sick call is commonly full of complaints less severe than hatch hand or other high-morbidity upper extremity conditions. Many of these injuries can be managed non-operatively with the supplies on board and without losing a crew member to a MEDEVAC. As above, the first steps with any hand injury include obtaining X-rays and a comprehensive clinical examination. No wrist or hand injury should be written off as a sprain without appropriate supporting evidence, even if the injury initially appears benign. Modern X-rays of the extremity provide extremely small radiation doses and are comparable with background exposure levels, so do not feel shy when ordering X-rays to evaluate suspected fractures, open wounds, masses, or foreign bodies.

Please keep in mind that the following section pertains to fractures that are stable and can be maintained within acceptable tolerances of alignment. Unstable fractures that fall out of tolerances and joints that subluxate, dislocate, or lose congruency likely require operative management and should get a MEDEVAC within 1 week to allow for appropriate treatment by an orthopedic surgeon.

Carpal, Metacarpal, and Phalangeal Fractures: Likely Nonoperative Management

In general, carpal, metacarpal, and phalangeal fractures or dislocations are common hand injuries seen in orthopedic practice, and they are extremely prevalent among the military population. As recent literature suggests, metacarpal fractures are the most common musculoskeletal injury treated by both civilian and military providers [36]. Even though most metacarpal fractures do not require surgery, they create significant problems for military units, given organizational human resource limitations and mission-related or deployment-readiness requirements [35].

Both pier-side and underway, sailors and marines are at high risk for these injuries. There are various subtypes and eponyms describing intraarticular fractures of the finger or thumb metacarpals and phalangeal heads and bases; however, simple overarching management principles apply and there is no need to memorize eponyms or classification schemes. As above, all open fractures should receive broad-spectrum antibiotics, tetanus prophylaxis, and urgent MEDEVAC to tertiary care. Any grossly contaminated wounds should undergo irrigation and debridement prior to MEDEVAC.

To simplify the decision-making algorithm for closed fractures, any fractures that extend into any joints with displacement or any non-avulsion injuries of carpal bones should get a MEDEVAC to tertiary care as soon as practical, but definitely within 2 weeks from the time of injury. Nondisplaced, minimally angulated, and stable fractures of the metacarpals or phalanges with a normal neurovascular exam can be splinted to support healing and definitively treated aboard the ship.

Treatment specifics vary slightly depending on the injured area and the healing potential of particular bones. Generally, the treatment algorithm for hand fractures involves looking at available X-rays and evaluating findings against acceptable anatomic tolerances. If the fracture measures within the allowable tolerances, the fracture can merely be immobilized, as described above. If the fracture falls outside of tolerances, a decision must be made to administer a hematoma block and attempt reduction of the fracture versus a MEDEVAC for the patient to receive specialty care.

A hematoma block is similar to a soft-tissue field block, except that it targets the evolving subcutaneous environment of the fracture hematoma. Using an appropriately sized needle and syringe, the needle can be directed through the skin and into the fracture hematoma, followed by aspiration of dark blood to confirm appropriate positioning and subsequent injection of up to 10 mL of the 50/50 mixture of 0.25% Marcaine plain and 1% Lidocaine plain (Fig. 19.11). Care should be taken to ensure

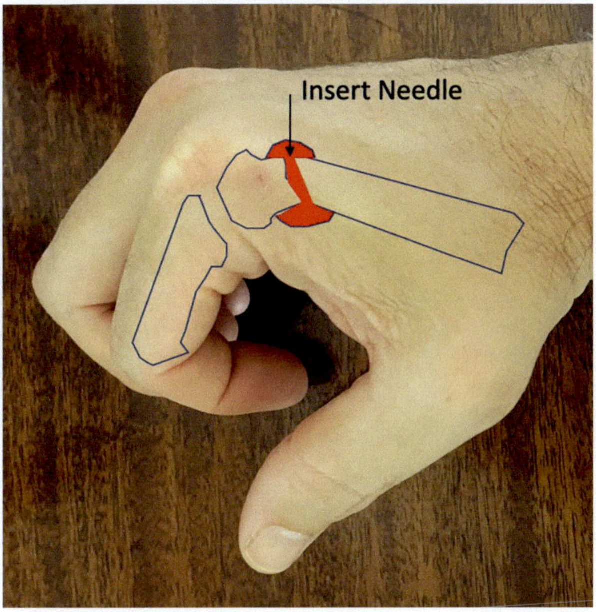

Fig. 19.11 A hematoma block can be a highly effective technique to facilitate fracture reduction and management of orthopedic injuries. An anesthetic-loaded syringe is prepared and a needle introduced transcutaneously into the fracture hematoma. Aspiration of dark blood confirms appropriate positioning, allowing subsequent infiltration of anesthetic medications directly to the fracture site. (Source: Photo courtesy of John P. Waggoner, MD)

that administration of the anesthetic agents occurs in the fracture hematoma and not directly in a vessel, to avoid any unwanted systemic side effects. A hematoma block is most effective within the first 24–48 h after injury, as a subacute hematoma has already started the consolidation and healing process, with local analgesia having poor diffusion through the solid mass of coagulated blood.

Another useful tool that can help with the reduction of fractures is a finger-trap device. Once the neurovascular exam is complete, analgesia should be provided and the patient can be placed in finger traps with the elbow at 90° for 15 min to allow gravity to overcome the intrinsic strength of the connective tissues. While various commercial finger-trap devices exist, makeshift versions can be easily created using cord and highly adhesive tape (Fig. 19.12). For a makeshift finger trap, manual countertraction can be applied using an assistant or by securing any 10-pound object to the brachium.

For all fractures, regardless of initial diagnostic or physical exam findings, X-rays should be repeated after 1 week, and splinting to immobilize the fracture should be in place for 3–4 weeks. Immobilization should be discontinued once the fracture is no longer tender to palpation. Once the splint comes off, early range of motion is critical to prevent stiffness; all hand and finger fractures benefit from gradual OT post-injury in the form of active range of motion exercises and gentle strengthening exercises to prevent stiffness. A soft wrap or padded sleeve that does not restrict motion may also be helpful, particularly if the sailor or marine works in particularly hazardous locations. Further region-specific tolerances and management tips are discussed in the following sections.

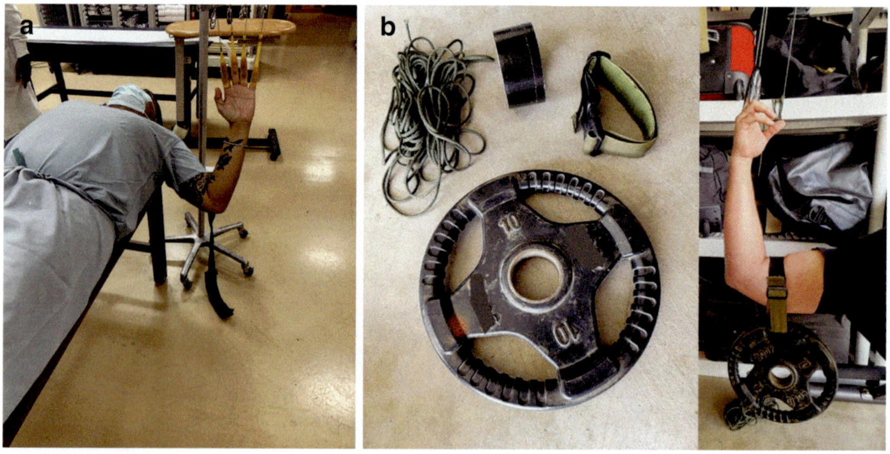

Fig. 19.12 Finger-trap devices are excellent adjuncts to fracture-reduction maneuvers. (**a**) Commercial device with polymer or metal finger sleeves and crank to provide counter traction. (**b**) Example of makeshift finger trap using parachute cord, rigger's tape, and nylon strap. A 10-pound weight applies counter-traction at the brachium. (Source: Photos courtesy of John P. Waggoner, MD)

Carpal Fractures: Likely Nonoperative Management Versus Routine Medical Evacuation (MEDEVAC)

Case 19.5

A 37-year-old male F/A/18 pilot tripped on a knee knocker while carrying a heavy box, falling onto an outstretched hand with pain at the base of his thumb and tenderness to palpation of the anatomic snuffbox. He immediately presented to his flight surgeon for evaluation as he was set to fly later that evening.

The majority of non-displaced, stable carpal fractures can be successfully treated in a nonoperative manner: full-time immobilization for 6 weeks in a short-arm plaster or commercial splint that immobilizes the wrist, discontinued after X-ray confirmation of healing and followed by range of motion OT. The most commonly fractured carpal bones include the scaphoid, triquetrum, and trapezium. Clinical suspicion for these injuries should be high if a patient exhibits persistent anatomic snuffbox tenderness, ulnar-sided wrist pain, or thumb-base pain, respectively, even in the face of normal-appearing X-rays.

Recent trends demonstrate that patients often return to work more rapidly and have superior functional outcomes with surgical treatment of certain carpal fractures. Delay in diagnosis results in high rates of lost productivity and can lead to medical separation for scaphoid fractures specifically [37]. If there is a concern for a possible scaphoid fracture in the setting of negative initial X-rays of the wrist based upon the mechanism of injury, such as a fall to an outstretched hand and tenderness to palpation over the anatomic snuffbox seen in Case 19.5, it is imperative to treat as if a fracture is present then obtain repeat X-rays of the wrist 2 weeks later to re-assess for a fracture that was not evident on initial studies. The overall morbidity associated with missed scaphoid fractures is significant! Known scaphoid fractures should be placed in a thumb-spica wrist splint to better immobilize the proximal thumb, allow for healing, and limit risks of further fracture displacement. Please note that fixation of acute, nondisplaced scaphoid fractures with percutaneous screw fixation has been shown to have improved outcomes over nonoperative management, specifically with regards to radiographic union and return to military duty [38].

For higher-energy mechanisms, carpal bone dislocation, compartment syndrome, and post-traumatic carpal tunnel syndrome are important conditions that must be ruled out with appropriate X-rays and physical examination. Carpal tunnel symptoms involving numbness, tingling, or pain in the radial three digits and compartment syndromes with pain out of proportion and pain with passive stretch are commonly acknowledged medical emergencies and familiar to most clinicians: both require emergent MEDEVAC for timely surgical treatment.

One particular type of carpal dislocation that may be less familiar and frequently missed during initial evaluation is a perilunate dislocation. Perilunate dislocations can be found with careful scrutiny of X-rays, looking for breaks in Gilula's arcs or overlapping bones on the AP view and loss of capitate-lunate-radius collinearity on the lateral view (see Figs. 19.4 and 19.13) [39]. While the ligament-disruption patterns for perilunate dislocations are complex, the injury basically occurs due to high-energy axial loading and hyperextension of the wrist joint, resulting in significant soft tissue injury and concomitant fractures of many bones. Perilunate dislocations should be treated as medical emergencies, and urgent/emergent MEDEVAC should be arranged.

Prior to MEDEVAC, reduction should be attempted to limit the risks of developing carpal tunnel syndrome during transfer. Once the neurovascular exam is complete, adequate analgesia and relaxation should be achieved necessary for success. Place the patient in finger traps as previously discussed to allow gravity to overcome the intrinsic strength of the connective tissues. The reduction maneuver involves hyperextending the wrist to recreate the mechanical deforming forces, followed by

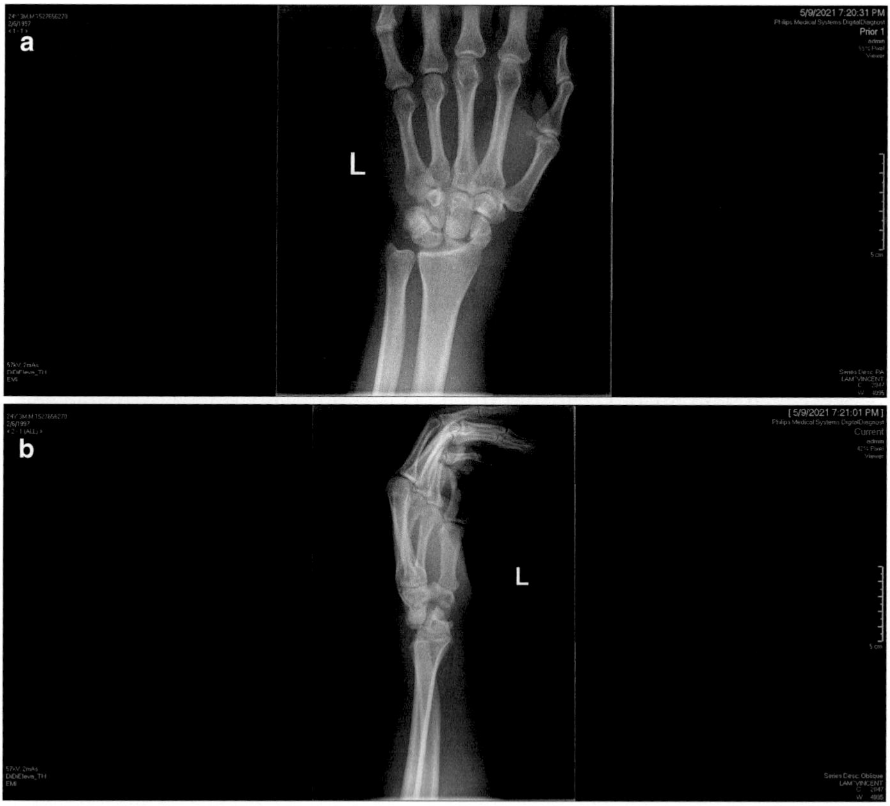

Fig. 19.13 (**a**) Anteroposterior (AP) and (**b**) lateral views of a complex carpal fracture-dislocation (trans-scaphoid peri-lunate dislocation) with X-ray findings diagnostic of perilunate dislocation. Note the loss of linear alignment of the carpal bones, with the capitate dorsally dislocated in relation to lunate, loss of continuity of Gilula's lines, and fracture of the scaphoid. (Source: Images courtesy of Navy Medicine Readiness and Training Command San Diego Radiology Department, used with permission)

traction and flexion of the distal hand back in a volar direction over the wrist with slight radial deviation. This maneuver often results in a palpable clunk as the carpal bones return to their anatomic positions. Do not attempt more than two reduction attempts to minimize additional trauma and possible iatrogenic carpal tunnel or compartment syndrome. Once reduction of a perilunate dislocation is achieved, the wrist can be treated as any nondisplaced injury, with immobilization in a wrist splint and elevation for transportation and soft tissue rest. Whether anatomic reduction is obtained or not, patients with perilunate dislocations should undergo urgent/emergent MEDEVAC for surgical treatment by a hand surgeon.

Metacarpal Fractures: Likely Nonoperative Management Versus Routine Medical Evacuation (MEDEVAC)

Case 19.6

A 37-year-old male Chief Petty Officer (CPO) had a particularly bad day at work and vented his frustration by punching one of the steel passageway walls. He noted immediate pain and swelling over the back of the hand and difficulty straightening his small finger. He came in to be evaluated by his friend from the Goat Locker, the Independent Duty Corpsman (IDC).

Metacarpal fractures are possibly the most common injuries to present to a shipboard medical clinic [36, 40, 41]; fortunately, most metacarpal fractures heal well without surgery and with splint immobilization for 4 weeks [40]. The fractured region of the metacarpal typically dictates its treatment, with metacarpal neck fractures allowing for greater angular tolerances than metacarpal shaft fractures with nonoperative management. Proximal metacarpal base fractures and distal head fractures with fracture lines extending into the corresponding joints should get a routine MEDEVAC to obtain specialist attention within 1–2 weeks.

Proximal base fractures are rare, but X-ray evaluation should include careful scrutiny of the MCPJ and consideration of metacarpal base appearance relative to the adjacent metacarpals to ensure that no MCPJ dislocation occurred. Base fractures of the second or third metacarpals are exceedingly rare due to stout intermetacarpal ligaments and low mobility in these areas, but metacarpal base fractures are more common in the ulnar side of the hand, particularly at the hamate-fifth metacarpal joint [42]. As with any hand fracture involving the joint, these base fractures or fracture-dislocations should get MEDEVAC for further care, especially if there is an associated, unstable dislocation.

Metacarpal shaft fractures are likely to result after higher axial loads or by a direct impact or smashing mechanism to the dorsal hand. As with any fractures of the diaphysis or shaft of tubular bones, the fracture pattern may be transverse, spiral, or oblique [42], with varying levels of stability depending on the affected metacarpal and location of the fracture line along the shaft. As described, more angular deformity tolerance is allowed moving in an ulnar direction across the metacarpals

Table 19.2 Metacarpal fracture tolerances. While different sources may allow greater tolerances, this table provides a conservative guide to metacarpal fracture management

Metacarpal	Acceptable shaft angulation (Degrees)	Acceptable neck angulation (Degrees)	Acceptable shortening (mm)
Index or Long	10	15	1–5
Ring	20	30	1–5
Small	30	60	1–5

because the greater mobility of the fourth and fifth metacarpals allows for greater post-injury functional accommodation. Acceptable tolerances for metacarpal fractures can be seen in Table 19.2. While angular deformities are often the most pronounced and visible features on X-rays, a provider should also carefully evaluate the X-rays and fingers during physical exam to detect any significant digital rotational or shortening deformities. These rotational or shortening deformities can be challenging to see on X-rays; however, they may be quite pronounced on physical examination. Rotational deformities manifest as digital scissoring when asking patients to flex their phalanges simultaneously while shortening deformities often manifests as inability to fully extend the affected phalange, also known as an "extensor lag."

Metacarpal neck fractures are typically called "boxer's fractures" because the mechanism leading to failure in the neck region often involves striking a solid object with a clenched fist as shown in Case 19.6 [36, 42], axially loading the metacarpal from the distal impact at the MCPJ and resulting in an apex-dorsal deformity. Historically, the term "boxer's fracture" specifically referred to the fifth metacarpal neck, which is most vulnerable to fracture given its mobility and the tendency for amateur fighters to strike with the ulnar sides of their fists [42]. As Green's text acknowledges, the term is actually a misnomer, as professional boxers are more likely to impact targets with their second and third knuckles, rarely fracturing their fifth metacarpal necks [42]. Patients often present to clinic stating that they fell onto a clenched fist and deny punching anything, which is probably less likely than the commonly accepted mechanism but also another way in which an axial load could transmit through the distal metacarpal to cause a neck fracture.

Treatment of metacarpal shaft and neck fractures is similar, generally involving careful clinical history, physical exam, and appropriate X-rays, followed by immobilization for 4 weeks. Fortunately, the metacarpals are uniquely positioned and "biologically splinted" by the intercarpal ligaments and interosseous musculature, making them amenable to closed reduction and nonoperative management [36]. For any fractures that fall within the tolerances listed in Table 19.2, the injured metacarpal can be splinted in situ without any attempt needed to better reduce the deformities visible on X-rays. For fractures displaced outside of those tolerances, reduction should be attempted prior to immobilization.

As with most hand fractures, finger traps can be extremely useful to assist with the restoration of length, alignment, and rotation. Often, appropriate additional reduction forces and splinting materials can be applied while the patient is hanging in the finger-trap device. In general, angular deformities are corrected by point-application of force at the apex of the angular deformity, rotational deformities are corrected by counter-rotation, and shortening deformities are corrected by axial traction.

Another maneuver that can be helpful for apex-dorsal deformities of metacarpal shafts or necks is the Jahss Maneuver. This maneuver involves flexing the patient's affected MCPJ while applying a dorsal axial pressure against the distal metacarpal head and neck and simultaneously providing counterpressure at the metacarpal aspect proximal to the fracture (Fig. 19.14) [42]. This maneuver relaxes the hand's intrinsic muscles and allows a clinician to create a dorsally directed force at the proximal end of the metacarpal that offers a mechanical advantage and facilitates reduction.

Once deformities are corrected to within acceptable tolerances, the hand should then be splinted in the safe hand position, also referred to as the intrinsic-plus position, which corresponds to 70° of wrist extension, full 90° of flexion at the MCPJ, and neutral position of the PIPJ and DIPJ (Fig. 19.14). This position relaxes the intrinsic musculature and tightens the collateral ligaments, without risking skin necrosis or undue stiffness of the fingers [42]. Many options for splinting metacarpal fractures exist that are not practical to discuss in this chapter; however, general

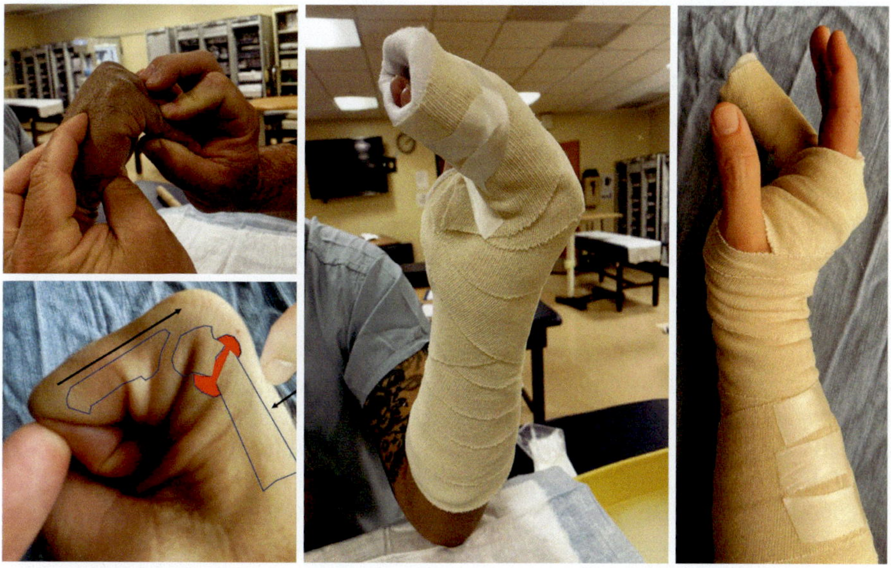

Fig. 19.14 Metacarpal fractures often heal well without surgery. Left: Images and cartoon overlay depicting the Jahss Maneuver, involving flexion at the metacarpophalangeal joint (MCPJ) with an axial force transmitted through the proximal phalanx to create a dorsal force on the distal metacarpal head and counterpressure applied at dorsal metacarpal shaft. Right: Examples of hand splinted in the safe position. In this case a 4, 5 Ulnar Gutter Splint, with 70° of wrist extension, 90° of MCPJ flexion, and neutral position of the proximal interphalangeal joint (PIPJ) and distal interphalangeal joint (DIPJ). (Source: Photos courtesy of John P. Waggoner, MD)

principles involve flexing the affected MCPJ(s) and the adjacent finger(s) for inclusion in the distal portion of the splint. For example, a fifth metacarpal fracture would best be treated in a 4, 5 "ulnar gutter" splint that flexes down the fourth and fifth MCPJ. A second metacarpal fracture would best be treated in a 2, 3 "radial gutter" splint that flexes down the second and third MCPJ. Third or fourth metacarpal fractures are best treated with a "clam digger" splint that flexes down all four of the fingers at the MCPJ.

Finally, thumb fractures are unique. The first, or thumb, metacarpal is vulnerable in ways that metacarpals of the hand proper are not. Eponyms exist for various types of thumb metacarpal base, head, or adjacent ligamentous injuries, and most of those special fractures require surgical care. Because of the thumb's unique anatomy, a best practice for dealing with thumb metacarpal fractures is to stick to the simplistic algorithm offered: If the thumb metacarpal base or head are fractured, with any portion of the fracture extending into the corresponding joints, and/or the fracture is unstable, the patient will be best served with MEDEVAC and follow-on care at a tertiary center (ideally within 1 week after injury) to optimize outcomes for surgical management. Thumb metacarpal shaft and neck fractures are relatively rare, but these can likely be treated definitively aboard the ship without MEDEVAC. Closed, stable fractures without any angular, rotational, or shortening deformities can effectively be treated in a plaster or commercial thumb spica splint for 4 weeks.

Phalangeal Fractures and Dislocations: Likely Shipboard Nonoperative Management

Phalangeal dislocations and fractures are less likely to be stable than metacarpal fractures due to their lack of adjacent supporting soft-tissue structures, greater degrees of freedom in motion, and their proximity to PIPJ and DIPJ; however, these fractures are often easily reducible, treated nonoperatively, and not requiring urgent MEDEVAC.

Dealing first with dislocations, the phalangeal joints can dislocate in any direction; however, dorsal dislocations are by far the most common [40]. While specific pathophysiological mechanisms and reduction maneuvers exist for MCPJ, PIPJ, and DIPJ dislocations, there are general principles to best manage these patients and hopefully save the significant expenses and associated readiness issues related to urgent/emergent MEDEVAC. Dorsal dislocations involve concomitant injury to the volar plate at the affected joint, so they can be reduced with axial traction and gradual volar pressure applied at the base of the proximal dorsal portion of the dislocated phalanx. Lateral dislocations can involve capsular and collateral ligamentous damage, but they can usually be reduced with axial traction and counter pressure at the base of the proximal portion of the dislocated phalanx: radially directed forces should be applied to an ulnarly dislocated phalanx and ulnarly directed forces should be applied to a radially dislocated phalanx. Volar dislocations are less common and can be harder to treat, as the dislocated phalanx may button-hole through the concomitantly injured central slip of the extensor tendon. Volar dislocations can be reduced by applying initial flexion to unlock the phalangeal base and subsequent axial traction with gradual dorsal pressure applied at the base of the proximal volar portion of the dislocated phalanx.

Simple dislocations that are successfully reduced can then be buddy-taped to the adjacent finger or fingers and splinted for definitive care or subsequent MEDEVAC. Dorsal dislocations should be splinted in slight flexion, while volar dislocations should be splinted in full extension [42], allowing the corresponding tissues an appropriate time to heal. Lateral dislocations should be splinted with the affected joint in a neutral position.

Mallet fingers involve traumatic rupture or avulsion of the distal extensor tendon off of the dorsal distal phalangeal base. Jersey fingers involve traumatic rupture or avulsion of the distal FDP tendon off the volar distal phalangeal base. Mallet fingers can be splinted with the DIPJ in extension, leaving the PIPJ free. An X-ray in the splint should be obtained to ensure the boney fragment is reduced. In general, a boney mallet finger (with a fracture of the distal phalanx) should be splinted for about 6 weeks, while a soft tissue mallet finger (where the extensor tendon has avulsed off the distal phalanx) should be splinting for 6–10 weeks full time with an additional 6 weeks of night-time splinting. Progressive flexion exercises should start around 6 weeks. On the contrary, a jersey finger is usually managed operatively by a hand surgeon and should get a more urgent MEDEVAC. A delay in the surgical treatment of a jersey finger, which is essentially a flexor tendon injury, can lead to loss of function and requires more invasive surgeries like a DIPJ fusion or two-stage flexor tendon reconstruction.

Phalangeal fractures come in many varieties, and their treatment is controversial; however, the general management principles for phalangeal fractures are similar to those of metacarpal fractures. Fractures involving the adjacent joints should get a routine MEDEVAC to be treated by a specialist within 1–2 weeks, while nondisplaced or stable phalangeal shaft fractures within tolerances may be definitively treated aboard the ship. While immobilization of the fracture to allow for healing is still the mainstay of treatment, immobilizing the wrist is typically not required to definitely treat these fractures.

Closed, stable fractures without any angular, rotational, or shortening deformities can effectively be immobilized in a plaster or commercial splint for 3–4 weeks. With regard to splinting, immobilization of the joint above and below the fracture is sufficient. For example, an isolated midshaft fracture of the long finger middle phalanx requires immobilization of the DIPJ above and PIPJ below the fracture. Leaving the other portion of the hand free is essential to avoid stiffness; the whole hand does not need to be immobilized. If there are multiple phalangeal fractures, as in the traditional presentation of a hatch hand, a full volar resting splint spanning the fingers, hand, and wrist may be appropriate, especially during the MEDEVAC process.

Immobilization should be discontinued once the fracture is no longer tender to palpation. Once the splint comes off, early range of motion exercises are critical to prevent stiffness. Stiffness of the immobilized joints is the most common complication following treatment, so active range of motion exercises and gentle strengthening exercises as soon as clinical healing is apparent are critical to ensure the best outcome. All hand and finger fractures benefit from gradual OT post-injury for this reason. One note regarding phalangeal fractures and radiographic appearances: Visual evidence of radiographic healing may take many months to manifest, so clinical examination and lack of tenderness to palpation on clinical examination is sufficient evidence of healing to begin range of motion recovery activities [42]. It is still beneficial to obtain X-rays to assess for the stability of the fracture early on and progression of healing later on in the recovery process. The patient can return to work once he or she is pain-free and has sufficient range of motion and strength recovery to perform primary duties.

In summary, given the likelihood of collateral ligament injury and the benefits associated with formal OT if none is available, routine MEDEVAC is recommended for all dislocations and mallet fingers for formal OT, which usually starts once the injury has healed. Jersey fingers, unstable fractures, fracture dislocations, and irreducible dislocations should get a MEDEVAC on a more urgent basis.

Fingertip Injuries: Likely Shipboard Nonoperative Management

Clinical Vignette 19.1

A 27-year-old male Sailor presented to the medical department in the middle of a pre-deployment underway after injuring the tip of his right long finger on his dominant hand when he dropped a large box on it moving cargo in the hangar bay. The nail was partially avulsed, the nail bed was lacerated, and there was a tuft fracture visualized on X-ray.

After digital block was performed, the remaining nail was removed, and the finger was copiously irrigated with sterile saline. Using sterile technique, the nailbed laceration was repaired with interrupted 5-0 chromic sutures. The sterile foil of the suture was molded into a fingernail shape and placed into the eponychial fold. A splint was placed. A 1-week course of oral Keflex was given, and the wound was monitored frequently. The foil was removed once the nail grew in again. He went on to make a full recovery with no issues for the remainder of deployment.

The fingertip includes the fingernail and adjacent specialized connective tissues, maintaining highly specialized anatomy that is also at high risk of injury (Fig. 19.15). According to some sources, distal finger injuries are the most commonly encountered injuries of the hand in clinical practice [42], and they often result in significant military-specific burdens affecting human resourcing and operational readiness [43]. Fingertip injuries can be purely soft tissue injuries, involving the nail bed or distal finger pulp only. They also include three types of fractures of the distal phalanx [42]:

- Tuft or crush injuries
- Shaft
- Articular

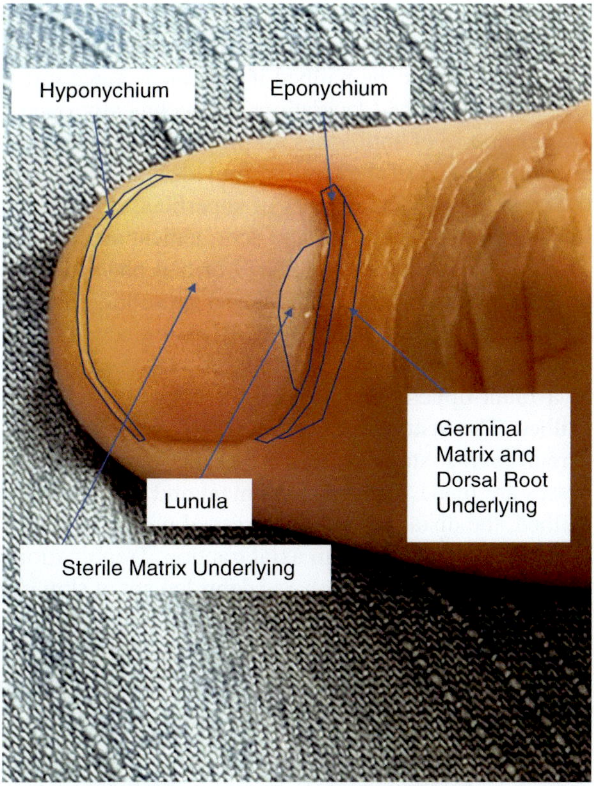

Fig. 19.15 Specialized fingertip anatomy. (Source: Photo courtesy of John P. Waggoner, MD)

As with all phalangeal fractures involving the joints, articular fractures near the tip of the finger, especially along the volar surface, should be considered for MEDEVAC within 1–2 weeks (though mallet fingers may get a MEDEVAC on a more routine basis if they are appropriately reduced and splinted as described previously). Distal phalangeal tuft and shaft fractures can likely be treated definitively onboard, depending on the degree of soft-tissue damage and nail matrix involvement.

For crushed fingertips with isolated subungual hematomas and no obvious fractures on X-rays, significant pain relief can be obtained with nail trephination or nail removal. For these isolated subungual hematomas, a good rule of thumb to help decide whether to remove the nail includes measuring the size of the underlying hematoma. For subungual hematomas that expand to more than 50% of the nail area, remove the nail to better inspect the underlying nail bed and perform necessary repairs. Hematomas covering less than 50% of the underlying nail are often amenable to trephination alone, which can be completed with a sterile drill, needle, electrocautery device, or even a heated paperclip, with the goal of relieving pain [42]. Cases painless subungal hematomas involving less than 50% of the nail bed do not necessarily require trephination.

Tuft fractures are commonly caused by crush mechanisms and frequently have associated nail bed or nail matrix lacerations, as seen in Clinical Vignette 19.1. The resultant subungual hematoma often causes significant pressure and pain, therefore decompression of the hematoma with fingernail removal is recommended to better inspect and repair the nailbed if indicated. Since tuft fractures with unroofed nails and existing nailbed lacerations are technically open fractures, consideration of a 1-week course of antibiotics for prophylactic treatment of skin flora should be made at the discretion of the treating provider. Empiric antibiotics have not been definitively shown to change rates of superficial infection in the peer-reviewed medical literature versus irrigation and debridement alone [44].

Any obvious injury to the nail or nail plate requires removal of the nail to perform necessary repairs and to aid in appropriate regrowth of the new nail. The nail is best removed in a sterile field after a digital nerve block is performed (previously described) by using a thin instrument such as one tong of a forceps, a freer elevator, or a blunt-tipped scissor blade to separate the nail surface from its underlying nailbed. The instrument should be advanced from distal to proximal under the fingernail until it stops at the base of the eponychial fold (Fig. 19.16). Once several passes are made with the instrument and the nail is sufficiently loosened from the nailbed, the distal nail can be grasped with a locking forceps or clamp and pulled straight out of its fold with axial traction. Trephination and nail-removal techniques can also aid decompression and debridement of skin infections surrounding the nail, including paronychia or adjacent abscesses.

As with the above injuries that require nailbed repair, thorough irrigation of the wound, tight closure of the laceration, and even approximation of skin edges help to improve patient outcomes. Recent literature suggests that nailbed repair with 2-octyl

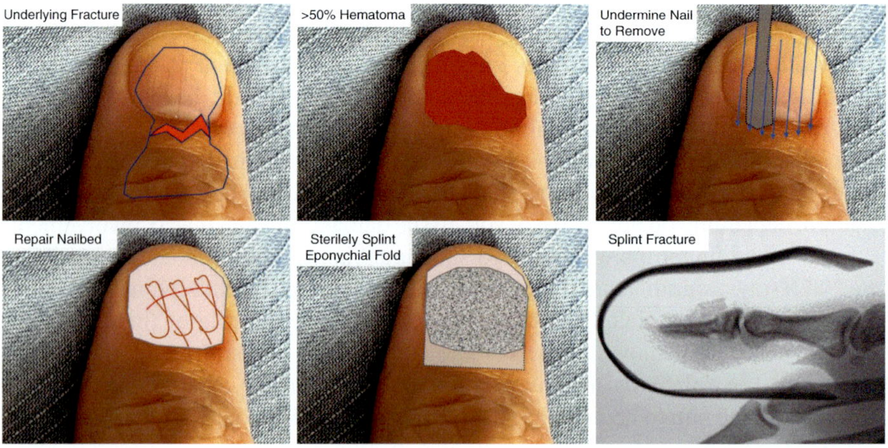

Fig. 19.16 Example of fingertip crush injury with underlying transverse distal phalangeal shaft fracture. From left to right, top to bottom: Initial crush injury and fracture; substantial subungual hematoma >50%; nail removal; repair of sterile matrix nailbed with chromic gut suture; splinting of eponychial fold with sterile foil suture container; lateral view of fluoroscopic image of the final splint and fracture reduction. (Source: Photos courtesy of John P. Waggoner, MD; Fluoroscopic Image courtesy of Navy Medicine Readiness and Training Command San Diego Orthopaedic Department, used with permission)

cyanoacrylate (brand name: Dermabond) yields comparable outcomes with absorbable suture materials [43], so use whatever method works best, given onboard supply availability and comfort/experience suturing wounds in this area. The use of absorbable suture, especially chromic gut if available, facilitates healing and minimizes repeated trauma and pain associated with subsequent suture removal.

Finally, the proximal aspect of the fingernail emanates from the matrix that lives beneath the eponychial fold. When the injured nail is removed, historical treatment protocols advocated "splinting" open this fold during the initial 1–2 weeks of fingertip immobilization to ensure that the eponychial fold does not scar down and limit future nail growth. While current studies challenge the utility of this practice, the authors do recommend stenting open the eponychial fold with the betadine-sterilized and trimmed original nail (if intact and not grossly contaminated) or the thin plastic or foil material from suture packaging as depicted in the vignette. This can be held in place with a steri-strip and does not necessarily need to be sutured in. The replacement nail or artificial material may help with fracture reduction and additional stability for the surrounding healing soft tissues [42]. All fingertip injuries benefit from 1 to 2 weeks of immobilization with splinting in a neutral DIPJ position. The eponychial fold splint can be removed after this period to facilitate future wound checks and eventual nail regrowth.

Distal phalanx fractures of the shaft or proximal metaphysis are generally transverse or, less commonly, longitudinal in nature and typically do not require significant reduction maneuvers or surgical management. These fractures should be immobilized for 3–4 weeks or until the distal phalanx is no longer tender to palpation. Although symptomatic non-unions of these fractures are rare, they can be successfully treated by hand surgeons after failed nonsurgical management. Therefore, there is little downside to attempting closed reduction and immobilization without MEDEVAC for shipboard patients presenting with non-articular distal phalanx fractures. Any severely open fractures, degloving injuries, digital amputations, or injuries with persistent exposed bones will likely do best with antibiotic administration, tetanus prophylaxis, and emergent MEDEVAC, but most finger injuries can be effectively treated with the supplies and facilities available on board the ship.

Supplies and Prevention

In terms of necessary supplies, most U.S. Navy warships already include medical loadouts adequate to definitively manage closed, nondisplaced injuries without surgery. Most ships now have the ability for onboard X-rays, with larger ships also having POCUS and other handheld adjunctive devices to assist with diagnosis and management. When preparing the medical department for deployment, ensure there is ample inventory of plaster, webril cotton wrapping for beneath the plaster, and some type of bias or ace wrap to overwrap the plaster; these materials alone allow splinting of virtually any type of upper extremity injury. While commercial splinting materials exist in the form of Velcro braces, SAM splints®, OrthoGlass®, and a myriad of orthotic finger devices like Alumafoam®, DigiSplints®, or Stax splints®, most hand and finger fractures can be appropriately stabilized with combinations of buddy taping, plaster and overwrap, or even by using popsicle sticks or tongue depressors in severely resource-constrained environments.

For hand and finger lacerations, use 4-0 nylon (or another non-absorbable suture) followed by careful removal after 10–14 days with steri-strip reinforcement. 3-0 Monocryl can be utilized for the deep layer if a layered closure is needed. 2-octyl cyanoacrylate (brand name: Dermabond) is also useful for rapid wound repair and as an alternative to suture closure of lacerations such as in the case of a nail bed repair (or 5-0 or 6-0 chromic gut with bacitracin lubrication can be used to repair the nail bed). Most abrasions, wounds, and surgical or suture repairs should be covered with an application of xeroform gauze to keep the skin moist and protected. As previously stated, a combination of 0.25% Marcaine plain and 1% Lidocaine plain for local anesthesia is recommended (no epinephrine) when performing procedures. Therefore, during preparation for deployment, ensuring sufficient inventory of these suture materials, laceration kits and instruments, local anesthetic vials, and dressing materials is recommended.

Finally, shipboard environments provide a plethora of alternative materials that might assist with wound care and splinting of orthopedic injuries. Readily available lines, raw metals, and other supplies for day-to-day operations can easily be substituted for commercially available products. For any patients presenting for orthopedic injuries that seem unsafe for transportation or for whom appropriate next treatment steps seem unclear, do not hesitate to use virtual telehealth (see Chaps. 5 and 12) or other shipboard communication systems to reach back to the duty orthopedist in the ship's catchment area. Someone is standing by the duty phone 24 h a day/7 days a week/365 days a year.

One final note regarding the importance of prevention of hand-related and other orthopedic injuries: while rapid diagnosis and time to treatment are important factors when dealing with shipboard injuries, the other critical role played by operational medical teams involves preventative medicine.

Many line officers and leaders may not be aware of the latest injury statistics or trends for musculoskeletal injuries occurring on the ship or battlefield; however, it is the job of the medical department leadership to assume total care for the unit. Based on the authors' experiences in a tertiary care center and familiarity with the orthopedic literature, it is imperative that the medical and surgical team puts the responsibility for injury prevention back on the key members of the line chain of command.

Orthopedic injuries are more likely to occur among enlisted personnel (97%) versus officers (3%), which could be related to inexperience, greater numbers, more frequent participation in hazardous duty, or higher susceptibility to operational fatigue [1, 35]. In general, shipboard injuries occur most frequently during air operations, at night, and in the middle of the deployment cycle during the highest operational tempo [1]. The civilian maritime force is aware of these trends and conducts mandatory safety briefs, lessons learned sessions, and critical incident stress debriefing for all crew members [45, 46]. Since the Navy is always focused on operational risk-assessment and risk-reduction measures, the surgical team initiating the discussion of similar policies with line leadership might significantly reduce shipboard orthopedic hand injuries and the need for costly urgent/emergent MEDEVAC if those processes are not already in place. Ensure that operations, executive, and commanding officers hold necessary medical and safety briefings when the operational tempo is high and before all high-risk evolutions. Do not hesitate to press these key decision-makers to obtain the appropriate, necessary medical supplies.

Conclusion

Know hand anatomy. Document a thorough and focused clinical exam prior to anesthesia, especially neurovascular status. Get appropriate X-rays. Hand urgencies include open or unstable fractures and tendon or nerve lacerations; hand emergencies include amputations, dysvascular limbs, and high-pressure injections. Thorough irrigation and debridement, reduction, splinting, early antibiotics, tetanus prophylaxis, and transfer to higher care in an appropriate time frame is key for contaminated and urgent/emergent injuries. The maritime surgical team is not expected to definitively manage complex hand trauma, however, they can significantly decrease future morbidity by appropriate assessment, diagnosis, and initial treatment.

Declaration of Interest The views expressed in this chapter are those of the authors and do not necessarily reflect the official policy or position of the Department of the Navy, Department of Defense, nor the US Government.

Funding This research did not receive any specific grant from funding agencies in the public, commercial, or not-for-profit sectors.

Conflict of Interest Statement The authors declare no conflict of interest.

References

1. Hebert DJ, Pasque CB. Orthopedic injuries during carrier battle group deployments. Mil Med. 2004;169(3):176–80. https://doi.org/10.7205/MILMED.169.3.176.
2. McNiesh LM. Injury pattern aboard the USS Enterprise. Mil Med. 1989;154(5):236–8. https://doi.org/10.1093/milmed/154.5.236.
3. Nealeigh MD, Kucera WB, Bradley MJ, et al. Surgery at sea: exploring the training gap for isolated military surgeons. J Surg Educ. 2019;76(4):1139–45. https://doi.org/10.1016/j.jsurg.2018.12.008.
4. Lin H, Ancheta A, Uzcategui L, Plurad D. Surgery in expeditionary strike group. Mil Med. 2009;174(3):241–4. https://doi.org/10.7205/MILMED-D-03-6307.
5. Wong K, Von Schroeder HP. Delays and poor management of scaphoid fractures: factors contributing to nonunion. J Hand Surg [Am]. 2011;36(9):1471–4. https://doi.org/10.1016/j.jhsa.2011.06.016.

6. Meals CG, Chang J. Ten tips to simplify the spaghetti wrist. Plast Reconstruc Surg Glob Open. 2018;6:1–8. https://doi.org/10.1097/GOX.0000000000001971.
7. Gilula LA. Carpal injuries: analytic approach and case exercises. Am J Roentgenol. 1979;133:503–17.
8. Auerbach DM, Collins ED, Kunkle KL, Monsanto EH. The radial sensory nerve. Clin Orthop Relat Res. 1994;308:241–9.
9. Bezerra A, Carvalho V, Nucci A. An anatomic study of the palmar cutaneous branch of the median nerve. Surg Radiol Anat. 1986;8:183–8.
10. Puna R, Poon P. The anatomy of the dorsal cutaneous branch of the ulnar nerve. J Hand Surg Eur. 2010;35E(7):583–5.
11. Johnson M, Ford M, Johansen K. Radial or ulnar artery laceration repair or ligate? Arch Surg. 1993;128:971–5.
12. Doscher W, Viswanathan B, Stein T, Margolis I. Physiologic anatomy of the palmar circulation in 200 normal hands. J Cardiovasc Surg. 1985;26(2):171–4.
13. Gellman H, Botte MJ, Shankwiler J, Gelberman RH. Arterial patterns of the deep and superficial palmar arches. Clin Orthop Relat Res. 2001;383:41–6.
14. Webster N, Saint-Cyr M. Flaps based on the dorsal metacarpal artery. Hand Clin. 2020;36(1):75–83. https://doi.org/10.1016/j.hcl.2019.09.001.
15. Dunlop RLE, Wormald JCR, Jain A. Outcome of surgical repair of adult digital nerve injury: a systematic review. BMJ Open. 2019;9(3):e025443. https://doi.org/10.1136/bmjopen-2018-025443.
16. Birch R, Quick T. Nerve injury and repair. In: Wolfe SW, Hotchkiss RN, Pederson WC, Kozin SH, Cohen MS, editors. Green's operative hand surgery. 7th ed. Philadelphia, PA: Elsevier; 2017. p. 979–1022.
17. Samora JB, Klinefelter RD. Flexor tendon reconstruction. J Am Acad Orthop Surg. 2016;24(1):28–36. https://doi.org/10.5435/JAAOS-D-14-00195.
18. Seiler JG III. Flexor tendon injury. In: Wolfe SW, Hotchkiss RN, Pederson WC, Kozin SH, Cohen MS, editors. Green's operative hand surgery. 7th ed. Philadelphia, PA: Elsevier; 2017. p. 183–230.
19. Colzani G, Tos P, Battiston B, Merolla G, Porcellini G, Artiaco S. Traumatic Extensor Tendon Injuries to the Hand: urgent/emergent hand injuries: clinical anatomy, biomechanics, and surgical procedure review. J Hand Microsurg. 2016;8(1):12. https://doi.org/10.1055/s-0036-1572534.
20. Strauch RJ. Extensor tendon injury. In: Wolfe SW, Hotchkiss RN, Pederson WC, Kozin SH, Cohen MS, editors. Green's operative hand surgery. 7th ed. Philadelphia, PA: Elsevier; 2017. p. 152–81.
21. Okur OM, Şener A, Kavakli H, et al. Two injection digital block versus single subcutaneous palmar injection block for finger lacerations. Eur J Trauma Emerg Surg. 2017;43(6):863–8. https://doi.org/10.1007/s00068-016-0727-9.
22. Yang E. Anesthesia. In: Wolfe SW, Hotchkiss RN, Pederson WC, Kozin SH, Cohen MS, editors. Green's operative hand surgery. 7th ed. Philadelphia, PA: Elsevier; 2017. p. 9–10.
23. Mackinnon SE, Dellon AL. Two-point discrimination tester. J Hand Surg. 1985;10A(6):906–7.
24. Dellon AL, Mackinnon SE, Crosby PM. Reliability of two-point discrimination measurements. J Hand Surg. 1987;12A(2):693–6.
25. Higgins JP. Replantation. In: Wolfe SW, Hotchkiss RN, Pederson WC, Kozin SH, Cohen MS, editors. Green's operative hand surgery. 7th ed. Philadelphia, PA: Elsevier; 2017. p. 1476–7.
26. Thai JN, Pacheco JA, Margolis DS, et al. Evidence-based comprehensive approach to forearm arterial laceration. West J Emerg Med. 2015;16(7):1127–34. https://doi.org/10.5811/westjem.2015.10.28327.
27. Friedrich JB, Vedder NB. Mangled upper extremity. In: Wolfe SW, Hotchkiss RN, Pederson WC, Kozin SH, Cohen MS, editors. Green's operative hand surgery. 7th ed. Philadelphia, PA: Elsevier; 2017. p. 1495–6.

28. Pappou IP, Deal DN. High-pressure injection injuries. J Hand Surg [Am]. 2012;37(11):2404–7. https://doi.org/10.1016/j.jhsa.2012.07.005.
29. Rosenwasser MP, Wei DH. High-pressure Injection Injuries to the Hand. J Am Acad Orthop Surg. 2014;22:38–45. https://doi.org/10.5435/JAAOS-22-01-38.
30. Bean B, Cook S, Loeffler BJ, Gaston RG. High-pressure water injection injuries of the hand may not be trivial. Orthopedics. 2018;41(2):e245–51. https://doi.org/10.3928/01477447-20180123-04.
31. ASSH. 4 degrees of burns. HANDCARE: American Society for Surgery of the Hand. Updated October, 2016. https://www.assh.org/handcare/blog/4-degrees-of-burns. Accessed 13 May 2021.
32. Ramos G, Cornistein W, Cerino GT, Nacif G. Systemic antimicrobial prophylaxis in burn patients: systematic review. J Hosp Infect. 2017;97(2):105–14. https://doi.org/10.1016/j.jhin.2017.06.015.
33. Latifi R, El-Hennawy H, El-Menyar A, et al. The therapeutic challenges of degloving soft-tissue injuries. J Emerg Trauma Shock. 2014;7(3):228–32. https://doi.org/10.4103/0974-2700.136870.
34. Roberts CS, Pape HC, Jones AL, Malkani AL, Rodriguez JL, Giannoudis PV. Damage control orthopaedics: evolving concepts in the treatment of patients who have sustained orthopaedic trauma. Instr Course Lect. 2005;54:447–62.
35. Parrish DK, Olsen CH, Thomas RJ. Aircraft carrier personnel mishap and injury rates during deployment. Mil Med. 2005;170(5):387. https://doi.org/10.7205/milmed.170.5.387.
36. Dichiera R, Dunn J, Bader J, et al. Characterization of metacarpal fractures in a military population. Mil Med. 2016;181(8):931. https://doi.org/10.7205/MILMED-D-15-00281.
37. Bond CD, Shin AY, McBride MT, Dao KD. Percutaneous screw fixation or cast immobilization for nondisplaced scaphoid fractures. J Bone Joint Surg Am. 2001;83A(4):483–8. https://doi.org/10.2106/00004623-200104000-00001.
38. Liu Peterson S, Donoughe JS, O'Neal D, et al. Streamlining definitive care for occult scaphoid fractures: a retrospective review of the workup of scaphoid nonunions and applying lessons learned. Mil Med. 2020;185(7–8):e958–62. https://doi.org/10.1093/milmed/usaa074.
39. Muppavarapu RC, Capo JT. Perilunate dislocations and fracture dislocations. Hand Clin. 2015;31(3):399–408. https://doi.org/10.1016/j.hcl.2015.04.002.
40. Meals C, Meals R. Hand fractures: a review of current treatment strategies. J Hand Surg. 2013;38(5):1021–31. https://doi.org/10.1016/j.jhsa.2013.02.017.
41. Carreño A, Ansari MT, Malhotra R. Management of metacarpal fractures. J Clin Orthop Trauma. 2020;11(4):554–61. https://doi.org/10.1016/j.jcot.2020.05.043.
42. Day CS. Fractures of the metacarpals and phalanges. In: Wolfe SW, Hotchkiss RN, Pederson WC, Kozin SH, Cohen MS, editors. Green's operative hand surgery. 7th ed. Philadelphia, PA: Elsevier; 2017. p. 231–77.
43. Wells ME, Scanaliato JP, Kusnezov NA, Nesti LJ, Dunn JC. The burden of fingertip trauma on the US Military. Hand Clin. 2021;37(1):155–65. https://doi.org/10.1016/j.hcl.2020.09.010.
44. Metcalfe D, Aquilina AL, Hedley HM. Prophylactic antibiotics in open distal phalanx fractures: systematic review and meta-analysis. J Hand Surg Eur. 2016;41(4):423–30. https://doi.org/10.1177/1753193415601055.
45. IMCA. Hand injury during closing of hatch. IMCA safety flash. International Marine Contractors Association. 2019. https://www.imca-int.com/safety-events/hand-injury-during-closing-of-hatch/. Accessed 11 Mar 2021.
46. Safety4Sea. Multiple injuries from falling hatch lid. n.d.. https://safety4sea.com/multiple-injuries-from-falling-hatch-lid/. Accessed 11 Mar 2021.

Further Reading

Orthobullets. An online resource that is like Wikipedia for Orthopaedic Surgeons. n.d. Provides basic overview of most topics in an outline format, including injury/pathology, work-up, and treatment. Free service, but it does require Internet access. Recommended.

Thompson JC. Netter's concise orthopedic anatomy. n.d. Comprehensive coverage of basic ortho-related anatomy. Small, high-yield book. Highly recommended.

Wolfe S, Pederson W, Kozin S, Cohen M. Green's operative hand surgery. n.d. In-depth resource for the orthopedic resident and hand surgeon. Has specifics for closed and open treatment of fractures of all individual bones. Includes more information than the shipboard medical officer may need, but an invaluable resource for hand surgery regardless. Recommended.

Zuckerman JD, Koval KJ. The handbook of fractures. n.d. Covers nearly the full spectrum of orthopedic fractures. Highly recommended.

Part IV
Critical Care, Trauma, and Burn Management

Chapter 20
The Floating Intensive Care Unit: Capabilities and Limitations

Gilbert Seda, Guy Jensen, Heather A. Hernandez, Kimberly Gerber, and Iliana Reyes

The basis of success in military medicine in the combat zone is an organized team, each member of which has been trained to accept the responsibilities of his assigned position and to be prepared to move to a new station, with different responsibilities, as new situations develop.

Emergency War Surgery NATO Handbook, 1958

Author deployment experience	
Gilbert Seda	Medical Director of Critical Care, NATO Role 3 Multinational Medical Unit, Operation Enduring Freedom, Kandahar Airfield, Afghanistan, 2011
	Director of Medical Services, USNS Mercy (T-AH-19), Pacific Partnership, Fiji, Papua New Guinea, Philippines, and Vietnam, 2015
	Director COVID-19 Team, USS Nimitz (CVN-68), Operation Inherent Resolve and Operation Freedom's Sentinel, CENTCOM and INDOPACOM Areas of Responsibility, 2020–2021
Guy Jensen	Ship's Surgeon, USS Nimitz (CVN-68), Operation Inherent Resolve and Operation Freedom's Sentinel, CENTCOM and INDOPACOM Areas of Responsibility, 2020–2021

G. Seda (✉) · K. Gerber · I. Reyes
Navy Medicine and Readiness and Training Command San Diego, San Diego, CA, USA
e-mail: gilbert.seda@gmail.com; kimberly.j.gerber.mil@health.mil; iliana.reyes.mil@health.mil

G. Jensen
USS Nimitz (CVN-68), Bremerton, WA, USA

H. A. Hernandez
Navy Medicine Readiness and Training Command Yokosuka, Yokosuka, Japan
e-mail: heather.a.hernandez8.mil@health.mil

M. D. Tadlock, A. A. Hernandez (eds.), *Expeditionary Surgery at Sea*,
https://doi.org/10.1007/978-3-031-21893-4_20

Author deployment experience	
Heather A. Hernandez	Individual Augmentee, Troop Medical Clinic, Operation Iraqi Freedom, Camp Virginia, Kuwait, 2007
	Squadron Lead Corpsman, Marine Fighter Attack Squadron-211 (VMA-211), Marine Aircraft Group-13, 13th Marine Expeditionary Unit, embarked on the USS *Boxer* (LHD-4), Operation Enduring Freedom, CENTCOM Area of Responsibility, 2010
	Squadron Lead Corpsman, Marine Fighter Attack Squadron-211 (VMA-211), Marine Aircraft Group-13, Operation Enduring Freedom, Camp Bastion, Helmand Province, Afghanistan, 2012
	Ship's Nurse, USS Nimitz (CVN-68), Operation Inherent Resolve and Operation Freedom's Sentinel, CENTCOM and INDOPACOM Areas of Responsibility, 2020–2021
Kimberly Gerber	Certified Registered Nurse Anesthetist, USS Nimitz (CVN-68), Operation Inherent Resolve and Operation Freedom's Sentinel, CENTCOM and INDOPACOM Areas of Responsibility, 2020–2021
Iliana Reyes	Critical Care Registered Nurse (COVID-19 Team), USS Nimitz (CVN-68), Operation Inherent Resolve and Operation Freedom's Sentinel, CENTCOM and INDOPACOM Areas of Responsibility, 2020–2021

BLUF (Bottom Line Up Front)

1. Similar to on shore, intensive care unit (ICU) level care in the maritime environment is resource- and staff-intensive. However, unlike shore-based facilities, there is minimal redundancy in staff to provide the necessary 24/7 care for the critically ill patient.
2. Tele-critical care consultation is always available.
3. The supply chain can be limited by ship location, outdated Authorized Medical Allowance Lists (AMALs), evolving government contracts, and inexperienced supply officers. The maritime surgical team members should know what resources are available on the platform they are on and plan ahead for critical care emergencies.
4. Caring for the critically ill patient at sea requires planning for patient movement via medical evacuation (MEDEVAC) to a higher level of care. Discussion about this should occur shortly after diagnosis, and all interventions performed on the ship should be tailored toward stabilizing patients and ensuring they will be as safe and stable as possible during the vulnerable period of transport.
5. The safe care and potential MEDEVAC of critically ill patients in the maritime environment requires excellent communication and planning not only within the ship's medical department but with the operational chain of command as well.
6. Providers should consider that practice patterns will likely differ than those at medical treatment facilities (MTFs) due to the lack of availability of specialized laboratory tests, cross-sectional imaging, specialty supplies, and onsite subspecialty care typically required for diagnosis and ongoing monitoring.

Introduction

Critical care at sea has similarities and differences to critical care on shore. In terms of similarities, critical care at sea is dependent on three simple things: staff, space, and supplies. In contrast, from the beginning of care of the critically ill patient on a ship, the team is immediately preparing to stabilize and safely transport the patient via medical evacuation (MEDEVAC) to the next level of care. Critical care at sea can also greatly vary with the type of platform where medical care is being rendered. Each platform is supported by designated medical staff, intensive care unit (ICU) bed capacity, and limited equipment and resources to provide critical care services. It is also dependent on world events like pandemics, natural disasters, and war. This chapter summarizes the capabilities and limitations of the floating ICU aboard United States (U.S.) Navy combatant and non-combatant vessels with emphasis on the operational setting, reviews MEDEVAC as it pertains to critical care, and provides a brief overview of critical care emergencies at sea.

Staff, Space, and Supplies

The floating ICU requires three essential components:

1. Non-critical care staff to care for the patient
2. ICU bed space to care for the patient
3. Adequate consumable and non-consumable supplies

Each of these components has unique challenges on board a U.S. Navy ship. Communication and coordination with medical and nonmedical staff are essential. In addition, the floating ICU must also MEDEVAC the patient to the next level of care which brings its own challenges.

Staff

With the exception of critical care registered nurses (CCRNs) and certified registered nurse anesthetists (CRNAs) who typically have spent years providing bedside patient care in a critical care setting, the majority of healthcare providers afloat have varying degrees of critical care experience. General surgeons, oral maxillofacial surgeons (OMFS), anesthesiologists, internists, family medicine physicians, and physician assistants have training in one or more rotations in adult medical, surgical, trauma, and/or neurocritical care. While they may also care for critical care patients in their clinical practice, that is not the assumed standard.

The available staff capable of providing critical care will depend on the designated platform. A non-combatant ship such as a hospital ship (T-AH) has the largest number of critical care staff with one or more critical care physicians, CCRNs, respiratory therapists (RTs), anesthesiologists, pharmacists, and surgical subspecialists. Many also have a trauma surgeon based on the mission requirements [1]. An aircraft carrier (CVN) carrier strike group (CSG) will have a senior medical officer (SMO), general surgeon, OMFS, family practitioner or internist, anesthesia provider, CCRN, and search air and rescue (SAR) corpsmen. Furthermore, CVNs underway are complemented with the medical staff from the air wings, which include flight surgeons. However, there is no perioperative nurse (CNOR) nor respiratory therapist (RT) [2]. An Expeditionary Strike Group (ESG) or Amphibious Readiness Group (ARG) has an embarked Fleet Surgical Team (FST) to enable surgical and critical care inpatient capability underway. FSTs include a medical officer in charge (i.e., Commander, Amphibious Task Force Surgeon (CATFS)), general surgeon, family practitioner or internist, anesthesia provider, CCRN, CNOR, and RT [2]. Independent duty corpsmen (IDC) with support from general duty corpsmen provide limited critical care support on guided missile cruisers (CG) and destroyers (DDG) and can transport patients to larger ships with surgical capabilities within the CSG or ESG/ARG.

The main challenge associated with providing critical care services afloat is the low number of complex critical care patients during deployment. For non-critical care providers, prior critical care experience is essential. The Society of Critical Care Medicine offers a course for the non-critical care provider called Fundamental Critical Care Support (FCCS) and FCCS-Resource Limited [3], but currently, neither course is a requirement. An underutilized resource is tele-critical care consultation. These consultations are done by phone or email and can be utilized for medical, surgical, or neurocritical care. While sometimes limited by operational security and internet bandwidth at sea, this resource is invaluable to the deployed maritime surgical team. See Chaps. 5 and 14 for further discussion of consultation methods and options. If requested, combatant ships can be also augmented with critical care providers. For example, during the coronavirus disease 2019 (COVID-19) pandemic, CSGs and ESG/ARGs were augmented with critical care physicians, additional CCRNs, and RTs to manage patients with acute hypoxemic respiratory failure [4].

However, if large numbers of Sailors or Marines require critical care services, the greatest limitation will then be nursing staff. Hospital corpsmen with proper supervision will have to serve as nurse extenders for large numbers of patients and will need training on the use of intravenous (IV) infusion pumps. A retrospective study that evaluated the ICU physician-to-ICU bed ratio found that a ratio of 1:7.5 to 1:15 had no difference in ICU or hospital mortality but the 1:15 ratio was associated with a longer length of stay [5]. Nursing-to-ICU bed ratios ideally range from 1:1 to 1:2. One study found that every additional patient per nurse was associated with a 9% increase in the odds of dying and was not associated with nurse experience [6].

Space

When considering critical care space, it is important to identify the number of ICU beds, non-ICU beds which can be converted to ICU beds if surge capacity is needed, and the space needed for ancillary service support such as laboratory,

Table 20.1 Afloat surgical spaces and capabilities

Platform	Space	Capability
Hospital ship (T-AH)	OR	12 beds
	ICU beds	80 beds + 20 PACU beds
	Ward beds—intermediate	400 beds
	Ward beds—minimal	500 beds
	Triage area	50 beds
	Ancillary capabilities	Laboratory, X-ray, CT scanner, blood bank
Amphibious assault ship (LHD/LHA)	OR	6 beds (LHD), 4 beds (LHA)
	ICU beds	15 beds
	Ward beds	42 beds
	Isolation beds	6 beds (LHD), 2 beds (LHA)
	Overflow capacity	528 beds (LHD), 300 beds (LHA)
	Ancillary capabilities	Laboratory, X-ray, biomedical repair, blood bank, and WBB
Aircraft carrier(CVN)	OR	1 bed
	ICU beds	3 beds
	Ward beds	52 beds
	Isolation beds	8 beds
	Overflow capacity	3 beds
	Ancillary capabilities	Laboratory, X-ray, biomedical repair, WBB only

OR operating room, *ICU* intensive care unit, *PACU* post-anesthesia care unit, *CT* computed tomography, *LHD* landing helicopter dock, *LHA* landing helicopter assault, *WBB* walking blood bank
Source: Government publication, not in copyright. Fleet Medicine Pocket Reference 2016, Surface Warfare Medical Institute, San Diego, California. Available at: https://www.med.navy.mil/sites/nmotc/swmi/Documents/Fleet%20Medcal%20Pocket%20Reference.pdf

X-ray, biomedical repair, and blood bank. Similar to staffing, the space dedicated to ICU beds depends on the ship's size and mission requirements (see Table 20.1). Non-combatant hospital ships (T-AH) have the largest ICU capability with four ICU wards of 20 ICU beds resulting in a total of 80 ICU beds [7]. Hospital ships also have a 20-bed post-anesthesia care unit (PACU), which can function as an additional ICU if there is a need for surge capacity during a humanitarian crisis, disaster, or war. In terms of combatant ships, the large deck amphibious assault ships [landing helicopter dock (LHD) and landing helicopter assault (LHA)] that FSTs deploy with have the next largest capacity for critical care support with four operating rooms (ORs), 15 ICU beds, and 45 ward beds. These platforms support 3000 Sailors and Marines who can disembark for ground operations. In contrast, CVNs have one OR, three ICU beds, and 52 ward beds [2] and support typically over 5000 Sailors and Marines. However, both CVNs and large deck amphibious assault ships also serve the Sailors and Marines on the other ships in the CSG or ESG (see Chap. 1).

Supplies

U.S. combatant ships do not have the ability to do computed tomography (CT) scanning. Therefore, clinical decisions are based on the history of present illness, medical and surgical history, review of systems, physical exam, basic laboratory studies, X-rays, and point-of-care ultrasound (POCUS). Patients may need to be reassessed over time if the diagnosis is uncertain.

Supplies for critical care can be both consumable and non-consumable items, including but not limited to ventilators, anesthesia machines, supplemental oxygen tanks, IV pumps, cardiac monitors, suction pumps, airway management supplies, portable X-ray machines, POCUS machines and supplies, laboratory supplies, central vein catheter (CVC) kits, personal protective equipment (PPE), antibiotics, and medications for sedation, analgesia, and prophylaxis (i.e., for venous thromboembolism (VTE) and stress ulcer prophylaxis). In particular, it is essential to know the platform's capacity to produce oxygen to refill empty oxygen tanks. See Chap. 31 for sample oxygen calculations.

At sea, the healthcare team has to constantly assess whether they have adequate supplies to care for the ICU patient and what medications can be substituted if necessary. For instance, ketamine can be used for rapid sequence intubation (RSI), procedural sedation, and sedation and analgesia for patients on mechanical ventilation [4].

Medical supply aboard combatant vessels are organized by numerous authorized medical allowance lists (AMALs) [8]. As stated in many other chapters (Chaps. 5, 8, 10, and 12), it is vital for the maritime surgical team and any other medical team members that could provide critical care at sea to assess supply inventory and deficiencies as early as possible in the deployment cycle to order, "tactically acquire," and/or make contingency plans to be able to provide effective critical care at sea. Ordering supplies at sea is challenging and often cannot be relied upon. If a ship's mission changes resulting in a change in ship's movement, medical supplies may be delivered to a location away from the ship. Furthermore, the staff ordering supplies may have limited training and experience in ordering medical supplies. To minimize supply errors, the Ship's or team Nurse and Surgeon should oversee all the supply orders for the ICU, ward, and OR. Moreover, the laboratory and pharmacy AMALs both need medical officer oversight as certain laboratory tests and medications for practicing critical care medicine may not be available (see Chaps. 8 and 16). Finally, the accession of narcotics can be challenged by sanctions or local customs and border control.

Medical Evacuation (MEDEVAC)

Discussion and planning regarding MEDEVAC are ongoing processes that can influence care and treatment decisions early in a patient's clinical course. Good decision-making and planning for the afloat ICU requires clinicians to be familiar with the developing operational picture including ship movements, MEDEVAC capability, and the proximity to shore-based Department of Defense (DoD) medical assets as well as civilian medical centers with the ability to care for critically ill patients. Additionally, patient movement not only to a higher level of care but within the ship itself requires the involvement of multiple departments (see Chaps. 11 and 31). Frequent communication throughout the entire chain of command is a must, given the variable environments of distributed maritime operations (DMO). *The decision to transport a patient is a medical intervention in and of itself; it should not be a "knee-jerk" or reflex decision by the provider* [9]. This is particularly true from a medical asset perspective, such as in a CSG or ESG/ARG, where the ability for prolonged care of critical ill patients is relatively robust compared to other austere environments.

The level of comfort providing ICU level of care on afloat platforms is based on the training experiences and shore side practice of the maritime surgical team. There is no requirement for recent ICU experience, completion of the FCCS course, or refresher training beyond residency training or nursing certification. Therefore, crews should try to refresh these skills prior to deployment. The typical air wing complement on a CVN usually contains SAR corpsmen, who can provide a valuable resource for the transport of patients. However, for patients on continuous infusions, particularly those requiring titrations, transport using a CCRN is essential. Though not required, anyone who may accompany a patient during transport should be encouraged to attend the Joint Enroute Care Course (JECC) which requires aircrew survival training, a swim qualification, and helicopter familiarization [10]. During recent deployments, several platforms have been outfitted with COVID-19 response teams that significantly increased the available manning to include an intensivist, an additional CCRN, and an RT [11]. However, it remains to be seen if these additional healthcare providers will continue to be part of the deployment manning for maritime platforms in the future. While many use the term Prolonged Casualty Care (PCC) to describe the care of critically ill or injured patients for prolonged periods beyond standard evacuation timelines, PCC by definition is a contingency capability typically provided in the pre-hospital environment. However, when taking care of critically ill patients aboard a CVN, LHA, LHD, or any austere maritime environment, a PCC mindset is often required. Chapter 30 discusses the PCC mindset needed to successfully manage critically ill patients at sea and offers a daily rounding checklist and minimum/better/best examples of critical care delivery for DMO.

Chapter 31 more thoroughly covers en route care (ERC), and it is also a topic too broad for the scope of this chapter; however, there are a number of challenges associated with the aeromedical transport of a critically ill patient. First, it is very difficult to provide any interventions while en route. Therefore, care should be taken to package patients as securely as possible for transportation. This means having a secure airway if any concern exists regarding airway protection or need for invasive mechanical ventilation. Additionally, the authors would recommend a low threshold for the use of sedation and paralytics during transport for the patient's own protection. This helps prevent ventilator dyssynchrony and reduces the risk of accidental self-extubation in flight. **However, this requires constant patient monitoring en route. While rare, equipment such as monitors and/or ventilators can fail, and have failed, in flight during MEDEVAC.**

In addition to the decisions to MEDEVAC and destination of MEDEVAC, decisions must also be made regarding both timing of MEDEVAC and the type of platform being used. Currently, both fixed wing and rotary wing transports are in use aboard CVNs; however, aeromedical evacuation is currently transitioning to all rotary wing assets as the fixed-wing C-2 Greyhound (i.e., COD) is being phased out of service and replaced with the MV-22 Osprey [12].

Critical Care Emergencies at Sea

Critical care emergencies at sea are infrequent occurrences that can happen at a moment's notice on both large platforms (i.e., CVN, LHD/LHA) with greater capacity and capability for critical care or small platforms (i.e., CG, DDG) with minimal capabilities. **The keys to effective management of critical care emergencies at sea are good teamwork and communication within the medical staff, early planning for MEDEVAC to the next level of care, and administrative coordination with medical and nonmedical staff.** Due to the size and depth of the field of critical care medicine, this chapter only briefly discusses critical care emergencies at sea. Suggested Reading and References are listed at the conclusion of the chapter with the reminder that teleconsultation is always available and should be used liberally.

Sepsis

Sepsis is a life-threatening organ dysfunction caused by a dysregulated host response to infection [13]. Sepsis and the inflammatory response that ensues can lead to distributive shock, multiple organ dysfunction syndrome (MODS), and death. At sea, there is always a possibility for sepsis due to one or more of the following: pneumococcal or meningococcal meningitis, severe community-acquired pneumonia (CAP), aspiration, pyelonephritis, acute cholecystitis, gallstone pancreatitis, soft tissue infections (including necrotizing soft tissue infections), septic arthritis, and severe pelvic inflammatory disease. Sepsis exists on a continuum of severity ranging from infection and bacteremia to sepsis and septic shock, which can lead to MODS and death. Sepsis has a hospital mortality of 17–26% based on severity [14]. The two most commonly used scores are the quick Sequential (Sepsis-related) Organ Failure Assessment (qSOFA) score and the National Early Warning Score (NEWS) [15]. Patients with sepsis present clinically with altered mental status, sinus tachycardia, hypotension, fever, and leukocytosis. As severity worsens, patients may develop septic shock and MODS (e.g., cyanosis, mental status changes, cool skin, acute kidney injury, oliguria) [16].

Care of the septic patient at sea involves immediate evaluation, resuscitation, and management. Supplemental oxygen should be supplied to all patients with sepsis, and oxygenation should be monitored continuously with pulse oximetry measuring of peripheral saturation of hemoglobin (SpO_2). Therapeutic priorities include securing the airway if needed, improving oxygen delivery by correcting hypoxemia, and establishing vascular access for the early administration of IV fluids and antibiotics [17]. While peripheral venous access may be sufficient for initial resuscitation, the majority of patients will require central venous access. However, the insertion of a CVC should not delay resuscitative fluids, vasopressors, and antibiotics. Current guidelines recommend the infusion of IV fluids (30 mL/kg), commencing within the first hour and completed within the first 3 h of presentation, and optimal doses of empiric broad-spectrum IV therapy with one or more antimicrobials within 1 h of presentation [18], see Chap. 16 for discussion of common disease processes and antimicrobials recommended and present on maritime platforms. Following initial investigations and empiric antimicrobial therapy, further efforts aimed at identifying and controlling the source(s) of infection should be performed in all patients with sepsis. Serum lactate (if available) can be used to guide the adequacy of the initial resuscitation but is a poor marker of tissue perfusion after resuscitation [19]. For patients who remain hypotensive despite fluid resuscitation, norepinephrine is the recommended first-line agent for septic shock [20] and is currently on the CVN AMAL. Similar to other critical care emergencies in this chapter, prompt MEDEVAC to the next level of care should be considered from the start when it can be performed safely.

Acute Coronary Syndromes (ACS)

Acute Coronary Syndrome (ACS), like many cardiac emergencies, can be a challenge to manage at sea. Patients with ST wave elevation myocardial infarction (STEMI) can receive tenecteplase (currently on CVN AMAL) but have to be monitored closely for bleeding and reperfusion arrhythmias [21] until MEDEVAC can be arranged. Cardiac catheterization is not possible at sea and often cannot be performed at shore-based facilities in a timely manner. Patients with non-ST elevation myocardial infarctions (NSTEMI) can be medically managed, but like STEMI patients should be moved to a higher level of care as soon as possible. All staff involved in advanced cardiac life support (ACLS) and cardiopulmonary resuscitation (CPR) should conduct regular drills and be familiar with the code cart. POCUS can be a useful tool to estimate left ventricular ejection fraction, identify wall motion abnormalities, and evaluate for a pericardial effusion.

On many larger deck platforms (CVN, LHD/LHA), it is possible to administer supplemental oxygen, nitroglycerin, morphine, statins, antiplatelets (Aspirin only), and beta-blockers. A modified, continuous telemetry service is all that can be provided. The Zoll Propaqs are the cardiac monitors used on ships [22]. They can only record a 10-s strip, so continuous telemetry is not possible. As there is typically only one dedicated CCRN on a platform, it is impossible to maintain 24/7 telemetry. Quantitative cardiac panels are not available. Only a qualitative troponin and creatinine kinase panel are available (provided in an iSAT) so serum enzyme levels cannot be followed over time. See Chap. 8 for available laboratory testing per platform.

Hypertensive Crisis

Acute hypertension or severe elevation in blood pressure (i.e., systolic pressure ≥180 mm Hg and/or diastolic pressure ≥120 mm Hg) can occur as a primary or secondary condition. This is differentiated into hypertensive urgency or hypertensive emergency, which is distinguished by signs of new or progressive acute end-organ injury (usually to the kidneys, brain, and/or heart) in hypertensive emergency [23]. Additional studies and laboratory tests that may be completed at sea include an electrocardiogram (ECG), chest X-ray, qualitative troponin, urinalysis, and chemistry panel. POCUS is a useful adjunct to evaluate for numerous signs of end-organ failure including increased intracranial pressure (ICP) by measuring for an optic nerve sheath diameter >5 mm, presence of pulmonary edema and/or increased pleural fluid indicated by B-lines and/or pleural effusion, and reduced left or right ventricular function (parasternal long and short-axis views may be the easiest to acquire) [24]. Chapter 9 discusses some of these POCUS evaluations.

Immediate but careful reduction in blood pressure is indicated in hypertensive emergencies as an excessive hypotensive response may lead to ischemic complications. If unable to lower blood pressure, or if excessive lability, MEDEVAC may be required.

Hyperglycemic Crisis

Hyperglycemic crisis is a metabolic emergency associated with new or preexisting diabetes mellitus, which includes diabetic ketoacidosis (DKA) and hyperosmolar hyperglycemic state (HHS). Management is similar for both conditions and includes correction of fluid and electrolyte abnormalities, including treatment of hyperglycemia, hyperosmolality, hypovolemia, metabolic acidosis (more common with DKA), hypokalemia, and possible hypophosphatemia [25]. These acute interventions are intended to avoid acute kidney injury, hypovolemia shock, severe metabolic acidosis, diabetic coma, or death [26]. Insulin, dextrose, and fluids are available to larger combatant platforms (CVN, LHD/LHA).

Frequent monitoring is essential. Although most larger shipboard medical departments have the ability to monitor glucose levels, ketones, and serial basic or comprehensive metabolic panels, they cannot typically check serum magnesium or phosphate levels. Urgent/emergent MEDEVAC is recommended since the laboratory tests and medications are limited.

Nonsurgical Neurologic Emergencies

There are different types of nonsurgical neurological emergencies that can happen at sea. Examples include acute ischemic or hemorrhagic stroke, refractory status epilepticus, acute polyneuropathies such as Guillain-Barre Syndrome (GBS) with respiratory depression, acute meningitis or encephalitis, and intracranial hypertension. Preserving brain tissue by optimizing supply and demand is fundamental to the treatment of all neurological emergencies. The prevention of secondary injury after the initial insult requires early recognition of the primary cause, proactive actions, and appropriate monitoring [27]. Table 20.2 lists the general principles of neurologic support in critical care. Expert consultation via tele-critical care is always advised, especially in the event of pending neurological deterioration or in situations that require urgent neurosurgical interventions (see Chap. 25). Assessing the root cause of neurological manifestations is difficult given the absence of electroencephalography (EEG) and neuroimaging (i.e., head or spine CT and magnetic resonance imaging (MRI)). Thus, the clinician will rely heavily on the clinical history and serial neurological exams. Vetted tools such as the Glasgow Coma Scale (GCS) can provide standardized and objective measurements of level of consciousness [28].

Table 20.2 General principles of neurologic support in critical care

Prevent abnormal oxygen demands
1. Avoid fever as it increases metabolic demand 2. Avoid seizures. Consider prophylactic antiepileptic drugs (AEDs) 3. Avoid anxiety, agitation, and pain 4. Avoid shivering 5. Minimize stimulation, particularly for the first 72 h
Promote oxygen delivery
1. Ensure systemic oxygen transport by adequate oxygenation, hemoglobin concentration, and cardiac output 2. Ensure optimal blood pressure 3. Avoid prophylactic or routine hyperventilation 4. Avoid hypotonic fluids 5. Ensure euvolemia to avoid brain hypoperfusion 6. Rapid-sequence intubation (RSI) for patients with increased intracranial pressure (ICP). Consider propofol or lidocaine to blunt the rise of ICP during intubation 7. Intubate patients with neuromuscular weakness with respiratory compromise

Source: Adapted from Killu, K, Sarani B. (Eds) *Fundamental Critical Care Support*, 6th Ed., Chapter 8, "Neurological Support," page 137. Copyright 2017, Society of Critical Care Medicine

Venous Thromboembolism (VTE)

While not common, VTE events can occur in the deployed setting; the team onboard a deployed maritime platform may be required to manage them. The shipboard and naval aviation environments provide ample opportunity for patients to be subjected to long periods of immobile standing, prolonged times in the seated position, as well as prolonged air travel, activities that have been shown to be associated with the development of deep venous thrombosis (DVT) [29, 30]. Postoperative patients recovering on board the ship are also at high risk for DVT, as postoperative ambulation may prove more difficult than at Military Treatment Facilities (MTF). In particular, maritime surgical personnel on casualty receiving and treatment ships (CRTS) like FSTs embarked on LHD/LHAs should be especially familiar with the care and prevention of deep venous thrombosis (DVT), given the high rates of DVT in trauma and burn patients [31].

Given the limitations in laboratory tests and lack of CT on expeditionary maritime platforms, the diagnosis of VTE is primarily based on history and physical examination. POCUS can also play a key role as an adjunct to the physical exam so embarked medical team members should become comfortable with this modality to evaluate for the presence of DVT prior to deployment (see Chap. 9) [32]. Patients being evaluated for leg pain or swelling should be specifically questioned about these risk factors.

The development of a hemodynamically significant pulmonary embolism (PE) in a deployed maritime environment is a life-threatening event, so prevention of DVT in high-risk patients is paramount. Immobilized patients without contraindications should be administered DVT prophylaxis as soon as safe and have the prophylaxis continued throughout their stay on the ship's ward or ICU. The CVN AMAL currently provides for lower extremity sequential compression devices (SCDs) that should be used as the primary prophylaxis, particularly in surgical patients. However, the team must ensure that the machine, tubing, and devices themselves are all compatible and in stock. The AMAL also provides for subcutaneous injections of unfractionated heparin as well as low molecular weight heparin (LMWH) that are suitable for chemoprophylaxis and should be administered as soon as deemed safe by the treating physician.

Patients diagnosed with a DVT regardless of cause should receive systemic therapeutic anticoagulation in the absence of any contraindications. For the CVN, functionally this treatment is limited to LMWH at therapeutic doses. The CVN AMAL does provide for adjusted dose heparin (ADH) also known as continuous heparin infusion; however, the laboratory does not have the ability to monitor partial thromboplastin time (PTT) as needed to adjust continuous heparin infusions. This may be corrected as AMALs are adjusted based on feedback from prior deployments.

In the event of a pulmonary embolism (PE) occurring prior to MEDEVAC, the risks of medical transport must be weighed against the patient's requirements for pulmonary and hemodynamic support. In the event of hemodynamic instability due to obstructive shock, consideration should be given to administration of tenecteplase for acute management of massive or sub-massive PE [33]. Systemic anticoagulation should be begun as soon as possible and not delayed for transport.

May-Thurner syndrome is a rarely diagnosed condition where patients develop a left-sided DVT secondary to an anatomic variant in which the right common iliac artery compresses the left common iliac vein against the spine. This anatomic variant is present in approximately 20% of the population, and the resulting DVT is rarely amenable to anticoagulation alone so this condition always deserves consideration. If suspected, patients should be moved toward shore-based medical facilities capable of providing confirmatory imaging [34].

Patients requiring systemic anticoagulation for DVT/PE should get a MEDEVAC to shoreside medical support as soon as is safe for the patient and feasible from an operational perspective. Supplemental oxygen and mechanical ventilation can be used in transport if required. Low-flying rotary-wing craft can also maintain a lower altitude for patients with increased oxygen requirements. Transport of a patient in this situation from the afloat ICU will require many resources and may require the ship to alter location in order to permit transport to shore-based medical or critical care transport assets, thus highlighting the importance of prevention and early diagnosis and treatment of patients with DVT/VTE.

Gastrointestinal (GI) Bleeding

Hemodynamically significant gastrointestinal (GI) bleeding is fortunately rare in the deployed maritime setting. In patients with concern for hemodynamically significant GI bleeding the first step is to resuscitate and stabilize the patient. Two large-bore IV catheters should be placed and if the need for blood or blood products exists, then the process of obtaining those should be initiated. Blood transfusion and blood banking is covered extensively in many different parts of this text (in particular Chap. 23), but both deglycerolization and activation of the walking blood bank (WBB) require time. Guidelines vary slightly but a goal hemoglobin of 7–9 gm/dL should be used as part of a damage control resuscitation strategy [35].

Once the patient is resuscitated, the management strategy can differ based on the availability of MEDEVAC. For stable patients with evidence of significant GI bleeding early MEDEVAC (if feasible) is recommended rather than initiating extensive management in the resource-constrained shipboard environment. In the absence of the ability to MEDEVAC then the next step in management (following resuscitation) should be to identify the source of bleeding. Both CVN and LHD/LHA platforms have surgical capabilities as well as endoscopic equipment (see Chaps. 14 and 18). Frequently, patient history can provide a potential source of bleeding; the importance of this, including a review of past medical records when possible, should not be overlooked. Lastly, in the patient with hematemesis and concern for possible aspiration, early controlled intubation should be strongly considered to protect the patient's airway. Chaps. 14 and 18 discuss the surgical and endoscopic management of GI bleeding in more detail.

Anaphylaxis

Early recognition and treatment of anaphylaxis are critical as cardiac arrest and death can occur. Although the vast majority of service members embarked on the ship are young and healthy, allergies are unpredictable and random. Common triggers are medications, insect venoms, and food reactions. Approximately 80% of patients are diagnosed through initial cutaneous signs and symptoms, such as angioedema, pruritus, flushing, dysphagia, and generalized urticaria. However, patients can rapidly progress into dangerous signs of respiratory distress, vomiting, abdominal pain, cardiac dysrhythmias, and anaphylactic shock [36].

Immediate management includes identifying and removing the allergen and the rapid administration of intramuscular (IM) epinephrine, IV crystalloid, and airway management. Epinephrine auto-injectors are available on the AMAL and should be used if available. If the patient is not responding to IM epinephrine, the clinician should consider an epinephrine infusion. It is imperative to note the dangers associated with IV administration of epinephrine. Careful titration and attention to detail of dosing of any high-risk vasoactive medications and drips should be double verified to avoid iatrogenic medication errors.

Angioedema and respiratory distress can quickly progress into a difficult airway; therefore, impending airway obstruction should trigger the call for a medical emergency to activate key members to assist. Multiple attempts to secure a difficult airway can exacerbate airway edema, so should be attempted by the most skilled providers; on most combatant maritime platforms, that is the anesthesia provider, however that includes OMFS on the CVN platform and critical care physicians on the non-combatant T-AH platform. Video laryngoscopes, flexible fiberoptic bronchoscopes, and gum elastic bougies can help navigate a difficult airway [37]. Supraglottic airway devices or laryngeal mask airway (LMA) devices (such as the I-gel and LMA Fastrach™, Telefelx) can also serve as conduits to bridge ventilation and oxygenation until a secured endotracheal airway is obtained. See Chap. 13 for a discussion of anesthesiology and airway management at sea. The patient should be observed until all symptoms have resolved as a biphasic anaphylactic reaction can occur in approximately 5% of patients. The patient should be provided with emergency action plans, a referral to an allergist upon return from sea, and an epinephrine auto-injector.

Conclusion

In summary, it is important to recognize that ICU capability is interdependent on dedicated ICU personnel, beds, and critical care equipment as all three components are necessary for safe, effective critical care in the floating ICU. In other words, good ICU care requires the staff, space, and stuff. After stabilization, the team must immediately assess options to move the patient to the next higher level of care via MEDEVAC. Teamwork is paramount with such limited clinical personnel. Careful communication with the line chain of command, consideration of mission requirements, and coordination with accepting facilities is imperative to provide warfighters with the safest and best critical care they deserve. Although it is not ideal to manage a critically ill patient in the middle of the ocean, it can be optimized with a greater understanding of its strengths and limited capabilities.

Declaration of Interest The views expressed in this chapter are those of the authors and do not necessarily reflect the official policy or position of the Department of the Navy, Department of Defense, nor the US Government.

Funding This research did not receive any specific grant from funding agencies in the public, commercial, or not-for-profit sectors.

Conflict of Interest Statement The authors declare no conflict of interest.

References

1. Boren D, Forbus R, Bibeau P, et al. Managing critical care casualties on the Navy's hospital ships. Crit Care Nurs Clin North Am. 2003;15(2):183–91. https://doi.org/10.1016/s0899-5885(02)00076-x. PMID: 12755184.
2. Surface Warfare Medical Institute. Fleet medicine pocket reference. 2016. https://www.med.navy.mil/sites/nmotc/swmi/Documents/Fleet%20Medcal%20Pocket%20Reference.pdf.
3. Society of Critical Care Medicine, Fundamental Critical Care Support course website. https://www.sccm.org/Fundamentals/FCCS.
4. Brown K, Tucker C. Ketamine for acute pain management and sedation. Crit Care Nurse. 2020;40(5):e26–32. https://doi.org/10.4037/ccn2020419.
5. Dara SI, Afessa B. Intensivist-to-bed ratio: association with outcomes in the medical ICU. Chest. 2005;128(2):567–72.
6. Cho SH, Hwang JH, Kim J. Nurse staffing and patient mortality in intensive care units. Nurs Res. 2008;57(5):322–30.
7. Provencher MT, Douglas TD. Humanitarian assistance and disaster relief aboard the USNS Mercy (TAH-19). J Surg Orthop Adv. 2011;20(1):38–43.
8. Evans J. Naval medical logistics command supports operational afloat and new construction platforms. 2019. https://www.dvidshub.net/news/printable/318319.
9. Walrath BD, Harper SA, Reno JL, et al. Joint theater trauma system clinical practice guideline: interfacility transport of patients between theater medical treatment facilities. 2018. https://jts.amedd.army.mil/assets/docs/cpgs/Interfacility_Transport_of_Patients_between_Theater_Medical_Treatment_Facilities_24_Apr_2018_ID27.pdf.
10. Joint Enroute Care Course website. https://medcoe.army.mil/saam-jecc.
11. Soares J. USAMMDA's Force Health Protection Division implements COVID-19 treatment protocol across multiple sites. 2020. https://www.army.mil/article/238219/usammdas_force_health_protection_division_implements_covid_19_treatment_protocol_across_multiple_sites.
12. Newdick T. The Warzone: this is our first look at the Navy's new CMV-22B Osprey flying from an Air Craft Carrier. 2020. https://www.thedrive.com/the-war-zone/37781/this-is-our-first-look-at-the-navys-new-cmv-22b-osprey-flying-from-an-aircraft-carrier.
13. Singer M, Deutschman CS, Seymour CW, et al. The third international consensus definitions for sepsis and septic shock (Sepsis-3). JAMA. 2016;315(8):801–10.

14. Fleischmann C, Scherag A, Adhikari NK, et al. International Forum of Acute Care Trialists. Assessment of global incidence and mortality of hospital-treated sepsis. Current estimates and limitations. Am J Respir Crit Care Med. 2016;193(3):259–72.
15. Usman OA, Usman AA, Ward MA. Comparison of SIRS, qSOFA, and NEWS for the early identification of sepsis in the Emergency Department. Am J Emerg Med. 2019;37(8):1490–7.
16. Gauer R, Forbes D, Boyer N. Sepsis: diagnosis and management. Am Fam Physician. 2020;101(7):409–18.
17. Rhodes A, Evans LE, Alhazzani W, et al. Surviving sepsis campaign: international guidelines for management of sepsis and septic shock. Intensive Care Med. 2017;43(3):304–77.
18. Malbrain MLNG, Van Regenmortel N, Saugel B, et al. Principles of fluid management and stewardship in septic shock: it is time to consider the four D's and the four phases of fluid therapy. Ann Intensive Care. 2018;8(1):66. https://doi.org/10.1186/s13613-018-0402-x.
19. Gattinoni L, Vasques F, Camporota L, et al. Understanding lactatemia in human sepsis. Potential impact for early management. Am J Respir Crit Care Med. 2019;200(5):582–9.
20. Tung M, Crowley JC. Norepinephrine for early shock control in sepsis. Am J Respir Crit Care Med. 2019;200(9):1192. https://doi.org/10.1164/rccm.201905-1083LE.
21. Melandri G, Vagnarelli F, Calabrese D, et al. Review of tenecteplase (TNKase) in the treatment of acute myocardial infarction. Vasc Health Risk Manag. 2009;5(1):249–56.
22. Zoll Propaq MD. https://www.zoll.com/products/defibrillators/propaq-md.
23. Ipek E, Oktay AA, Krim SR. Hypertensive crisis: an update on clinical approach and management. Curr Opin Cardiol. 2017;32(4):397–406.
24. Soni NJ, Arntfield R, Kory P, editors. Point-of-care ultrasound. 2nd ed. Philadelphia: Elsevier; 2020.
25. Dhatariya KK, Vellanki P. Treatment of Diabetic Ketoacidosis (DKA)/Hyperglycemic Hyperosmolar State (HHS): novel advances in the management of hyperglycemic crises (UK Versus USA). Curr Diab Rep. 2017;17(5):33. https://doi.org/10.1007/s11892-017-0857-4.
26. Goguen J, Gilbert J. Hyperglycemic emergencies in adults. Can. J Diabetes. 2018;42(Suppl 1):S109–14. https://doi.org/10.1016/j.jcjd.2017.10.013.
27. Germans MR, Boogaarts HD, Macdonald RL. Neuroprotection in critical care neurology. Semin Neurol. 2016;36(6):642–8.
28. Rutledge R, Lentz CW, Fakhry S, Hunt J. Appropriate use of the Glasgow Coma Scale in intubated patients: a linear regression prediction of the Glasgow verbal score from the Glasgow eye and motor scores. J Trauma Sep. 1996;41(3):514–22.
29. Samama M-M, Group SS. An epidemiologic study of risk factors for deep vein thrombosis in medical outpatients: the Sirius study. Arch Intern Med. 2020;160(22):3415–20.
30. Scurr JH, Machin SJ, Bailey-King S, Mackie IJ, McDonald S, Smith PDC. Frequency and prevention of symptomless deep-vein thrombosis in long-haul flights: a randomised trial. Lancet. 2001;357(9267):1485–9.
31. Grabo DJ, Seery JM, Bradley M, et al. Prevention of deep venous thromboembolism. Mil Med. 2018;183:133–6.
32. Shiloh AL, McPhee C, Eisen L, et al. Better with ultrasound: detection of DVT. Chest. 2020;158(3):1122–7.
33. Igneri LA, Hammer JM. Systemic thrombolytic therapy for massive and submassive pulmonary embolism. J Pharm Pract. 2020;33(1):74–89.
34. Peters M, Syed RK, Katz M, et al. May-Thurner syndrome: a not so uncommon cause of a common condition. Proc (Bayl Univ Med Cent). 2012;25(3):231–3. https://doi.org/10.1080/08998280.2012.11928834.
35. Stanley AJ, Laine L. Management of acute upper gastrointestinal bleeding. BMJ. 2019;364:l536. https://doi.org/10.1136/bmj.l536.
36. Pflipsen MC, Vega Colon KM. Anaphylaxis: recognition and management. Am Fam Physician. 2020;102(6):355–62.
37. Heidegger T. Management of the difficult airway. N Engl J Med. 2020;384(19):1836–47.

Further Reading

Bridges EJ, Schmelz J, Kelley PW. Military nursing research: translation to disaster response and day-to-day critical care nursing. Crit Care Nurs Clin North Am. 2008;20(1):121–31.
Joint Enroute Care Course website. https://medcoe.army.mil/saam-jecc.
McLarnon CO, Wise JH. Blue water nursing: the role of Navy nurses on board US Navy combatant ships. Crit Care Nurs Clin North Am. 2003;15(2):233–43.
Neurocritical Care Society Guidelines. https://www.neurocriticalcare.org/resources/guidelines.
Schmelz JO, Bridges EJ, Duong DN, Ley C. Care of the critically ill patient in a military unique environment. Crit Care Nurs Clin North Am. 2003;15(2):171–81.
Society of Critical Care Medicine, Fundamental Critical Care Support course website. https://www.sccm.org/Fundamentals/FCCS.
Society of Critical Care Medicine Guidelines. Clinical Resources Guidelines. https://www.sccm.org/Clinical-Resources/Guidelines/Guidelines.
Soni NJ, Arntfield R, Kory P, editors. Point-of-care ultrasound. 2nd ed. Philadelphia: Elsevier; 2020.
Surface Warfare Medical Institute. Fleet medicine pocket reference. 2016. https://www.med.navy.mil/sites/nmotc/swmi/Documents/Fleet%20Medcal%20Pocket%20Reference.pdf.

Chapter 21
Acute Respiratory Failure and Ventilator Management Afloat

Ian Grasso and Jeannette Collins

Even so quickly may one catch the plague?
Methinks I feel this youth's perfections
With an invisible and subtle stealth
To creep in at mine eyes. Well, let it be.

The Twelfth Night, Shakespeare

Author deployment experience	
Ian Grasso	Surface Warfare Officer, USS Lake Champlain (CG-57); 3 WESTPAC deployments, INDOPACOM and CENTCOM Areas of Responsibility, 2003–2007
	Director COVID-19 Team, USS Nimitz (CVN-68), Operation Inherent Resolve and Operation Freedom's Sentinel, CENTCOM and INDOPACOM Areas of Responsibility, 2021
	Staff Intensivist, Federal Emergency Management Agency (FEMA) and Defense Support of Civilian Authorities (DSCA), COVID Medical Response Team One, Lafayette, LA, USA, 2021
Jeannette Collins	Staff Intensivist (COVID-19 team), 32nd Marine Expeditionary Unit, embarked on the USS America (LHD-6), training operation, Seventh Fleet Area of Responsibility, 2020–2021

BLUF (Bottom Line Up Front)

1. Acute respiratory failure has multiple etiologies. Determining the cause can be even more difficult in an austere environment with limited resources.
2. Having a basic understanding of the available equipment and resources for the diagnosis and treatment of respiratory failure is paramount in the

I. Grasso (✉) · J. Collins
Navy Medicine Readiness and Training Command Portsmouth, Portsmouth, VA, USA
e-mail: iangrassomd@gmail.com

M. D. Tadlock, A. A. Hernandez (eds.), *Expeditionary Surgery at Sea*,
https://doi.org/10.1007/978-3-031-21893-4_21

deployed setting, in particular arterial blood gas (ABG), chest X-ray, and point-of-care ultrasound (POCUS).
3. Patients in the deployed environment will likely require mechanical ventilation earlier in their course due to limitations in adjunctive treatment modalities.
4. It is imperative to establish plans specific to the deployed platform for monitoring and filling tanks in an epidemic outbreak or a mass casualty incident (MCI) ahead of time for patients requiring medical oxygen.
5. There are simple noninvasive methods that can be utilized for detecting and monitoring acute hypoxemic respiratory failure when more advanced testing is not available such as monitoring end-tidal carbon dioxide ($ETCO_2$) or utilizing the S/F ratio: pulse oximetry measuring of peripheral saturation of hemoglobin/fraction of inspired oxygen (SpO_2/FiO_2).
6. An S/F ratio of 235 correlates with a partial pressure of oxygen in the arterial blood (PaO_2)/FiO_2 ratio of 200 and an S/F of 315 correlates with a PaO_2/FiO_2 ratio of 300.
7. There are evidence-based tenets that should be followed for the treatment of acute hypoxemic respiratory failure, even when the etiology remains unclear. On a ship, the available modalities include low tidal volume (LTV) ventilation, proning, Dexamethasone, and aggressive euvolemia.
8. Hypercapnic or mixed respiratory failures are usually due to toxic overdose, status asthmaticus, or chest wall injury in the young, healthy, military-age population. To treat hypercapnia, ventilate the patient with the appropriate minute ventilation.
9. When presented with a patient with mixed respiratory failure, there is little downside to giving a trial of Naloxone. The most common cause of hypercapnic respiratory failure in the military-age population is the illicit use of sedative agents (see #10).
10. Do not discount the ability for illicit substances to make it into the deployed environment; this can cause a delay in the diagnosis of drug-induced obtundation.

Introduction

In the age of coronavirus disease 2019 (COVID-19), there has been increased recognition of the importance of skilled management of medical critical illnesses, to include respiratory failure, in the deployed environment. The rapid spread of COVID-19 through the ranks of the USS Theodore Roosevelt (CVN-71) in 2020 brought into shocking clarity the fact that a pandemic respiratory illness could actually cripple a national strategic asset more rapidly than any theoretical near-peer tactical engagement or imagined traumatic or battle-related mass casualty incident (MCI). Operational experience in the pandemic quickly made clear that previous medical evacuation (MEDEVAC) capability to civilian hospitals in friendly host nations, a common option for newly medically ill individuals on ships with limited critical care capability, was no longer guaranteed. With the increasing diplomatic restrictions, afloat operational units need increased capability not only to assess and stabilize, but also to provide sustained critical care support until safe MEDEVAC can be facilitated. This chapter is meant to familiarize the surgical team with the recognition, pathophysiology, diagnosis, and treatment of the critically ill patient in respiratory failure in a resource-constrained operational maritime unit.

Respiratory Failure in the Operational Environment

Respiratory failure has many causes, and it can sometimes be difficult or even impossible to determine the exact etiology. Respiratory failure is generally characterized as hypoxemic, hypercapnic, or mixed, but it can also be secondary to other underlying disease processes, such as traumatic brain injury (TBI), toxic overdose, or even iatrogenic causes. As the COVID-19 pandemic has made clear, deployed clinicians must be familiar with the identification and management of severe pulmonary disease secondary to viral and/or bacterial pneumonia. Severe pneumonia has the potential to progress to acute respiratory distress syndrome (ARDS). While pneumonia is the leading cause of ARDS, there are other causes that must be considered as well. These include trauma and burns, smoke inhalation, transfusion-related acute lung injury (TRALI), sepsis, and pancreatitis, all of which could occur in young, otherwise healthy deployed personnel.

Diagnosis of Respiratory Failure with Limited Equipment

Oxygenation, and thus hypoxemia, is difficult to assess by physical exam. It is similar to shock, anxiety, and tachypnea, which are sensitive but non-specific signs of respiratory failure. Late signs of respiratory failure are retractions of intercostal muscles and paradoxical breathing, sometimes referred to as “belly breathing,” often seen as the diaphragm tires. Cyanosis and livedo reticularis can be seen in severe advanced disease, often in patients with impending respiratory and/or cardiac arrest. The altered mental status of carbon dioxide (CO_2) narcosis is a sensitive sign of hypercapnic failure, and it is generally confirmed with either arterial or venous blood gas analysis.

An arterial blood gas (ABG) is classically used to define the type of respiratory failure. Hypoxemia is defined as partial pressure of oxygen in the arterial blood (PaO_2) <60 mm Hg. Hypercapnia is defined as partial pressure of CO_2 in the arterial blood ($PaCO_2$) >45 mm Hg. However, ABG testing may not be readily available on all maritime platforms (see Chap. 8). Pulse oximetry measuring peripheral saturation of hemoglobin (SpO_2) is the most commonly used point of care measurement of oxygenation. SpO_2 is considered abnormal if it remains sustained <95%, and it is consistent with hypoxemia if saturations are sustained at less than 88–90%.

Pulse oximetry has the advantage of ease of use and acceptable accuracy in most cases; however, it does have disadvantages to a traditional ABG. First, pulse oximetry cannot detect levels greater than 100%; a saturation of 100% may be seen with any PaO_2 >65 mm Hg. Therefore, to avoid hyperoxia (often defined as PaO_2 >100 mm Hg), it is generally recommended that clinicians not allow patients receiving fraction of inspired oxygen (FiO_2) to be maintained at 100% SpO_2. Second, pulse oximetry is inaccurate in the setting of carbon monoxide toxicity (carboxyhemoglobinemia). Carboxyhemoglobinemia could certainly occur on a dynamic battlefield or aboard a ship, especially in a blast, fire, or large engineering casualty. In this case, co-oximetry (a four-sensor device instead of a two-sensor device) should be utilized to distinguish between oxy- and carboxyhemoglobin, if available. This tool is not currently on maritime platforms, but when considering current and future distributed maritime operations where prolonged casualty care (PCC) by Role 1 medical departments and prolonged holding of critically ill patients by maritime surgical teams will be required, operational medical leaders should consider adding this to shipboard AMALs. Finally, recent research has shown that melanotic skin pigmentation can overestimate saturation by up to 5%, leading to the possible underdiagnosis of significant hypoxemia in patients with darker skin tones.

Laboratory and Monitoring

ABG analysis is utilized for the identification, classification, and monitoring of acute respiratory failure. It is an accurate and easily obtained laboratory test, and it forms the basis of multiple treatment decisions in respiratory failure. While there is typically at least one i-STAT blood gas analyzer onboard larger platforms, there may be limitations in the number of test cartridges available. With limited storage space, in particular refrigerator space, i-STAT cartridges are typically in short supply. Therefore, it is necessary to become comfortable relying on alternate monitoring devices, such as end-tidal CO_2 ($ETCO_2$) and SpO_2, both of which provide continuous, though sometimes less accurate, values. While not always accurate, $ETCO_2$ monitoring is useful in detecting changes in $PaCO_2$. Ideally, the $ETCO_2$ value should be compared with an ABG at the initiation of monitoring.

Diagnostic Imaging

Aircraft carriers (CVNs) and large-deck amphibious assault ships like landing helicopter dock/landing helicopter assault (LHDs/LHAs) are equipped with the capability to perform simple chest X-rays. While hospital ships (T-AH) have computed tomography (CT) capability, CT is not available on United States (U.S.) Navy fleet combatant ships. Deployed clinicians should have a working knowledge of simple diagnoses that can be found on plain chest films, including pneumothorax, hemothorax, consolidative pneumonia, and diffuse alveolar filling processes, such as pulmonary edema from both cardiogenic and noncardiogenic causes.

Most CVNs, LHDs/LHAs, and mobile surgical units will also have a portable point-of-care ultrasound (POCUS) machine available. In the age of increased provider comfort with POCUS, this tool can also be utilized to identify the etiology of respiratory failure. POCUS can be combined with chest X-ray to gather "3D" information about specific lesions, not available via flat plate films alone. For example, pleural effusions can easily be localized and safely intervened upon with direct visualization; one can also readily identify trapped lung or loculations within the effusion for additional diagnostic information (Fig. 21.1). Additionally, specific localization of a consolidation can be difficult with X-ray alone, but in combination with POCUS, the pathology within the right middle versus right lower lobe can be more readily distinguished [1].

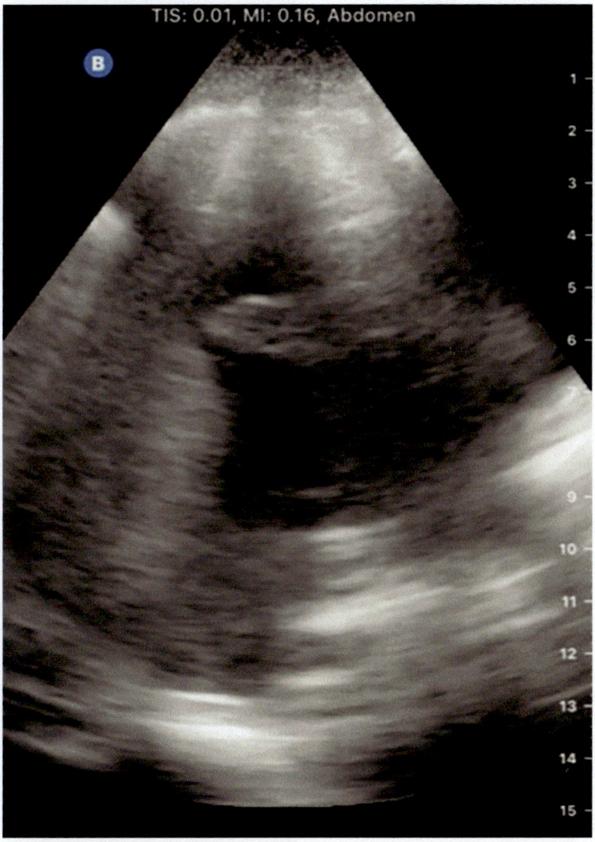

Fig. 21.1 Pleural effusion on thoracic ultrasound. (Source: Image courtesy of Ian Grasso, MD)

Differentiating between distinct disease processes using POCUS can be simple. For example, pneumothorax can be easily identified by the absence of lung sliding and detection of a lung point (see Chap. 9 for explanation and examples). Pulmonary consolidation or significant contusion can be identified by increased echodensity of the lung, loss of the bright pleural line, and air bronchograms, sometimes referred to as "hepatization" of the lung. Pulmonary edema can be identified by the increase in B-lines throughout the chest (Fig. 21.2). In combination with POCUS cardiac views, one can distinguish between cardiogenic versus noncardiogenic etiologies of respiratory failure. *In fact, POCUS evaluation of lungs, heart, and inferior vena cava (IVC)/deep veins in conjunction with chest X-ray can be utilized to diagnose most etiologies of acute respiratory failure.*

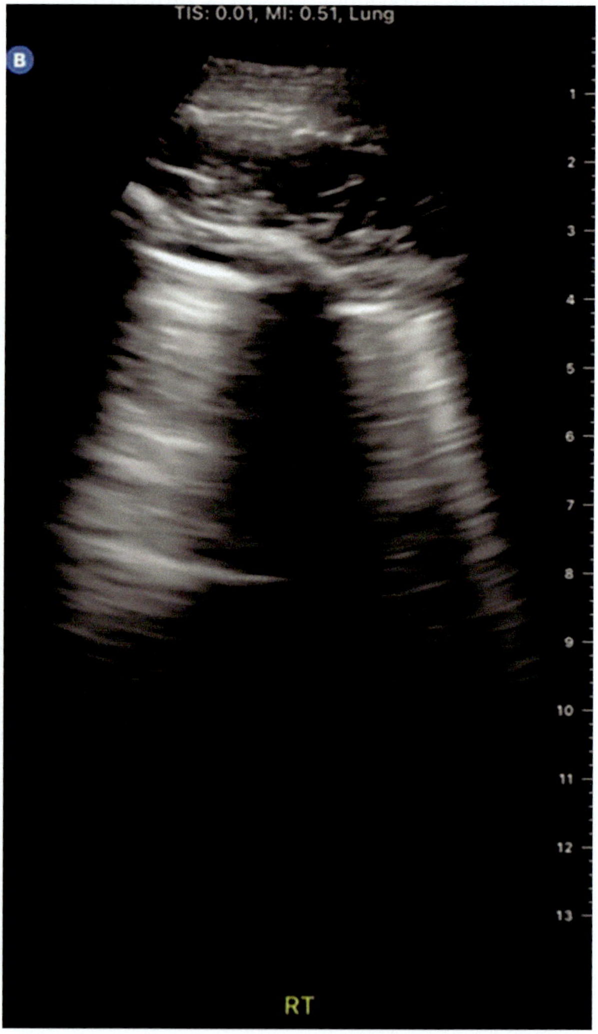

Fig. 21.2 B-lines seen in pulmonary edema on thoracic ultrasound. (Source: Image courtesy of Ian Grasso, MD)

Airway and Ventilator Management in the Operational Theater or Deployed Unit

Airway management equipment and ventilators are part of deployed units', ships', and surgical teams' Authorized Medical Allowance Lists (AMALs). The primary ventilator utilized in theater by the U.S. Navy is the Zoll EMV+ (Figs. 21.3 and 21.4). Anesthesia machines may also be available as additional or emergency ventilators on larger platforms, should the EMV+ ventilators become exhausted or have a failure. A full range of induction and sedative medications, video and direct laryngoscopes, endotracheal tubes, and airways adjuncts are available (see Chap. 13 for discussion of anesthesia and airway management). However, some forms of noninvasive positive pressure ventilation (NIPPV) like continuous positive airway pressure (CPAP), bi-level positive airway pressure (BIPAP), or high flow humidified oxygen are not readily available in the deployed maritime environment. If encountering actual or impending respiratory failure in a maritime operational unit, a definitive airway via endotracheal intubation should generally be attained.

While most patients intubated for airway protection due to blast injury, altered mental status, TBI, or maxillofacial injuries may not require high levels of FiO_2, nearly all patients with medical respiratory failure will. An important limitation of almost all deployed units on land and sea is medical oxygen. In general, one can expect to have no inline oxygen system to provide high levels of FiO_2. Instead, oxygen will need to be supplied by pressurized canisters of various sizes. Given the rates at which patients in ARDS can consume oxygen (rates around 10–20 L or more per minute), oxygen supplies can be readily depleted, so plans must be in place for bottles to be transported and continuously filled [2]. For this reason, high flow humidified oxygen delivery, a staple treatment for early hypoxemic respiratory

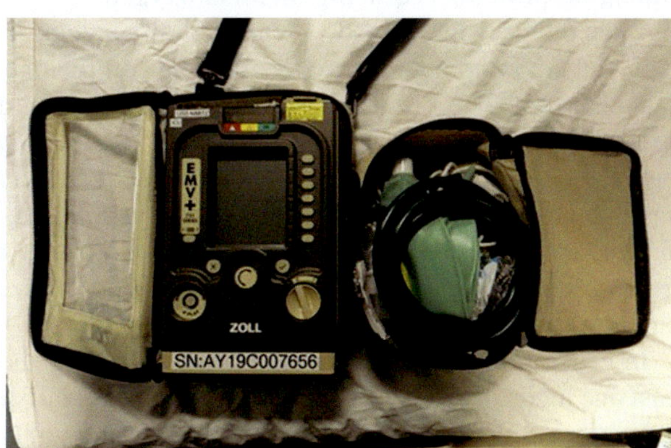

Fig. 21.3 Zoll EMV+ Ventilator and associated equipment in travel case. (Source: Photo courtesy of Ian Grasso, MD)

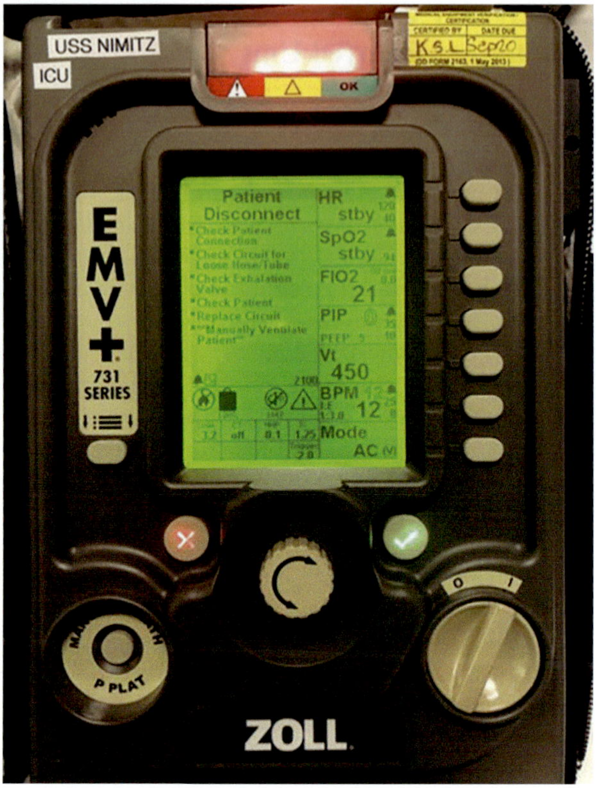

Fig. 21.4 Zoll EMV+ Ventilator in use. (Source: Photo courtesy of Ian Grasso, MD)

failure, is not available afloat. **Plans specific to the deployed platform for monitoring and filling tanks in an epidemic outbreak or MCI are imperative while managing patients requiring medical oxygen.**

Once the decision is made to take definitive control of a patient's airway in the deployed environment, one must utilize the ventilator as both a stabilization and a treatment tool. The EMV+ can provide the following modes during positive pressure invasive ventilation: assist-control (AC) ventilation, either volume or pressure regulated; synchronized intermittent mandatory ventilation (SIMV); and pressure support (PS) and CPAP. Adaptive modes of ventilation, such volume-targeted pressure modes (Marketed as autoflow, APV, and VC+ by manufacturers), and airway pressure release ventilation (APRV), commonly utilized in the hospital intensive care unit (ICU) setting, are not available.

In general, the maritime surgical team providers should be comfortable with at least one mode of AC ventilation and be able to identify changes in lung compliance and patient effort based on the flow, pressure, and volume curves for that particular mode. A full review of ventilator waveform analysis is beyond the scope of this chapter.

Acute Hypoxemic Respiratory Failure

Pulmonary contusions related to trauma and acute bacterial/viral pneumonia are among the most common causes of acute hypoxemic respiratory failure that may be encountered on deployed units. While the etiology of each is quite different, many of the treatment principles are similar and focus on maintaining adequate oxygenation and ventilation while minimizing iatrogenic lung injury. By better understanding normal lung physiology and the underlying pathophysiologies behind hypoxemia, one can better understand how to best treat hypoxemic respiratory failure.

Clinical Vignette 21.1

A 35-year-old Sailor with a past medical history of obesity (body mass index (BMI) of 30 kg/m^2) presented to the ship's medical department with dyspnea and nonproductive cough. The patient was onboarded 2 days prior to presentation. For the past week, the patient had been experiencing loss of taste and smell and mild rhinorrhea, which had been attributed to seasonal allergies. Vitals were significant for a respiratory rate (RR) of 24 and SpO_2 of 86% on ambient air. Exam was notable for coarse breath sounds bilaterally but otherwise unremarkable. Chest X-ray demonstrated diffuse bilateral peripheral opacities. Thoracic POCUS showed lungs with diffusely increased B-lines, scattered areas of increased echodensity, and air bronchograms with the cardiac exam notable for normal ejection fraction, no significant valvular abnormality, no pericardial effusion, and 50% collapsibility of the IVC on sniff test. SpO_2 improved to 92% on 4 L oxygen via nasal cannula. The following day, the patient was noted to have sustained SpO_2 in the mid-80s despite an increase in supplemental oxygen to 15 L via non-rebreather mask and attempts at self-proning.

Pathophysiology of Hypoxemia

Hypoxemia is defined as abnormally low oxygen level or reduced PaO_2. Hypoxemia can be caused by hypoventilation, ventilation/perfusion mismatch, right-to-left shunt, diffusion impairment, or a low partial pressure of oxygen in the environment. Of these causes, ventilation/perfusion mismatch, right-to-left shunt, and diffusion impairment are associated with an increased Alveolar-arterial (A-a) gradient, which is the differential between the oxygen available at the alveoli and the oxygen that ends up in the blood. The A-a gradient is calculated based on the results of the alveolar gas equation:

$$PAO_2 = FiO_2\,(Patm - Pwater\ vapor) - PaCO_2/R;$$

PAO_2: Alveolar oxygen, Patm: atmospheric pressure, Pwater vapor: water vapor pressure, R: the respiratory quotient and is generally 0.8, though may approach 1 in those with high carbohydrate diets.

To get the A-a gradient, the PaO_2 is then subtracted from the product of the alveolar gas equation (PAO_2). A normal A-a gradient is between 8 and 14, though it often increases with age [3].

While the A-a gradient is frequently utilized in the evaluation of hypoxemia in the hospital setting, it may not always be available in the deployed environment because an ABG is required for its calculation. Additionally, commonly used methods for calculating the degree of hypoxemia, such as PaO_2/FiO_2 (P/F) ratio and oxygenation index (OI), also utilize ABG for their calculation. Therefore, becoming comfortable with readily available noninvasive methods like SpO_2/FiO_2 (S/F) ratios is necessary and have been validated to correlate with P/F ratios, in that an **S/F ratio of 235 correlates with a P/F ratio of 200 and an S/F of 315 correlates with P/F ratio of 300**. In recognizing this correlation, S/F ratio can be utilized in the diagnosis of acute hypoxemia and ARDS.

Ventilation/perfusion (V/Q) mismatch and shunting are also important concepts in understanding hypoxemia. The apical portions of the lung receive relatively more ventilation than perfusion, and thus have a V/Q that is >1. The basilar portions of the lung receive relatively higher perfusion than ventilation, and thus have a V/Q < 1. Diseases such as chronic obstructive pulmonary disease (COPD) and pulmonary embolism (PE) cause a high V/Q ratio, or a significant amount of dead space. High V/Q hypoxemia is responsive to oxygen therapy or increases in FiO_2 (follows the molecular gradient). A low V/Q ratio is seen in alveolar filling processes such as pneumonia, pulmonary edema, severe atelectasis, and lobar collapse due to mucus plugging; in these disease states, deoxygenated blood travels through areas of the non-ventilated lung, thus causing hypoxemia. This type of hypoxemia, also called shunt physiology, is nearly impossible to correct with increases in FiO_2 as demonstrated in Clinical Vignette 21.1, and generally requires an increase in positive end-expiratory pressure (PEEP) or correction of the underlying blockage.

Acute Respiratory Distress Syndrome (ARDS)

ARDS is a complex medical condition that could be discussed over multiple chapters in itself. In the age prior to COVID-19, ARDS due to medical illness would rarely need mention in regard to downrange medical care [4]. ARDS is not a single disease entity; it has multiple causes and etiologies. At its most basic level, ARDS is a *research definition* for severe noncardiogenic hypoxemic respiratory failure leading to diffuse alveolar damage and ultimately scarring and fibrosis. That being said, the mortality of critically ill patients meeting the Berlin Criteria for severe ARDS is nearly 50% (Table 21.1). Additionally, the huge body of research for ARDS has led to usable constructs for the treatment of all types of respiratory failure.

Table 21.1 Berlin criteria for acute respiratory distress syndrome (ARDS)

Timing	Onset *within 1 week* of known insult or new or worsening respiratory symptoms
Imaging	Bilateral opacities *not fully explained* by effusions, lobar or lung collapse, or nodules
Origin	Respiratory failure *not fully explained* by heart failure or fluid overload
Oxygenation (Level of Severity)	
Mild	200 mm Hg < $PaO_2/FiO_2 \leq$ 300 mm Hg *with* PEEP or CPAP $\geq$5 cm H_2O
Moderate	100 mm Hg < $PaO_2/FiO_2 \leq$ 200 mm Hg *with* PEEP $\geq$5 cm H_2O
Severe	$PaO_2/FiO_2 \leq$ 100 mm hg *with* PEEP $\geq$5 cm H_2O

PaO_2 partial pressure of oxygen in the arterial blood, FiO_2 fraction of inspired oxygen, *PEEP* positive end-expiratory pressure, *CPAP* continuous positive airway pressure, H_2O water
Source: Adapted from Definition Task Force ARDS. Acute respiratory distress syndrome: the Berlin definition. JAMA. 2012; 307:2526–33

Treatment of Acute Hypoxemic Respiratory Failure

There are basic evidence-based tenets summarized in Table 21.2 that should be followed for the treatment of acute hypoxemic respiratory failure, even when the etiology remains unclear. Depending of the platform some of these treatments may not be available in the middle of the ocean; those that are available are discussed below. Each ship, mission, and team must have contingency plans in place with medical and line leadership for either the prolonged casualty care (PCC) or the MEDEVAC of patients with high levels of critical care required, as these resources are typically constrained on maritime platforms (see Chap. 20 for discussion of the maritime ICU resources and Chap. 30 for PCC).

Low Tidal Volume (LTV) Ventilation

In the era prior to the seminal ARDSnet trial in 2000, large tidal volume ventilation was the norm. In fact, the control group in the ARDSnet trial used a tidal volume of 12 mL/kg (or 960 mL/breath for an average 80 kg man); this high of a tidal volume would be unheard of today. Instead, as demonstrated by that trial, a tidal volume of 4–6 mL/kg should be utilized in patients with ARDS. In fact, a tidal volume of 8 mL/kg should be the absolute maximum used in any mechanically ventilated patient for any reason. There is over 20 years' worth of literature and practical experience proving the benefits of low tidal volume (LTV) ventilation in respiratory failure for critically ill patients [5].

The downside of LTV ventilation is twofold. One, younger patients generally do not easily tolerate the low flow states demanded by LTV ventilation. These patients

Table 21.2 Acute respiratory distress syndrome (ARDS) treatments

P/F ratio	Standard of care	Considerations
200–300	• Low tidal volume (LTV) ventilation • Lowest FiO_2 necessary to achieve SpO_2 >95%	• Self-proning • Aggressive euvolemia (target CVP <4 cm H_2O) • High flow nasal cannula (HFNC) • Noninvasive positive pressure ventilation (NIPPV)
150–200	• LTV ventilation • Proning • Dexamethasone (DEXA-ARDS protocol)	• Aggressive euvolemia • APRV (for experienced clinicians and RTs only) • ECMO consult
0–150	• LTV ventilation • Proning	• VV-ECMO • Paralysis • Inhaled vasodilators
Never do	Oscillator	

P/F ratio of partial pressure oxygen in arterial blood/Fraction of inspired oxygen (PaO_2/FiO_2), *SpO_2* pulse oximetry measuring of peripheral saturation of hemoglobin, *CVP* central venous pressure, *H_2O* water, *APRV* airway pressure release ventilation, *RT* respiratory therapist, *ECMO* extracorporeal membrane oxygenation, *VV-ECMO* veno-venous extracorporeal membrane oxygenation

often try to overcome the ventilator, inducing the phenomenon of "double triggering," which effectively doubles their set tidal volume. Allowing patients to manage their own flow with either a pressure control or spontaneous mode may sometimes be effective; however, these patients often surpass the upper limits of safe tidal volumes [6]. Therefore, dyssynchrony and double triggering mandate an increase in sedation in order to increase passivity on the ventilator.

Second, utilizing LTV ventilation will typically decrease minute ventilation. Minute ventilation (VE) is equal to RR multiplied by tidal volume (TV); VE = RR × TV. Normal minute ventilation is generally 5–8 L per minute. A significant reduction in the tidal volume without the ability to compensate with RR can lead to respiratory acidemia. In ARDS, permissive hypercapnia is generally well tolerated, as long as the pH remains >7.20–7.25. However, in patients with poor lung compliance or in those with concurrent metabolic acidosis, such as those in shock or renal failure, worsening hypercapnia will lead to profound acidemia and ultimately hemodynamic collapse.

Proning

Patients who meet criteria for ARDS and who have a P/F ratio <150 and are requiring FiO_2 greater than 60% should be proned. Proning is thought to derive its physiologic benefit by improving V/Q mismatch by opening posterior and basilar lung units. The PROSEVA trial, which showed a clear mortality benefit, used a 16-h/8-h prone/supine ratio [7]. This is the standard ratio used for ARDS, with allowances made for patient comfort and facial skin breakdown.

It is often thought that patients who are proned must be paralyzed. While this may ease the process of proning, it is not required in a deeply sedated patient. Furthermore, based on the 2019 ROSE trial, continuous neuromuscular blockade provides no significant mortality benefit in ARDS. However, many clinicians may choose to paralyze (either continuously or in bolus doses) in ARDS in order to improve lung compliance, decrease metabolic demand, and allow for complete synchrony with the ventilator.

Throughout the COVID-19 pandemic, there has been an increase in clinician and nurse comfort with proning ventilated patients on a set schedule. The pandemic has also clearly shown the benefit of awake self-proning in patients on BIPAP or humidified high flow nasal cannula; unfortunately, those forms of oxygen delivery are not available on board a ship as previously stated.

Dexamethasone

Regardless of the etiology, patients with ARDS are suffering from an acute inflammatory state, ultimately leading to diffuse alveolar damage. In order to combat this widespread inflammation, patients should be treated with intravenous (IV) steroids. Prior to the COVID-19 pandemic, the DEXA-ARDS trial showed a mortality benefit in patients treated with protocolized dexamethasone (IV 10 mg twice daily for 5 days followed by IV 10 mg daily for 5 days). This data was extrapolated into treating COVID-induced ARDS with better success. Multiple trials to date have now shown benefit of both dexamethasone and methylprednisolone in the most severe COVID-19 respiratory failure cases [8]. Even patients at high risk of steroid-induced complications should receive a trial of these medications. Close attention to maintaining euglycemia is necessary. Additionally, mineralocorticoids can cause fluid retention so diuresis may be necessary to achieve euvolemia. Dexamethasone is currently available on the CVN AMAL as well as on small ships in the fleet.

Aggressive Euvolemia

Aggressive euvolemia is a cornerstone of management of all forms of respiratory failure, in particular ARDS. The literature supports diuresis to maintain a central venous pressure (CVP) of <4 cm H_2O (FACTT trial). Since CVP monitoring is no longer commonly utilized, noninvasive measures of fluid status, such as using POCUS to assess the IVC (as an estimate of right atrial pressure), are more commonly used. Some degree of worsening in renal function can be expected, so many intensivists will sacrifice some degree of renal function in order to avoid entering the fibrotic phase of ARDS. However, this is a clinician-dependent practice preference [9–11].

Hypercapnic and Mixed Respiratory Failure

Clinical Vignette 21.2

A 23-year-old Marine was found acting strangely and brought to the medical department. The patient was carried through the entrance on a stretcher, where he was found to be unresponsive and incoherent with a Glasgow Coma Scale (GCS) of 10. While monitors were connected and vital signs taken, the patient became completely obtunded. GCS was reassessed at 6. SpO_2 was 94% on room air. While the airway cart was brought over in preparation for endotracheal intubation, a venous blood gas (VBG) was quickly drawn, showing a pH of 7.12, $PaCO_2$ of 140 mm Hg, and PaO_2 of 20 mm Hg. Intubation was complicated by bradycardia and hypotension. About 100 mcg pushes of IV phenylephrine were required to maintain a perfusable blood pressure. After successful intubation and ten minutes on the ventilator, he had to be restrained and sedated. ABG showed a pH 7.38, $PaCO_2$ of 38 mm Hg, and PaO_2 of 340 mm Hg. After 12 h of mechanical ventilation, the patient awakened and followed commands. After successful extubation, the patient admitted to consuming unknown pills sent by friends in a care package.

Pathophysiology of Hypercapnia

pH and $PaCO_2$ are under incredibly tight physiologic control involving multiple chemoreceptors. From an evolution standpoint, they are the most highly conserved cerebral structures in mammals, including humans. Therefore, hypercapnia, defined as a $PaCO_2 > 45$, is always abnormal, even if metabolically compensated. Compensated chronic reespiratory acidosis is not uncommon, but will rarely be witnessed in a young deployed population.

The end result of pure hypercapnia is hypoxemia, as defined by the alveolar oxygen equation [$PAO_2 = FiO_2$ (Patm − Pwater vapor) − $PaCO_2/R$]. The hypoxemia of apnea is easily corrected by FiO_2. To fix hypercapnia, the patient must be ventilated [4].

As in Clinical Vignette 21.2, the most common cause of hypercapnic respiratory failure in the military-age population is illicit use of sedative agents, including but not limited to narcotics and alcohol. Narcosis from well-intentioned pain control in trauma patients can also occur. When presented with a patient in mixed respiratory failure, there is little downside to giving a trial of Naloxone. Depending on the half-life of the ingested agent, the patient may initially respond, but then again become obtunded.

In older populations, COPD is the most common cause of hypercapnic respiratory failure. This is usually acute on chronic respiratory acidosis. While COPD is not a typical shipboard presentation, patients with other obstructive airway diseases can have a similar presentation, like asthma seen in younger military populations;

however, their respiratory acidosis is typically strictly acute. In order to maintain a deployable status, a patient's asthma must generally be well controlled. However, acute exacerbations are not uncommon and can lead to death downrange. Common potential triggers of asthma exacerbations in the deployed environment include smoke, airborne particles, and solvents used in maintenance and cleaning.

An additional cause of hypercapnia important to note in military populations is hypoventilation due to severe abdominal or spinal injuries. While these patients may already have a secured airway due to the extent of their injuries, an occult injury leading to hypoventilation should be considered.

Mixed respiratory failure can be complex, but the most common cause in younger populations is hypoventilation due to toxic ingestion as in the vignette. Do not discount the ability for illicit substances to make it into the deployed environment; this can cause a delay in the diagnosis of drug-induced obtundation. Patients with TBI and a GCS less than eight will often breathe unless there is damage to the brain stem. However, they will not protect their airway from secretions and aspiration. Finally, if left untreated, blunt force trauma leading to rib fractures, large lung contusions, and thoracic weakness will inevitably lead to mixed respiratory failure.

Treatment of Acute Hypercapnic Respiratory Failure

The treatment of hypercapnic respiratory failure is relatively simple: use the mechanical ventilator to generate an appropriate minute ventilation. In most young patients, the ventilator will be able to appropriately pressurize the chest to ventilate the patient. There are a few exceptions, most notably severe chest wall trauma and burns. These conditions may require surgical intervention to allow for effective ventilation.

Conclusion

Respiratory failure can be diagnosed in the operational environment with history, clinical exam, and simple diagnostic tools. Become comfortable with alternative, validated, noninvasive methods of continuous monitoring, such as the S/F ratio and $ETCO_2$ monitoring, in patients with acute respiratory failure. Some of the most effective literature-supported treatments for ARDS and acute hypoxemic respiratory failure are available in the deployed setting and have been used successfully by maritime teams in the recent COVID-19 pandemic. Members of the maritime surgical team, with their knowledge and experience in the care of critically ill patients, will likely be asked to play a role in the care of patients in acute respiratory failure on the maritime platform.

Declaration of Interest The views expressed in this chapter are those of the authors and do not necessarily reflect the official policy or position of the Department of the Navy, Department of Defense, nor the US Government.

Funding This research did not receive any specific grant from funding agencies in the public, commercial, or not-for-profit sectors.

Conflict of Interest Statement The authors declare no conflict of interest.

References

1. Wallbridge P, Steinfort D, Ren Tay T, Irving L, Hew M. Diagnostic chest ultrasound for acute respiratory failure. Respir Med. 2018;141:26–36.
2. Narendra DK, Hess DR, Sessler CN, et al. Update in management of severe hypoxemic respiratory failure. Chest. 2017;152(4):867–79.
3. Pisani L, Corcione N, Nava S. Management of acute hypercapnic respiratory failure. Curr Opin Crit Care. 2016;22:45–52.
4. Lentz S, Roginski MA, Montrief T, et al. Initial emergency department mechanical ventilation strategies for COVID-19 hypoxemic respiratory failure and ARDS. Am J Emerg Med. 2020;38:2194–202.
5. Marini JJ. Mechanical ventilation: past lessons and the near future. Crit Care. 2013;17(Suppl 1):S1. https://doi.org/10.1186/cc11499. Epub 2013 Mar 12. PMID: 23514222; PMCID: PMC3603465.
6. Thompson BT, Chambers RC, Liu KD. Acute respiratory distress syndrome. N Engl J Med. 2017;377(6):562–72. https://doi.org/10.1056/NEJMra1608077. PMID: 28792873.
7. Guérin C, et al. Prone positioning in severe acute respiratory distress syndrome. N Engl J Med. 2013;368(23):2159–68.
8. Villar J, et al. Dexamethasone treatment for the acute respiratory distress syndrome: a multicentre, randomised controlled trial. Lancet Respiratory Med. 2020;8(3):267–76.
9. Wiedemann HP, et al. Comparison of two fluid-management strategies in acute lung injury. N Engl J Med. 2006;354(24):2564–75.
10. Rice TW, et al. Comparison of the SpO_2/FIO_2 ratio and the PaO_2/FIO_2 ratio in patients with acute lung injury or ARDS. Chest. 2007;132(2):410–7.
11. Venkatesh B, et al. Adjunctive glucocorticoid therapy in patients with septic shock. N Engl J Med. 2018;378(9):797–808.

Chapter 22
Damage Control Surgery at Sea

Benjamin T. Miller, Pamela M. Choi, and Joseph DuBose

> *Penetrating wounds of the abdomen should be treated definitively at the very earliest point where reasonable surgical facilities and staff exist.*
>
> *A.B. Carson, Senior Medical Officer aboard LST(H)-931 during operations off Iwo Jima, February 1945*

Author deployment experience	
Benjamin T. Miller	Staff Surgeon, Fleet Surgical Team-6, embarked on the USS Bataan (LHD-5), Operation Inherent Resolve, Fifth Fleet Area of Responsibility, 2017
	Staff Surgeon, forward deployed Naval Hospital Guam, 2018–2020
Pamela M. Choi	Ship's Surgeon, USS Harry S. Truman (CVN-75), Operation Inherent Resolve, Sixth Fleet Area of Responsibility, 2017–2018
Joseph DuBose	Chief of Trauma, 332nd EMDOS, Role 3 Air Force Theater Hospital, Operation Iraqi Freedom, Balad, Iraq, 2009
	Chief of Trauma, NATO Role 3 Multinational Medical Unit, Operation Enduring Freedom, Kandahar Airfield, Afghanistan, 2010
	Chief of Trauma, Role 3 AFTH, Operation Enduring Freedom, Bagram Air Base, Afghanistan, 2011–2012
	Surgical Support Missions, Joint Special Operations Medical Command, 2016, 2017, 2018, 2019

B. T. Miller (✉)
Cleveland Clinic, Cleveland, OH, USA
e-mail: millerb35@ccf.org

P. M. Choi
Navy Medicine Readiness and Training Command San Diego, San Diego, CA, USA
e-mail: pamela.m.choi.mil@mail.mil

J. DuBose
University of Texas-Austin, Dell Seton School of Medicine, Austin, TX, USA

M. D. Tadlock, A. A. Hernandez (eds.), *Expeditionary Surgery at Sea*,
https://doi.org/10.1007/978-3-031-21893-4_22

BLUF (Bottom Line Up Front)

1. Damage control surgery (DCS) is a three-stage, planned management strategy for critically injured patients with the "lethal triad" of hypothermia, acidosis, and coagulopathy.
2. Drill Tactical Combat Casualty Care (TCCC) compressible hemorrhage control with all shipboard personnel and Zone 1 Resuscitative Endovascular Balloon Occlusion of the Aorta (REBOA) as applicable with the surgical team for noncompressible torso hemorrhage.
3. DCS is a clinical decision.
4. DCS is NOT a procedure of last resort once irreversible coagulopathy begins to manifest clinically. Commit to DCS early.
5. Heat the ship's medical spaces before casualties arrive.
6. Anticipate any surgical instruments, supplies, and consumables needed for DCS before going underway.
7. Fresh whole blood (FWB) is ideal for casualty resuscitation at sea. Activate the walking blood bank (WBB) early.
8. Delay definitive surgical repairs until normal metabolism and physiology are restored. Many times this will be at a higher level of care but can be on the ship during times of prolonged casualty care (PCC) such as during distributed maritime operations (DMO).
9. Drill trauma activations, including WBB activation with the ship's medical company and any/all embarked surgical teams.
10. In times of PCC, create teams to staff the intensive care unit (ICU) in shifts to prevent fatigue.

Introduction

Clinical Vignette 22.1

*While deployed to the United States (U.S.) Fifth Fleet Area of Responsibility in 2017, the USS Bataan (LHD-5) had a mass casualty incident (MCI) when it received six critically injured patients simultaneously by tilt rotor aircraft (*Table 22.1*). One patient with severe facial injuries lost vital signs in the aircraft en route to the ship, so the surgical team on the aircraft performed a resuscitative thoracotomy with aortic cross-clamping. On arrival to the USS Bataan (LHD-5), the patient was immediately taken to the operating room (OR) for resuscitation and to identify other sources of bleeding.*

In the OR, blood component therapy with packed red blood cells (PRBCs) and fresh frozen plasma (FFP) was rapidly transfused. When his vital signs returned, the aortic cross-clamp was removed. As expected, after 30 min of aortic cross-clamping he was profoundly acidotic (pH 6.74, lactate 14.9 mmol/L) and hypothermic (core body temperature of 34 °C). At laparotomy, he was found to have a mesenteric

Table 22.1 Patients and their injuries treated in the mass casualty incident (MCI) in 2017 on board Wasp class amphibious assault ship, the USS Bataan (LHD-5)

Patient	Injuries	Treatment	Units PRBC	Units FFP	Units FWB
1	• Pelvic fracture • Pulmonary contusion	• Pelvic binder • Subclavian CVC • Femoral arterial line • ET intubation	4	2	6
2	• Left comminuted tibia and fibula fractures • Pulmonary contusion	• Left lower extremity four-compartment fasciotomy • Fasciotomy washout with splint placement • Bilateral tube thoracostomy • Subclavian CVC • Radial arterial line • ET intubation	0	0	4
3	• Facial fractures and lacerations • Cardiac arrest • Mesenteric avulsion • Right ulna fracture • Suspected spine injury	• Left anterior thoracotomy with aortic cross-clamp • Exploratory laparotomy • Small bowel resection • Bilateral tube thoracostomy • Temporary abdominal closure • Abdominal and chest re-exploration with mesenteric and chest wall vessel ligation • Abdominal washout • Entero-enterostomy • Right upper extremity splint • Subclavian CVC • Right groin cut-down for femoral arterial line • ET intubation • Repair right femoral artery • Radial arterial line • Tracheostomy	8	8	28
4	• Suspected spine injury	• Spine precautions	0	0	0
5	• Suspected spine injury	• Spine precautions	0	0	0
6	• Left open tibia and fibula fractures • Suspected spine injury	• Left lower extremity four-compartment fasciotomy • Left tibia external fixation • Fasciotomy washout • Spine precautions	0	0	1

PRBC packed red blood cells, *FFP* fresh frozen plasma, *FWB* fresh whole blood, *CVC* central venous catheter, *ET* endotracheal

avulsion with intraperitoneal hemorrhage. The bleeding mesenteric vessels were ligated, and approximately 20 cm of devascularized small bowel was resected. Damage control surgery (DCS) was performed to get him out of the OR as soon as possible: the small bowel was left in discontinuity, a temporary abdominal dressing was created, and bilateral chest tubes were placed. He was then brought to the intensive care unit (ICU) for further resuscitation [1].

All U.S. Navy Sailors are required to learn how to fight shipboard fires and seal flooding compartments. These efforts, known as "damage control" since World War II, maintain mission integrity even after the ship absorbs considerable damage. Emulating the Navy's principles of rapid repairs to save the ship, trauma surgeons pioneered "damage control surgery" in the early 1990s, which urged quick hemorrhage control and a truncated initial operation to prevent patient death from metabolic failure [2]. DCS is a three-stage approach to treating patients in hemorrhagic shock before the "lethal triad" of hypothermia, acidosis, and coagulopathy is irreversible [3].

1. Injured patients are quickly taken to the OR to arrest bleeding, control contamination, and restore extremity perfusion with vascular shunts.
2. Patients are then moved to the ICU for resuscitation, rewarming, and correction of coagulopathy.
3. After normal physiology is restored, patients are returned to the OR for definitive surgical repairs and abdominal closure.

Indications for DCS afloat are similar to those on land, but include special considerations unique to the maritime environment. This chapter aims to review guidelines and practical recommendations for DCS at sea for the maritime surgical team.

"Damage Control Zero" and Advanced Resuscitative Care Afloat

Compressible hemorrhage control, part of Tactical Combat Casualty Care (TCCC) training, saves lives in both the pre-hospital and hospital settings [4]. TCCC is now required for all shipboard providers and corpsmen, but it is important to refresh the TCCC "damage control zero" maneuvers used to stop bleeding with all embarked medical personnel (see Chap. 10 discussing the likely nursing-driven Fleet-wide TCCC rollout). These straightforward maneuvers include the application of direct pressure on wounds, appropriate placement of tourniquets on injured extremities, placement of pelvic binders for hemodynamically unstable patients with pelvic fractures, the use of advanced hemostatic dressings (e.g., Combat Gauze®, North American Rescue), early tranexamic acid (TXA) administration and blood-based hypotensive resuscitation (goal SBP $\geq$100 mm Hg) [5].

However, noncompressible torso hemorrhage is more difficult to control and remains a leading cause of death among combat casualties [6]. Efforts to save these casualties with early fresh whole blood (FWB) transfusion and Zone 1 Resuscitative Endovascular Balloon Occlusion of the Aorta (REBOA), or Advanced Resuscitative Care, is gaining traction. If REBOA is a part of the ship's combat casualty care or algorithm, make sure that all critical personnel have appropriate REBOA training. Review the indications and contraindications to REBOA with the team. Drill REBOA exercises following the Joint Trauma System (JTS) Clinical Practice Guidelines (CPGs).

Indications for Damage Control Surgery (DCS)

When considering DCS at sea, several factors should be taken into account: injury type and severity, available resources, sea states, time to medical evacuation (MEDEVAC), patient physiology, and surgeon expertise. If the decision is made to perform DCS, do it early in the patient's course before physiologic derangements are irreversible. DCS may even be the decision before reaching the OR. DCS should be strongly considered for casualties presenting with systolic blood pressures (SBP) less than 90 mm Hg and for patients with the "lethal triad" of hypothermia, acidosis, and coagulopathy (Table 22.2). However, while laboratory results and vital signs can guide decision-making, DCS remains a clinical decision [7].

Hypothermia

Hemorrhage and exposure cause hypothermia, or core body temperature less than 35 °C (95 °F). Hypothermia is an indication for DCS to prevent worsening coagulopathy [3]. Casualties can lose heat at the point of injury (POI) and/or en route to the ship. Sea water immersion, especially at extreme latitudes, causes profound convective heat loss (see Chaps. 27 and 28). Air transport may also expose casualties to frigid elements. Remove wet clothing and use rewarming blankets en route to the ship to prevent further heat loss. After arrival, casualties in the ship's resuscitation and OR areas can shed even more heat. The ship's medical spaces tend to be cold with minimal temperature control measures, with some OR temperatures as low as 50 °F. Work with the engineering department to learn how to warm the medical spaces before casualties arrive. See Chap. 28 for discussion of hypothermia rewarming methods.

Table 22.2 Indications for damage control surgery (DCS) at sea

Indications for Damage Control Surgery (DCS) at sea
Penetrating or Blunt injury with Systolic Blood Pressure (SBP) <90 mm Hg
Core Body Temperature <35 °C
Serum pH <7.2 or lactate >5 mmol/L
International Normalized Ratio (INR) >50% of normal and/or diffuse nonsurgical bleeding

Acidosis

Global tissue hypoperfusion from hypovolemia leads to acidosis. In a vicious cycle, increasing lactic acidosis further depresses cardiac output, worsens coagulopathy, decreases peripheral resistance, and may cause fatal cardiac dysrhythmias. Arterial pH of less than 7.2 or serum lactate greater than 5 mmol/L is an indication for DCS [3].

Coagulopathy

Hemorrhage and hypothermia worsen coagulopathy by depleting clotting factors and retarding the coagulation cascade. DCS is considered for patients with an international normalized ratio (INR) greater than 50% of normal [3]. However, many warships lack INR measurement capabilities (see Chap. 8). Platelet count can be used as a surrogate for INR, as thrombocytopenia may indicate consumption of other clotting factors. Alternatively, DCS can be considered if there is diffuse non-surgical bleeding from tissue surfaces.

Abdominal Damage Control Surgery (DCS)

Enter the abdomen quickly and pack bleeding areas with laparotomy pads. For patients with profound coagulopathy, diffuse packing may be all that can be done during damage control laparotomy. If the patient's physiology permits, look for and control intra-abdominal injuries [8]. If there is a splenic injury, splenectomy, NOT splenorrhaphy, should be performed. Arterial embolization for spleen and liver injuries is not an option at sea. Most liver injuries can be controlled with careful packing that restores normal liver anatomy and contour. When managing liver trauma, remember the principles of Pringle, pack, and pray; furthermore, if the liver is not bleeding, don't mess with it [9].

A brief Pringle maneuver with a vascular clamp may slow hepatic bleeding to help plan the best approach. Another option is to fashion a Red Rubber Robinson catheter into a Rummel tourniquet around the portal triad (Fig. 22.1). Maritime surgical technologists (STs) and surgeons can be unfamiliar with how to put together a Rummel tourniquet because it is used infrequently. At the proximal end of the catheter funnel where the caliber changes a small hole is cut in the side of the catheter. The distal end of the catheter is then threaded through the cut hole and out the proximal funnel (around the hepatoduodenal ligament) and tightened. Once hepatic inflow is stopped, a clamp is placed around both ends of the red rubber.

If packing fails to stop hepatic hemorrhage, catheter balloon tamponade, vessel ligation, hepatorrhaphy with large sutures, or electrocautery are other options

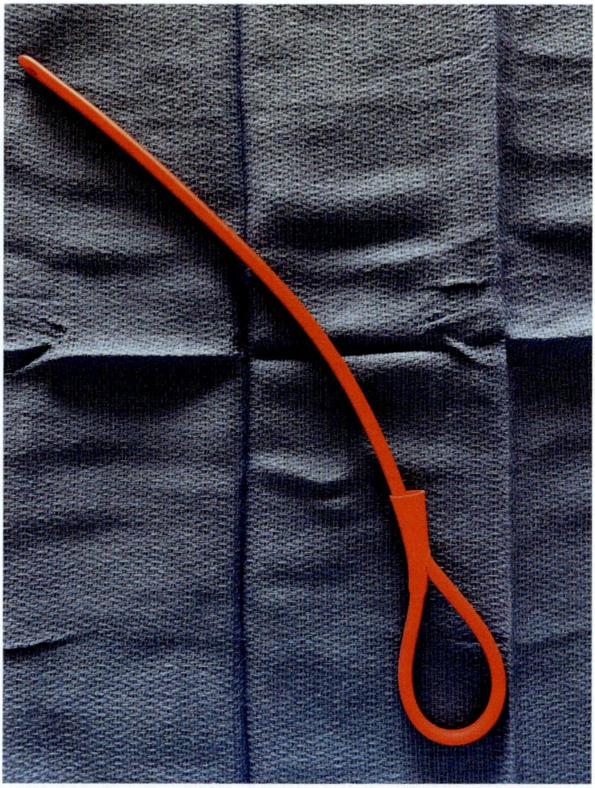

Fig. 22.1 Red Rubber Robinson catheter fashioned into a Rummel tourniquet. (Source: Photo courtesy of Matthew D. Tadlock, MD)

depending on the injury. Use hemostatic agents (e.g., SURGICEL® or SURGIFLO®, Johnson & Johnson) to slow bleeding from raw liver surfaces. Avoid liver resections unless non-anatomic resectional debridement is required for hemorrhage control. An improvised catheter balloon tamponade device for deep parenchyma injury tracts can be fashioned by cutting several holes in a Red Rubber Robinson catheter and passing it through a Penrose drain; tie both ends of the Penrose drain to the Red Rubber Robinson catheter with heavy silks. After placing the tamponade device through the injury tract, clamp the distal end of the red-rubber catheter, and instill with normal saline to create a tamponade effect and then clamp the proximal end of the catheter [9]. Pancreas injuries should be packed and drained [7].

Close gastric and duodenal injuries with sutures or a stapling device. Bowel resections should be performed for mesenteric injuries or to control contamination. Leave the bowel in discontinuity and make a temporary abdominal dressing. For the shipboard temporary abdominal closure, create a negative-pressure dressing using a plastic drape (e.g., 1010 Steri-Drape™, 3 M or a sterile Mayo table cover), blue towels, drains, and a plastic adherent drape dressing (e.g., Ioban™, 3 M). Cut several small holes in the plastic drape, and then cover the bowel with this fenestrated sheet, tucking the edges under the fascia all the way down each paracolic gutter and into the pelvis. Place blue towels over the drape, and then lay closed-suction drains over the towels. Finally, cover the drains and towels with the plastic adherent dressing. Attach the drains to suction to remove pooled peritoneal fluid.

Explore expanding retroperitoneal hematomas for major vascular or solid organ injuries. Nephrectomy may be performed for a kidney injury; however, confirm a contralateral kidney before committing. Drain ureteral injuries by placing a tube in the ureter and then exteriorizing it through the skin [7]. Or simply clip the end of the ureter, which will cause it to dilate to facilitate later repair at a tertiary facility.

Controlling hemorrhage from pelvic fractures at sea without available angioembolization or pelvic external fixation expertise may be challenging. First, wrap the unstable pelvis with a pelvic binder or sheet (see Chap. 24 for a step-by-step guide). If this fails to stop the bleeding, try pelvic preperitoneal packing. If the pelvic bleeding persists despite preperitoneal packing, Zone 3 REBOA deployment or external fixation of the pelvis can be used if the surgical team has the necessary expertise and equipment (again see Chap. 24). The last resort for major pelvic bleeding is exploratory laparotomy. Common and external iliac artery injuries can be controlled with vascular shunts, and the internal iliac artery injuries can be temporarily occluded with vessel loops or clips. Major venous injuries can be ligated in an emergency [3].

Vascular Damage Control Surgery (DCS)

Restoring flow is the goal for all vascular injuries, but some may be best treated with ligation in a damage control situation. After obtaining proximal and distal control of the vessel, decide if the injury needs to be repaired, shunted, or ligated [10]. Approach suspected aortic injuries via a left medial visceral rotation and inferior vena cava (IVC) injuries via a right medial visceral rotation [11]. Small aortic injuries are repaired primarily with 3–0 or 4–0 polypropylene suture. For larger injuries, restore flow with a vascular shunt (e.g., Argyle™ shunt, Cardinal Health) or even a chest tube. Similarly, the IVC may be repaired with 4–0 or 5–0 polypropylene suture. The infrarenal IVC can be ligated if absolutely necessary.

For extremity vascular injuries, use tourniquets for initial hemorrhage arrest. A tourniquet may be all that is needed if early MEDEVAC is possible; however, tourniquet times greater than 6 h are not conducive to limb salvage. In a damage control situation, injury repair with a vascular anastomosis is a time-consuming effort, ill-advised in the context of the "lethal triad." Instead, restore flow with a vascular shunt. Most ships have vascular shunts on their Authorized Medical Allowance List (AMAL), but ensure that the OR is stocked with these consumables prior to deployment (see Chap. 12). Traditional vascular shunts are preferable, but if they are not available, improvised shunts of IV tubing, small nasogastric tubes (NGTs), or small chest tubes (based on vessel size) can be used.

After obtaining control of the injured vessel, proximal and distal thrombectomy is performed. An appropriately sized vascular shunt is then placed across the injury. Be careful not to damage the vessel intima, especially if the shunt has been revised.

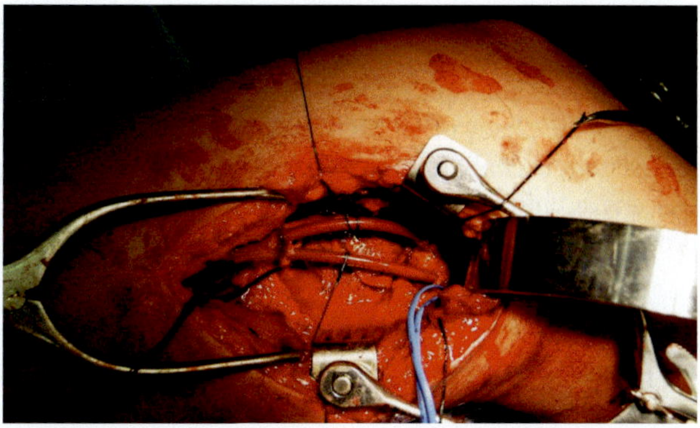

Fig. 22.2 Vascular shunts placed in the left popliteal artery and vein (above knee) secured with silk ties. (Source: Photo courtesy of Joseph DuBose, MD)

Secure the shunt in place with silk ties or Rummel tourniquets (Fig. 22.2). If silk sutures are used, tie them close to the edge of the injury because the vessel edges will need to be debrided during definitive repair. Use a Doppler device to evaluate for distal flow if no pulse is palpated. Consider a four-compartment fasciotomy in any patient with a lower extremity vascular injury, especially if prolonged follow-on transport is expected. Don't forget that all peripheral veins, except for the popliteal veins, can be ligated in emergent situations. Avoid traumatic amputations at sea when possible, because limb salvage capabilities are more likely at higher echelons of care.

Damage Control Resuscitation (DCR)

No chapter on DCS would be complete without the discussion of damage control resuscitation (DCR); see Chap. 23 for a more thorough review of this topic. DCR occurs before and during all phases of DCS until normal physiology is restored. Prior to definitive control of hemorrhage DCR begins during "Damage Control Zero," with blood-based hypotensive resuscitation (goal SBP $\geq$100 mm Hg) and minimizing crystalloid. In brief, the resuscitative phase of damage control aims to restore normal metabolism and physiology. Correct hypothermia with aggressive rewarming techniques, including forced-air warming blankets (e.g., Bair Hugger™, 3 M) and warming crystalloids and colloids.

The goal of DCR is to treat and/or prevent the coagulopathy of trauma by minimizing crystalloids and resuscitating with or approximating FWB with component therapy. Transfusing a balanced ratio of blood components—packed red blood cells (PRBCs), fresh frozen plasma (FFP), and platelets—will be impossible afloat unless deployed on a hospital ship. Most of the PRBCs and FFP are frozen, there are no apheresis machines to generate platelets, nor is cryoprecipitate available. FWB, drawn from the walking blood bank (WBB) is the only way to provide a balanced resuscitation at sea. Warm FWB transfusion is also ideal because it corrects hypothermia and improves acidosis by increasing oxygen delivery to tissues. FWB also best corrects coagulopathy underway [1]. Activate the WBB early if a massive transfusion is anticipated, as it may take almost an hour to generate the first unit of FWB. In the chaos of an MCI at sea, getting a type-specific unit of FWB to the correct patient is challenging. To avoid confusion, prepare patient labels before casualties arrive, and then assign labels to each patient to identify them and their blood products.

Definitive Surgical Repairs

After resuscitation to correct hypothermia, acidosis, and coagulopathy, return patients to the OR for definitive surgical repairs and to look for missed injuries. At sea, this is a luxury and may depend on the timing of available MEDEVAC opportunities. However, prolonged casualty care (PCC) at sea, defined as 96 h or more, during Distributed Maritime Operations (DMO) may be required [12]. Only perform a bowel anastomosis, colostomy, or abdominal closure if the team has the available resources, as discussed in the conclusion of the vignette. Otherwise, MEDEVAC the patient to a higher echelon of care if possible. Do not perform a vascular anastomosis or repair ureters at sea unless the surgical team has the necessary resources and expertise.

Clinical Vignette 22.1 Conclusion

*An hour into the patient's resuscitation in the ICU, there was brisk bleeding from the temporary abdominal dressing and chest tubes, likely worsened by his acidosis and thrombocytopenia (70,000 platelets/microliter). He was quickly taken back to the OR where bleeding mesenteric and chest wall vessels were found and ligated. Warm FWB became available and was transfused during the second operation, correcting the patient's thrombocytopenia and acidosis. He was then taken back to the ICU for further resuscitation. In total, he received 28 units of FWB, 8 units of PRBCs, and 8 units of FFP (*Table 22.1*).*

*There were delays in patient evacuation, giving the embarked surgical teams time to perform definitive surgical repairs. After correcting physiologic and metabolic abnormalities, the patient with intestinal discontinuity underwent a bowel anastomosis and definitive abdominal closure (*Fig. 22.3*). However, another patient with a tibia fracture who had undergone lower extremity four-compartment fasciotomy with tibia external fixation (*Fig. 22.4*) did not undergo tibia repair because no orthopedic expertise beyond "damage control orthopedic surgery" was available (see Chap. 24). All patients treated aboard the USS Bataan (LHD-5) survived to MEDEVAC transfer after more than 36 h afloat.*

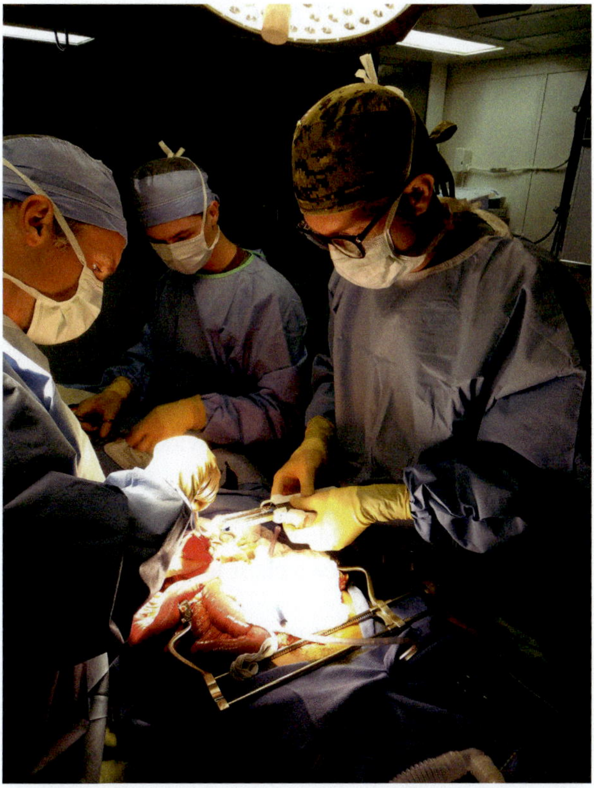

Fig. 22.3 Patient #3 from mass casualty incident (MCI) (see Table 22.1 and Clinical Vignette 22.1) undergoing a bowel anastomosis and definitive abdominal closure on board Wasp class amphibious assault ship, the USS Bataan (LHD-5), 2017. (Source: Photo courtesy of Benjamin T. Miller, MD)

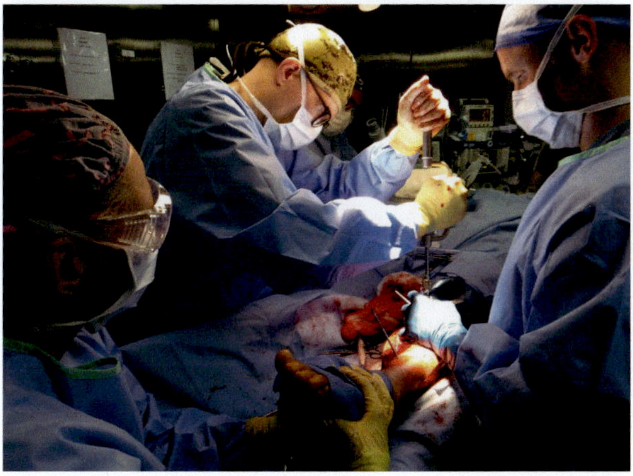

Fig. 22.4 Patient #6 from mass casualty incident (MCI) (see Table 22.1) undergoing a left tibia external fixation on board Wasp class amphibious assault ship, the USS Bataan (LHD-5), 2017. (Source: Photo courtesy of Benjamin T. Miller, MD)

Aircraft Carrier (CVN) Considerations

Aircraft carriers (CVN) are not casualty receiving and treatment ships (CRTS) by design, so their surgical capabilities are more limited. The surgical team consists of one surgeon, one anesthesia provider (typically a certified registered nurse anesthetist (CRNA)), and two STs. During routine surgical operations, the surgeon is typically assisted by the oral maxillofacial surgeon (OMFS), family practitioner, or flight surgeon. However, in a true MCI the surgeon will likely be assisted by general duty corpsmen as the physicians fill other roles.

Appropriate triage and early identification of surgical needs are crucial (see Chap. 7). Activate the WBB early because CVNs do not have stored blood component therapy available. For injury identification, a small portable point-of-care ultrasound (POCUS) is available to perform Focused Assessment Sonography for Trauma (FAST). Most shipboard providers on the CVN will likely not have formal or comprehensive ultrasound training, so these skills should be reviewed. See Chaps. 8 and 9 for a discussion about shipboard radiology and POCUS. There may not be portable or available radiography equipment, depending on the ship and situation, so be ready to place a chest tube based only on physical exam findings in an unstable patient.

The surgeon must also understand the ship's surgical equipment and supplies. Equipment availability is limited during instrument sterilization, so always have extra laparotomy packs and a chest set available. Often the surgeon works closely with the enlisted personnel assigned to the OR to ensure that all needed equipment is available and functional (see Chap. 12). Additionally, the ICU has only three beds with a single critical care registered nurse (CCRN) as the only nurse on board so plan for early MEDEVAC if prolonged postoperative patient care is anticipated. See Chaps. 1, 5, 6, 10, 12, and 14 for discussion of the capabilities and limitations of the maritime surgical team and communication about MEDEVAC.

Large Deck Amphibious Assault Ship Considerations

Large deck amphibious assault ships deploy with the ship's company, medical personnel from a Marine Expeditionary Unit (MEU), and a Fleet Surgical Team (FST). For the USS Bataan (LHD-5) in 2017, four trauma teams were created that integrated the embarked units with the ship's company during pre-deployment exercises. Each team member had a defined role for every resuscitation: trauma team leader, airway management, exposure and secondary survey, vital signs, intravenous (IV) access, and recorder. Frequent casualty-receiving drills familiarized each member with their role and improved the trauma readiness, which paid off when a true MCI occurred.

During certain missions, ships may be augmented with an Expeditionary Resuscitative Surgical System (ERSS) or a Surgical Resuscitation Team. It is critical to drill with these embarked units as they are added to ensure smooth team integration. Embarked teams will likely have already rehearsed resuscitations together during pre-deployment exercises, so it may be easier for them to run individual trauma resuscitations.

It is also useful to train in exercises where casualties are received from aircraft on the flight deck, taken to the resuscitation areas, and then to the OR. It may feel silly, but it truly helps every member of the maritime surgical team individually and as a whole to perform notional operations like vascular exposures and thoracotomies. Be sure to drill the WBB activation during training events too, even going so far as to exercise it to completion by drawing blood from donors and then auto-transfusing their unit of blood back into them. See Chap. 7 regarding Triage, Chapter 23 regarding WBB, and Chaps. 11 and 31 for patient transport.

Amphibious assault ships are designed to be CRTS and receive several casualties at once, so be ready to run multiple operations simultaneously. If more than one casualty is expected, give the OR assignments before patients arrive and "pre-stage" the ORs with anticipated surgical instruments. At one point during the MCI on the USS Bataan (LHD-5), the patient from Clinical Vignette 22.1 was undergoing re-exploration for bleeding in one OR while another patient was undergoing lower extremity four-compartment fasciotomy in an adjacent OR. Both ORs were appropriately staffed for concurrent operations because there were three embarked surgical teams. Also, all embarked teams had trained in notional exercises together, so members from different teams were smoothly integrated in the ORs. However, there was not enough time to autoclave some of the surgical instruments, so they were dipped in jugs of povidone-iodine solution, or "battlefield sterilized" instead.

During an otherwise routine deployment, an MCI rallies all personnel to contribute. In the excitement, it is easy to forget that the crew still needs rest. Even though casualties will be evacuated as soon as possible, they may end up embarked longer than anticipated. Establish teams early to work in shifts in the ICU to prevent excessive personnel fatigue, and consider rounding twice daily on ICU patients during PCC (see Chap. 30).

Austere Resuscitative Surgical Team Considerations

The ERSS platform is the Navy's austere resuscitative surgical team (see Chap. 1). As described throughout this chapter, the ERSS can augment FSTs on larger amphibious warships including landing helicopter deck (LHD) or landing helicopter assault (LHA) ships. The ERSS can also augment naval vessels with Role 1 medical departments with a formal operating room (e.g., landing platform docks, LPDs) or without formal operating rooms (e.g., destroyers, cruisers, expeditionary sea bases). The ERSS capability and capacity are limited by the severity of injury, the platform being augmented, and **blood availability**. A WBB capability is not currently routine on smaller naval warships with Role 1 medical departments and sometimes, ERSS teams only have the blood they can carry. No matter how austere the environment is, the principles of DCS are the same, however, for the ERSS definitive surgery will typically occur after patients undergo MEDEVAC to a higher level of care.

Conclusion

The principles of DCS, whether on land or at sea, are the same: a truncated operation to prevent irreversible physiologic abnormalities, resuscitation in the ICU, and delayed definitive surgical repairs. Maritime surgeons and surgical teams need to be aware of their equipment and technical limitations to prepare for DCS. Consumable resources are quickly depleted and difficult to replace. Hypothermia from immersion or heat loss en route will worsen coagulopathy, so warm the ship's medical spaces before casualties arrive. Warm FWB is ideal for transfusions afloat, so activate the WBB early. Drill with the ship's medical company and embarked surgical teams for smooth integration. Rehearse patient movement from the casualty-receiving areas to the resuscitation areas and then the OR. As a team, DCS can be successful in the maritime environment to save critical lives.

Declaration of Interest The views expressed in this chapter are those of the authors and do not necessarily reflect the official policy or position of the Department of the Navy, Department of Defense, nor the US Government.

Funding This research did not receive any specific grant from funding agencies in the public, commercial, or not-for-profit sectors.

Conflict of Interest Statement The authors declare no conflict of interest.

References

1. Miller BT, Lin AH, Clark SC, Cap AP, Dubose JJ. Red tides: mass casualty and whole blood at sea. J Trauma Acute Care Surg. 2018;85(Suppl 2):S134–9.
2. Rotondo MF, Schwab CW, McGonigal MD, Phillips GR III, Fruchterman TM, Kader DR, et al. 'Damage control': an approach for improved survival in exsanguinating penetrating abdominal injury. J Trauma. 1993;35(3):375–83.
3. Wyrzykowski AD, Feliciano DV. Trauma damage control. In: Feliciano DV, Mattox KL, Moore EE, editors. Trauma. 6th ed. New York: McGraw Hill; 2008. p. 851–70.
4. Butler WJ, Smith JE, Tadlock MD, Martin MJ. Initial assessment and resuscitation of the battlefield casualty—an overview. Curr Trauma Rep. 2020;6:194–206.
5. 2022 Tactical Combat Casualty Care Guidelines for Medical Personnel. 2021. Available at: https://deployedmedicine.com/market/11. Accessed 31 Jan 2022.
6. Butler F, Holcomb JB, Shackelford S, Barbella S, Bailey J, Baker J, et al. Advanced resuscitative care in Tactical Combat Casualty Care: TCCC guidelines change 18-01. J Spec Oper Med. 2018;18(4):37–55.

7. Hicks CW, Haider A. Damage control operation. In: Cameron J, Cameron A, editors. Current surgical therapy. 11th ed. Philadelphia: Elsevier; 2014. p. 1061–7.
8. Shapiro MB, Jenkins DH, Schwab CW, Rotondo MF. Damage control: collective review. J Trauma. 2000;49:969–78.
9. Eastridge B, Blackbourne LH, McBride KM, Dunne JR. Liver and spleen injury management combat. In: Martin MJ, Beekley AC, Eckert MJ, editors. Front line surgery: a practical approach. 2nd ed. Cham: Springer; 2017. p. 131–43.
10. Starnes BW, Beekley AC, Sebesta JA, Anderson CA, Rush RM. Extremity vascular injuries on the battlefield: tips for surgeons deploying to war. J Trauma. 2006;60(2):432–42.
11. Kobayashi LM, Costantini TW, Hamel MG, Dierksheide JE, Coimbra R. Abdominal vascular trauma. Trauma Surg Acute Care Open. 2016;1:1–7.
12. Day WG, Cooper E, Phung K, Miller B, DuBose J, Lin AH. Prolonged stabilization during a mass casualty incident at sea in the era of distributed maritime operations. Mil Med. 2020;185(11–12):2192–7.

Chapter 23
Damage Control Resuscitation and the Walking Blood Bank

James Wallace, Guy Jensen, Monica Camelo, and Diego A. Vicente

The tree of liberty must be refreshed from time to time with the blood of patriots and tyrants.

Thomas Jefferson

Author deployment experience	
James Wallace	General Medical Officer, Charlie Surgical Company, Operation Enduring Freedom, Afghanistan, 2012
	Resident Surgeon, USNS Mercy (T-AH-19), Pacific Partnership, Philippines, 2016
	Ship's Surgeon, USS Nimitz (CVN-68), Operation Inherent Resolve and Operation Freedom's Sentinel, Third Fleet Area of Responsibility, 2020–2021
Guy Jensen	Ship's Surgeon, USS Nimitz (CVN-68), Operation Inherent Resolve and Operation Freedom's Sentinel, CENTCOM and INDOPACOM Areas of Responsibility, 2020–2021
Monica Camelo	Staff Surgeon, Fleet Surgical Team-9, 2019–2020; embarked on the USS Somerset (LPD-25), Arctic Expeditionary Capabilities Exercise, Arctic Circle, 2019; embarked on the USS John P. Murtha (LPD-23) and the USS Portland (LPD-27), multiple contingency operations, INDOPACOM Area of Responsibility, 2019; embarked on the USS Tripoli (LHA-7), sail around South America, 2020

J. Wallace (✉)
MedStar Washington Hospital Center, Washington, DC, USA

G. Jensen
USS Nimitz (CVN-68), Bremerton, WA, USA

M. Camelo
1st Medical Battalion, Camp Pendleton, CA, USA

D. A. Vicente
Navy Medicine Readiness and Training Command San Diego, San Diego, CA, USA
e-mail: diego.a.vicente.mil@health.mil

M. D. Tadlock, A. A. Hernandez (eds.), *Expeditionary Surgery at Sea*,
https://doi.org/10.1007/978-3-031-21893-4_23

Author deployment experience	
Diego A. Vicente	Ship's Surgeon, USS Harry S. Truman (CVN-75), Operation Inherent Resolve, AFRICOM Area of Responsibility, 2015–2016
	Officer in Charge, Role 2 Light Maneuver team, embarked on the USS Hershel "Woody" Williams (ESB-4), 2020; Provided embarked Role 2 Surgical Support, AFRICOM Area of Responsibility, 2020

BLUF (Bottom Line Up Front)

1. Damage control resuscitation (DCR) involves rapid triage, hemorrhage, and sepsis control, as well as targeted blood product resuscitation in severely injured patients.
2. In a patient dying from hemorrhagic shock from any cause, the best resuscitative product is fresh whole blood (FWB).
3. A comprehensive understanding of the limitations associated with various shipboard platforms and assets is critical for maritime surgical teams, particularly in austere environments.
4. Shipboard component blood products can be utilized in patients requiring transfusions; however, available blood products may be limited by storage times and safe infusion of blood products may be limited by preparation and thawing times.
5. The process of thawing and deglycerolizing Packed Red Blood Cells (DRBC) is a perishable skill that needs to be practiced routinely during deployment.
6. Walking blood banks (WBBs) have been implemented on large deck ships and utilized in the management of mass casualty incidents (MCIs) at sea. In the event the WBB is activated, rapid identification of potential donors is critical. To do this, pre-deployment preparation is key.
7. Activating and implementing a WBB is also a perishable skill, but more complex and dynamic involving multiple members of the deployed team. Therefore, all aspects involved need to be practiced routinely during deployment.
8. While application of WBB protocols is feasible in smaller ships for austere Role 2 surgical teams, the eligible pool of blood donors may be significantly limited and insufficient for the management of even a single severely injured patient, so having component blood products is essential.
9. Development of a maritime strategy and surgical team mindset that accounts for limited resources in an environment constrained by geography is critical for an effective medical mission dedicated to preventable loss of life.

Introduction

Clinical Vignette 23.1

A United States (U.S.) warship was in the Seventh Fleet area of operations performing routine freedom of navigation patrols and flight operations. An arresting cable snapped during aircraft recovery causing severe injury to five different Sailors. Two of the Sailors sustained open tibia/fibula fractures, one Sailor sustained an open femur fracture with significant soft tissue trauma and blood loss. The final two Sailors were crouching at the time of the accident and were struck in their abdomens by the cable resulting in obvious bruising, abdominal tenderness, and hypotension with positive Focused Assessment with Sonography in Trauma (FAST) examinations. Expected rotary wing medical evacuation (MEDEVAC) of casualties could only take place in 48 h.

The Walking blood bank (WBB) was quickly activated. Three units of low titer O whole blood (LTOWB) were collected from the prescreened donor pool. One unit each was given to the Sailor with the open femur fracture and the two Sailors with blunt abdominal trauma. Damage control resuscitation (DCR) was continued for the two Sailors with blunt abdominal trauma using a total of nine units of type-specific blood: one Sailor required three units of AB− blood and the other six units of A+. The two Sailors with open tibia/fibula fractures were treated with splinting and pain control. Fresh whole blood (FWB) resuscitation allowed the surgical team time to rotate the other three Sailors through the ship's one operating room (OR) for definitive surgical control of the bleeding. All five Sailors eventually got a MEDEVAC and ultimately survived their injuries.

Years of ongoing conflicts in Iraq and Afghanistan have shaped a military medical system that has made great strides in improving the survival of service members injured in conflict despite increases in injury severity scores. These improvements have come in part due to improved resuscitation strategies, including the use of warm FWB, the increase in the availability of surgical care inside the "Golden Hour," and MEDEVAC systems that rapidly move patients toward progressively higher levels of care.

As the U.S. begins to consider the implications of a possible future "great power competition," novel management strategies for casualty care and transport should be considered. For instance, the ability to rapidly move patients toward higher levels of care may be limited or absent due to either geography or lack of clear air superiority. As described in Chap. 22, multiple critically injured patients were cared for aboard the USS Bataan (LHD-5) for over 38 h prior to MEDEVAC [1, 2].

Moreover, these transportation constraints may be further strained as the U.S. Navy evolves a distributed maritime operations (DMO) strategy. In these instances, providers could find themselves caring for patients for days. Therefore maritime surgical teams will require a prolonged casualty care (PCC) mindset focusing on the best care possible, using the resources available. A PCC mindset dictates that maritime medical departments and surgical teams need to be well versed in the management of blood products as well as DCR techniques. See Chap. 30 for a more thorough discussion of PCC.

Table 23.1 Principles of damage control resuscitation (DCR) [5]

1. Avoid crystalloid resuscitation to prevent dilutional coagulopathy
2. Component blood products should be used in a 1:1:1 ratio or fresh whole blood (FWB) should be used
3. Avoid over-resuscitation. Resuscitate to a goal systolic blood pressure (SBP) of 100 mm Hg or 110 mm Hg if traumatic brain injury (TBI) is suspected
4. Resuscitation is not a replacement for surgery; hemorrhage control is vital
5. Tranexamic Acid (TXA) can reduce mortality if given within 3 h of injury. One 2 gram dose is the current recommendation
6. Intravenous (IV) calcium should be supplemented during ongoing blood transfusion. 1 gram should be given with the first transfused unit and repeated after every four subsequent units
7. Use in-line blood warmers whenever possible to avoid hypothermia
8. Having donors prescreened to be Low Titer O whole blood (LTOWB) donors decreases time to transfusion and the likelihood of severe transfusion reaction compared to type-specific blood

Damage Control Resuscitation (DCR)

DCR is an adjunct to damage control surgery (DCS), but can be applied to any hemodynamically unstable patient requiring blood product resuscitation. DCR refers to the principles of restoring homeostasis, limiting tissue hypoxia, and limiting coagulopathy [3–5]. In the injured and bleeding patient this should be managed with a blood-based resuscitation strategy (i.e., "replace what was lost") [5].

Given the frequent geographic isolation of U.S. Navy vessels, DCR efforts afloat are frequently referred to as remote damage control resuscitation (RDCR). **Limited resources with significant constraints in equipment, training, personnel, and supply chains complicate medical care at sea. Providers must have an understanding of the limitations associated with various shipboard assets when embarking, particularly in austere environments**. The principles of DCR are summarized in Table 23.1.

Platform-Specific Capabilities

Aircraft Carrier (CVN)

Aircraft carriers (CVNs) are the largest warships in the U.S. Fleet with a crew of more than 5000 Sailors when the Air Wing is embarked. When deployed, the CVN's associated carrier strike group (CSG) may include an additional 2000 Sailors. While the CVN's medical department is the primary MEDEVAC facility for the CSG, CVNs are not considered Casualty Receiving and Treatment Ships (CRTS), as they are equipped with only one OR, three intensive care unit (ICU) beds, 52 ward beds, and no stored blood products and therefore must rely on the WBB. The Senior Medical Officer (SMO) is responsible for the medical department; when a medical emergency requires activation of the WBB the SMO and Commanding Officer (CO) should be notified. See Chaps. 1 and 6 for a deeper discussion about the CSG, CVN capabilities, and communication required of medical leadership.

Fleet Surgical Team (FST)

Amphibious warships include landing helicopter dock (LHD), landing helicopter assault (LHA), landing platform dock (LPD), and dock landing ships (LSD) which are essential for United States Marine Corps (USMC) power projection from the sea. An Amphibious Squadron (PHIBRON) typically consists of three warships: LHD/LHA, LPD, and LSD; altogether, they comprise an amphibious ready group (ARG).

The LHD class of ship has a Navy crew of 1100 and Marine troops up to 1800, 6 ORs, up to 14 ICU beds, 45 ward beds, a blood bank capacity of more than 400 units of frozen packed red blood cell (PRBC) and fresh frozen plasma (FFP) along with a WBB. With a similar blood-carrying capacity, the LHA class has a Navy crew of 1100 and Marine troops up to 1800, only 2 ORs, 3 ICU beds, and 24 hospital beds. The LPD class has a Navy crew of 400 and up to 800 Marine troops with 2 ORs, 24 hospital beds, a blood bank capacity of more than 50 units of frozen blood products along with a WBB. The LSD class has no ORs, no blood products, and only up to 11 hospital beds [6].

Fleet Surgical Teams (FSTs) are the augmented medical assets afloat for the ARG. Each FST is assigned to a PHIBRON to augment the medical department with surgical care, intensive care, en route care, and blood bank services [7]. The Commander Amphibious Task Force (CATF) Surgeon is the officer in charge of the FST. The CATF surgeon works closely with the SMO in charge of the medical department of each ship; however, the CATF surgeon is ultimately responsible for coordinating all medical care, surgical support, and blood bank resources to all the CRTS and medical battalions attached to the ARG [8]. Again, refer to Chaps. 1 and 6.

Expeditionary Resuscitative Surgery System (ERSS)

Expeditionary Resuscitative Surgery System (ERSS) teams are single surgeon seven-person austere resuscitative surgical teams composed of a general surgeon, emergency department physician, certified registered nurse anesthetist (CRNA), critical care registered nurse (CCRN), surgical technologist (ST), respiratory therapist (RT), and a physician assistant (PA). Teams integrating onto smaller vessels (e.g., cruisers or destroyers) augment existing medical assets (i.e., Independent Duty Corpsmen (IDC)), and work with medical and line leadership to coordinate casualty movement. The goal is for the team to be able to deliver care to trauma

Table 23.2 Storage temperatures and shelf lives for different types of blood products [9]

Product	Storage	Shelf life
FWB	Room temperature	24 h
FWB	1–6 °C	If refrigerated within 8 h of collection, then 21–35 days
Frozen PRBCs (FRBC)	−65 °C or colder	10 years
Deglycerolized PRBCs (DRBC)	1–6 °C or colder	14 days after thawing
Fresh PRBCs	1–6 °C	Up to 42 days
Frozen FFP	−65 °C or colder	1 year
Thawed FFP	1–6 °C	24 h after thawing
Fresh FFP	1–6 °C	5 days
Platelets	1–6 °C	5 days

FWB fresh whole blood, *PRBC* packed red blood cells, *FFP* fresh frozen plasma

patients in austere environments. They are equipped with modular medical equipment packs in order to be highly mobile and able to deliver DCR and DCS close to the point of injury (POI) in pre-designated host nation facilities or aboard available sub or surface vessels in any space of opportunity. Again, please refer to Chaps. 1 and 6 for the discussion of the complex missions and interfaces with the line community these teams face.

Practical limitations of these teams regarding the WBB include their provisional nature, the limited number of Sailors aboard smaller vessels, as well as the potentially limited investment from the ship's crew due to the temporary nature of the teams. Furthermore, a WBB capability (including pre-screening the crew before deployment) is not a routine exercise. Therefore, augmentation of the WBB with stored component blood products is particularly important for these teams in the setting of those issues. They are typically equipped with a blood refrigerator with settings for both freezing and refrigerating components. In the absence of deglycerolization equipment on the Authorized Medical Allowance List (AMAL) on the ERSS platform, blood products must be stored at 1–6 °C in the refrigerator (Table 23.2).

Frozen Blood Product Capabilities

During Vietnam, when inventories of transfusable units dwindled, component therapy was instituted to maximize the utility of each donated unit. The first use of frozen red blood cells (FRBC) was reported at the Naval Station Hospital, Danang, Republic of South Vietnam, in 1966. However, it was not until 2005 that the Automated Cell Processor (ACP)®215 (Haemonetics Cell Processing System) was developed, leading to the use of 860 deglycerolized PRBC (DRBC) units transfused within the CENTCOM Area of Responsibility (AOR) during 2008–2012 with no transfusion reactions or complications [8].

Table 23.3 Tactical Combat Casualty Care (TCCC) guidelines resuscitative fluids of choice for casualties in hemorrhagic shock listed from most to least preferred [10]

1. Cold stored Low Titer O whole blood (LTOWB)
2. Pre-screened LTOWB
3. Fresh Frozen Plasma (FFP), red blood cells (RBCs), and platelets in a 1:1:1 ratio
4. FFP and RBCs in a 1:1 ratio
5. FFP or RBCs alone
6. Unscreened group O fresh whole blood (FWB) or type-specific FWB should only be performed under appropriate medical direction by trained personnel

The Armed Service Blood Program (ASBP) assigns an Area Joint Blood Program Office (AJBPO) as a point of contact for managing and distributing all available blood products within Department of Defense (DoD) service. During an outside the continental United States (OCONUS) deployment, certain units can request frozen blood products from frozen depots located in Sigonella, Sicily, and Okinawa. Each depot can store up to 40,000 units of frozen blood products [6]. A daily report from ships carrying blood products of all available fluids and blood products is submitted to the AJBPO for accountability and readiness. Small deck amphibious assault ships (LPD) may rely on resupplying their blood storage from larger deck ships (LHD/LHA). Table 23.3 lists common forms utilized for blood product acquisition during deployment, however, each team should review current processes relative to their platform and area of responsibility.

Frozen blood products must be maintained at a temperature of −65 °C or colder [9]. FRBCs have an approved shelf life of ten years. In optimal conditions, two FRBC units can be deglycerolized using the ACP®215. Therefore, on an LHD/LHA class ship equipped with four ACP®215 units, a technician can thaw and deglycerolize 36 units in 12 h [9]. However, as emphasized in several chapters throughout the book, this process can take 45 min for the first batch of unit(s) to be available, thus maritime surgical teams need to plan for this delay during resuscitative efforts. Often DRBC units are prepared ahead of time to have some blood products readily available depending on the operational environment. This decision is typically made after discussion with the key members of the surgical team (e.g., surgeon and CRNA), the CATF surgeon, and the ship's SMO. DRBC units are stored at 1–6 °C for up to 14 days in a closed system. For FFP, shelf life for frozen units is 1 year, but they will only last 24 h post-deglycerolization (Table 23.2) [11].

FWB: Fresh Whole Blood; PRBC: Packed Red Blood Cells; FFP: Fresh Frozen Plasma

Massive transfusion with DRBC showed no difference in mortality outcomes when compared to a control population transfused with non-DRBC in Afghanistan. To ensure its efficacy, the DRBC must contain more than 80% of RBC from the original unit.

Shipboard blood acquisition is coordinated with the local medical treatment facility (MTF) to acquire blood products 15–30 days before deployment and 10–15 days before arrival OCONUS. The WBB provides FWB and is considered a tertiary source of blood only to be used after U.S. Food and Drug Administration (FDA)-approved blood sources are no longer available (see the next section).

Blood components must be maintained under specific storage conditions to maintain the integrity of the products for transfusion (Table 23.2). There must be an apparent organization of storage areas indicating locations for storage of both usable and unusable blood components to avoid staff confusion and prevent transfusion errors. Freezers and refrigerators need to have a functional alarm system installed for both power and temperature. Frozen blood products close to expiring within 3 months need to be rotated to the nearest MTF. Strict adherence to these blood product storage and dates is critical given that use of "older" blood has been associated with increased mortality in trauma patients and can alter cardiac function [12, 13].

Amphibious ships are required by instruction (OPNAVINST 6530.4) to maintain the capability to store and process frozen blood products. The process of thawing and deglycerolizing units of FRBC should be routinely tested before and periodically during deployment. Maritime mass casualty incidents (MCIs) are often unpredictable and like any skill, the process of thawing and deglycerolizing FRBC units must be routinely practiced to ensure blood is available when needed. FRBC units that are group "O" can be used for transfusion to all groups/types without the need for crossmatching [7].

Walking Blood Bank (WBB)

Table 23.3 lists the Tactical Combat Casualty Care (TCCC) recommended resuscitative fluids for casualties in hemorrhagic shock listed from most to least preferred [10]. Options 1–3 are not currently routinely available on any maritime platform. Options 4 and 5 are not ideal during DCR and DCS, particularly in casualties requiring a massive transfusion protocol-based resuscitation as coagulopathy will occur without whole blood or approximating whole blood with component therapy. Furthermore, many ships do not have the capabilities to store component blood products; however, the lack of component blood products need not have a negative effect on patient outcomes. When the embarked medical assets on the USS Bataan Bataan (LHD-5) needed to treat six severely injured trauma patients simultaneously, they found that the use of the WBB to provide FWB provided a more effective supply than component blood products [2]. Actually, the FWB was preferred since it did not require deglycerolizing as in the case of FRBC or thawing as in the case of FFP, and it already contained platelets and fibrinogen that would not otherwise have been available. However, for a WBB to function as needed during a MCI such as the one on the USS Bataan (LHD-5) or in Clinical Vignette 23.1, surgical and medical teams must both prepare and routinely drill the process of collecting blood for transfusion. Like preparing DRBC units, **activating and accurately implementing a**

WBB during a MCI is a perishable skill. However, the WBB is a much more complex and dynamic process than preparing DRBC units.

Preparation

Preparation for deployment and contingency operations should start by reviewing the After Action Reports (AAR) and challenges presented in previous deployments [6] along with the local ship-specific WBB Standard Operating Procedure (SOP). Refer to current instructions (OPNAVINST 6530.4) and the Joint Trauma System (JTS) Clinical Practice Guidelines (CPG) when creating a WBB SOP, specifically CPG 18: damage control resuscitation, CPG 21: whole blood transfusion, and CPG 82: prehospital blood transfusion [7, 14, 15].

Next, freezers and ACP®215 units on amphibious assault ships and blood refrigerators on all ships should undergo functional testing prior to any pre-deployment operations. WBB collection kits have a short expiration window and should be checked to assure they will be functional throughout the deployment and reinforcements ordered with plenty of buffer time because of all the issues with the supply system. For platforms with this equipment, the maritime surgical team needs to ensure that all the required maintenance and inspections are occurring for both the equipment and alarm systems by the biomedical technicians along with the maintenance of the equipment used for ORs discussed in Chap. 12.

Per instruction (COMNAVAIRINST 6000.1, COMNAVSURINST 6000.1) all ship's medical departments are required to maintain a current printed listing of each crewmember's blood type, RH factor, and donor eligibility. Refer to current guidelines from the platform and area of responsibility, but typically a minimum of 10% of the crew are required to be pre-screened for WBB donation. However, the ideal goal should be to screen 30% of the crew. Per the ASBP (DODI 6480.04), whole blood donor screening is required for any deployment greater than 30 days. It is essential to keep updating the list to ensure the accuracy of the roster. Asking all potential donors to fill out an ASBP Form 572 (Pre-Screen/Emergency Whole Blood Donation Record) through the Birth Month Recall (BMR) process is an efficient way to maintain a qualified donor pool. Potential donors for all possible blood types should be sought out. It is best that the donor pool mimics the overall U.S. distribution of blood types: 45% O, 40% A, 11% B, and 4% AB [16]. Potential donors that have been pre-screened using the ASBP Form 572 are termed "qualified donors."

The ASBP can be utilized to host blood drives while in port and prior to deployment. Blood drive coordination helps assure a ready pool of donors, confirms blood type (which may be incorrect in the service member's medical record), and testing for transfusion-transmitted disease (TTD) (e.g., human immunodeficiency virus (HIV), syphilis, hepatitis B, and hepatitis C). For maritime platforms, blood drives should be held 90 days before deployment to ensure all results are back before deployment. Sailors who have donated blood in an ASBP-sponsored blood drive and whose blood was found to be safe upon analysis are designated as "prime donors."

If requested, the ASBP can test crew members found to have type O blood for titers. LTOWB comes from type O donors who have donated blood in an ASBP-sponsored blood drive and whose blood was tested for anti-A and anti-B antibody titers and was found to be fully safe upon analysis. Only units containing a low titer of antibody (i.e., <1:256 saline dilution, immediate spin method) are designated LTOWB. Ideally, WBB donors should be re-titered every 90 days in conjunction with TTD testing. However, since the availability of titer testing is extremely limited, every effort should be made to ensure that donors are titered at least annually and prior to each deployment.

In the event the WBB is activated, rapid identification of potential donors is critical. In addition to recruiting a donor pool and coordinating blood drives, a roster of potential donors must be maintained. Theater Medical Data Store (TMDS) is a web-based information storage system that is used to maintain blood inventories at OCONUS hospitals and forward operating bases (FOBs). Unfortunately, due to connectivity issues, TMDS is often unavailable while out to sea. At the time of this publication, the Bureau of Medicine and Surgery (BUMED) Maritime Blood Strategy Sub-Community was working on novel tracking solutions. Most medical departments have created electronic logs to track all eligible donors when they were tested and when they will need to be retested. The donor log tracker (typically a spreadsheet) should be maintained and regularly updated by the laboratory technicians. Hard copies of the tracker along with completed ASBP Forms 572 should also be maintained.

Activation/Screening

When a medical emergency requires WBB activation, the quarterdeck should be contacted and the Officer of the Deck (OOD) should announce over the 1-MC "Activate the Walking Blood Bank." Ideally, the evolution takes about 45 min total to screen, collect, and deliver blood products, but to achieve that amount of time takes practice and preparation.

The *muster point* should be a location that can accommodate a large group of potential donors and should not be located within the medical department to avoid high traffic areas during an MCI. Often the mess deck provides a fitting location large enough to separate potential donors based on their blood type. Designated corpsmen are in charge of screening potential donors using ASBP Form 572, taking initial vitals, and directing donors to collection points. Per FDA guidance, donors must meet donor criteria specified in FM 4-02.70/NAVMED P-5120/AFMAN 41-111.

At the same time, the WBB team as indicated in the Watch Quarter Station Bill, will begin preparing to receive donors and collect blood at the *collection point*. Blood collection is also not often performed in the medical spaces for the same reasons that the muster point is not there. Often the dental spaces are designated as collection points. The blood drawing equipment is located in the WBB Portable Medical Locker (PML), which should be pre-staged at the collection point.

Although laboratory technicians should be members of the WBB team, additional personnel must be called upon as the task is too much for a few people.

Personnel most commonly assigned and trained to be phlebotomists are dental technicians. During the collection, 450 mL ± 10% of FWB will be collected. Phlebotomists should be aware that each bag should weigh approximately 485 gm or measured by use of 10-inch 550 paracords (wrapping around the unit, with both ends touching), included in WBB collection kit [7]. If it is less or more than the desired amount, clotting secondary to not enough or toxicity secondary to too much citrate can occur. Once the collection is complete, the phlebotomist labels the unit: blood type, date, time, and unit number [7]. Sample tubes with the correct donor/unit number also need to be saved, labeled with the unit number/donor, and double-checked for correct labeling to be sent for testing retrospectively; a request to the nearest MTF is sent at the next port call to test the donor's blood for blood-borne pathogens if those tests are not available on the platform (which it typically is not).

The WBB team should have access to the donor log tracker and completed ASBP Forms 572. Based on the type of blood requested, prescreened donors will have their blood drawn per ship-specific WBB SOP. Additionally, many ships use prepackaged WBB collection kits. WBB teams should be familiar with the local SOP, the available WBB collection kits, and documentation requirements on the ASBP Form 572.

Delivery

The blood sample tubes, bag of donated blood, and ABSP Form 572 are then transported to the medical department laboratory, where the laboratory technician performs rapid testing for blood-borne pathogens (if testing is available), completes a crossmatch, and sets aside required samples for shipment for retrospective testing. When the sample is determined to be safe and the crossmatch is confirmed, the results should be annotated on the ASBP Form 572, and the unit transported to the recipient for transfusion. Form 151 (Whole Blood Transfusion Checklist) and SF 518 (Medical Record-Blood or Blood Component Transfusion) can be used to assist in and properly record the transfusion of blood. Table 23.4 provides a summary of some of the forms involved in the acquisition and delivery of blood products.

Table 23.4 Forms involved in the acquisition and delivery of blood products in the maritime environment

Forms for Requesting/Shipping Component Blood Products
DD Form 573: Shipping Inventory of Blood Products
DD Form 1502N: Notice for Frozen Medical Materiel Shipments (Perishable Keep Frozen)
DD Form 1502-1N: Notice for Chilled Medical Materiel Shipment (Perishable Keep Chilled)
Forms for Screening/Collection/Delivery of Fresh Whole Blood (FWB)
ASBP Form 572 (previously DD 572): Pre-Screen/Emergency Whole Blood Donation Record
Form 151: Whole Blood Transfusion Checklist
SF 518: Medical Record-Blood or Blood Component Transfusion

However, forms and platforms evolve with time, so it is always best to check the current protocols during the pre-deployment period.

Proper blood typing and infectious screening requires time, time that may not be available depending on the recipient's clinical status. In such circumstances, if the surgeon deems it necessary to obtain FWB at a faster rate, they may authorize the emergency release of FWB from the WBB without the completion of all infectious screening tests and or crossmatching. This is to be meticulously documented by laboratory personnel. All FWB units released in this fashion will be documented as such in the WBB Log. (Note: FWB may be kept stored at room temperature for up to 24 h. If FWB is refrigerated within 8 h of collection it becomes stored whole blood (SWB), where citrate-phosphate-dextrose (CPD) bags may be stored for 21 days and citrate-phosphate-dextrose-adenosine (CPDA-1) bags may be stored for 35 days between 1–6 °C (Table 23.2) [7].

Per General Naval Air Training and Operating Procedures Standardization (NATOPS), aircrew personnel will not be able to participate in any flight duties for at least 4 days after donation, sometimes longer. All donors will be monitored post-donation and will be given a light-duty chit for a minimum of 72 h [17].

Post-delivery

After completion of the WBB, all donor blood units or donor unit blood bags post-transfusion should be returned to the laboratory. Laboratory personnel verify the disposition of all donor units and document this in the WBB log. Regular contact should be maintained with the Blood Support Detachment to obtain follow-up results on confirmatory testing of donor blood samples. Upon notification of confirmed positive results, a licensed clinical provider should be notified to ensure that the donor is notified and counseled. If a patient received a confirmed FWB unit from a donor confirmed to be positive for a blood-borne pathogen, the ASBP should be notified, who will initiate patient notification and respective evaluation of both donor and patient. In accordance with HA Policy 10-002, Policy on the Use of Non-US Food and Drug Administration, all recipients of FWB shall receive follow-up infectious disease testing as soon as possible along with 3, 6, and 12 months' testing post-transfusion.

Evaluation of the efficacy of a successful WBB is validated by drilling, and it is crucial to integrate all afloat medical and dental assets. Ideally, formal training classes with the local blood donation center (BDC) should be arranged pre-deployment. The WBB should be a part of all mass casualty drills, which should be regularly practiced (see Chap. 7). It is best that the documentation of the entire sequence of events, including the actual drawing of units, rapid disease testing, crossmatching, auto-transfusion, is practiced during WBB drills for the most accurate simulation.

Documentation of all shipboard transfusions and collections, blood component therapy or the WBB, including ABSP Form 572 or alternate blood donation record, Form 151, SF 518 or alternate transfusion record, and/or any shipping or receiving of blood products documents must be forwarded to the Navy Blood Program Office and the homeport blood bank. Copies of all blood bank records should also be maintained by the ship's laboratory.

Special Considerations for Austere Role 2 Surgical Teams

ERSS teams are not currently assigned to an operational Navy Type Command (TYCOM), unlike the previously described CVN (TYCOM: Commander, Naval Air Forces) and FST (TYCOM: Commander, Naval Surface Forces) maritime surgical teams. Therefore, while these teams are intended to function independently, their support is currently directed through the Naval Component Commander and Combatant Commander who may have a variable understanding of medical needs and support requirements. A comprehensive review of AARs from prior shipboard ERSS teams suggests that the barriers to delivering effective damage control care to avoid preventable loss of life include limited trauma experience of the individual augmentee, lack of pre-deployment clinical trauma training, limited familiarity with the equipment, and lack of medical logistics and infrastructure support beyond the vessel of opportunity [18]. Contrasting the expected capabilities relative to existing resources merits some contemplation and equipoise beyond the scope of this chapter; however, given the evolution of DMO, members of these teams will need to be aware of these issues prior to deployment in order to mitigate risks to patient care and optimize available resources.

In order to apply the DCR principles described previously to an ERSS team, pre-deployment development of trauma management protocols should be established within the team to clearly define roles during resuscitation compatible with vessel and space of opportunity. Further, the team roles should also be established to prepare shipboard protocols for resuscitation products, WBB, controlled substances, and patient movement, as these protocols may not exist in the designated vessel.

Once these roles have been established, the blood bank officer (typically the CRNA) should immediately begin to coordinate with regional ASBP blood banks to develop pre-deployment blood drives to accurately identify the ship's crew blood type O donors and specifically test for the LTOWB preferred donors. These blood donation events for the ship allow for testing the ship's crew and also provide much-needed resources to regional blood banks.

Due to limitations discussed previously in this chapter, augmentation of the WBB with stored component blood is particularly important. Coordination between the regional ASBP blood banks and the team blood bank officer to optimize components of blood products for balanced resuscitation while considering the duration of the mission and shelf life of blood products is an important first step to developing an effective DCR strategy. Of note, strict maintenance of blood products in the refrigerator is critical given the mortality risks of transfusing expired blood [12]. Additional considerations for re-supply while on mission include international laws for transport of blood products across borders and maintenance of designated cool temperatures for blood products in transit. Further, the appropriate disposal of unused blood products by the team should be coordinated with the regional ASBP blood bank.

Finally, the key to any successful DCR strategy in an austere environment is patient transport and re-supply of expended equipment and blood products. ERSS teams should develop MEDEVAC plans prior to reaching the AOR. These plans include comprehensive knowledge of medical assets to accept patients, fixed and rotary wing assets to transport the patient, as well as contingency plans for PCC at sea in the event that transportation is not available. While these topics are discussed in separate Chaps. 20, 21, 30, and 31, it is important to note that interactions for MEDEVAC may not take place with well-informed medical personnel, and the ERSS leadership can mitigate communication issues by identifying capable personnel in the AOR prior to activation of patient transports.

Once teams have established trauma and WBB protocols, team roles, resuscitation strategies, and MEDEVAC plans, team training with drills is even more critical to prepare to receive casualties. Major deficits may include team flow and dynamics in absence of pre-deployment clinical trauma training and redundancy in capabilities (i.e., IV and airway placements) given limited trauma experience. Teams should continue to undergo development as the DMO strategy is rolled out. Surgeons leading these teams need to be aware of existing deficits in team experience, training, equipment, and logistics support in order to develop deployment strategies for patient care and team training.

Conclusion

As the U.S. Navy continues to develop a DMO strategy, medical departments will find themselves further strained. MCIs like the one in the clinical vignette will require providers to care for injured Sailors and Marines for long periods of time. To save lives during DMO and after MCIs, maritime surgical teams be knowledgeable in blood product administration and DCR techniques. Moreover, they must have a keen understanding of platform-specific limitations of personnel, training, equipment, and supply so that an effective strategy for blood product procurement and utilization can be developed and associated training and drilling can be performed so preventable loss of life can be avoided.

Declaration of Interest The views expressed in this chapter are those of the authors and do not necessarily reflect the official policy or position of the Department of the Navy, Department of Defense, nor the US Government.

Funding This research did not receive any specific grant from funding agencies in the public, commercial, or not-for-profit sectors.

Conflict of Interest Statement The authors declare no conflict of interest.

References

1. Day WG, Cooper E, Phung K, Miller B, DuBose J, Lin AH. Prolonged stabilization during a mass casualty incident at sea in the era of distributed maritime operations. Mil Med. 2020;185(11–12):2192–7.
2. Miller BT, Lin AH, Clark SC, Cap AP, Dubose JJ. Red tides: mass casualty and whole blood at sea. J Trauma Acute Care Surg. 2018;85(1S):S134–S9.
3. Bjerkvig CK, Strandenes G, Eliassen HS, et al. "Blood failure" time to view blood as an organ: how oxygen debt contributes to blood failure and its implications for remote damage control resuscitation. Transfusion. 2016;56:S182–S9.
4. Woolley T, Thompson P, Kirkman E, et al. Trauma Hemostasis and Oxygenation Research Network position paper on the role of hypotensive resuscitation as part of remote damage control resuscitation. J Trauma Acute Care Surg. 2018;84(6S):S3–S13.
5. Glaser J. Damage control resuscitation (CPG ID: 18). 2019.
6. Fleet medical pocket reference. San Diego, CA: Surface Warfare Medical Institute; 2016. p. 120.
7. Chief of Naval Operations CotMC. OPNAVINST 6530.4 Series, Department of the Navy Blood Program. In: Dot N, editor. Washington DC: Department of the Navy; 2007. p. 96.
8. TM 8-227-11/NAVMED P-5123/AFI 44–118, OPERATIONAL PROCEDURES FOR THE ARMED SERVICES BLOOD PROGRAM ELEMENTS. In: Defense Do, editor. Washington, DC: Departments of the Army, Navy, and Air Force; 2007.
9. Standard VC, Procedure O. Glycerolization and Deglycerolization of Red Blood Cells in a closed system using the Haemonetics ACP 215. Boston: National Blood Research Laboratory; 2003.
10. 2022 Tactical Combat Casualty Care Guidelines for Medical Personnel. 2021. Available at: https://deployedmedicine.com/market/11. Accessed 1 Jan 2022.
11. Berséus O, Boman K, Nessen SC, Westerberg LA. Risks of hemolysis due to anti-A and anti-B caused by the transfusion of blood or blood components containing ABO-incompatible plasma. Transfusion. 2013;53:114S–23S.
12. Wang D, Sun J, Solomon SB, Klein HG, Natanson C. Transfusion of older stored blood and risk of death: a meta-analysis. Transfusion. 2012;52(6):1184–95.
13. Reilly M, Bruno CD, Prudencio TM, et al. Potential consequences of the red blood cell storage lesion on cardiac electrophysiology. J Am Heart Assoc. 2020;9(21):e017748.
14. Cap AP, Beckett A, Benov A, et al. Whole blood transfusion. Mil Med. 2018;183(suppl 2):44–51.
15. Shackelford CSA. Prehospital blood transfusion (CPG ID: 82). 2020.
16. About blood. 2020. https://www.militaryblood.dod.mil/donors/about_blood.aspx. Accessed 12 Apr 2021.
17. US navy aeromedical reference and waiver guide. San Diego, CA: Navy Operational Training Command; 2021. p. 429.
18. Vicente DA, Ugochukwu O, Johnston MG, Craft C, Damin V, Tadlock MD. Preparing austere maritime surgical teams for deployment during the COVID-19 global pandemic: is it time to change the training pipeline? Mil Med. 2021;186(9–10):e873–8.

Chapter 24
Orthopaedic Damage Control at Sea

Sean G. Sheppard, Bradley Deafenbaugh, Lucas S. McDonald, and James R. Bailey

Never was so much owed by so many to so few.

Winston Churchill

Author deployment experience	
Sean G. Sheppard	Orthopaedic Resident Surgeon, Navy Medicine Center Readiness and Training Command San Diego, San Diego, CA, USA, 2018–present
Bradley Deafenbaugh	Battalion Surgeon, 2nd Marine Division, Operation Iraqi Freedom, Ar Ramadi, Anbar Province, Iraq, 2007
	Orthopaedic Trauma Surgeon, Navy Medicine Center Readiness and Training Command San Diego, San Diego, CA, USA, 2015–present
Lucas S. McDonald	Flight Surgeon, HMH 462, Operation Iraqi Freedom, Al Asad Air Base, Iraq, 2008
	Orthopaedic Surgeon, Expeditionary Resuscitative Surgical System, 2018; Provided Role 2 Surgical Support, 2018
	Orthopaedic Surgeon, NATO Role 3 Multinational Medical Unit, NATO Resolute Support and Operation Freedom's Sentinel, Kandahar Airfield, Afghanistan, 2019
James R. Bailey	U.S. Marine Corps Logistics Officer, Brigade Service Support Group-1, Kenya, 2000
	Orthopaedic Surgeon, NATO Role 3 Multinational Medical Unit, NATO Resolute Support, Kandahar Airfield, Afghanistan, 2015
	Orthopaedic Surgeon, NATO Role 3 Multinational Medical Unit, NATO Resolute Support and Operation Freedom's Sentinel, Kandahar Airfield, Afghanistan, 2017–18

S. G. Sheppard · B. Deafenbaugh · L. S. McDonald · J. R. Bailey (✉)
Navy Medicine Readiness and Training Command San Diego, San Diego, CA, USA
e-mail: seangsheppard@gmail.com; braddeafenbaugh@gmail.com; lucas.s.mcdonald@gmail.com; jamesbailey98@gmail.com

M. D. Tadlock, A. A. Hernandez (eds.), *Expeditionary Surgery at Sea*,
https://doi.org/10.1007/978-3-031-21893-4_24

BLUF (Bottom Line Up Front)

1. Damage control orthopaedic surgery temporizes injuries until the next echelon of care is reached and contributes to lifesaving measures.
2. Orthopaedic injuries benefit from timely reduction and stabilization. Priority should be placed on a focused physical exam to identify acute limb deformities and neurovascular abnormalities. Reduction of a fracture or dislocation can reverse neurovascular discrepancies and should be attempted; it may require local or general anesthesia with muscle relaxation.
3. Stabilization of fractures should be performed with splinting and should include the joint above and below the zone of injury. Plaster splints are preferred by most surgeons, but often the only splinting material available is prefabricated (i.e., SAM™ splints).
4. External fixation is a treatment option for fractures/dislocations that cannot be stabilized in a splint or for patients who require prolonged transport.
5. Open fractures require additional care, including early antibiotic administration (within 3 h), surgical debridement, and temporary or definitive stabilization.
6. Pelvic fractures can cause extensive blood loss and should be identified quickly. Circumferential pelvic antishock sheeting (CPAS) should be performed for an unstable pelvic ring injury that is contributing to hemodynamic instability. Providers should be suspicious of an open pelvic fracture if concomitant rectal or genital injuries are present.
7. Infections of bone and soft tissue can lead to permanent disability and should be managed with timely, thorough irrigation and debridement and appropriate antimicrobial coverage.
8. Acute compartment syndrome (ACS) is a clinically diagnosed orthopaedic emergency that should be identified quickly and treated with early (less than 6–8 h) fasciotomy to prevent further permanent damage.
9. When performing a two-incision four-compartment lower leg fasciotomy, beware of the common pitfalls of missing the anterior (incorrectly identifying the intermuscular septum) and the deep posterior muscle compartments (not freeing the soleus from the tibia and identifying the posterior tibial neurovascular bundle).
10. The axillary nerve is the nerve most injured following a shoulder dislocation and should be checked for function to include sensation over the lateral shoulder and motor function of the deltoid muscle.

Introduction

Damage control orthopaedics is performed daily in Level 1 trauma centers across the country. Protocol-driven life- and limb-saving principles are developed with the input from large trauma teams, advanced equipment, rapid access to operating rooms (ORs), and trained orthopaedic surgeons. This same standard can be difficult to achieve in the austere shipboard environment, especially during armed conflict.

During mass casualty incidents (MCIs), damage control principles save lives and temporize injuries until the next echelon of care is reached. Cap et al. [1] calculated that between 2001–2014, 76% of United States (U.S.) service members who were killed in action died before reaching a military medical treatment facility (MTF). The medical community responded to this statistic by improving point of injury (POI) care and en route care (ERC). Training such as Trauma Combat Casualty Care (TCCC) is now an integral part of medical training for all deploying military personnel. After two decades of continuous combat, damage control principles are well established, but integrating these "lessons learned" to the shipboard environment remains challenging.

In 2017, the USS Bataan (LHD-5) experienced a mass casualty incident (MCI) while at sea following a land-based helicopter crash. Miller et al. [2] reported the event, describing six simultaneous casualties arriving via MV-22 Osprey tilt-rotor aircraft. The medical team aboard the ship successfully demonstrated expertise in trauma resuscitation and the use of the Walking Blood Bank (WBB), discussed in Chaps. 22 and 23. Additionally, they highlighted the value of damage control orthopaedics. In this specific incident, one patient sustained an unstable pelvis fracture that was treated with a pelvic binder, and three other patients presented with long bone fractures requiring upper extremity splinting, lower extremity four-compartment fasciotomy, and external fixation. All six of these patients were stabilized and remained on board for over 30 h until transport to Landstuhl Regional Medical Center (LRMC). This case study clearly demonstrates that knowledge of basic damage control orthopaedic techniques can ensure proper care of the injured patients while improving the overall resuscitation efforts and outcomes.

Fracture Care

Immediate fracture care includes obtaining a neurovascular exam and determining the extent of the soft tissue injury (also discussed in detail in Chap. 19). Open fractures are treated with early antibiotic administration and irrigation and debridement. Closed fractures can be treated with early reduction and immobilization. Unstable and grossly deformed fractures should be reduced to the best of one's ability. When accessible, the use of X-ray can guide reduction; however, if no X-ray capability exists, correction of obvious deformity should be guided by simply making the limb straight through longitudinal traction, rotation, and manipulation.

Extremity Fractures

In extremity fractures, the motor, sensory, and vascular exam is crucial in determining immediate post-injury function. Patients with limb deformities following high-energy trauma can present with neurovascular compromise. Closed reduction should be performed in a timely manner with reexamination after fracture stabilization, as this can normalize exam findings and once absent pulses distal to the fracture may be palpable. While anatomic reduction may not be possible, the establishment of length and alignment with splinting should be performed. If a post-reduction examination demonstrates continued abnormal exam findings, the presence of a neurovascular injury should be considered.

Thorough irrigation and debridement should be performed in open fractures. In some settings where facilities do not allow thorough debridement, a bedside debridement should be performed to remove large debris from the fracture site. Joint Trauma System (JTS) Clinical Practice Guidelines (CPGs) highlight the importance of open fracture care debridement [3]. All viable tissue should be maintained to provide the best definitive reconstructive options. Tagging damaged neurovascular structures can assist subsequent surgeons in identifying structures of interest. Open fractures should be treated with prophylactic antibiotics (a first-generation cephalosporin) as well as a tetanus booster as soon as possible. Time from injury to the administration of antibiotics is the most important factor in determining the rate of infection for open fractures [4–8].

Fracture immobilization improves the overall stability of the patient. Long bone fractures can contribute a high percentage of overall blood loss, soft tissue damage, and respiratory splinting due to pain in the polytrauma patient [3]. In the acute setting, most extremity fractures are amenable to splinting, which can be accomplished quickly, affording more time to focus on life-threatening injuries in the damage control setting. Splinting is appropriate for most low energy upper extremity and distal lower extremity fractures (to include foot and ankle fractures). Proper splinting consists of immobilizing the bone or joint above and below the zone of injury. Care should be taken to adequately pad bony areas to avoid skin breakdown.

The most appropriate splint for most foot and ankle fractures is an appropriately padded posterior slab with stirrups, commonly called a “Seattle splint” or “U and L” (Fig. 24.1). If splinting a tibia shaft fracture, the splint should cross the knee, traditionally with a posterior slab that spans from the upper thigh to the foot with stirrups. Femoral fractures are often treated with traction or external fixation until definitive fixation can be performed.

Upper extremity fractures from the elbow to the distal radius can be safely splinted in a “Sugar tong” splint (Fig. 24.2). Though often challenging to apply effectively, humeral shaft fractures are best treated provisionally in a coaptation splint (Fig. 24.3), while proximal humerus fractures can often be treated in a simple sling. Fractures of the distal humerus or elbow are treated in a posterior slab splint (Fig. 24.4). Splints are typically constructed from laminated plaster material readily

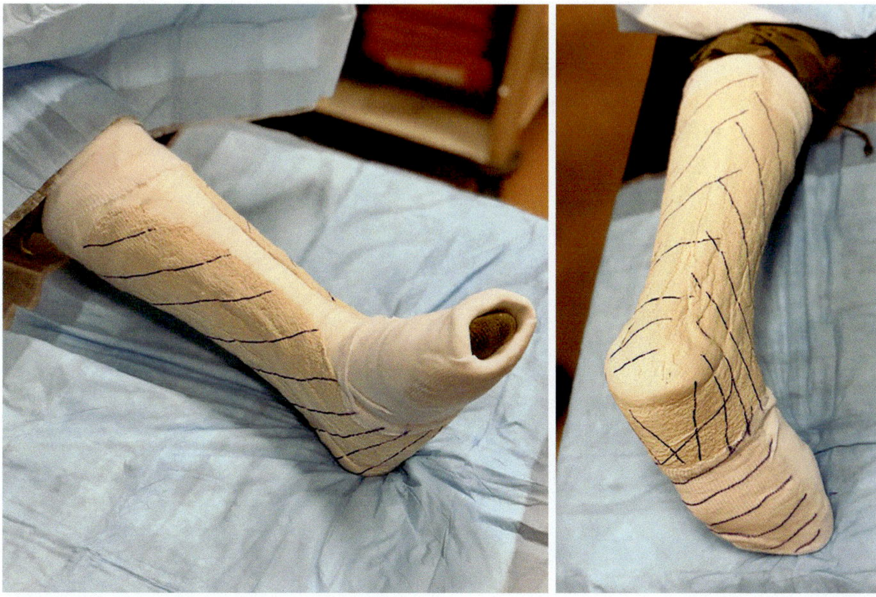

Fig. 24.1 Two views of the "Seattle splint" or "U and L" used in the treatment of most foot and ankle fractures. (Source: Photos courtesy of Sean G. Sheppard, MD)

Fig. 24.2 Two views of the "Sugar tong" splint used in the treatment of upper extremity fractures from the elbow to the distal radius. (Source: Photos courtesy of Sean G. Sheppard, MD)

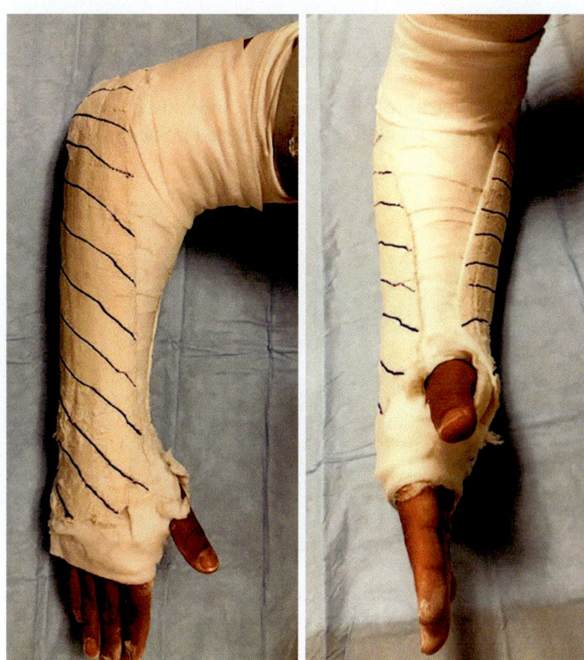

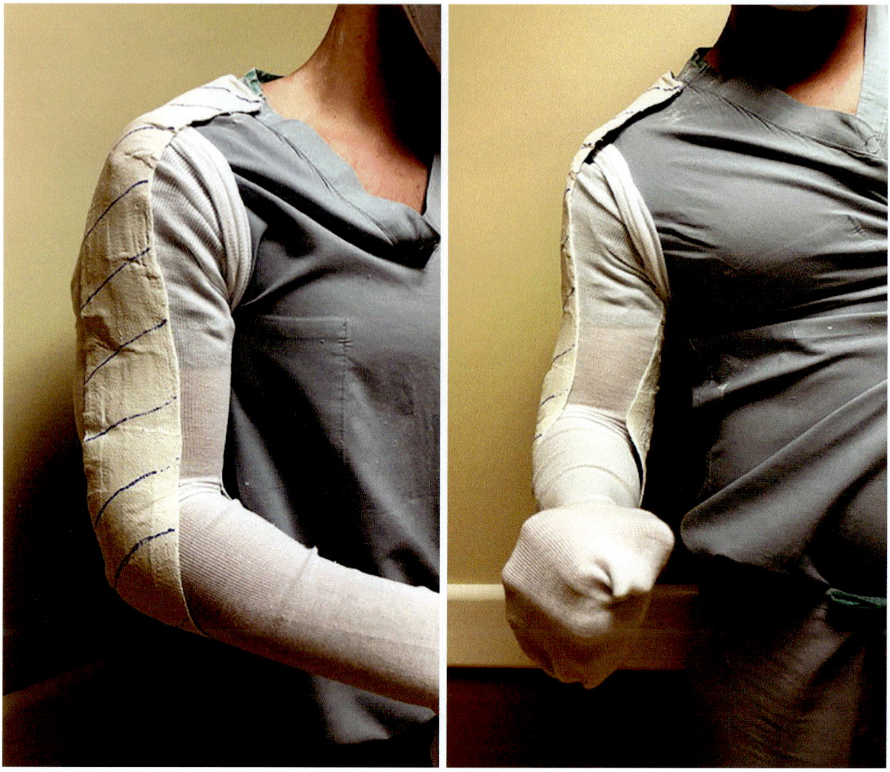

Fig. 24.3 Two views of the coaptation splint used in the provisional treatment of humeral shaft fractures. (Source: Photos courtesy of Sean G. Sheppard, MD)

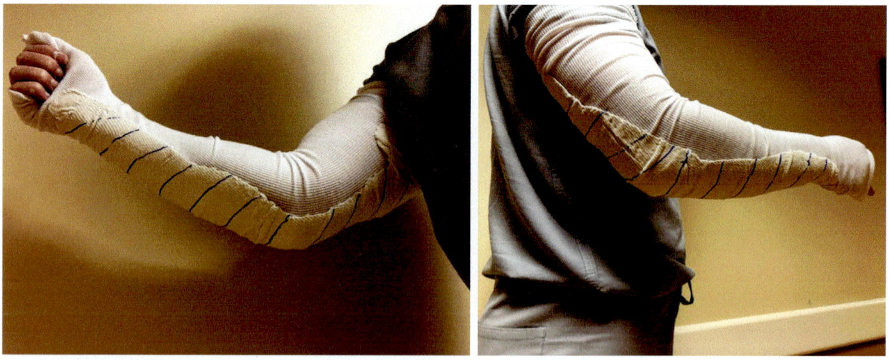

Fig. 24.4 Two views of the posterior slab splint used in the treatment of distal humerus or elbow fractures. (Source: Photos courtesy of Sean G. Sheppard, MD)

found in hospital settings. The plaster undergoes an exothermic reaction upon immersion in water, which allows the plaster slab to be molded into place and then harden into a rigid splint. It is critical to place two layers of cast padding (i.e., Webril) between the skin and wet plaster to prevent burns to the skin from the exothermic reaction. Premade fiberglass rolls are often available for temporary use in trauma or damage control settings. If no plaster or fiberglass rolls available, pliable aluminum precut splinting material such as SAM™ splints can be used for stabilization. Splints should be non-circumferential to allow for swelling and prevent circulation compromise distal to the zone of injury. Repeat physical exam should be performed after splinting to determine neurovascular status of the appendage [3].

If a splint is insufficient to maintain alignment of an extremity or reduction of a joint, or the patient is to undergo a long and possibly rough transport by air, land, or sea, external fixation may be a better option. External fixation is also a helpful tool in the setting of a concomitant extensive soft tissue disruption and/or vascular injury. JTS CPG fracture guidelines highlight various options for external fixation constructs [3]. If an extremity requires vascular shunting or repair, surgical teams should coordinate sequence of external fixation and vascular intervention. Considerations include ischemia time, degree of deformity, surgeon comfort, speed of external fixation application, and indications for direct arterial repair versus initial shunting. If vascular shunting or repair is performed first, limb shortening due to injury must be accounted for to prevent vascular repair/shunt compromise when the limb is subsequently reduced and brought out to length with external fixation. However, when the clinical decision is made to perform damage control surgery (see Chap. 22) there is no role for definitive repair of vascular injuries and it is generally best to shunt them prior to external fixation.

The goal of external fixation is to maintain length, alignment, and rotation of long bone fractures or reduce injury to cartilage surfaces after intra-articular fracture extension. Additionally, external fixation facilitates patient transport and aids in soft tissue monitoring and recovery before definitive fixation. Application of external fixation can be performed in austere environments without fluoroscopic guidance. Safe pin placement requires an understanding of osseous and neurovascular anatomy. Commercially available, self-contained sterile kits with hand-powered drills and self-drilling, self-tapping pins are commonly available for forward deployed units. If the equipment to perform external fixation is not available, or if the surgeon is not trained to perform the procedure, splinting can be used for temporary stabilization as detailed previously.

External fixator construct stability can be improved by maximizing osseous apposition at the fracture, placing connecting bars closer to the skin, increasing the distance between pins within the same fracture fragment, and using the largest diameter pin possible as dictated by basic fracture management principles. Standard pin size for long bone external fixation constructs is 5.0 mm, though downsizing may be required for upper extremities. External fixation constructs can span an entire bone or span the injured joint based on fracture location. For example, in the case of a middle third tibial shaft fracture, pins can be placed entirely in the tibia, with two pins proximal and two pins distal to the fracture. However, a distal femur

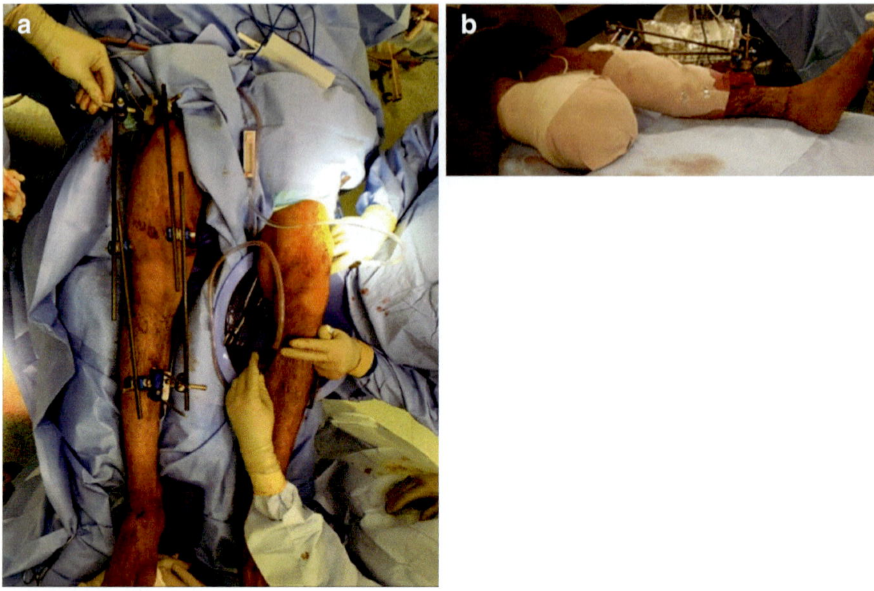

Fig. 24.5 Examples of knee-spanning external fixator with two pins in the tibia and two pins in the femur (**a**) across the right knee joint (**b**) across the left knee joint. (Source: Joint Trauma System Clinical Practice Guidelines (JTS CPG): Orthopaedic Trauma: Extremity Fractures (CPG ID:56). 26 Feb 2020, used with permission)

or tibial plateau fracture generally requires a knee-spanning external fixator with two pins in the tibia and two pins in the femur, as seen in Fig. 24.5. A "Delta frame" can be used as external fixation for fractures about the ankle such as unstable trimalleolar or pilon fractures, seen in Fig. 24.6. These pins are connected by bars to stabilize across the joint once the fracture has been better aligned and length regained.

The safe zone for placement of pins in the tibia includes the entire subcutaneous anteromedial aspect of the tibia seen in Fig. 24.7. The anterior and posterior edges of this region are easily palpated, even in the swollen extremity. Placing the pins centered and perpendicular to this surface will ensure bicortical fixation of the pins into the near and far cortex. For the femur, the safe zone extends from directly anterior to directly lateral in the femoral shaft. If possible, the distal pin should be placed no more distal than two finger breadths above the superior pole of the patella in order to avoid placement of the pin directly into the knee joint. When placing a pin into the calcaneal tuberosity as part of a "Delta frame" construct to span the ankle joint, the pin should be placed medial to lateral and in the posterior/inferior aspect of the tuberosity so as to avoid neurovascular injury.

Pins should be placed both "near and far" in the fragment in relation to the fracture. In a closed fracture, fracture location estimation is performed by direct palpation with a goal of placing the "near" pin approximately 2–3 cm away from the fracture. The "far" pin should be placed as far away as safely possible based on anatomy and fracture site. After identifying the pin site, a 1-cm longitudinal incision

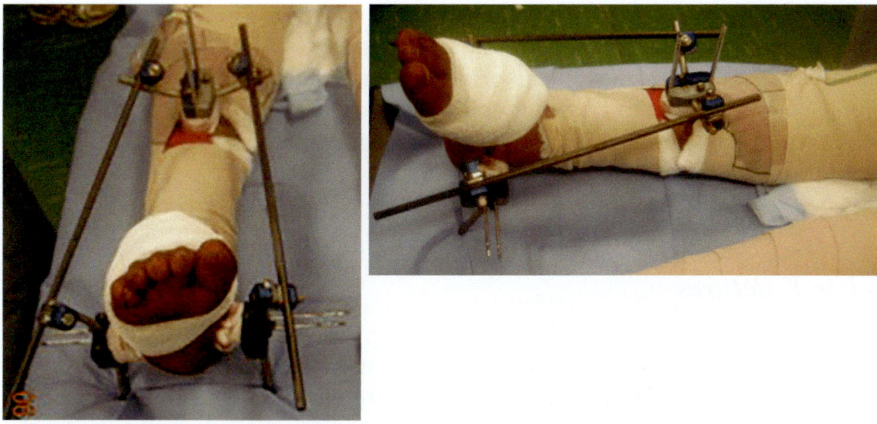

Fig. 24.6 Two views of the ankle-spanning "Delta frame" for external fixation across the right ankle joint for fractures about the ankle with two transfixation calcaneal pins necessary to connect bars to the pin clamps with no pin-to-bar connectors available. Two pins may lessen the need for a posterior splint, but a splint can be useful for additional soft tissue protection and to prevent forefoot plantarflexion. Note the addition of the two short "kickstand" bars posteriorly that decrease direct pressure on the heel. (Source: Joint Trauma System Clinical Practice Guidelines (JTS CPG): Orthopaedic Trauma: Extremity Fractures (CPG ID:56). 26 Feb 2020, used with permission)

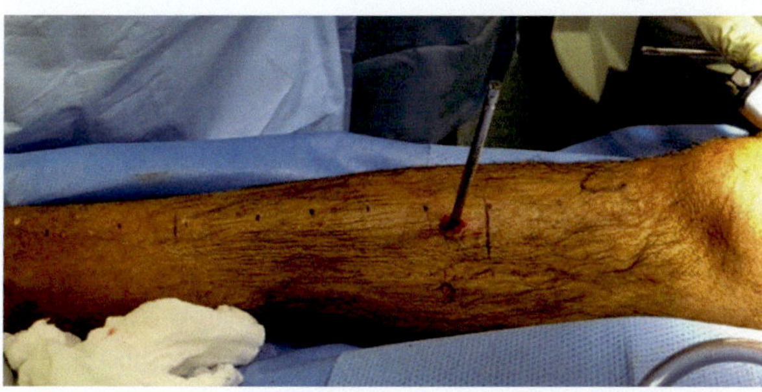

Fig. 24.7 Demonstration of safe zone for placement of pins along the anteromedial aspect of the tibia. (Source: Joint Trauma System Clinical Practice Guidelines (JTS CPG): Orthopaedic Trauma: Extremity Fractures (CPG ID:56). 26 Feb 2020, used with permission)

is made, and blunt dissection performed to identify the bone. The pin is loaded into a manual or power drill and the pin is used to palpate the bone to ensure it is placed centrally on the bone. The pin is advanced through the near cortex to the far cortex, identified by an increase in resistance, and then 6–8 turns across the far cortex to ensure cortical engagement. If X-ray capability exists, confirm that the pin tip is completely across the cortex with multiple screw threads engaging the far cortical bone [3].

Once the pins are placed, bars and clamps are used to connect the pins, and the fracture is reduced through traction and manual manipulation. Once adequate reduction is achieved, the clamps are subsequently tightened to secure the external fixator device and rigidly maintain the reduction. Pin sites can be dressed using a petroleum jelly bandage followed by sterile gauze and a kerlix roll to protect the skin with movement or transport. While keeping the connecting clamps and bars close to the skin will increase the rigidity of the construct, it is important to allow enough room between the skin and clamps/bars to allow for subsequent swelling.

Pelvic Fractures

The prevalence of pelvic trauma drastically increased with the advent of improvised explosive device (IED) attacks experienced throughout Operations Iraqi and Enduring Freedom (OIF/OEF) [1]. Pelvic fractures create unique challenges for the trauma team as they can be a major source of blood loss, are associated with visceral and neurovascular injuries, and have a high rate of mortality [9, 10]. Pelvic fracture stabilization principles are similar to extremity fractures, focusing on reduction and immobilization to help stabilize the patient.

Thorough examination of the pelvis and perineum is critical as open fractures can be easily masked as genital or rectal trauma [11]. If concerned, a rectal and genitourinary/gynecologic exam should be performed to assess for wounds, and if identified, antibiotic prophylaxis administered. Over 70% of pelvic-associated hemorrhage is associated with venous injury and can be controlled with maneuvers to reduce pelvic volume, including placement of pelvic binders or external fixators [12]. Pelvic hemorrhage that is associated with arterial bleeding may require surgical procedures, to include pelvic packing, endovascular embolization (which is not available on maritime platforms), or exploratory laparotomy with temporary ligation of the internal iliac arteries bilaterally. Pelvic packing is ideally performed through a midline incision inferior to the umbilicus over the pubic symphysis taking care not to enter the peritoneal cavity. Carefully separate the rectus muscles in the midline to enter the pre-vesicular space of Retzius. Bluntly open the space and remove any blood clots. Usually at least three laparotomy pads are packed tightly into the preperitoneal space on either side (total six laparotomy pads). Up to five laparotomy pads can be packed on either side, for a total of ten. It is important to close the midline anterior rectus fascia over the packing to maintain the tamponade effect. If exploratory laparotomy is required, typically the peritoneal cavity can be entered from a midline incision superior to the preperitoneal packing incision; take care not to enter the preperitoneal space and disrupt the tamponade effect [13]. Pelvic packing through an exploratory laparotomy has been described, but it is not as effective as preperitoneal packing.

It may be performed via the same incision as exploratory laparotomy although with retroperitoneal packing or through a suprapubic incision, with retroperitoneal packing focusing on the sacral plexus, iliac vessels, and corona mortise [13].

Initial stabilization for unstable pelvic ring injuries consists of accurate placement of a pelvic binder. An "open book" pelvis fracture, in which there is anterior pubic symphysis widening as the result of ligamentous and/or bony pelvic disruption, can result in significant hemorrhage. **A pelvic binder is used to decrease the potential volume of the pelvic cavity that occurs in open book pelvic injuries and therefore serves to tamponade the bleeding vessels**. When there is no X-ray capability, or when the provider is in doubt as to whether a pelvic ring injury exists or would benefit from a pelvic binder, the provider should err on the side of caution and apply the binder. A number of commercially available pelvic binders can be used; alternatively, a folded bed sheet secured with clamps can be utilized, known as circumferential pelvic antishock sheeting (CPAS) [14]. To properly perform CPAS, as outlined by Routt et al., start with the patient in a supine position as they would be found on a trauma board or bed. The sheet is folded to permit wrapping fully around the waist region with extra material to spare. It is critical that the sheet must be placed under the patient with the center of the sheet directed over the greater trochanters. While removing the slack from the sheet, tightly wrap the sheet around the greater trochanters and overlap the sheet at the proper tension to close down the pelvis. Once properly tensioned, clamps can be used to maintain sheet reduction (Fig. 24.8) [14]. Post-reduction X-ray should be obtained of the pelvis to ensure adequate reduction of the rotational pelvis injury (Fig. 24.9). Additional stabilization can be performed by internally rotating and taping the feet together. The binder or sheet may stay in place for 24 to 48 h, but it is critical to keep the binder free of wrinkles or pressure points that can, and will, necrose the skin. When the binder is placed for an extended period of time, skin checks should be performed every 12 h. To perform a skin check, one member of the team should hold the pelvis reduced while other members of the team loosen the binder and examine the underlying skin then reapply the CPAS. Alternatively, for prolonged care, pain control, and stability during transport, pelvic external fixation can be performed.

External fixation of the pelvis can be performed by either the iliac crest or supra-acetabular techniques. Both require an adequate knowledge of anatomy and understanding of the spatial relationships of the pelvis. In the acute trauma setting at sea, a pelvic binder or sheet is the treatment of choice due its effectiveness and ease of application. If pelvic external fixation is performed, the preferred technique in the austere environment is to place pins into the iliac crest as it can be performed quickly through manual palpation without fluoroscopic guidance, which is not typically available. With direct palpation, identify the iliac wing region that is approximately 4 cm posterior to the anterior superior iliac spine (ASIS), the most anterior and prominent portion of the iliac crest. A 2–4 cm incision is made along each iliac crest centered on this location [15]. This region of the ilium and iliac crest is known as the gluteal pillar and is the thickest portion of the ileum. To assist with spatial orientation, Kirschner wires (if available although not typically found on most naval vessels) can be placed on the inner and outer tables of the iliac wings to assist with the trajectory of the external fixation pin; alternatively, the index and thumb of the

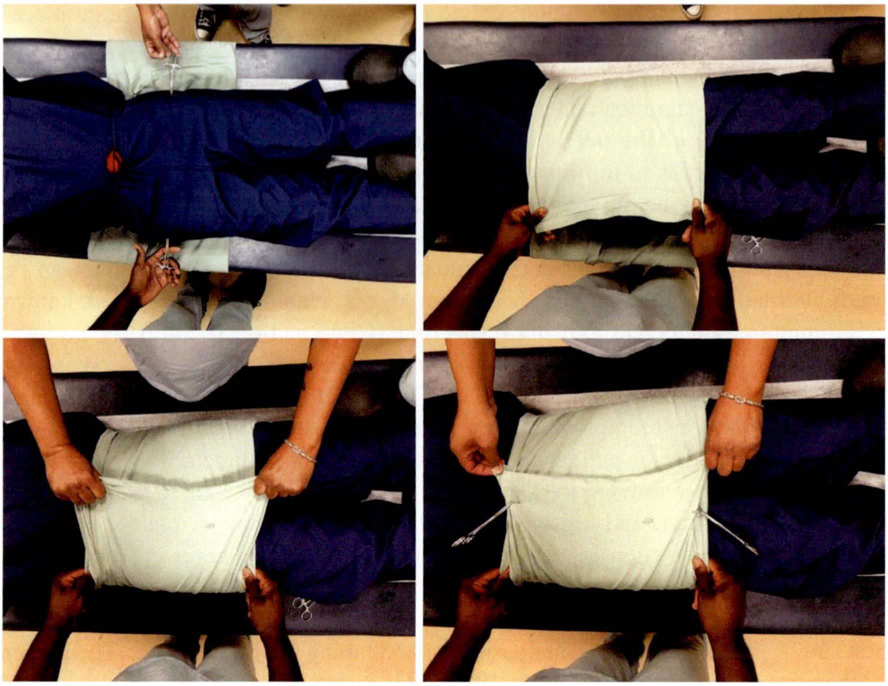

Fig. 24.8 Demonstration of circumferential pelvic antishock sheeting (CPAS) for pelvic fracture stabilization. From left to right, top to bottom: Patient supine with bed sheet centered over greater trochanters as marked by towel clamps; tension one side of the sheet from across the patient taking care to keep wrinkles out of the sheet; while holding tension of the first side of the sheet, pull the other side of the sheet and apply force to rotationally reduce the pelvis; once adequately reduced, apply clamps to the sheet and ensure proper tension maintained. (Source: Photos courtesy of James R. Bailey, MD)

opposite hand can be placed on the inner and outer table to guide the pin trajectory. If available, the cortex of the iliac crest is perforated by a drill and the pin is inserted between the inner and outer tables of the iliac wing. The general vector of the pin's insertion should be toward the patient's contralateral greater trochanter of the hip, but tactile feedback is an important component of accurate placement. The second pin is inserted in a similar fashion approximately 1 cm posterior to the first pin and then repeated on the opposite side. Once the pins are placed, the pelvis is manually reduced (each hemipelvis is internally rotated through a medially directed force) and the pins are subsequently connected via anteriorly based rods.

Key Points

- Basic fracture care requires careful neurovascular exam of the appendage and reduction of fracture with immobilization. Adequate immobilization involves splinting of the joint/bone above and below the zone of injury.

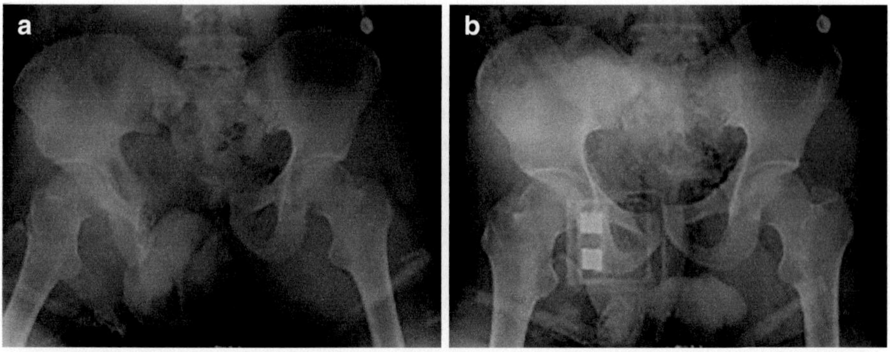

Fig. 24.9 Anteroposterior (AP) X-ray of an "open book" pelvic fracture (**a**) before and (**b**) after appropriate reduction. (Source: Images courtesy of Sean G. Sheppard, MD)

- The most critical aspect of open fracture treatment is administering antibiotics (first-generation cephalosporin) as soon as possible. Open fractures additionally require timely irrigation and debridement and tetanus coverage.
- External fixation can be considered for unstable fractures in patients requiring prolonged transport.
- Pelvic ring fractures can be a major source of bleeding. Timely stabilization of unstable pelvic injuries or injuries that may be contributing to blood loss can significantly improve hemodynamic stability. This can be done with either CPAS or external fixation.

Infection Control

Wartime infections have long been a cause of death and disability. In recent OIF/OEF conflicts, IEDs, complex dismounted blast injuries, and fungal super-infections made treatment of wartime injuries challenging. Multiple JTS CPGs guide treatments in hopes of achieving improved clinical outcomes [4, 16–18]. Ultimately, the hallmarks of treatment of open wounds and open fractures include early and appropriate administration of antibiotics and early and thorough wound debridement of contamination and devitalized tissue with frequent reevaluation and debridement of contaminated wounds [4, 17, 18]. Refer to Chap. 16 for a more in-depth discussion of antimicrobial agents' availability on maritime platforms.

Civilian studies demonstrate that early administration of antibiotics may be the single most important treatment to prevent long-term infection in open fractures [7]. The JTS CPG for Infection Prevention in Combat-Related Injuries recommends that all **trauma patients with penetrating injuries or open wounds (including open fracture or open joint injuries) receive antibiotics within 3 h of injury** [4]. While the mainstay of antibiotic treatment for these injuries is intravenous (IV) Cefazolin, many forward-deployed non-medical combat forces are only equipped with oral antibiotics. While shipboard injuries may not face these same constraints, the possibility of Prolonged Casualty Care (PCC), previously called Prolonged Field Care (PFC), does exist if safe medical evacuation (MEDEVAC) to the next level of care is not possible. In this case, knowledge of antibiotic treatment algorithms is required. Civilian literature for open fractures often recommends broad coverage with gram-negative microorganisms as well as the addition of penicillin for certain types of contamination. Through years of recent U.S. conflict and data from the JTS, reflexive empiric broad-spectrum coverage antibiotics are not recommended in these war injuries. The Infection Prevention in Combat-Related Injuries CPG provides an excellent Table for Post-Injury Antimicrobial Agent Selection and Duration included here as Table 24.1 [4].

In a shipboard environment, it may be necessary to provide additional coverage for waterborne bacteria if wounds were exposed to either fresh or salt water [19]. Oral Levofloxacin 750 mg daily with oral Doxycycline 100 mg twice a day as second-line coverage can be used to treat suspected or known exposure to *Aeromonas* and *Vibrio* species [17].

In blast injuries superimposed fungal infection should be considered. These types of infections often occurred in servicemembers wounded during the Iraq and Afghanistan wars with associated increased morbidity, mortality, and prolonged hospitalizations [18, 20–31]. Diagnosis usually involves histopathology which is not available in many deployed settings so suspicion should be high if risk factors for fungal infection exist. The JTS CPG for Invasive Fungal Infection in War Wounds lists four key risk factors for invasive fungal infections [18]:

- Dismounted blast injury
- Above knee immediate traumatic amputation or progressive transition from below knee to through knee to above knee amputation
- Extensive perineal, genitourinary, and/or rectal injury
- Massive transfusion (>20 units packed red blood cells (PRBC)) within 24 h of injury

If three or more of these risk factors exist, it is recommended to start topical antifungal treatment [18, 32–34]. This can easily be accomplished with 0.025% Dakins solution used in irrigation and/or placed directly into wounds with Dakins-soaked dressings [18, 32–35]. IV antifungals, including amphotericin B, are typically reserved for use at tertiary referral centers with infectious disease (ID) consultation; however, in PCC this may need to be considered if it is even available in the deployed maritime environment. Thorough and meticulous sharp debridement must be performed and often requires serial attempts to remove the large amount of dirt, foreign material, and clothing that can be found in high-energy blast wounds. These multiple "washouts" are also instrumental in documenting the progression and evolution of the zone of injury in these wounds, often requiring more tissue to be removed with each debridement.

Table 24.1 Post-injury antimicrobial agent selection and duration based upon injury pattern

Injury	Preferred agent(s)	Alternate agent(s)	Duration
Extremity wounds (includes skin, soft tissue, and bone)			
Skin, soft tissue, no open fractures	Cefazolin, 2 gm IV q6-8h[b,c]	Clindamycin (450 mg PO TID or 900 mg IV q8h)	24 h
Skin, soft tissue, with open fractures, exposed bone, or open joints	Cefazolin, 2 gm IV q6-8h[b,c,d]	Clindamycin 900 mg IV q8h	24 h initially and repeat with each subsequent I&D until soft tissue coverage.
Thoracic wounds			
Penetrating chest injury without esophageal disruption	Cefazolin, 2 gm IV q6-8h[b,c]	Clindamycin (450 mg PO TID or 900 mg IV q8h)	1 day
Penetrating chest injury with esophageal disruption	Cefazolin, 2 gm IV q6-8h[b,c] PLUS metronidazole 500 mg IV q8-12h	Ertapenem 1 gm IV x 1 dose, OR Moxifloxacin 400 mg IV x 1 dose	Stop 24 h after definitive closure
Abdominal wounds			
Penetrating abdominal injury with suspected/known hollow viscus injury and soilage; may apply to rectal/perineal injuries as well	Cefazolin, 2 gm IV q6-8h[b,c] PLUS metronidazole 500 mg IV q8-12h	Ertapenem 1 gm IV x 1 dose, OR Moxifloxacin 400 mg IV x 1 dose	Stop 24 h after control of contamination
Maxillofacial and neck wounds			
Open maxillofacial fractures or maxillofacial fractures with foreign body or fixation device	Cefazolin, 2 gm IV q6-8h[b,c]	Clindamycin 900 mg IV q8h	24 h
Central nervous system wounds			
Penetrating brain injury	Cefazolin 2 gm IV q6-8h. [b,c]Consider adding metronidazole 500 mg IV q8-12h if gross contamination with organic debris	Cetriaxone 2 mg IV q24h. Consider adding metronidazole 500 mg IV q8-12h if gross contamination with organic debris. For patients with a history of anaphylaxis or allergies to cephalosporins, vacomycin 15-20mg/kg IV q 8-12h PLUS ciprofloxacin 400 mg IV q8-12h	5 days or until CSF leak is closed, whichever Is longer
Penetrating spinal cord injury	Cefazolin, 2 gm IV q6-8h. [b,c]ADD metronidazole 500 mg IV q8-12h if abdominal cavity is involved	As above. ADD metronidazole 500 mg IV q8-12h if abdominal cavity is involved	
Eye wounds			
Eye injury, burn or abrasion	Topical: Erythromycin or Bacitracin ophthalmic intment QID and PRN for symptomatic relief. Systemic: No systemic treatment required	Fluoroquinolone 1 drop QID	Until epithelium healed (no fluoroescein staining)
Eye injury penetrating	Levofloxacin 750 mg IV/PO once daily+ vancomycin 15-2 0 mg/kg IV q8-12h. Prior to primary repair, no topical agents should be used unless directed by ophthalmology	Moxifloxacin 400 mg IV/PO once daily	7 days or until evaluated by an ophthalmologist
Burns			
Superficial burns	Topical antimicrobials with daily dressing changes (include mafenide acetate[e] or silver sulfadiazine; may alternate between the two), OR silver impregnated dressing changed q3-5d, OR Biobrane	Silver nitrate solution applied to dressings	Until healed
Deep partial thickness burns	Topical antimicrobials with daily dressing changes, OR silver impregnated dressing changed q3-5d, PLUS excision and grafting	Silver nitrate solution applied to dressings PLUS excision and grafting	Until healed or grafted
Full thickness burns	Topical antimicrobials with daily dressing changes PLUS excision and grafting	Silver nitrate solution applied to dressings PLUS excision and grafting	Until healed or grafted
Point of Injury/delayed evacuation			
Expected delay to reach surgical care	Moxifloxacin 400 mg PO x 1 dose. Ertapenem 1 g IV or IM if penetrating abdominal injury, shock, or unable to tolerate PO medications	Levofloxacin 500 mg PO x 1 dose. Cefotetan 2 g IV or IM q12h if penetrating abdominal injury, shock, or unable to tolerate PO medications	Single dose therapy

[a]*Post-injury antimicrobial agents ore recommended to prevent early post-traumatic infectious complications, including sepsis, secondary to common bacterial flora. Selection is based on narrowest spectrum and duration required to prevent early infections prior to adequate surgical wound management. This narrow spectrum is selected to avoid selection of resistant bacteria. The antimicrobials listed are not intended for use in established infections, where multidrug-resistant (MOR) or other nosocomiof pathogens may be causing infection*

[b]*Cefozolin may be dosed based on body moss: 1 gram if weight< 80kg (176 lbs), 2 grams if weight81.160 kg (177-352 lbs), 3 grams if weight > 160kg (>352 lbs); doses up to 12 grams daily are supported by FDA-approved package insert*

[c]*Pediatric dosing: cefozolin, 20-30 mg/kg IV q6-8h (maximum, 100 mg/kg/day); metronidozole, 7.5 mg/kg IV q6h; clindomycin 2540mg/kg/doy IV divided q6- 8h; ertopenem, 15 mg/kg /Var IM q12 (children up to 12 years) or 20 mg/kg IV or IM once daily (children over 12 years; maximum, 1 gm/day); ceftrioxone, 100 mg/kg/day IV divided q12-24h (dosing for CNS injury); levofloxocin, 8 mg/kg IV or PO q12h (levofloxodn is only FDA-approved in children for prophylaxis of inhalational anthrax in children > 6 months of age, but this dose is commonly used for other indications); vancomycin 60 mg/kg/day IV divided q6h (dosing for CNS injury); ciprofloxocin, 10mg/kg IV (or 10.20mg/kg PO) q12h*

[d]*These guidelines do not advocate adding enhanced Grom negative bacteria coverage (i.e., addition of fluoroquinolone or aminoglycoside antimicrobials) in type III fractures*

[e]Mofenide acetate is contraindicated in infants less than 2 months of age

[f]*Post-injury antimicrobial therapy as suggested by the Acute Traumatic Wound Management in the Prolonged Field Core Setting CPG*

IV intravenous, *PO* oral, *TID* three times daily, *I&D* incision and drainage, *CSF* cerebrospinal fluid, *PRN* as needed, *QID* four times daily

Source: Joint Trauma System Clinical Practice Guideline (JTS CPG): Infection prevention in combat-related injuries (CPG ID:24). 27 Jan 2021, used with permission

Key Points

- The hallmarks in the treatment of open wounds and open fractures include early and appropriate administration of antibiotics as well as early and thorough wound debridement of contamination and devitalized tissue with frequent reevaluation and debridement of contaminated wounds.
- Infection prophylaxis should avoid empiric broad-coverage antibiotics. IV Cefazolin is the mainstay treatment recommendation, but attention should be paid to special scenarios including waterborne/aquatic injuries and fungal super-infections.
- The importance of a thorough and meticulous sharp debridement cannot be understated. Wounds will evolve and multiple washouts often require interval removal of tissue and significant blood loss. Be prepared to manage these wounds; they will require significant resources and take a toll on medical logistics, OR availability, and medical personnel.

Acute Compartment Syndrome (ACS)

Pathophysiology

Muscles of the upper and lower extremity are grouped in strong fascial compartments with a limited capacity to expand. When excess fluid (blood, interstitial fluid, etc.) enters a compartment, intra-compartmental pressure rises. When the intra-compartmental pressure rises to a certain level, capillary perfusion is impeded and the contents of the compartment become ischemic, a process known as acute compartment syndrome (ACS). If the intra-compartmental pressure is not lowered, the ischemic changes become irreversible, cell death ensues, and the consequences are devastating. An untreated ACS will lead to an ischemic contracture of the affected compartments and can potentially result in life-threatening rhabdomyolysis with acute kidney injury and/or renal failure.

Associated Conditions

ACS is a surgical emergency, and timely diagnosis of the condition is crucial. There are a variety of injuries and clinical scenarios that can cause the condition, and the maritime surgical team should be familiar with them to have the appropriate level of suspicion for its potential development. ACS is most commonly seen in the lower leg and typically associated with a tibial shaft fracture but is also frequently seen in the forearm as the result of both-bone forearm fractures or distal radius fractures [36]. While areas such as the thigh, gluteal region, upper arm, hand, and foot are less common locations for the development of ACS, it can still occur in these regions so they must be monitored for signs and symptoms. Besides long bone fractures, ACS can occur following crush injuries, direct blows to a compartment, prolonged traction, patient malpositioning during surgery, prolonged tourniquet use, tight circumferential dressings, direct arterial injury, snakebites, fluid over-resuscitation, burns, and electrocutions. Even relatively benign mechanisms of injury, such as an ankle sprain or IV catheter infiltration, can cause ACS. Finally, ACS can commonly be attributed to reperfusion of an extremity after a vascular repair or shunting. In these situations, prophylactic compartment releases should be performed prior to definitive revascularization, particularly in the deployed setting.

Signs and Symptoms

Classically, the "5 Ps" were used to describe the signs and symptoms of ACS: pain, pallor, pulselessness, paralysis, and poikilothermia (decreased temperature of the extremity). However, most of these signs are considered late findings of an already established ACS; therefore, the clinical utility of these findings is questionable since the goal is to provide timely intervention and prevent complications. The most reliable early symptom of ACS is pain. The pain is often "out of proportion" to the injury, though this can be confusing and unhelpful when trying to determine how much pain a patient should have with a high-energy open fracture. Providers should pay close attention to escalating pain medication requirements, as this can signal rising compartment pressures. An additional sign used in diagnosis is pain with passive stretch of the muscles contained within the compartment. For example, in a patient with developing ACS of the lower leg, passive dorsiflexion and plantarflexion of the ankle will stretch the muscles contained within the compartments and result in significantly increased pain. Additional signs of early ACS include a tense, swollen compartment that is extremely tender to palpation. Examining the contralateral extremity can be helpful for comparison. Subtle, early paresthesias can often be identified with a careful neurologic exam (e.g., decreased sensation in the superficial peroneal nerve distribution in a patient with suspected lower leg ACS) and should further heighten suspicion. Patients with pain with passive stretch have up to a 68% chance of having ACS, and this increases to 93% with the additional finding of paresis [37].

Establishing a diagnosis of ACS in the obtunded patient can be extremely challenging, as the team cannot rely on patient-reported symptoms (particularly pain). In this scenario, a portable device that measures compartment pressure can be utilized. A variety of commercial devices can be purchased; if the ship is equipped with such a device (unlikely), it is imperative that the members of the maritime surgical team be comfortable with its use. While specific, step-by-step instructions are beyond the scope of this chapter, the provider must be familiar with the concept of delta-P: the difference between the compartment pressure and the patient's diastolic pressure. A delta-P of less than 30 mm Hg (i.e., the compartment pressure measurement is within 30 mm Hg of the patient's diastolic blood pressure) is considered diagnostic of ACS [38].

If a commercial compartment pressure-measuring device is not available (a likely scenario on most ships), compartments can be measured by using a 16- or 18-gauge IV catheter attached by arterial line or central venous catheter (CVC) tubing to a pressure transducer and syringe filled with saline all connected via a three-way stopcock [39]. The device is zeroed and the needle is introduced into each compartment no more than 5 cm from the fracture. Infuse 1 mL of saline to create a small area of "space" around the needle. On the monitor, the pressure will rise and the wave will flatten when the pressures equalize. Move the needle back 1–2 mm to see if the pressure falls to a lower level, which can happen if the needle has material in it or it is lodged in the muscle. The lower reading is the correct reading. Higher readings with a waveform that is flatlined is a similar situation as to when an arterial line that is up against the arterial wall and needs to be pulled back 1–2 mm. With the catheter in the muscle, gently squeeze the extremity and record if there are changes in the pressure commensurate with the squeeze. If the measurement is within 30 mm Hg of the patient's diastolic blood pressure, the obtunded patient should be considered to have a diagnosis of ACS and immediate fasciotomy is required. Appendix A discusses another makeshift device that utilizes a blood pressure manometer instead of an electronic transducer.

It is important to stress that compartment pressure-measuring devices are not recommended for routine care in the awake patient, as the diagnosis is largely driven by history and a non-invasive physical examination [40]. In obtunded patients, if no compartment pressure-measuring devices are available, fasciotomy should be performed in patients with high clinical suspicion.

Treatment

Any patient with concern for a developing ACS must be closely managed. Serial examinations should be performed with the involved limb at the level of the heart and any circumferential or tight dressings should be immediately loosened. **Once diagnosed, ACS is managed through urgent operative intervention**. To prevent irreversible tissue necrosis, which can occur within 6–8 h of an established ACS, a complete surgical release of the involved compartments is required. In the lower leg, this is accomplished through a two-incision, four-compartment fasciotomy, with complete release of the anterior, lateral, superficial posterior, and deep posterior compartments. Surgeons must be familiar with this technique and ensure that all compartments are adequately released, as incomplete release can be associated with devastating complications. In combat casualties requiring compartment release, the two most commonly missed compartments in the lower leg when attempting a four-compartment fasciotomy are the anterior and deep posterior compartments [41].

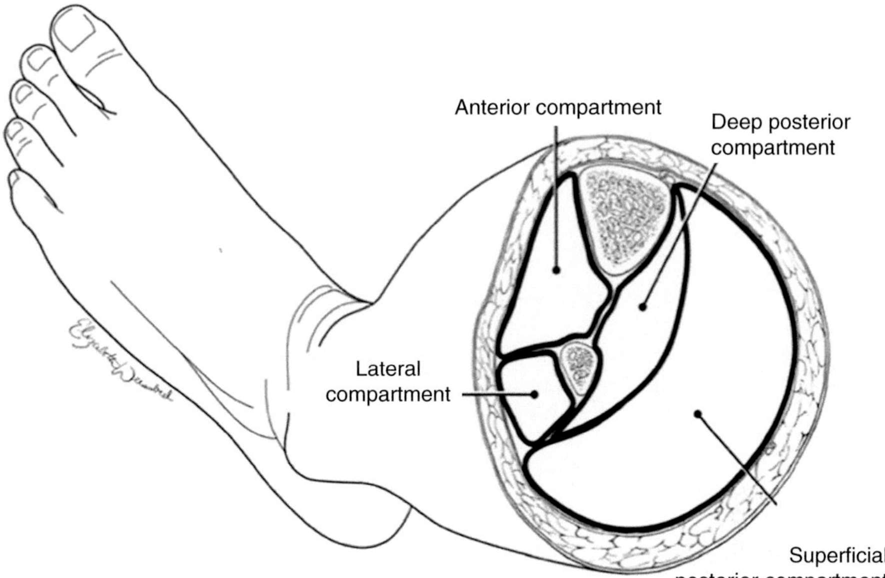

Fig. 24.10 Cross sectional anatomy of mid-portion of left lower leg. (Source: Lower Extremity Fasciotomy: Indications and Technique. Bowyer MW. Current Trauma Reports, 2015, used with permission)

A cross-sectional diagram of the pertinent compartments of the lower leg is best demonstrated in Fig. 24.10 [42]. The skin incisions should be essentially the length of underlying fascial incisions. The lateral incision is made one finger breadth anterior to the fibula starting three finger breadths distal to the head of the fibula down to three finger breaths proximal to the lateral malleolus (Fig. 24.11) [42]. Once skin flaps are raised, an intermuscular septum should be visualized (Fig. 24.12) or palpated representing the separation between anterior and lateral compartments. However, this may be difficult to palpate or visualize in a patient with swollen compartments, therefore a transverse incision is made to definitively identify the septum. Both compartments can then be decompressed longitudinally completing the "H-type" incision as seen in Fig. 24.13. A common pitfall is making the initial skin incision too far posterior and the lateral and superficial posterior compartments are confused for the intermuscular septum separating the anterior and lateral compartments.

The medial incision is made one finger breadth below the palpable medial ridge of the tibia (Fig. 24.14). After getting through the skin and subcutaneous tissue, the fascia to the superficial posterior compartment will be visualized and exposed longitudinally. Common pitfalls are to split gastrocnemius and soleus and not get deep to the soleus to decompress the deep posterior compartment, properly demonstrated in Fig. 24.15. The key to getting into the deep posterior compartment is dissecting the soleus bridge completely free from the underside of the tibia (Fig. 24.16).

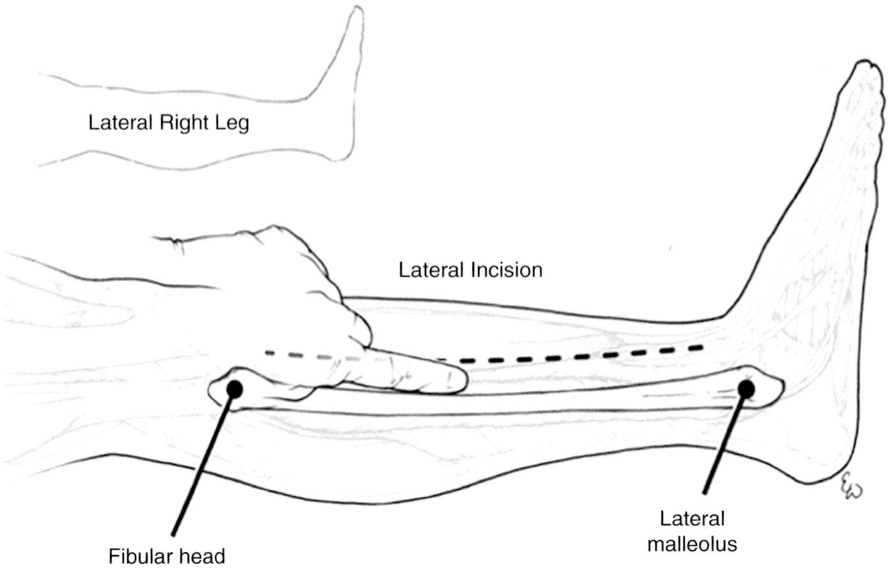

Fig. 24.11 Lateral incision depicted one finger breadth anterior to fibula. (Source: Lower Extremity Fasciotomy: Indications and Technique. Bowyer MW. Current Trauma Reports, 2015, used with permission)

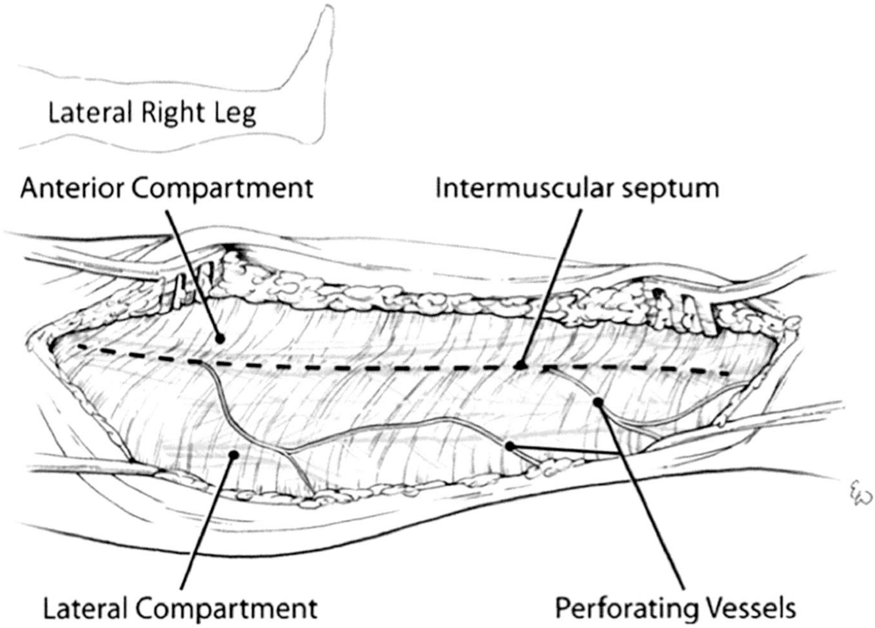

Fig. 24.12 Intermuscular septum separating anterior and lateral compartments. (Source: Lower Extremity Fasciotomy: Indications and Technique. Bowyer MW. Current Trauma Reports, 2015, used with permission)

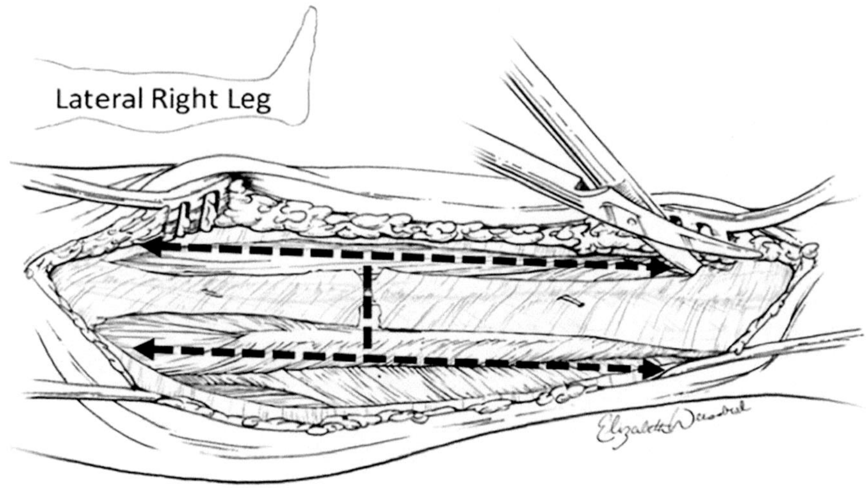

Fig. 24.13 Longitudinal fascial release with H-type incision connecting compartments through intermuscular septum. (Source: Lower Extremity Fasciotomy: Indications and Technique. Bowyer MW. Current Trauma Reports, 2015, used with permission)

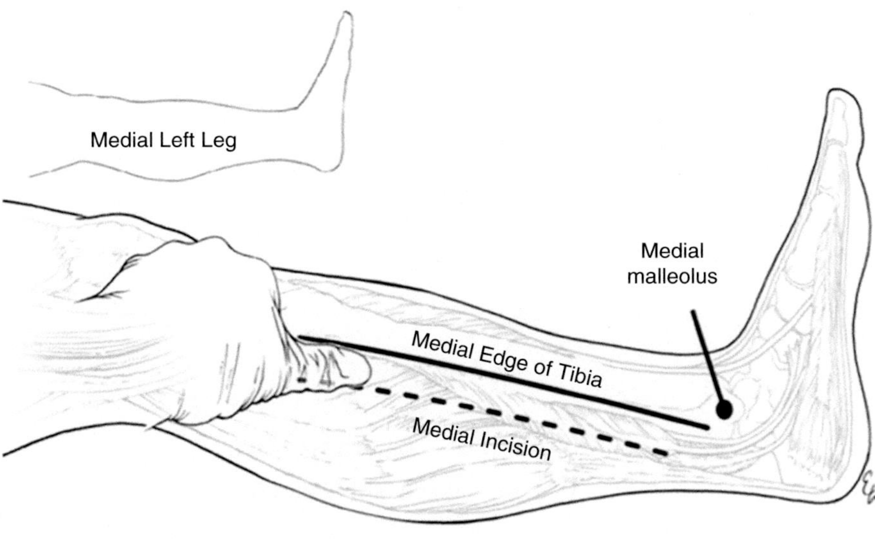

Fig. 24.14 Medial incision one finger breadth posterior to medial edge of tibia. (Source: Lower Extremity Fasciotomy: Indications and Technique. Bowyer MW. Current Trauma Reports, 2015, used with permission)

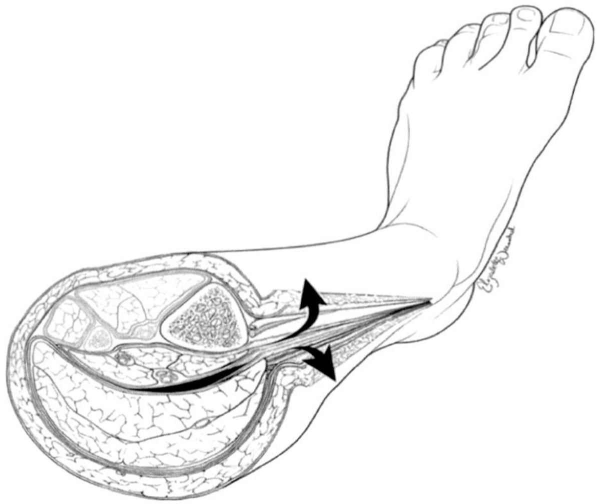

Fig. 24.15 Entry into deep posterior compartment requires separating superficial posterior compartment from underside of tibia demonstrated here in cross-section. (Source: Lower Extremity Fasciotomy: Indications and Technique. Bowyer MW. Current Trauma Reports, 2015, used with permission)

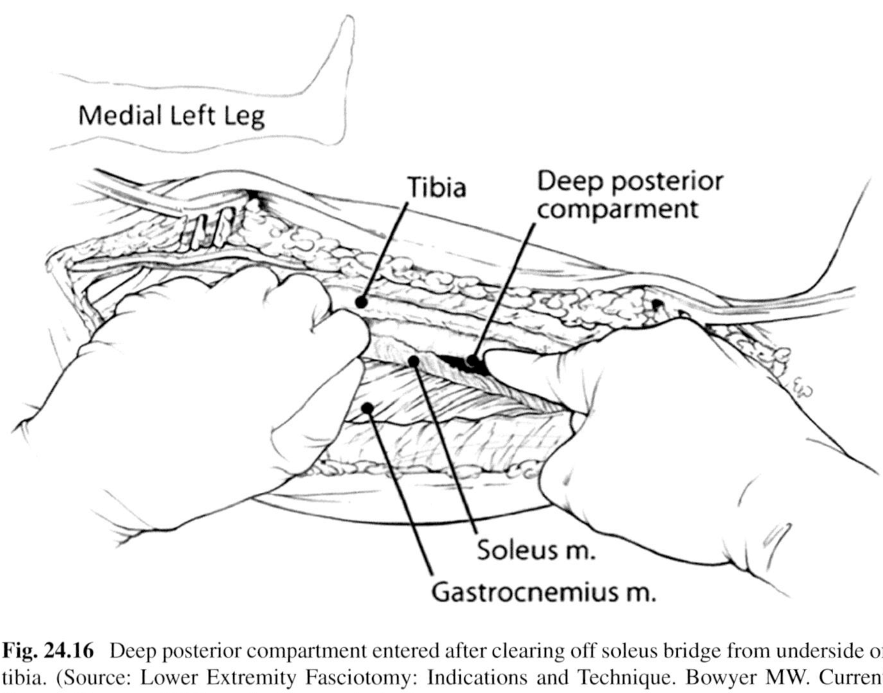

Fig. 24.16 Deep posterior compartment entered after clearing off soleus bridge from underside of tibia. (Source: Lower Extremity Fasciotomy: Indications and Technique. Bowyer MW. Current Trauma Reports, 2015, used with permission)

Visualizing the posterior tibial neurovascular bundle confirms the release of the deep posterior compartment [42]. These wounds are not generally closed at the initial procedure given the amount of tissue swelling and serial procedures are needed utilizing negative pressure therapy to get the wounds closed. If the wounds cannot be primarily closed within 7–10 days, then split-thickness skin grafts (STSG) may be considered (see Chap. 26 for technique). **Prophylactic fasciotomy is recommended in a patient at high risk for developing ACS during subsequent MEDEVAC**. While this is an extremely challenging scenario, patients with crush injuries, high energy tibia, or forearm fractures, or patients with prolonged limb ischemia time and subsequent reperfusion are indicated for prophylactic compartment release [40].

Key Points

- Early diagnosis of ACS is critical and almost exclusively relies on a high index of suspicion combined with recognition of escalating pain, pain with passive stretch, and painful, tense compartments.
- Established ACS is a surgical emergency and requires operative intervention with full release of all involved compartments.
- Prophylactic fasciotomy is recommended in high-risk patients requiring MEDEVAC.
- Beware of the common pitfalls of missing the anterior (incorrectly identifying the intermuscular septum) and the deep posterior muscle compartments (not freeing the soleus from the tibia and identifying the posterior tibial neurovascular bundle).

Dislocations

Traumatic dislocations are a common cause of injury in young healthy adults, though the exact incidence is difficult to determine as many are treated in prehospital care. Epidemiological studies note the most common site of dislocation is the shoulder (50.6%) [43]. In the U.S., the estimated incidence of shoulder dislocations is 23.9 per 100,000 person-years with young age and male gender identified as additional risk factors [44]. Isolated ankle dislocations are rare [43], and fracture dislocations are more common. While other dislocation patterns may be encountered in a shipboard setting, the management of traumatic shoulder dislocation and ankle fracture-dislocations are key skills covered in this chapter.

Shoulder

The shoulder is inherently unstable with a small glenoid and relatively larger humeral head facilitating wide ranges of motion in the shoulder. Secondary stabilization is provided by soft tissue structures including the labrum, capsule, ligaments, and rotator cuff muscles. The axillary nerve is the nerve most injured following a shoulder dislocation and should be checked for function to include sensation over the lateral shoulder and motor function of the deltoid muscle.

Anterior shoulder dislocations are the most common type of shoulder dislocation and often result from a blow to an abducted and externally rotated arm [45]. Posterior shoulder dislocations can be traumatic in nature or following electrocution or a seizure. Inferior shoulder dislocations (luxation erecta) occur with an axial load to an abducted arm or a forceful hyperabduction of the arm such as catching oneself with the arm overhead after falling down a ladder or stairwell.

Anteriorly dislocated shoulders rest in the abducted and externally rotated position and the shoulder often appears squared. Patients typically resist any movement. In hospital settings, X-rays are commonly obtained before and after reduction. Injury radiographs ensure there are no associated fractures and post-reduction X-rays confirm successful reduction [46]. If injury X-rays are not available, treatment should not be delayed. However, when available, post-reduction radiographs, specifically an axillary lateral radiograph (patient's arm abducted with the radiograph plate placed on the shoulder and the beam projected through the axilla) should be performed. If this cannot be completed due to pain, a Velpeau axillary view can be obtained (the patient leans back 15° over the table edge and the beam is directed from above the shoulder to the plate placed on the table edge).

Posterior shoulder dislocations are less common. Examination demonstrates a flattened anterior arm held in the adducted and internally rotated position. Radiographic evaluation with a standard anteroposterior (AP) view often results in missed injuries and an axillary lateral radiograph will confirm the diagnosis. In the case of inferior dislocations (luxation erecta), the patient presents with the involved arm above their head and an inability to adduct the arm. This injury presents with axillary or other nerve palsy in up to 60% of cases and associated rotator cuff tear or greater tuberosity fracture in up to 80% of cases [47, 48].

Reduction should be performed as quickly and safely as possible. Specific risks for the procedure are rare, but include humerus, glenoid, or coracoid fractures, rotator cuff tears (though likely present prior to the reduction), and axillary nerve or artery injury. Reduction can often be obtained without analgesia in relatively atraumatic dislocations or recurrent dislocations that are less than 24 h post-injury and is most successful with techniques that do not require significant traction, to include the scapular manipulation, external rotation, and the Milch technique [49, 50]. Intraarticular lidocaine is often effective in providing pain relief and facilitating reduction, though it fails more often if employed more than 6 h after injury [51, 52]. It is best performed through the lateral approach with 20 mL of 1% lidocaine and an 18- or 20-gauge needle. Starting 1 cm inferior to the acromion process the needle is directed inferomedial 2.5–3 cm [52]. If available, procedural sedation may assist in the completion of the reduction maneuver, especially in heavily muscled individuals or in delayed presentations as it effects a relaxation of spasmed rotator cuff musculature.

There are multiple methods for reducing an anterior shoulder dislocation without evidence demonstrating the superiority of one method over another. One algorithm is to start with an attempt at scapular manipulation and if not successful, transition to the external rotation technique (with or without the Milch technique) and if necessary, transition to the Stimson technique or traction-countertraction [53].

1. Scapular Manipulation-Upright
   (a) Place the head of the bed at 90° with the patient seated with their legs off the edge of the bed and the uninjured shoulder leaning against the upright part of the bed [54].
   (b) Standing behind the patient, push the tip of the acromion inferiorly, rotating the scapula while an assistant is providing gentle forward or downward arm traction.
2. Scapular Manipulation-Prone
   (a) With the patient lying prone, the injured arm hangs off the side of the stretcher with 10 to 15 pounds of weight on a splint acting as traction.
   (b) The scapula is manipulated by pushing the acromion inferiorly and rotating it medially [54].
3. External Rotation Technique
   (a) This method can be completed with only one clinician and is successful in up to 90% of attempts, often without sedation [55].
   (b) The patient lies supine with elbows flexed to 90°. The provider grasps the elbow with one hand to keep it adducted against the body and holds the wrist with the other hand.
   (c) The patient is asked to let their arm fall to the side (externally rotate) slowly (over 5–10 minutes) until reduction occurs (typically between 70° and 100°).
4. Milch Technique
   (a) If the External Rotation Technique is unsuccessful, this can be added.
   (b) The fully externally rotated arm is abducted to the overhead position, maintaining external rotation through the maneuver.
   (c) Gentle traction is performed with direct pressure over the humeral head using the provider's thumb in the axilla until reduction is obtained.
5. Stimson Technique
   (a) The patient is placed prone with 10 to 15 pounds of weight attached to the injured extremity.
   (b) As the spasmed muscles fatigue, reduction typically occurs within 30 minutes.
6. Traction-Countertraction
   (a) A sheet is wrapped under the axilla. One assistant provides gentle continuous traction at the wrist or elbow and another provides countertraction with the sheet.

Posterior shoulder dislocations are reduced with gentle traction to an adducted arm with the elbow flexed. The arm is internally rotated and adducted while direct pressure is applied to the posterior humeral head or gentle lateral traction is applied to unlock the dislocated humerus. Inferior shoulder dislocations are achieved by traction-countertraction in line with the abducted humerus.

Following reduction of the anteriorly dislocated shoulder it should be immobilized in the position of adduction and internal rotation for 1–3 weeks with early, though not emergent, consultation to an orthopaedic surgeon for surgical evaluation.

Ankle

While isolated ankle dislocations are rare, ankle fractures with associated ankle (tibiotalar) dislocations are more common and seen in up to 36% of ankle fractures [56]. Ankle fractures most often occur through rotational mechanisms transmitted through the foot to the talus and then the malleoli. Grossly identifiable ankle fracture-dislocations should be reduced as soon as possible to limit soft tissue tension. While injury X-rays may identify concomitant injuries, gross reduction attempts should not be delayed to minimize cartilage damage and prevent skin necrosis.

Tibiotalar reductions are commonly performed with either an intra-articular block or procedural sedation. Both are viable options and head-to-head comparisons provide advantages of each, including faster reduction with intra-articular block, though lower rates of reduction on initial tries when performed by a non-orthopaedic surgeon [57].

Classically, the fracture-dislocation is reduced utilizing the Quigley maneuver. The knee is flexed, thereby relaxing the gastrocnemius-soleus complex, then the foot is adducted and supinated. In short, after obtaining adequate analgesia, the great toe on the injured foot can be lifted, placing the foot in the position described above. Following reduction, a short leg splint should be applied with the foot in 90° of flexion and an appropriate three-point mold in place. Occasionally, the fracture-dislocation is too unstable to hold the foot at 90° of flexion and must be splinted in slight plantarflexion.

Post-reduction X-rays, to include AP, lateral, and mortise views, should be obtained to ensure the reduction is stable. If unstable, it should be re-reduced and if it remains unstable, consideration should be made for placement of an external fixator for stability. After initial stabilization, planning for transfer off the ship should commence as this is an injury best definitively stabilized within the first couple of weeks of injury.

Key Points

- Early identification and treatment of dislocations is recommended.
- Shoulder dislocation reductions can be performed with a range of anesthetic options ranging from no anesthesia to conscious sedation. A tiered approach is recommended for the reduction of dislocated shoulder joints, with confirmation reduction X-rays when available.

- Ankle fracture-dislocations are common and should be reduced and splinted in a timely manner to prevent skin breakdown and cartilage damage. Reduction is typically accomplished via the Quigley maneuver.
- When treating ankle fracture dislocations, both intra-articular/hematoma block and procedural sedation provide effective analgesia, however, intra-articular block provides long-lasting pain relief.

Conclusion

Although the typical maritime surgical team does not have an orthopaedic surgeon, significant orthopaedic injuries are common in isolated presentations or in combination with other injuries. Damage control orthopaedic surgery temporizes injuries until the next echelon of care is reached and contributes to lifesaving measures. Orthopaedic injuries benefit from timely identification, physical exam, reduction, treatment and stabilization, and sometimes MEDEVAC. Utilizing the premises in this chapter, the maritime surgical team can prepare to manage these injuries at sea.

Declaration of Interest The views expressed in this chapter are those of the authors and do not necessarily reflect the official policy or position of the Department of the Navy, Department of Defense, nor the US Government.

Funding This research did not receive any specific grant from funding agencies in the public, commercial, or not-for-profit sectors.

Conflict of Interest Statement The authors declare no conflict of interest.

References

1. Cap AP, Pidcoke HF, DePasquale M, Rappold JF, Glassberg E, Eliassen HS, Bjerkvig CK, Fosse TK, Kane S, Thompson P, et al. Blood far forward: time to get moving! J Trauma Acute Care Surg. 2015;78(6):S2–6.
2. Miller BT, et al. Red tides: mass casualty and whole blood at sea. J Trauma Acute Care Surg. 2018;85(1S Suppl 2):S134–9.
3. Osborn, et al. Joint Trauma system clinical practice guideline (JTS CPT): orthopaedic trauma: extremity fractures (CPG ID: 56), 26 Feb 2020.
4. Barsoumian, et al. Joint trauma system clinical practice guideline (JTS CPT): infection prevention in combat-related injuries (CPG ID: 24). 27 Jan 2021.
5. Gustilo RB, Anderson JT. Prevention of infection in the treatment of one thousand and twenty-five open fractures of long bones: retrospective and prospective analyses. J Bone Joint Surg Am. 1976;58:453–8.
6. Gustilo RB, Mendoza RM, Williams DN. Problems in the management of type III (severe) open fractures: a new classification of type III open fractures. J Trauma. 1984;24:742–6. https://insights.ovid.com/pubmed?pmid=773941 Accessed Feb 2020.

7. Yun HC, Murray CK, Nelson KJ, Bosse MJ. Infection after orthopaedic trauma: prevention and treatment. J Orthop Trauma. 2016;30:S21–6.
8. Lack WD, Karunakar MA, Angerame MR, et al. Type III open tibia fractures: immediate antibiotic prophylaxis minimizes infection. J Orthop Trauma. 2015;29:1–6.
9. Bailey JR, Stinner DJ, Blackbourne LH, Hsu JR, Mazurek MT. Combat-related pelvis fractures in nonsurvivors. J Trauma. 2011;71(1):58–61. https://doi.org/10.1097/TA.0b013e31822154d8.
10. Davis JM, Stinner DJ, Bailey JR, Aden JK, Hsu JR, Skeletal Trauma Research Consortium. Factors associated with mortality in combat-related pelvic fractures. J Am Acad Orthop Surg. 2012;20:S7–S12. https://doi.org/10.5435/JAAOS-20-08-S7.
11. Copeland CE, Bosse MJ, McCarthy ML, MacKenzie EJ, Guzinski GM, Hash CS, Burgess AR. Effect of trauma and pelvic fracture on female genitourinary, sexual, and reproductive function. J Orthop Trauma. 1997;11(2):73–81.
12. Gordon, et al. Joint trauma system clinical practice guideline (JTS CPT): pelvic fracture care (CPG ID: 34), 15 Mar 2017.
13. Polk TM, Martin MJ, Eckert MJ. Dismounted complex blast injury mangement. In: Martin MJ, Beekley AC, Eckert MJ, editors. Front line surgery: a practical approach. 2nd ed. Cham: Springer; 2017. p. 229.
14. Routt MLC, Falicov A, Woodhouse E, Schildhauer TA. Circumferential pelvic antishock sheeting: a temporary resuscitation aid. J Orthopaedic Trauma. 2002;16(1):45–8.
15. Höntzsch D. AO surgery reference, Pelvis external fixation.
16. Gordon, et al. Joint Trauma system clinical practice guideline (JTS CPT): high bilateral amputations and dismounted complex blast injury (CPG ID: 22). 06 Aug 2016.
17. Rapp, et al. Joint Trauma system clinical practice guideline (JTS CPT): acute traumatic wound management in the prolonged field care setting (CPG ID: 62). 24 July 2017.
18. Rodriguez, et al. Joint trauma system clinical practice guideline (JTS CPT): invasive fungal infection in war wounds (CPG ID: 28). 04 Aug 2016.
19. Noonburg GE. Management of extremity trauma and related infections occurring in the aquatic environment. J Am Acad Orthop Surg. 2005;13(4):243–53. https://doi.org/10.5435/00124635-200507000-00004. PMID: 16112981.
20. Trauma Infectious Diseases Outcomes Study Group: Department of Defense Technical Report - invasive fungal infection case investigation. Bethesda, MD: Infectious Disease Clinical Research Program, Uniformed Services University of the Health Sciences; April 11, 2011. [Not publically available].
21. Warkentien T, Rodriguez C, Lloyd B, Wells J, Weintrob A, Dunne J, et al. Invasive mold infections following combat-related injuries. Clin Infect Dis. 2012;55(11):1441–9.
22. Weintrob AC, Weisbrod AB, Dunne JR, Rodriguez CJ, Malone D, Lloyd BA, et al. Combat trauma-associated invasive fungal wound infections: epidemiology and clinical classification. Epidemiol Infect. 2015;143(1):214–24.
23. Paolino KM, Henry JA, Hospenthal DR, Wortmann GW, Hartzell JD. Invasive fungal infections following combat-related injury. Mil Med. 2012;177(6):681–5.
24. Evriviades D, Jeffery S, Cubison T, Lawton G, Gill M, Mortiboy D. Shaping the military wound: issues surrounding the reconstruction of injured servicemen at the Royal Centre for Defence Medicine. Philos Trans R Soc Lond Ser B Biol Sci. 2011;366(1562):219–30.
25. Tribble DR, Rodriguez CJ. Combat-related invasive fungal wound infections. Curr Fungal Infect Rep. 2014;8(4):277–86.
26. Fares Y, El-Zaatari M, Fares J, Bedrosian N, Yared N. Trauma-related infections due to cluster munitions. J Infect Public Health. 2013;6(6):482–6.
27. Lundy JB, Driscoll IR. Experience with proctectomy to manage combat casualties sustaining catastrophic perineal blast injury complicated by invasive mucor soft-tissue infections. Mil Med. 2014;179(3):e347–50.
28. Tully CC, Romanelli AM, Sutton DA, Wickes BL, Hospenthal DR. Fatal Actinomucor elegans var. kuwaitiensis infection following combat trauma. J Clin Microbiol. 2009;47(10):3394–9.

29. Radowsky JS, Strawn AA, Sherwood J, Braden A, Liston W. Invasive mucormycosis and aspergillosis in a healthy 22-year-old battle casualty: case report. Surg Infect. 2011;12(5):397–400.
30. Mitchell TA, Hardin MO, Murray CK, Ritchie JD, Cancio LC, Renz EM, et al. Mucormycosis attributed mortality: a seven-year review of surgical and medical management. Burns. 2014;40(8):1689–95.
31. Hospenthal DR, Chung KK, Lairet K, Thompson EH, Guarro J, Renz EM, et al. Saksenaea erythrospora infection following combat trauma. J Clin Microbiol. 2011;49(10):3707–9.
32. Lewandowski L, Purcell R, Fleming M, Gordon WT. The use of dilute Dakin's solution for the treatment of angioinvasive fungal infection in the combat wounded: a case series. Mil Med. 2013;178(4):e503–7.
33. Barsoumian A, Sanchez CJ, Mende K, Tully CC, Beckius ML, Akers KS, et al. In vitro toxicity and activity of Dakin's solution, mafenide acetate, and amphotericin B on filamentous fungi and human cells. J Orthop Trauma. 2013;27(8):428–36.
34. Vick LR, Propst RC, Bozeman R, Wysocki AB. Effect of Dakin's solution on components of a dermal equivalent. J Surg Res. 2009;155(1):54–64.
35. Kheirabadi BS, Mace JE, Terrazas IB, Fedyk CG, Estep JS, Dubick MA, et al. Safety evaluation of new hemostatic agents, smectite granules, and kaolin-coated gauze in a vascular injury wound model in swine. J Trauma. 2010;68(2):269–78.
36. Shore BJ, et al. Acute compartment syndrome in children and teenagers with tibial shaft fracture: incidence and multivariable risk factors. J Orthop Trauma. 2013;27(11):616–21.
37. Ulmer T. The clinical diagnosis of compartment syndrome of the lower leg: are clinical findings predictative of the disorder? J Orthop Trauma. 2002 Sep;16(8):572–7.
38. McQueen M, et al. The estimated sensitivity and specificity of compartment pressure monitoring for acute compartment syndrome. J Bone Joint Surg Am. 2013;95(8):673–7.
39. Wilson SC, Vrahas MS, Berson L, Paul EM. A simple method to measure compartment pressures using an intravenous catheter. Orthopedics. 1997;20(5):403–6.
40. Gordon W, et al. Joint trauma system clinical practice guideline (JTS CPT): acute extremity compartment syndrome and the role of fasciotomy in extremity war wounds (CPG ID: 17). 2016.
41. Ritenour AE, Dorlac WC, Fang R, et al. Complications after fasciotomy revision and delayed compartment release in combat patients. J Trauma. 2008;64(2 Suppl):S153–61.
42. Bowyer MW. Lower extremity fasciotomy: indications and technique. Curr Trauma Rep. 2015;1:35–44.
43. Nabian NH, et al. Epidemiology of joint dislocations and ligamentous/tendinous injuries among 2,700 Patients: Five-year Trend of a Tertiary Center in Iran. Arch Bone Jt Surg. 2017;5(6):426–34.
44. Zacchilli MA, Owens BD. Epidemiology of shoulder dislocations presenting to emergency departments in the United States. J Bone Joint Surg Am. 2010;92:542–9.
45. Sherman SC. Shoulder Dislocations and reduction. UpToDate. https://www.uptodate.com/contents/shoulder-dislocation-and-reduction. Accessed 02 May 21.
46. Chong M, Karataglis D, Learmonth D. Survey of the management of acute traumatic first-time anterior shoulder dislocation among trauma clinicians in the UK. Ann R Coll Surg Eng. 2006;88(5):454.
47. Ameh V, Crane S. Nerve injury following shoulder dislocation: the emergency physician's perspective. Eur J Emerg Med. 2006;13(4):233.
48. Mallon WJ, Bassett FH III, Goldner RD. Luxatio erecta: the inferior glenohumeral dislocation. J Orthop Trauma. 1990;4(1):19.
49. Wen DY. Current concepts in the treatment of anterior shoulder dislocations. Am J Emerg Med. 1999;17(4):401.
50. O'Connor DR, Schwarze D, Fragomen AT, Perdomo M. Painless reduction of acute anterior shoulder dislocations without anesthesia. Orthopedics. 2006;29(6):528.

51. Miller SL, Cleeman E, Auerbach J, Flatow EL. Comparison of intra-articular lidocaine and intravenous sedation for reduction of shoulder dislocations: a randomized, prospective study. J Bone Joint Am. 2002;84-A(12):2135.
52. Kosnik J, Shamsa F, Raphael E, Huang R, Malachias Z, Georgiadis GM. Anesthetic methods for reduction of acute shoulder dislocations: a prospective randomized study comparting intraarticular lidocaine with intravenous analgesia and sedation. Am J Emerg Med. 1999;17(6):566.
53. Sagarin MJ. Best of both (BOB) maneuver for rapid reduction of anterior shoulder dislocation. J Emerg Med. 2005;29(3):313.
54. Kothari RU, Dronen SC. Prospective evaluation of the scapular manipulation technique in reducing anterior shoulder dislocations. Ann Emerg Med. 1992;21(11):1349.
55. Eachempati KK, Dua A, Malhotra R, Bhan S, Bera JR. The external rotation method for reduction of acute anterior dislocations and fracture-dislocations of the shoulder. J Bone Joint Surg Am. 2004;86-A(11):2431.
56. Lawson KA, Ayala AE, Morin ML, Latt JD, Wild JS. Ankle fracture-dislocations: a review. Foot Ankle Orthopaedics. 2018:1–8.
57. MacCormick LM, Baynard T, Williams BR, Vang S, Xi M, Lafferty P. Intra-articular hematoma block compared to procedural sedation for closed reduction of ankle fractures. Foot Ankle Int. 2018;39(10):1162–8.

Chapter 25
Austere Neurosurgical Emergencies

Jonathon Cooke

Neurosurgery is far too important to be taken seriously.

Dr. Philip Villanueva

Author deployment experience	
Jonathon Cooke	Battalion Surgeon, United States Marine Corps Marine Expeditionary Unit 11, Tarawa Expeditionary Strike Group, embarked on the USS Germantown (LSD-42), maritime operations, CENTCOM Area of Responsibility, 2007–2008
	Neurosurgeon/Neurointensivist, forward deployed Naval Hospital Okinawa, 2015–2017
	Director of Surgical Services, NATO Role 3 Multinational Medical Unit, NATO Resolute Support and Operation Freedom's Sentinel, Kandahar Airfield, Afghanistan, 2020

BLUF (Bottom Line Up Front)

1. Hypotension must be avoided in severe traumatic brain injury (TBI); systolic blood pressures (SBPs) should not fall below 100 mm Hg.
2. Consider seizure, including non-convulsive status epilepticus, in the differential diagnosis of a TBI patient with an unexplained persistently low Glasgow Coma Scale (GCS).
3. An unexplained depressed level of consciousness (LOC), sudden hypertension, lateralizing neurological exam, or posturing may be signs of elevated intracranial pressure (ICP).

J. Cooke (✉)
Navy Medicine Readiness and Training Command San Diego, San Diego, CA, USA
e-mail: jonathon.cooke.mil@health.mil

M. D. Tadlock, A. A. Hernandez (eds.), *Expeditionary Surgery at Sea*,
https://doi.org/10.1007/978-3-031-21893-4_25

4. Cushing's triad (bradycardia, hypertension, irregular respirations) does not always present together and any one of the triad elements should alert a clinician to the potential of elevated ICP.
5. Management of elevated ICP should follow an algorithmic approach tailored to the individual patient and initiated emergently if ICP elevation is suspected without delay for imaging, consultation, or transport.
6. Pain and agitation can elevate ICPs and should be treated aggressively. However, be aware that this may eliminate the neurological exam as an assessment tool.
7. Hyperventilation should be only used as a short-term temporizing measure as prolonged or profound hypocapnia can precipitate ischemia and further brain injury.
8. Hypertonic saline has emerged as the treatment of choice for hyperosmolar therapy.
9. The most common placement error for external ventricular drains (EVDs) is anterior and lateral trajectory.
10. For the non-neurosurgeon to perform a decompressive craniotomy forward deployed in an austere environment it is ultimately a personal choice involving many competing factors, including but not limited to the time/distance to medical evacuation (MEDEVAC), appropriate equipment to perform the procedure, and the non-neurosurgeon's experience.

Introduction

Management of severe traumatic brain injury (TBI) in the austere setting remains a challenge among forward deployed providers. There are not enough neurosurgical resources to adequately cover all areas of operation where injury may occur. Stabilization and prompt medical evacuation (MEDEVAC) remain best practice. Yet MEDEVAC may not be practical or even possible due to geographic location, operational tempo, or lack of MEDEVAC assets. Therefore, it is imperative that all forward deployed maritime surgical teams have a basic understanding of the principles of both medical and salvage surgical management of these patients. This chapter will present the pathophysiology of TBI and provide best practice-based guidelines for austere TBI medical management. Finally, a step-by-step approach to external ventricular drain (EVD) placement, burr hole placement, and decompressive hemicraniectomy will be covered.

Traumatic Brain Injury (TBI) Pathophysiology

Intracranial Dynamics

The skull is a non-expansile structure containing a fixed volume of brain, minimum requirement of arterial blood, as well as variable volumes of venous blood and cerebrospinal fluid (CSF). Through a process called autoregulation, these variable volumes (arterial blood, venous blood, and CSF) are kept sufficient to need. Autoregulation is the subconscious homeostatic process by which cerebral blood flow is maintained to supply the brain with adequate perfusion across a range of hemodynamic states [1]. This functions normally between systolic blood pressure (SBP) of 50–150 mm Hg and cerebral perfusion pressure (CPP) of 60–160 mmHg. CPP is the intracranial pressure (ICP) subtracted from the mean arterial pressure (MAP). The mechanism behind this is unknown. Outside of these parameters autoregulation may not occur or may be delayed, thus maintaining adequate CPP is essential to prevent potentially disastrous consequences. Goal CPP is 60–70 mm Hg [2].

Primary and Secondary Brain Injury

Primary brain injury is the initial mechanism of harm such as a projectile, blunt, or explosive force. The damage caused by primary brain injury cannot be reversed. However, there will be some tissue not irreversibly damaged but only threatened. This area will reduce metabolic activity to preserve itself. Known as the penumbra, this threatened area has the potential to reactivate and lead to return of function. Secondary brain injury is injury to this penumbra caused by aberrations in hemodynamic and metabolic activity from the primary brain injury. Secondary brain injury can potentially be prevented with judicious and prompt neurocritical care.

Neurocritical Care

Evaluation

Prompt recognition of patients with neurological injury is critical but not always simple. While patients with depressed Glasgow Coma Scale (GCS) (Table 25.1) and signs of neurological trauma are easily diagnosed, those with a depressed GCS without those signs or with an unknown mechanism of injury may be missed. It should be noted that motor score is most predictive of a good prognosis but is less reliable in the acute setting. In addition to traumatic injury, metabolic, endocrine,

Table 25.1 Glasgow Coma Scale (GCS) [3]

Points	Response
Eye opening	
4	Spontaneous-open with blinking at baseline
3	To verbal stimuli, command, speech
2	To pain only (not applied to face)
1	No response
Verbal	
5	Oriented
4	Confused conversation, but able to answer questions
3	Inappropriate words
2	Incomprehensible speech
1	No response
Motor	
6	Obeys commands for movement
5	Purposeful movement to painful stimulus
4	Withdraws in response to pain
3	Flexion in response to pain (decorticate posturing)
2	Extension response in response to pain (decerebrate posturing)
1	No response
Total points = GCS score	*Head injury classification*
13–15	Mild
9–12	Moderate
8 or less	Severe

infectious, autoimmune, vascular, and toxic exposures may mimic a severe TBI. Primary and secondary surveys should be performed under the tenets of Advanced Trauma Life Support (ATLS) and Tactical Combat Casualty Care (TCCC), depending on the role of care. Once the diagnosis of a severe TBI is established, it is important to rapidly begin interventions that maintain supportive parameters to the penumbra.

Medical Management

Full spine precautions are to be maintained at all times. The caveat to this is a non-explosive, isolated, penetrating skull injury which does not require spinal immobilization [4]. Continuous monitoring of SBP, heart rate, cardiac rhythm, and oxygenation should be initiated if available. Large bore intravenous (IV) access should be established and basic laboratory tests, including chemistry panel, complete blood count, and coagulation assay, should also be sent if available. An advanced airway should be placed if the patient has a GCS <9, a rapidly declining neurological exam, or other concerns about the ability to protect their airway. Oxygen administration should be titrated to maintain pulse oximetry measuring of peripheral saturation of hemoglobin (SpO_2) >90% while preventing hyperoxia. End tidal carbon dioxide ($ETCO_2$) should be normal to mildly hypercapnic; a goal of 35–40 mm Hg is reasonable, and hyperventilation should be avoided in the absence of concern for herniation (which will be covered further below). Body temperature should be normalized; hyperthermia should be avoided and treated aggressively with antipyretics and external cooling if required. Electrolytes should be replenished and normalized. Avoiding hypo- and hyperglycemia is important, and a range of 140–180 mg/dL should be maintained. See Chap. 20 for more discussion of critical care at sea.

As with any trauma, both crystalloid and blood products should be utilized judiciously per guidelines with transfusion threshold hemoglobin <7 gm/dL without other cardiac or end organ perfusion concerns. In patients in hemorrhagic shock with multiple traumatic injuries and a suspected TBI, fresh whole blood (FWB) is preferred; however, permissive hypotension with a 90 mm Hg SBP target is not appropriate or adequate. When performing resuscitation in casualties with suspected TBI, a higher SBP goal of 100–110 mm Hg is critical to avoid hypoperfusion to the penumbra of salvageable brain tissue and consistent with current TCCC guidelines and Joint Trauma System (JTS) Clinical Practice Guidelines (CPGs), including https://jts.amedd.army.mil/assets/docs/cpgs/Neurosurgery_and_Severe_Head_Injury_02_Mar_2017_ID30.pdf. Maintain SBP above 100 mm Hg for ages 49–70 at all times utilizing crystalloid, blood products, and vasopressors as indicated; for ages 15–49 and over 70, aim for SBP greater than 110 mm Hg [2]. In patients with severe TBI not requiring blood resuscitation, normal saline is the preferred crystalloid resuscitation and hypotonic fluids should be avoided.

Hypotension is an independent risk factor for poor outcome in severe TBI [2]. As mentioned previously, the CPP must be maintained to support neurologic function and recovery. Each instance of SBP <100 mm Hg increases the risk of poor outcome. Therefore, it is important to support SBP through control of hemorrhage, prompt resuscitation, and early vasopressor use. There is much debate about the ideal range of SBP, and it is more commonly accepted that each patient has a unique ideal SBP. While the guidelines listed above support keeping SBP greater than 100 mm Hg for ages 49–70, it is ideal to elevate it even more toward a "normal" 120 mm Hg. If invasive monitoring is available to provide an ICP, then MAPs should be augmented to ensure a CPP of 60–70.

Neurological Exam

A baseline neurological exam including GCS (Table 25.1) or Full Outline of UnResponsiveness (FOUR) score (Table 25.2) is important in the austere setting. Not only will this guide providers as to the localization of the injury but it will serve

Table 25.2 Full Outline of UnResponsiveness (FOUR) score [5]

Points	Response
Eye	
4	Eyelids open or opened, tracking, or blinking to command
3	Eyelids open or opened but not tracking
2	Eyelids closed but open to loud voice
1	Eyelids closed but open to pain
0	No response to pain, eyelids remain closed
Best motor	
4	Thumbs-up, fist, or peace sign
3	Localizing to pain
2	Flexion response to pain
1	Extension response to pain
0	No response to pain or generalized myoclonus status
Brainstem reflexes	
4	Pupil and corneal reflexes present
3	One pupil wide and fixed
2	Pupil or corneal reflexes absent
1	Pupil and corneal reflexes absent
0	Pupil, corneal, and cough reflexes absent
Respiration	
4	Not intubated, regular breathing pattern
3	Not intubated, Cheyne-stokes breathing pattern
2	Not intubated, irregular breathing
1	Breathes above ventilator rate
0	Breathes at ventilator rate or apnea

as a marker of change when repeated over time. Additionally, the GCS and FOUR score are likely equally prognostic with the FOUR score providing different tools to help evaluate patients who are intubated or have incomplete neurological lesions. The exam is even more important when imaging adjuncts are not readily available, such as on a maritime platform. A thorough exam should be performed if possible. In patients presenting in extremis, an exam should be attempted at the earliest opportunity once resuscitated and practical. This exam should be repeated hourly and as necessary if a change is suspected. Pupillometry is another adjunct to the physical exam that can be utilized in the austere settings. Many manufacturers make products that can measure the rate of reactivity of the pupils and the difference between the eyes. This has been shown to predict impending ICP event. Optic nerve sheath diameter can be established with ultrasonography and has been validated as a method detecting elevated ICP [6]. Diameter ranges from 4.8–5.9 mm have been suggested as cutoffs. However, neither pupillometry nor optic nerve sheath diameter provides information to the degree of ICP elevation.

Anti-epileptic Drugs (AEDs)

Patient with a witnessed seizure or clinical suspicion of a seizure should be placed on anti-epileptic drugs. Active seizures should be broken with ablative drugs including benzodiazepines, propofol, and anti-epileptic drugs (AEDs) administered concurrently (all available currently on the aircraft carrier (CVN) Authorized Medical Allowance List (AMAL)). Prophylactic seizure management remains a controversial topic. AEDs have been shown to prevent early (<7 days) but not late seizures, and seizure prophylaxis is indicated in certain lesions. It is reasonable to administer prophylactic AEDs to patients with an imaging diagnosis of a subdural or supratentorial intraparenchymal lesion (either traumatic subarachnoid or intraparenchymal hemorrhage). Posterior fossa and epidural lesions are not epileptogenic by themselves and should not receive prophylactic AEDs. Common AEDs are IV Levetiracetam 500–1000 mg (maintenance dosing is 500–1000 mg twice daily with adjustments needed for renal dysfunction) or IV phenytoin 20 mg/kg (maintenance dose 5 mg/kg/day with the dose broken up into three equal doses). Both of these AEDs are available on the CVN AMAL. Consider seizure, including non-convulsive status epilepticus, in the differential diagnosis of a TBI patient with an unexplained persistently low GCS. In the austere setting where axial imaging is not available, AEDs are generally not recommended unless there is a suspected or witnessed seizure. Without imaging, AEDs could be considered in patients with a concern for elevated intracranial pressure on physical exam, but the interventions discussed in the next section are the first priority.

Elevated Intracranial Pressure (ICP)

Diagnosing ICP elevation may be simple when **classic exam (fixed and dilated pupil and Cushing's triad of bradycardia, hypertension, and irregular respirations)** or imaging findings are present. However, recognition of occult signs of herniation requires a higher index of suspicion in the austere setting where adjuncts and imaging may not be available. An unexplained depressed level of consciousness (LOC), sudden hypertension, lateralizing neurological exam, or posturing may be signs of elevated ICP. One should also note that Cushing's triad does not always present together and any one of the triad elements should alert a provider to the potential of elevated ICP.

Management of elevated ICP can be complex and therefore should follow an algorithmic approach tailored to the individual patient's overall clinical status. If ICP elevation is suspected it should be treated immediately. Do not delay intervention for imaging, consultation, or transport. Initial treatment begins with optimizing position. The head should be midline and head of bed elevated to at least 30 degrees (reverse Trendelenburg position in patients with concomitant thoracic or lumbar spine injuries). If a cervical collar is present ensure that it is not too tight and compressing jugular venous outflow.

Pain and agitation can elevate ICP and should be treated aggressively. However, be aware that this may eliminate a neurological exam as a tool. Short acting opioids like fentanyl are first line agents for analgesia. Propofol and dexmedetomidine (on the CVN AMAL) are the sedatives of choice given their rapid onset and metabolism. Ketamine is also an option at dissociative doses and likely does not elevate ICPs as much as previously thought. Dexmedetomidine and ketamine have the added benefits of not suppressing respiratory drive. Benzodiazepines and barbiturates are second-line agents but may be effective. The clinician should be ready to augment hemodynamics, as these agents are myocardial suppressants. The optimal choice in the austere setting depends on the patient and the available resources as well as the knowledge, comfort, and experience of the maritime surgical team (see Chaps. 13 and 20).

Hyperventilation is an effective but short-term solution that may temporize an ICP crisis. Long-term hyperventilation is not recommended as it may be deleterious and precipitate ischemia and elevation in ICP. As mentioned previously, maintaining an $ETCO_2$ of 35–40 mm Hg will help mitigate elevated ICP. In a crisis this may be decreased to 30 mm Hg while other measures are being instituted.

Fever may also precipitate ICP elevation and should be treated aggressively with antipyretics and external cooling if available. However, cooling may cause shivering that can also elevate ICP, so this should also be treated. Common methods include counter-warming by placing warm (not too hot that would cause thermal injury) saline bags under the arms, in the palms, groin, and on the soles of the feet. Acetaminophen and magnesium (on the CVN AMAL) with buspirone and meperidine (not currently on the CVN AMAL) may be effective in limiting shivering. Paralytics should be used as a last resort and for as short a duration as possible as they have deleterious effects on critically ill patients and will eliminate the neurological exam. Be sure to check both the platform's AMAL and the medications that are actually available prior to deployment.

Hyperosmolar Therapy

Osmolar augmentation is perhaps the most effective medical treatment method for elevated ICP. Though controversy exists as to the ideal treatment, rapid initiation of hyperosmolar therapy has been shown to lower ICP. Many regimens exist and the treatment used should be one with which the practitioner is most comfortable and familiar that is also available on the platform. Some of the more common methods are outlined below.

Mannitol is an osmotic diuretic that improves red blood cell rheology currently available on the CVN AMAL. Peak action occurs 30 minutes after administration. It can readily be given through a peripheral IV or central venous catheter (CVC). Bolus doses of 1 g/kg IV push should be given. As this is a diuretic, it should be used cautiously in patients in whom volume resuscitation is ongoing. Doses can be repeated every 4–6 hours using laboratory data to guide therapy or given based on clinical exam change.

Hypertonic saline has emerged as the treatment of choice for hyperosmolar therapy. Many preparations exist, but the two most common are 3% and 23.4%, 500 cc of 3% is currently on the CVN AMAL. 3% is bolused at 2.5 cc/kg over 15–30 minutes. A 3% drip may be started at 15–30 cc/h and titrated by 15 cc/h based on laboratory data. It may be given through a peripheral IV above the wrist or elbow, CVC, or intraosseous (IO) line. 23.4%, should only be administered in 30 cc aliquot boluses administered over 5 minutes into a CVC or IO line. Both of these preparations can precipitate hypotension and pulmonary edema so providers should be prepared to treat both when these therapies are considered.

Baseline sodium levels should be determined with acid-base status and serum osmolality if available. Sodium or chemistry laboratory tests should be repeated every 6 hours while undergoing osmolar augmentation. Goal serum sodium range remains controversial, but ranges from 145–155 mmol/L are reasonable. Serum osmolality should not exceed 320 mOsmol/kg to prevent renal injury.

Surgical Management

External Ventricular Drain (EVD) and Intracranial Pressure (ICP) Monitor Placement

External ventricular drains (EVD) and ICP monitors can offer valuable information in the management of the critically ill severe TBI patient. They can be placed with a shallow learning curve and reasonable risk by most surgeons. Indications for monitoring include GCS <9 and an abnormal head CT scan or in patients with a normal CT scan (or when one is not available like on a maritime platform) and two out of the following three conditions: age > 40 years, unilateral/bilateral motor posturing, and SBP <90 mm Hg [2]. However, placement to help guide ICP management is also reasonable though whether it improves outcomes remains controversial. The decision to place one of these devices should be based upon patient's clinical status and the comfort and experience of the provider with expert consultation if possible. See Chaps. 5 and 14 for a discussion of how to gain access to 24/7 virtual consultation.

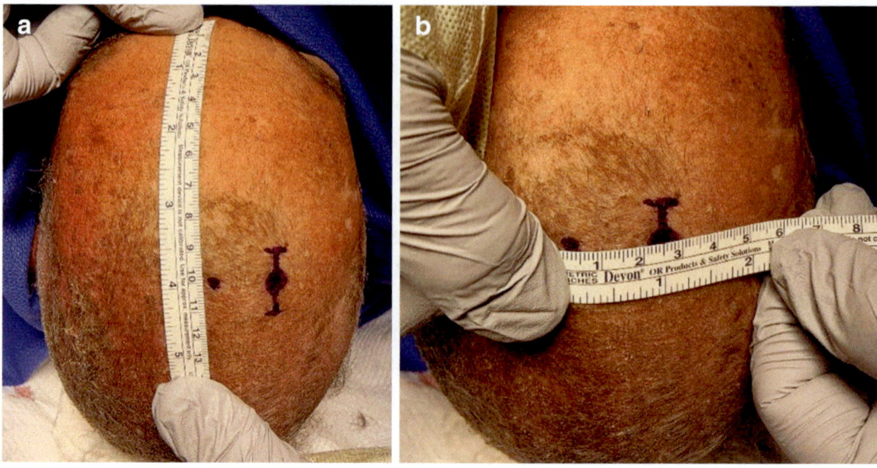

Fig. 25.1 Kocher right frontal entry point measurement for placement of external ventricular drain (EVD)/intracranial pressure (ICP) monitor. The patient's head is positioned neutrally and the planned entry point is (**a**) 10 cm measured back from the glabella and (**b**) 2.5–3 cm from midline, or in the mid-pupillary line. (Source: Photos courtesy of Jonathon Cooke, MD and Matthew D. Tadlock, MD)

Intracranial access for placement of both devices is same. The head is positioned in neutral orientation. A wide shave of hair should be done to allow for adequate sterilization as well as to permit adhesion of the dressing to the scalp. An appropriate antibiotic (see Chap. 16 for discussion of antimicrobials available on maritime platforms) should be dosed 30 minutes prior to skin incision when possible. A Kocher right frontal entry point is ideal; however, the left side may also be utilized with low additional risk. Kocher entry point is measured 10 cm back from the glabella (the smooth, high prominence between the eyebrows and above the nose) and 2.5–3 cm off the midline (Fig. 25.1). Alternatively, the mid-pupillary line is a good reference for how far lateral the incision should be. The area should be marked, prepped, and draped in a normal sterile fashion. Enough room should be left in draping for tunneling of the drain or monitor at least 2.5 cm away from the incision to minimize infectious risk.

Local anesthetic may be used if desired. A 1.5–2 cm straight incision is made in the sagittal plane. The periosteum is dissected off the bone. The tunneler is passed posteriorly out the incision to a point at least 2.5 cm away from the incision. A twist drill or pneumatic drill is brought on and aimed for a point to the ipsilateral medial canthus of the eye in the sagittal plane and a line parallel to the external auditory meatus in the coronal plane (Fig. 25.2). The drill is advanced through the inner table to the intracranial cavity and then withdrawn. Bone fragments should be swept away to allow access to the dura. The dura is then pierced with an 18-gauge needle. There may be some venous ooze if a cortical vein is encountered. Usually this does not result in any significant intracranial bleeding.

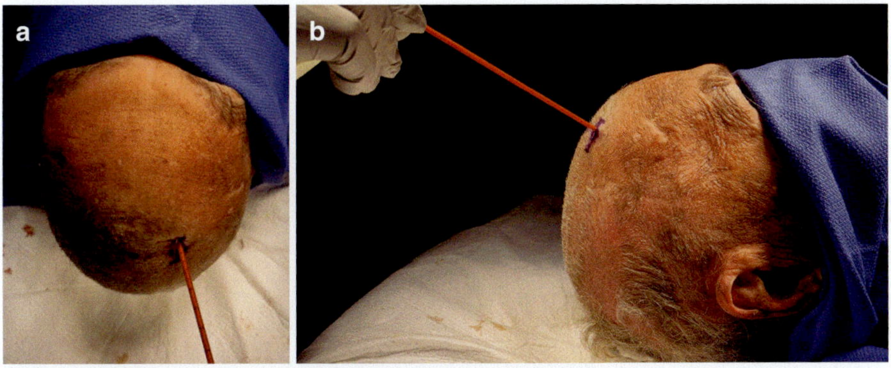

Fig. 25.2 Trajectory for external ventricular drain (EVD) placement, including (**a**) anterior-posterior EVD trajectory and (**b**) lateral EVD trajectory. The EVD is aimed at the ipsilateral medial canthus in the coronal plane and in line with the tragus in the sagittal plane. The EVD is advanced to no more than 6.5 cm at the bone edge to avoid injury to deep structures. The most common error is an anterior-lateral trajectory; if cerebrospinal fluid (CSF) is not encountered after two passes, the third pass should correct for this. (Source: Photos courtesy of Jonathon Cooke, MD and Matthew D. Tadlock, MD)

All, some, or none of this equipment may be available to the maritime surgical team, depending on the platform and the mission. It is best to check ahead of time to see what is available and "tactically acquire" if necessary (see Chap. 12). If placing an ICP monitor, it is usually placed to 2 cm of depth or if using a bolt-based system according to manufacturer's instructions. If placing an EVD, the drain is then lined up in the same orientation as described for the drill. Advance slowly into the ventricle to a depth no greater than 6.5 cm at the skull to avoid injury to deep structures. Once the ventricle is accessed, brisk CSF flow will be seen if the intracranial contents are under pressure. However, in a low CSF pressure environment, drop the drain or place gentle suction with a syringe to obtain CSF. If no CSF return is present then slowly remove the drain and irrgate it to remove blood and other contents that may occlude the pores and attempt replacement. If the second attempt is unsuccessful, it would behoove the surgeon to double-check all of the landmarks as well as location of the burr hole to ensure ideal location and trajectories. If these are all in correct placement, there may be a shift of intracranial contents away from the side of pathology. Aiming slightly more medial and posterior can usually yield results. The most common placement error is being too anterior and lateral. Once the drain is in position, tunnel posteriorly taking care not to dislodge its position (Fig. 25.3). Place a single purse string suture at the exit site of the drain taking care not to occlude the drain. The excess drain is then coiled and three staples or sutures are placed to prevent dislodgement. This is then sterilely attached to a pre-flushed CSF collection system. It is important to only flush the intracranial contents in the CSF drainage collection system with preservative-free irrigations. The CSF collection system should be zeroed at the tragus and set to 10 mm Hg and open.

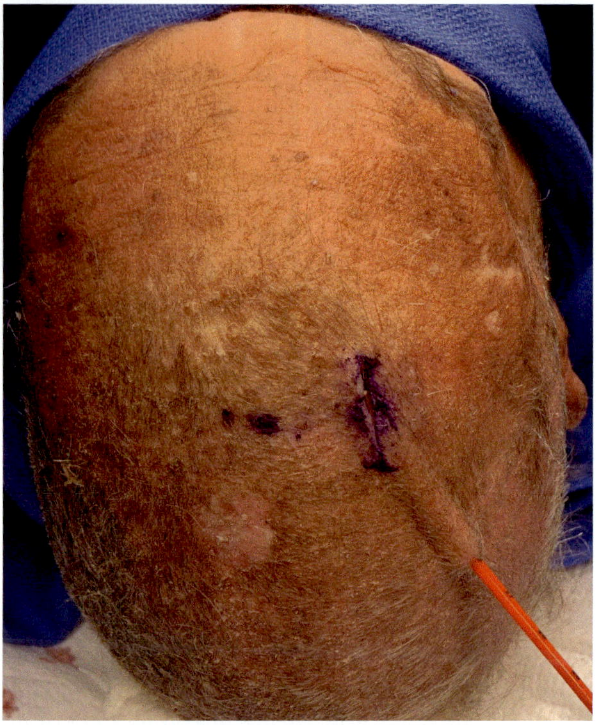

Fig. 25.3 External ventricular drain (EVD) tunnel. The EVD is then tunneled 2.5 cm away from the incision to lower the risk of infection. (Source: Photo courtesy of Jonathon Cooke, MD and Matthew D. Tadlock, MD)

Decompressive Hemicraniectomy

Non-neurosurgeons performing neurosurgical procedures remains a topic of controversy. Exploration of the issue is outside the scope of this chapter. That being said, there is perhaps no lonelier feeling than being faced with an unfamiliar surgical emergency in an austere setting. The decision to proceed with surgical intervention is at this stage a personal one. The non-neurosurgeon and maritime surgical team should make all attempts to seek expert consultation and guidance (again, see Chaps. 5 and 14). However, if none is available then the clinical urgency, time to transport, local resources, available surgical equipment, surgeon and team experience, and a realistic assessment of the risks and benefits of not intervening should all be taken into account prior to proceeding. **Ideally, the decision for a non-neurosurgeon to perform this procedure on deployment should be made *before* the deployment.** Therefore, the surgeon should gain experience performing the procedure with a neurosurgeon in garrison. The JTS also has a CPG on this topic and it is worth reviewing prior to deployment (available at: https://jts.amedd.army.mil/assets/docs/cpgs/Emergency_Life-saving_Cranial_Procedures_by_Non-Neurosurgeons_in_Deployed_Setting_23_Apr_2018_ID68.pdf)

Whether or not to perform a decompressive craniectomy in the absence of CT imaging is also of ongoing debate. Without imaging guidance there is a high risk of incorrect side surgery or even an unnecessary surgery. If patient movement is impossible within a reasonable timeframe and the patient's clinical condition continues to worsen then it may be reasonable to perform a hemicraniectomy. A skull X-ray may show an underlying skull fracture or air in a penetrating lesion that may guide localization. Physical exam findings may also assist in localizing pathology. Unilateral fixed and dilated pupil, outward signs of trauma, and/or hemiparesis are all helpful in localizing pathology to one side or the other. Consultation with a neurosurgeon should be pursued if possible. Current JTS CPGs suggest it is reasonable to perform a decompressive craniectomy for a patient with severe TBI (GCS <8) and lateralizing signs with progressive neurological decline despite maximal medical management and signs of elevated ICP (e.g., Cushing's triad) if a patient cannot be transferred to a higher level of care within 4 hours and surgeon training and resources are adequate. The guidelines recommend against a craniectomy if the patient has a post-resuscitation GCS of 3 with bilateral fixed and dilated pupils as this injury is likely to be non-survivable or if surgeon training or resources are not adequate to perform the decompression.

Prior to decompression, antibiotics should be administered. Also, optimization of ICP should be performed. The patient should get a dose of either mannitol or hypertonic saline with the ability to give more. $ETCO_2$ should be kept 30–35 mm Hg. The head of bed should be elevated slightly to assist with venous drainage. Also ensure that the head is not too rotated kinking the jugular venous outflow. A bump of rolled blankets may be placed under the ipsilateral shoulder and the head rotated contralaterally 90 degrees to expose the side and back of the head. The head may rest on a jelly doughnut or stack of towels. Pin fixation may also be used but is not necessary and likely not available.

To perform a decompressive hemicraniectomy the head should be completely shaved past the midline and a curvilinear reverse question mark incision planned and marked (Fig. 25.4). This incision should allow for a minimum 15 cm diameter craniotomy. The inferior limb of the craniotomy incision should be within 1 cm of the tragus to prevent iatrogenic injury to the terminal facial nerve branches. The area is then prepped and draped in sterile fashion allowing enough room for placement of drains at the end of the case. The proposed incision should be infiltrated with local anesthetic with epinephrine to assist with hemostasis.

In 3–5 cm sections, the skin should be incised down to the periosteum and Raney clips applied to minimize blood loss. Without Raney clips (probable on some maritime platforms) there is the potential for significant blood loss from the scalp so the surgeon should try to mitigate this with direct pressure and cautery. Once the incision has reached the inferior limb, the temporalis fascia will be encountered. The skin incision should be superficial to the fascia to minimize bleeding from the temporalis muscle as well as iatrogenic transection of the superficial temporal artery (Fig. 25.5).

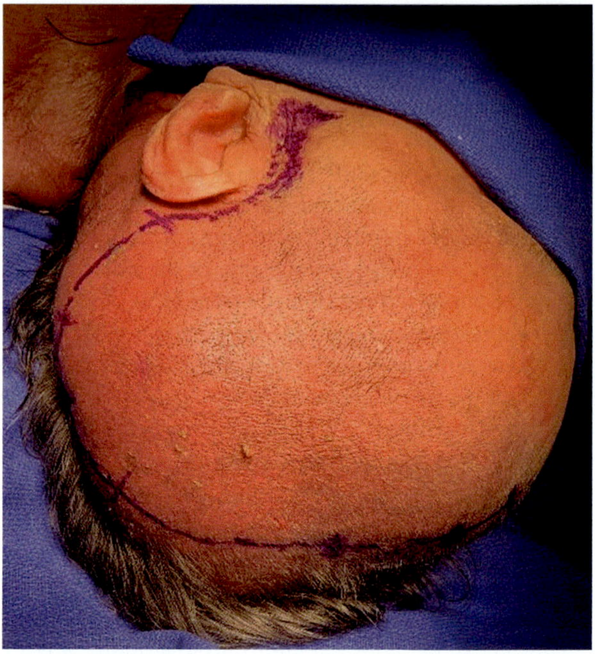

Fig. 25.4 Skin incision for hemicraniectomy. The root of the zygoma is palpated and the midline of the skull is identified. A curvilinear reverse question mark incision is planned and made large enough to allow for a 15-cm diameter craniotomy. The inferior limb of the incision should be kept within 1 cm of the tragus to prevent iatrogenic injury to facial nerve branches. (Source: Photo courtesy of Jonathon Cooke, MD and Matthew D. Tadlock, MD)

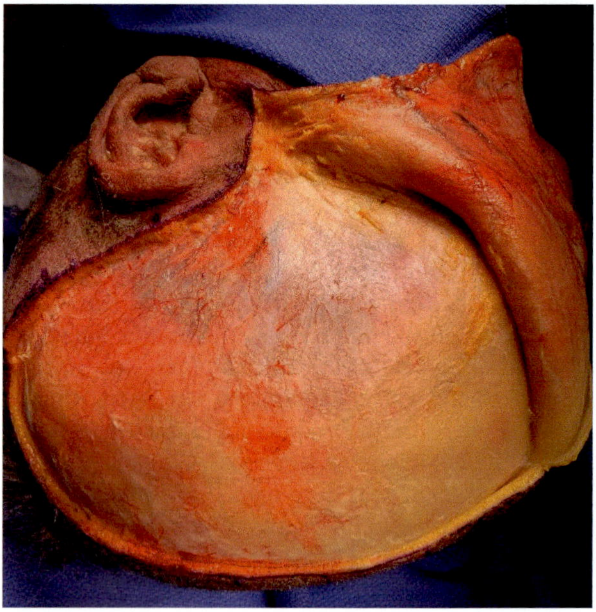

Fig. 25.5 The cranial incision has been opened to expose the temporalis muscle. This may be taken down in a separate layer or with the skin to create a myocutaneous flap. (Source: Photo courtesy of Jonathon Cooke, MD and Matthew D. Tadlock, MD)

When the skin incision is complete, the root of the zygoma should be palpated and exposed using electrocautery. Electrocautery is then used to transect the temporalis muscle and periosteum throughout the entirety of the incision. Next, with

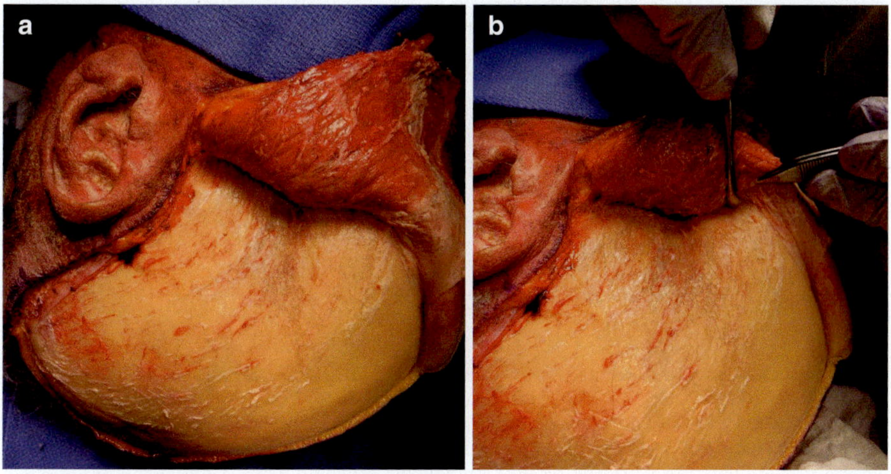

Fig. 25.6 (**a**) The temporalis muscle has been transected and removed to expose the underlying skull. (**b**) An instrument marks the zygomaticofrontal suture (marking the floor of the anterior fossa) and posterior to this the root of the zygoma is seen just in front of the ear (marking the floor of the middle fossa). (Source: Photos courtesy of Jonathon Cooke, MD and Matthew D. Tadlock, MD)

traction on the temporalis muscle, this should be cut away from the calvarium using electrocautery, creating a myocutaneous flap with a pedicle on the zygoma (Fig. 25.6).

Once the flap is created, traction should be placed on the muscles using either perforated towel clips or Allis clamps and fishhooks. This tension on the temporalis muscle will help with hemostasis from any muscle bleeding. There may be small emissary veins oozing from the calvarium and these can be cauterized or waxed over with bone wax.

At this time attention is turned to planning the craniotomy. Burr holes should be planned at the root of the zygoma as well as the anatomic keyhole, which is the junction of the squamosal temporal bone, the greater wing of the sphenoid, and the frontal and parietal bones (Fig. 25.7a). A third burr hole may be planned 2–3 cm off midline above the superior temporal line to help prevent iatrogenic injury to the superior sagittal sinus or large bridging veins during craniotomy (Fig. 25.7b). Once these burr holes are planned the hole should be created with pneumatic burr or twist drill to expose the underlying dura.

A small blunt curved instrument such as a 4 Penfield dissector should be placed into the burr hole and the dura stripped circumferentially as far as possible around this opening. If possible, a pneumatic drill with a B-1 bit and footplate should be brought on. If no pneumatic drill is available, a Gigli saw may be used to create a craniotomy. The craniotomy is made taking care to avoid the frontal air sinus anteriorly and the superior sagittal sinus medially. It may be difficult to connect the burr holes at the keyhole and root of zygoma due to the anatomic morphology of the sphenoid wing. Techniques to assist in this include coming from either burr hole toward the middle and meeting there or using the B1 bit without the footplate to

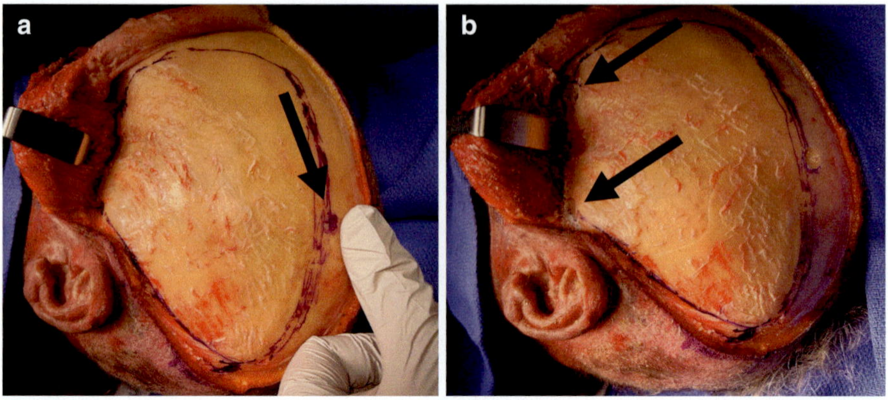

Fig. 25.7 (**a**) Ensure that burr holes placed superiorly (black arrow) are 2 cm off midline to avoid potentially catastrophic injury to the superior sagittal sinus. (**b**) Burr holes planned at the root of the zygoma and the keyhole (black arrows) straddle the sphenoid wing. Additional burr holes can also be placed. (Source: Photos courtesy of Jonathon Cooke, MD and Matthew D. Tadlock, MD)

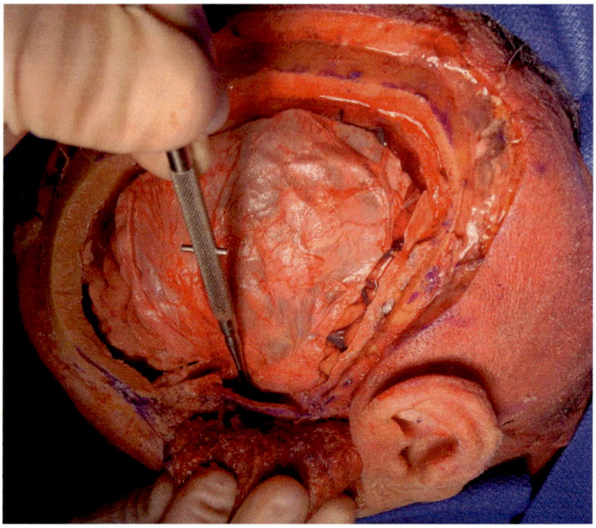

Fig. 25.8 The bone flap has been removed and the underlying dura is encountered. An instrument is placed on the floor of the middle fossa to show that further temporal bone must be removed down to the floor of the middle fossa to allow room for the temporal lobe to swell. (Source: Photo courtesy of Jonathon Cooke, MD and Matthew D. Tadlock, MD)

carefully thin out the bone to an eggshell consistency and then gently fracturing it. Care must be taken not to use too much force to fracture the sphenoid bone, as a fracture may extend medially into important medial vascular structures. Creating the craniotomy with only the Gigli saw can be *very challenging*, particularly if the non-neurosurgeon has never performed the procedure before. Therefore, as stated multiple times, the available equipment in addition to the maritime surgical team experience with the procedure should be part of the pre-deployment calculus in deciding to perform a craniotomy.

Once the outline of the craniotomy is completed, the bone flap should be gently elevated by scraping the inner surface of the bone to separate the dural attachment

(Fig. 25.8). Once the bone is free, any bleeding dural vasculature may be coagulated with bipolar or sparing monopolar cautery. Monopolar cautery should never be used on the brain parenchyma as the field of current spreads out from the tip and damages surrounding tissues. It is also common for there to be brisk bleeding from the middle meningeal artery at the sphenoid wing. This may be coagulated with bipolar cautery or more commonly will need to be tamponaded with either bone wax or some type of hemostatic agent.

Once hemostasis is achieved the dura is opened by using a 15 blade to make a small incision carefully through the dura while trying to leave the arachnoid intact. The dura is transparent so the initial incision should be made in an area absent of vascular structures. A half-centimeter opening is all that is necessary to then transition to Metzenbaum scissors to complete a semi-circular opening almost to the width of the craniectomy with pedicle based at the zygoma, in the same orientation as the myocutaneous flap (Fig. 25.9).

If a hematoma is encountered then it can be *gently freed* from the brain with suction, irrigation, or blunt instruments. If a bleeding vessel on the brain is encountered, it should be tamponaded with a piece of gelfoam or cotton. Cautery should be used only if tamponade is unsuccessful as overzealous cautery can lead to ischemia, infarction, edema, and further hemorrhage. Hemostasis should be achieved and the wound should be irrigated.

The dura can then be laid back over the surface of the brain without reapproximating it with any type of suture. If available, a sheet of Seprafilm may be placed over the dura at this time which may help prevent adhesions that may complicate a future cranioplasty. A flat drain of some type should be placed over the dura into the inferior-most aspect of the wound and tunneled 2.5 cm away from the wound edge. Suture the temporalis muscle back together and close the galea with inverted

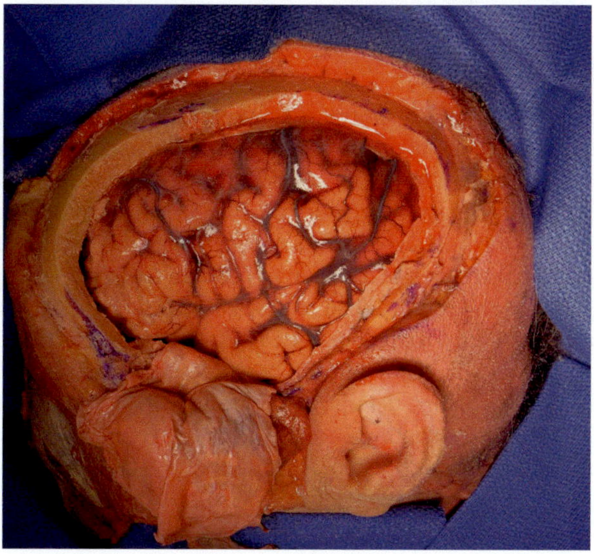

Fig. 25.9 The dura is incised and opened with the pedicle based on the myocutaneous flap. (Source: Photo courtesy of Jonathon Cooke, MD and Matthew D. Tadlock, MD)

interrupted 2–0 Vicryl or other absorbable suture. The skin may be stapled or closed with running suture.

If the patient will undergo MEDEVAC to a coalition hospital or country, then the bone flap may be discarded as synthetic flaps may be fashioned with great accuracy. If the patient is to remain in a theater without advanced medical technology, then the flap may be soaked in iodine, wrapped in a sterile bag (e.g., a c-arm drape), and either placed in a −80 °C freezer or placed into the peritoneum as a last resort.

The decompressive craniotomy for trauma is not the most eloquent of neurosurgical operations but there are a few nuances:

- Take time to control extracranial bleeding on the way in. This will save time on the way out, especially if the brain is very swollen and there is a need to close quickly. This may save the patient from a postoperative epidural hematoma and ultimate poor outcome.
- Control any arterial bleeding immediately. The extracranial superficial temporal artery and the intracranial middle meningeal artery will be encountered; be prepared!
- While the dura may be coagulated at will, be cautious using electrocautery on the surface of the brain. Only bipolar cautery should be used intracranially. Additionally, sections of the brain are drained by single veins. Injury to these veins and subsequent cautery will create venous congestion, infarct, swelling, and possible hemorrhage.
- Be prepared to move quickly once the dura is opened. The brain can swell quickly and if the next moves are not ready to be made, it can swell and herniate on the field! Do all of your bony work prior to opening the dura, especially biting down the temporal bone to allow maximum room for the brain to swell. The brain needs room lower down, not as much higher up.

Conclusion

Ever-increasing operational commitments around the globe increase the potential for a neurological catastrophe in the austere setting. Current neurosurgical resources are insufficient to permit expertise at each site of injury and some missions preclude the ability to rapidly transport patients. The maritime surgical team should be familiar with medical stabilization and management of severe TBI, and non-neurosurgeons may be faced with a decision to perform a CSF-diverting procedure or even decompressive craniotomy. The mantra of operational forces to train as they fight should also be applied to medical assets. The more comfortable providers are with the challenges of TBI, the better the outcomes for patients will be. This chapter offers the bread-and-butter details for the maritime surgical team dealing with severe TBI. More in-depth information can be found in the JTS CPGs pertaining to this subject and expert virtual consultation is available 24/7.

Declaration of Interest The views expressed in this chapter are those of the authors and do not necessarily reflect the official policy or position of the Department of the Navy, Department of Defense, nor the US Government.

Funding This research did not receive any specific grant from funding agencies in the public, commercial, or not-for-profit sectors.

Conflict of Interest Statement The authors declare no conflict of interest.

References

1. Armstead WM. Cerebral blood flow autoregulation and dysautoregulation. Anesthesiol Clin. 2016;34(3):465–77.
2. Carney N, Totten AM, et al. Guidelines for the management of severe traumatic brain injury 4th edition. Neurosurgery. 2017;80:6–15.
3. https://www.cdc.gov/masstrauma/resources/gcs.pdf.
4. Joint Trauma System. Clinical practice guidelines: cervical and thoracolumbar spine injury evaluations, transport, and surgery in the deployed setting. 05 August 2016.
5. Sadaka F, Patel D, Lakshmanan R. The FOUR score predicts outcome in patients after traumatic brain injury. Neurocrit Care. 2012;16:95–101.
6. Wang LJ, Yao Y, et al. Noninvasive and quantitative intracranial pressure estimation using ultrasonic graphic measurement of optic nerve sheath diameter. Sci Rep. 2017;7:42063.

Chapter 26
Burn, Inhalation, and Electrical Injuries

Bruce M. Potenza

The deepest lessons come out of the deepest waters and the hottest fires.

Elisabeth Elliot

Author deployment experience	
Bruce M. Potenza	Trauma Surgeon, Fleet Surgical Team-6, embarked on the USS *Kearsarge* (LHD-3), Kosovo Force, EUCOM Area of Responsibility, Operation Noble Anvil, 1999
	Ship's Surgeon, USS *Kitty Hawk* (CVN-63), contingency operations, Third Fleet Area of Responsibility, 1995
	Ship's Surgeon, USS *Carl Vinson* (CVN-70), contingency operations, Third Fleet Area of Responsibility, 2011
	Staff Surgeon, USNS *Mercy* (T-AH-19), contingency operations, Third Fleet Area of Responsibility, 2002
	Director, University of California San Diego Regional Burn Center, San Diego, CA, USA, 2003–2016
	Chief of Trauma, NATO Role 3 Multinational Medical Unit, NATO Resolute Support and Operation Freedom's Sentinel, Kandahar Airfield, Afghanistan, 2019–2020
	Chief of Surgery, San Diego Veteran Administration Healthcare System, San Diego, CA, USA, 2021–present

B. M. Potenza (✉)
Division of Trauma, Critical Care, Acute Surgery and Burns-UC, San Diego, CA, USA
e-mail: Bruce.Potenza@va.gov

M. D. Tadlock, A. A. Hernandez (eds.), *Expeditionary Surgery at Sea*,
https://doi.org/10.1007/978-3-031-21893-4_26

BLUF (Bottom Line Up Front)

1. The depth of a burn wound is characterized by the level of injury to the epidermis, dermis, and deeper structures. Burn depth determines wound healing potential and treatment options.
2. The Rule of Nines and/or using the palm of the patient's hand (approximately 1% total body surface area (TBSA)) can be used to initially estimate TBSA to begin fluid resuscitation but may overestimate. Recalculate using the Lund and Browder Chart both after wounds are cleaned and at each role of care to ensure accurate resuscitation. First-degree burns are not included in the TBSA calculation.
3. Look for traumatic etiologies of hypotension in a combined burn/trauma patient exhibiting early hypotension. Hypotension from burn injury is not present in the first few hours after the injury.
4. Airway patency, not hypotension is a potential threat to life during the "Golden Hour" in major burn patients. Large burns with a >40% TBSA may require prophylactic intubation as the large volume resuscitation required may result in upper airway edema and airway compromise.
5. Soot in the hypopharynx is a good indicator of upper airway insult or injury. Anticipate the patient trying to cough up copious amounts of soot. They may develop a transient reactive airway problem that can be treated with beta agonist nebulizers (Albuterol).
6. Burn patients with significant facial edema WILL have posterior pharyngeal and supraglottic edema, making intubation more difficult. An edematous face portends a difficult airway to manage. Establish a definitive airway as soon as practicable.
7. When indicated, a surgical cricothyrotomy should be performed before the burn patient decompensates, not when the patient is in extremis! In a patient with difficult anatomy, the four-finger technique will aid in determining where to make an incision.
8. Burns with >20% TBSA require intravenous (IV) fluid resuscitation to combat the third spacing associated with the systemic inflammatory response syndrome (SIRS) to avoid hypotension and improve visceral organ perfusion.
9. Both the Parkland formula and the Rule of Tens are useful tools to estimate the initial rate of fluid resuscitation.
10. Resuscitate with lactated Ringer's (LR) preferentially over normal saline (NS). NS can be used if that is all that is available, but it can cause a hyperchloremic metabolic acidosis. Follow serum electrolytes closely with large volume resuscitations.
11. When resuscitating burn casualties, the Goldilocks strategy is best—"just right"! Under-resuscitation will lead to poor tissue perfusion, end-organ damage (particularly acute kidney injury (AKI)), and progression of the burn injury. Over-resuscitation may result in pulmonary edema and extremity and/or abdominal compartment syndrome.

12. The key to a successful burn resuscitation is close monitoring of urine output (UOP), systolic blood pressure (SBP), and heart rate. UOP is a reliable surrogate of adequate fluid resuscitation.
13. DO NOT give IV fluid boluses to burn patients! This will only drive more fluid out of the intravascular space! Instead, increase the hourly IV fluid rate.
14. If access to IV fluids is limited, oral rehydration therapy (ORT) may be an alternative in burn patients with 20–40% TBSA.
15. Burn wound bandaging uses an inner layer to keep topical antibiotic on the burn to prevent infection and desiccation while the outer layer protects the wound from the environment.
16. Patient transport via medical evacuation (MEDEVAC) to a higher level of care is the goal. Packaging a burn patient adds an extra level of complexity as securing the airway can be more difficult, there may be ongoing resuscitation, and wounds may require attention.
17. Burn sepsis is a surgical emergency which requires source control (burn excision), resuscitation and systemic antibiotics.
18. Any patient who is in a closed space fire should be assumed to have some degree of carbon monoxide (CO) exposure. Patients at risk for CO poisoning may have a normal or falsely elevated pulse oximetry—don't be misled! Initiate high flow oxygen therapy as soon as possible. (Simple field oximeters cannot distinguish between carboxyhemoglobin and oxyhemoglobin).
19. Steam and electrical burns can be deceiving. A small electrical entry burn wound may be hiding significant internal soft tissue injury. Deep partial or full thickness steam burns appear white, feel rubbery and are dry.
20. Deep partial or full thickness circumferential extremity burns may develop a compartment syndrome during a large volume fluid resuscitation. Monitor the patient closely as this may develop anytime during the resuscusitation. Escharotomies should be performed in the operating room (OR).
21. Tightly shut eyelids from facial edema may result in elevated intraocular pressures (IOP). A significant elevation of IOP pressure (>40 mmHg) or there is a high clinical suspicion decompress the orbit with a lateral orbital canthotomy and inferior cantholysis.

Introduction

Burn care in the deployed setting can be challenging. Thankfully, the majority of burn injuries are small and partial-thickness; if managed appropriately, they will heal with conservative treatment leading to a return to duty of the servicemember. Deeper burns may require excision and grafting. Large burns (>20% total body surface area (TBSA)) require resuscitation, extensive wound care, and likely excision and grafting. They are labor and resource intensive. Inhalation injuries and deep burns that involve the face, hands, or perineum should be transferred to a Role 3 or 4 medical treatment facility (MTF) or the United States Army Institute of Surgical Research (USAISR) Burn Center in San Antonio, TX, for definitive care if possible.

Traditional shipboard deployment of United States (U.S.) Navy medical personnel was expanded to multiple land-based medical facilities during the Iraq and Afghanistan conflicts. There were many instances where local nationals received definitive burn care at these facilities. Therefore, it is important for the maritime surgical team to have a reasonable knowledge and skillset to provide burn care in various austere settings. Second, there may be instances where a forward-deployed shipboard medical unit may not have the ability to provide for a timely medical evacuation (MEDEVAC) to a higher level of care. Shipboard medical departments and surgical teams should be prepared to render burn care until such time the patient can be safely transported.

Definitive surgical care shipboard may also be necessary if a patient with a large, deep burn is not able to get a timely MEDEVAC. The larger the burn, the more important this becomes. Resuscitation starts when the patient enters the medical system and is completed within 48-hours (h). Excision should normally be done starting at 3–5 days post-injury and be completed by day 5–7. Without excision of full-thickness large burns, the patient will run the risk of developing a burn wound infection or burn sepsis. Communication via satellite phone or asynchronously via email to the USAISR Burn Center will provide prudent advice on the management of large burns when rapid transfer is not likely. There is no reason to "go it alone"! The USAISR Burn Center should be contacted as soon as possible when caring for a significant burn casualty. Contact information for USAISR Burn Center:

- *DSN 312-429-2876 (429-BURN)*
- *Commercial (210) 916-2876 or (210) 222-2876*
- *Email burntrauma.consult.army@mail.mil*

This chapter is arranged with the deployed surgical teams in mind. It will attempt to describe a systematic approach for the initial evaluation and management of burn injuries. It also expands into definitive care of burn wounds as well as pitfalls that one may encounter. The initial visual impression of a patient with a large burn can cause the inexperienced surgical team to flounder. Do not get caught up in the emotional distress that affects many who see a bad burn for the first time. The patient's life may hang in the balance, so the team must focus on the tasks at hand and start treating the patient. **There are many skilled burn and plastic surgeons who can do amazing things for this patient in the future, but only the efforts of the maritime surgical team in the first 48 h can give the patient that opportunity.**

Key factors to the successful treatment of these injuries include the following:

- Understanding of the mechanism of injury and its pathophysiology
- Determining of the severity of the wound in terms of depth and TBSA
- Evaluating and managing concomitant traumatic injury
- Managing the airway
- Determining resuscitation requirement
- Providing burn wound care including cleaning, debridement, topical antibiotics, bandaging, and pain control

- Preparating for transfer
- Performing emergent surgical interventions and definitive surgical care when applicable

The primary focus of this chapter will be the nonoperative care of the burn patient for both definitive care and for patients pending transfer to a higher echelon of care. However, surgeons deployed at sea or at combat casualty hospitals may need to perform simple operative procedures. The arrangement of this chapter is a little unorthodox starting with the mechanism of burn injury followed by the initial evaluation and management of the burn patient. Next there will be a discussion of pathophysiology and ending with a description of definitive (operative) care.

Mechanism of Injury

The mechanism of burn injury is as important to burn patients as it is to trauma patients; it can give clues to the extent, location, and types of injuries patients may have. The estimation of the depth of the burn and likelihood of inhalation injury, rhabdomyolysis, or compartment syndrome can be aided by understanding the clinical implications of the mechanism of the burn. Common mechanisms of burn injury include thermal (scald, steam, flame, and contact/conduction), friction, electrical, chemical, and radiation.

While military burn injuries tend to follow civilian burn injury epidemiology of scald, flame, friction, and contact, there are higher incidences of:

- combined burn and trauma injuries,
- high-pressure steam burns from equipment powered by steam propulsion, facility heating, and hot water generation,
- burns due to explosions from an improvised explosive devices (IED), bomb, or demolition,
- burns due to jet blasts,
- electrical injuries from direct contact with an active power source, arching flash burns due to equipment that holds an electrical charge such as radar units, and large equipment panels,
- chemical burns due to incendiary material,
- radiation burns from prolonged radiation exposure.

Severity of Burn Injury

The severity of the burn injury is determined by several factors, including the "energy or heat" of the exposure, length of time of the exposure, area of the body that is injured, and the physiology of the host. The depth of a patient's skin varies depending on location, making some areas more resilient to burn injury. The bigger the burn, the more difficult it becomes to perfuse the injured areas and surrounding "at-risk" tissue resulting in deeper burns. Poor tissue perfusion due to inadequate resuscitation or hemorrhagic shock due to trauma will also result in a deeper burn injury.

Anatomy

Skin is made up from two distinct layers: epidermis and dermis. The epidermis is the outermost layer of skin and functions as a semipermeable membrane that separates the patient from the environment. The epidermis ranges from 0.05–1.5 mm thick. Important cellular components within the epidermis include keratinocytes, squamous epithelium, and melanocytes. The dermis depth ranges from 1.5–4 mm thick. Important structures include sweat and sebaceous glands, blood and lymph vessels, nerves, and hair follicles. The latter, if uninjured, is one of the epidermal cell germinal centers for the skin. The "skin buds" seen when a partial-thickness burn is healing are epithelial cells migrating up from the base of the hair follicle upward onto the surface of the wound and away from the hair follicle. If there are enough epithelial buds, the new epithelium will coalesce on the surface and form an intact epidermis.

Skin depth varies by anatomic location. The best example of an area with thin skin is on the face: eyelids, nares, and ears. Some of the thickest areas of skin are found on the posterior torso and buttocks as well as palmar hand and plantar feet surfaces. The thicker the skin, the more heat injury it can sustain and the higher likelihood of healing with nonoperative management.

Depth of Burn Injury and Corresponding Treatment Modalities

The depth of burns is characterized by the level of injury to the epidermis, dermis, or structures deep to the dermis (Fig. 26.1). They are classified in the following manner corresponding to modalities of treatment:

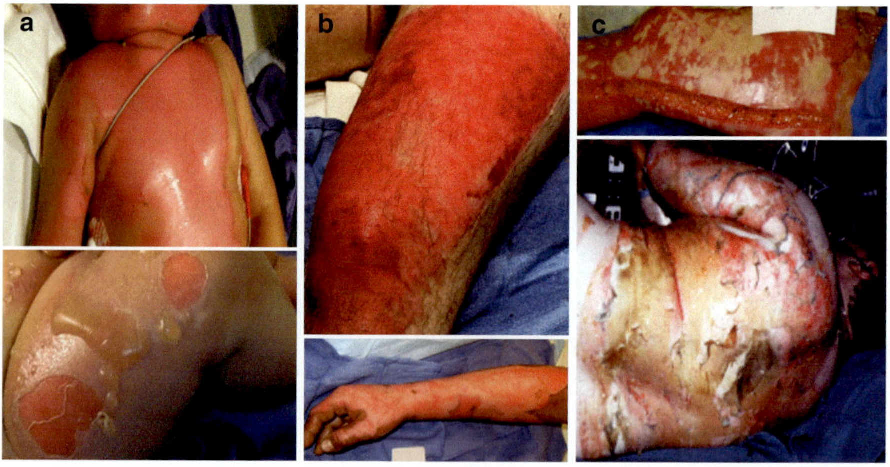

Fig. 26.1 Examples of burn depth. (**a**) Superficial partial-thickness (second degree) burn due to scalding on a child (pink and moist). (**b**) Deep partial-thickness (second degree) burn to the right thigh and right forearm (dry, red, and pale). (**c**) Full-thickness (third degree) burn with escharotomy on the right leg and posterior torso (dry and leathery). (Source: Photos courtesy of Bruce Potenza, MD, MPH)

1. *First degree*: Superficial burn

   (a) This burn injury only involves the epidermis.
   (b) They are erythematous, painful to some degree, and may be pruritic. A good example of this is a sunburn.
   (c) Treatment includes cleaning and oral pain relief with non-narcotics like acetaminophen or non-steroidal anti-inflammatory drugs (NSAIDs). Twice daily application of topical, over the counter, moisturizing agents may provide a soothing feeling to reduce pain and itching. They require no bandaging and can be exposed to the air. They will heal in 7–10 days on average.

2. *Second degree*: Superficial partial-thickness burn

   (a) This burn injury involves the epidermis and superficial dermal layer of skin. The skin appendages and areas of dermal regeneration are left intact resulting in the skin being able to regenerate and repair the injured area.
   (b) They blanch, are moist, and typically develop blisters. They are quite sensate and painful as the nerve endings are intact.
   (c) Treatment includes cleaning, local wound care (to include debridement of bullae if >2 cm), bandaging, re-evaluation, and pain relief with non-narcotic and narcotic agents, especially for burn wound care. With proper wound care most of these burns will heal with time. Bandaging involves application of topical antibiotics, non-adherent covering, and a clean bandage to cover the wound. Wound care and bandage changes ideally are done daily. Alternatively, a silver-impregnated bandage can be applied directly to a clean burn wound and covered with a clean bandage and left in place for 3–5 days. Caution should be taken with the initial care of the burn injury to make sure that it is progressing in a favorable direction.

3. *Second degree*: Deep partial-thickness burn

   (a) This burn injury involves the deeper layers of the dermis, including cutaneous nerves, skin appendages and hair follicles. Therefore, the skin has little capacity to regenerate or repair itself.
   (b) They are dry, appear whitish in color, don't blanch well, and the skin (epidermis) may already be sloughing. They may have diminished sensation.
   (c) Treatment includes cleaning, local wound care (to include mechanical debridement), bandaging, re-evaluation, and pain relief. Left to conservative management, the wound heals by typical methods of inflammation, granulation, contraction, remodeling, and in many cases scarring. A better treatment modality is excision and grafting for definitive care. If small in size they can be managed conservatively, especially if <10% TBSA and/or they are located on areas of the body with a thick dermal layer. They can undergo future excision and grafting at a Role 3 or 4 facility if they do not heal. Splinting and daily physical therapy should be performed if the burn crosses a joint or involves the hands.

4. *Third degree*: Full-thickness burn

    (a) This burn injury involves all layers of the skin and usually the immediate subcutaneous adipose tissue.
    (b) They are dry, leathery, do not blanch, and are insensate.
    (c) Initial treatment includes local wound care, bandaging, re-evaluation, and pain relief. Definitive treatment of these wounds requires excision of the burn wound and grafting. A notable exception is a small area no larger than 2–4 sq. cm.

5. *Fourth degree*: Burn involving structures deep to the skin including soft tissue and bone.

    (a) This burn injury involves all areas of a full-thickness burn with an additional component of muscle, bone, or other deep tissues. They are seen with prolonged exposure to a heat source or a short exposure to an intense heat source (e.g., being trapped in a burning structure or explosions from IEDs).
    (b) They are dry, appear lifeless or may be severely charred, and are insensate.
    (c) Initial treatment includes cleaning, local wound care, bandaging, and re-evaluation along with escharotomies or fasciotomies if indicated. Definitive treatment will involve extensive surgical excision of the burn wound, including skin and damaged soft tissue, prolonged wound care, and eventual grafting. Definitive treatment is best left to burn surgical subspecialists and centers, as the patients are often complex, time consuming, and best served by a multidisciplinary approach to burn care and rehabilitation.

Total Body Surface Area (TBSA) of Burn Injury

The TBSA of burn wounds is important for several reasons. It is part of the "common language" used by burn surgeons to describe burn injury. The remaining descriptors include relative depth of burn wound, anatomic location, and if there was an inhalation component. First-degree burns are not included in the TBSA calculation. The TBSA and a breakdown of the percentages of partial-thickness and full-thickness burns is charted and reported when discussing the patient with other physicians.

The TBSA also guides resuscitation efforts. Burn injuries that are <20% TBSA rarely need intravenous (IV) fluid resuscitation. Burns >20% TBSA will manifest a systemic inflammatory response syndrome (SIRS) leading to third spacing of fluids, decreased circulating volume, poor visceral organ perfusion, and eventually hypotension. These patients need precise burn resuscitation. While the TBSA can be calculated in several ways, a formal calculation using a **Lund and Browder Chart** is most accurate (Fig. 26.2). This is undertaken once the patient's burn wounds are cleaned and precise "eyes on the burn wound" can be undertaken and recorded for each body area.

BURN AREA CHART

Patient Identification

Shade images accordingly: 2° 3°

Lund & Browder Chart - estimate to the nearest 10th%											
Area	% 2°	% 3°	Area	% 2°	% 3°	Area	% 2°	% 3°	Area	% 2°	% 3°
Head			R. buttock			RL arm			L thigh		
Neck			L. buttock			LL arm			R leg		
Ant. trunk			Genitalia			R hand			L leg		
Post. trunk			RU arm			L hand			R foot		
			LU arm			R thigh			L foot		

Total % 2° _____ + Total % 3° _____ = Total % Burn _____

Age	A	B	C	D	E	F
0 - 1 yr	10	9	3.3	2.2	2.5	2.5
1 - 5 yrs	9	8	3.8	2.7	2.5	2.5
5 - 10 yrs	7	6	4.5	3.5	2.8	2.7
10 - 15 yrs	6	5	4.5	4	3	3
Adult	4	3	5	4.5	3.5	3.5

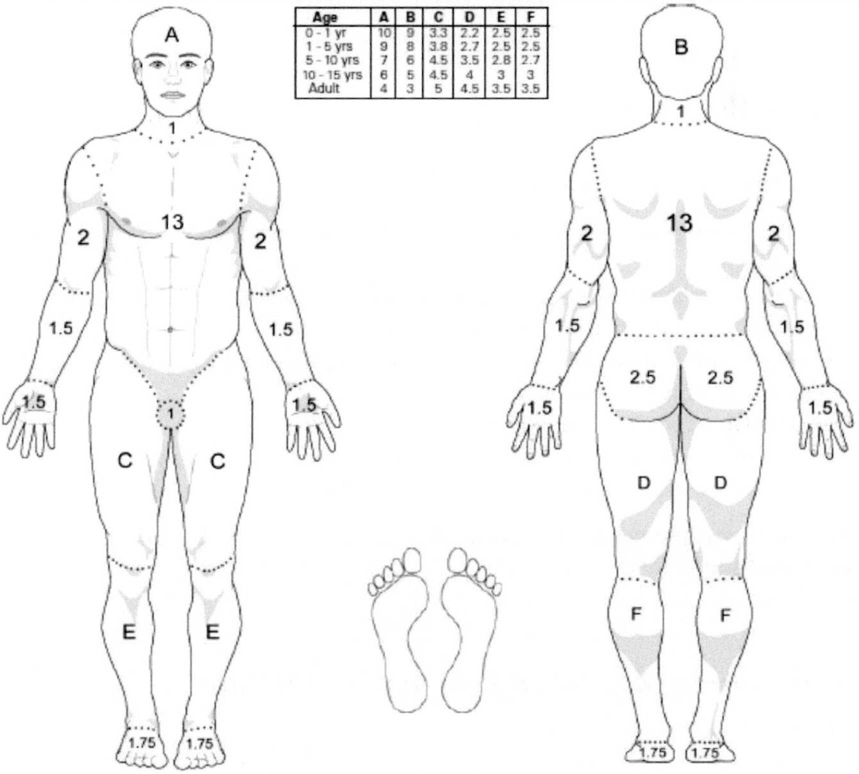

Physician Signature/PID# Date & Time

Fig. 26.2 Lund and Browder Burn Estimate Chart (diagram to be filled out documenting burn injury and depth). Second-degree burn shading \\\\\\\\\\. Third-degree burn shading XXXXXXXXXX. (Source: Adapted from the University of California—San Diego Burn Center, used with permission)

The Lund and Browder chart is age-specific so that younger children's anatomic differences are considered in the calculation of TBSA. When a Lund and Browder chart is not available or the patient is in the field the Rule of Nines can be quickly applied. The **Rule of Nines** estimates the TBSA of the bilateral upper extremities as 9% each, the legs 18% each, the anterior and posterior torso are 18% each, and the head is 9%. Smaller burns can rapidly be estimated by looking at the patient's palmar surface area and estimating the combined size of the palmar surface of the digits (all digits opposing each other) and palm, representing approximately 1% of their TBSA. A more rigorous estimate should be done when the patient arrives at a medical facility.

Unfortunately, in the field or at initial evaluation, the calculation of the depth and TBSA of the burn wound are oftentimes overestimated because it is difficult to determine these quantities in large burn wounds with soot and burned clothing on the patient. As the patient moves up the echelons of care, the depth and TBSA calculations should be recalculated during each initial evaluation and treatment phase in order to get a more accurate appraisal since accurate resuscitation depends upon an accurate estimation of the depth and TBSA of the burn injury.

Phases of Burn Care

There are five phases of burn care:

1. Stop the burning and initial first aid "buddy care" in the field (0–30 min plus transport time).
2. Initial evaluation and management, to include airway and resuscitation management, at a medical facility (1–48 h).
3. Definitive burn wound care, which could include nonoperative and/or operative management of the burn wound (2–14 days).
4. Rehabilitation (weeks to months).
5. Remodeling or revision; where the complications of scarring, contractures, or ulcerations are addressed (months to 1–2 years).

This chapter addresses the first three phases, which could occur on the maritime surgical platform.

Stop the Burning and Initial First Aid "Buddy Care" in the Field

Immediate cessation of the burning process is imperative to lessen the burn injury. Burn victims on fire must stop, drop, and roll. Oftentimes a "buddy" will need to assist to get them to the ground and cover them with clothing or a blanket to smother the flames. Some clothes will retain heat despite the flames being extinguished such as, synthetic materials (nylon), work boots that have become superheated from fighting a fire, and metal objects on the clothes of the patient. Remove all as soon as possible! Patients who are found lying on a hot surface (e.g., the street or a flight deck) are also at risk for contact burns. Move them off these surfaces to prevent this from occurring. Chemical burns should be lavaged immediately to reduce the contact time of the chemical to the skin. Electrical power should be disabled prior to approaching a patient in contact with a live power source. The action of a "buddy" can be lifesaving to the burn victim.

Initial Evaluation and Management at a Medical Facility

Evaluation

Once the patient arrives at a medical facility, they should be assessed using Advanced Trauma Life Support (ATLS) protocols. Perform the primary and secondary surveys to exclude significant traumatic injuries and then concentrate on the burn injuries.

Combined trauma and burn patients will often need additional fluid for the traumatic injury in addition to the burn fluid resuscitation. Hypotension in burn patients with a concomitant traumatic injury must raise the possibility of hemorrhagic shock rather than burn under resuscitation. **Hypotension from trauma can occur at any time; hypotension from a burn injury takes time to develop and is not present in the first few hours after the injury.**

Approach the burn examination in a systematic fashion. All burns need to be evaluated to determine the depth of the injury and TBSA. Record the findings, list the TBSA, and break it down into TBSA due to second- or third-degree burns. Drawing a picture can be quite helpful (see Fig. 26.2). For example: "40-year-old male servicemember with a 36% TBSA flame burn affecting the bilateral lower extremities. The right leg sustained an 18% second-degree burn and the left leg an 18% third-degree burn." Then list vital signs, other injuries, interventions, and transport method to help the receiving medical team to have a better appreciation of the patient's injuries.

If multiple casualties arrive, triage patients appropriately (Chap. 7). For burn patients, quickly determine the depth and TBSA. Determine need for airway management. If the burn is >20% TBSA, calculate the resuscitation rate and begin with crystalloid. Cover the burns with clean gauze or a sheet. Move onto the next seriously injured patient and reassess in 30 min. If the patient has circumferential extremity burns, there will be 2–3 h before the escharotomies may be needed to be performed in the OR. (See remaining part of chapter for discussions of airway, resuscitation, and escharotomy).

If this is the only patient in the trauma bay, it is reasonable to also begin burn care with gentle cleaning and bandaging. If the patient is going to move up the medical echelon quickly, definitive burn wound care can be delayed. IV pain medications may be needed, but be sure to recover the patient. Once the burns are covered, the lack of stimulation may result in oversedated patient.

Airway

This section discusses the evaluation and management of an acute airway injury, which is a subset of the broader category of inhalation injury. One major risk factor for airway injury is being exposed to fire while in a closed space environment, which could be a room, compartment, workspace, cockpit, auto, or truck. These situations expose the victims to superheated temperatures, low oxygen levels, and the toxic byproducts of combustion. If the patient ran while their chest clothing was on fire, they likely inhaled hot toxic fumes.

On examination look for evidence of burns to the face or chest. Signs and symptoms of airway injury include tachypnea, shallow breathing, hoarseness, stridor, wheezing, and use of accessory muscles. Patients may speak in short sentences, sit upright in the gurney, and look anxious. Examine the patient for facial burns, soot in the mouth and/or nares, or the presence of carbonaceous sputum. Specifically, look for soot in the posterior area of the mouth (hypopharynx). Soot deposited this far posterior in the oral cavity is likely to be found in the lower respiratory tract. Follow pulse oximetry trends and maintain (SpO_2) >90%. In the deployed environment, oxygen may be in short supply (see Chaps. 13, 20, 21, 30, and 31). Always be cognizant of capabilities and resupply. Supplemental oxygen via nasal cannula or mask with intubation per ATLS protocols should be followed. If intubation on presentation is not indicated, closely monitor the patient over time. If the patient demonstrates clinical deterioration, move forward with establishing a definitive airway. Don't wait too long! If there is significant facial edema, there WILL be posterior pharyngeal and supraglottic edema. An edematous face portends an edematous and difficult airway.

A thoughtful clinical decision to intubate needs to be made considering all these factors. Burn care is dynamic and a good airway may deteriorate with time with edema formation in the upper airway. **Constantly reassess the patient for signs of respiratory compromise.** Large burns with a >40% TBSA may require prophylactic intubation as the large volume resuscitation required may result in upper airway edema leading to eventual airway compromise. While it is possible to intubate the patient to do wound care and extubate at the completion of the procedure similar to any other surgical procedure, consideration of anticipated analgesic and sedative requirements for the burn care of a large burn (>40% TBSA) is also a factor in the decision to intubate.

The Difficult Surgical Airway

If a difficult intubation is anticipated, use any adjuncts available (see Chap. 13). A glidescope can be lifesaving. A laryngeal mask airway (LMA) can buy some time but is not a definitive airway and is subject to tissue edema and eventual loss of the airway if not changed over to a definitive airway.

Move to a surgical airway when indicated, preferably not when the patient is in extremis. If there is a need to obtain a surgical airway in a patient with full-thickness neck burns, it will be challenging to palpate the landmarks for a cricothyrotomy since the skin will be firm and leathery. For patients with difficult anatomy, the four-finger technique will aid in determining where to make the incision. With an outstretched palm, place a small finger in the suprasternal notch; where the tip of the index finger falls will estimate the location of the cricothyroid membrane in the midline of the patient's neck. Make a 3-4 cm vertical full thickness midline incision into the unburned soft tissue. Palpating the cricothyroid membrane is much easier through the unburned soft tissue. Place a non-dominant index finger on the cricothyroid membrane and use a scalpel or the cricothyrotomy needle kit to secure a surgical airway. **Do not let a full-thickness neck burn prevent a surgical airway! Remember, the full-thickness neck burn will be excised and grafted at a later setting.**

Resuscitation

ORAL: IV resuscitation is not needed in patients with <20% TBSA burns. Oral rehydration therapy (ORT) can be used in these situations as the fluid loss from this size of burns is small and there is no systemic capillary leak syndrome. Any oral fluids can be used for these smaller burns.

If access to IV fluids is limited, ORT may be an alternative in patients with burns of 20–40% TBSA. A nasogastric tube could be placed if needed to assist. Avoid additional "sweet/sugar" oral drinks as they may induce an osmolar diuresis. Some sample ORT formulas for large burns include:

- One liter of water, one teaspoon of table salt (3 g), three tablespoons of sugar (36 g)
- Gatorade® with 1/4 teaspoon salt and 1/4 teaspoon baking soda per quart

IV: Larger burns will require IV resuscitation to keep up with the intravascular fluid loss. This is due to the burn capillary leak syndrome resulting in interstitial edema. There are common resuscitation formulas that can be used as guides to the resuscitation such as the Parkland Formula and the Joint Trauma System (JTS) Clinical Practice Guidelines (CPGs) Rule of Tens formula. Resuscitate with lactated Ringer's (LR) preferentially as normal saline (NS) could result in a hyperchloremic metabolic acidosis. However, if no LR is available, use what is on hand! Always follow serum electrolytes closely with large volume resuscitations.

The key to a successful resuscitation is close monitoring of the effectiveness of that resuscitation with dynamic hourly fluid adjustments. The larger the TBSA, the deeper the burn, the higher the fluid requirements. Urine output (UOP), systolic blood pressure (SBP), and heart rate are important indicators to monitor resuscitation. Large burns cause a hypermetabolic response with a resting heart rate of 100–120 in a patient with adequate pain control. A heart rate >120 should raise a suspicion that the resuscitation is falling behind and there is a fluid deficit. Under-resuscitation will lead to poor tissue perfusion and potential end-organ damage, particularly with acute kidney injury (AKI) and progression of the burn injury depth. Over-resuscitation may result in pulmonary edema or compartment syndrome of the extremity or abdomen.

The **Parkland formula** is calculated as (2–4 mL/kg) × TBSA with the total to be administered in a 24-hour period. Smaller burns (20–40% TBSA) start out at the 2 mL/kg rate, and larger burns (>40% TBSA) at the 4 mL/kg rate. In the first 8 h, half of this fluid amount is administered with the remaining half over the next 18 h. Titration of surrogate endpoints cannot be emphasized enough.

Example of **Parkland formula**:

1. An 80 kg patient has a 50% TBSA.
2. Choose a rate of 4 mL/kg, as this is a large burn. 4 mL × 80 kg = 320.
3. Calculate total 24-hour resuscitation volume: 320 × 50% TBSA = 320 × 50 = 16,500 mL.
4. Give half of this fluid over the first 8 h: 16,500 mL/2 = 8250 mL.
5. Hourly rate: 8250 mL/8 = 1031 mL/h.
6. Give the remaining half over the ensuing 18 h.
7. Hourly rate: 8250 mL/18 = 458 mL/h.

The USAISR Burn Center resuscitation formula **Rule of Tens** is less specific than the Parkland formula and groups patients into two baseline weight categories to calculate hourly rate of IV fluid resuscitation.

- Patients weighing 40–80 kg: 10 mL × % TBSA.
- Patients weighing >80 kg: 10 mL × % TBSA baseline plus 100 mL/h for every 10 kg >80 kg.

Examples of **Rule of Tens**:

1. A 60 kg adult with a 50% TBSA burn would require

$$10\,\text{mL} \times 50\%\text{TBSA} = 10 \times 50 = 500\,\text{mL} / \text{h}.$$

2. A 90 kg adult with a 50% TBSA burn would require

$$10\,\text{mL} \times 50\%\text{TBSA} = 10 \times 50 = 500 + 100 = 600\,\text{mL} / \text{h}.$$

Burn resuscitations requiring >6 mL/kg × % TBSA are considered extremely large volume resuscitations. Patients requiring this volume of resuscitation are demonstrating an aggressive SIRS and may need vasoactive medications to maintain SBP and a reduction in the volumes being resuscitated. They appear physiologically to behave like a septic patient, and the orientation of the resuscitation of the patient will mirror that physiology.

IV access is similar to trauma with two large-bore peripheral IVs for the resuscitation. If the percentage of TBSA is large (>40% TBSA) or IV access is compromised due to the burn location, then a central venous catheter (CVC) should be considered. This central access will also permit basic laboratory testing during the resuscitation. A consistent surrogate measurement of adequate fluid resuscitation is UOP. Target UOPs are:

- 0.5–1 mL/kg/h for adult patients
- 1–1.5 mL/kg/h for pediatric patients >2 years old
- 1.5–2 mL/kg/h for pediatric patients <2 years old.

Therefore, accurate hourly intake and output are essential for large burn resuscitations. In the **early phase of the burn,** there is not significant fluid loss through the burned skin. The UOP is an accurate marker of clinically significant output. If the UOP is below the desired amount in the adult, increase the rate by 10–20% in the next hour. For example, an 80 kg patient with an IV fluid resuscitation rate of 800 mL/h is not making the target UOP. Increase the rate by 10% (80 mL/h). However, to make the flow sheet easier to follow, round up to the nearest 100 mL and increase the rate to 900 mL/h. Check the next hour and go up another 10% or stay at this rate depending on response. It is not a good practice to bolus these patients. The loss of the bolus fluid is accelerated by the capillary leak problem, and the increase in hydrostatic pressure from the fluid bolus will drive more fluid into the interstitium. **The net intravascular fluid gain is less with a bolus approach than by increasing the fluid rate.**

Burn Wound Care

The main principles of burn wound care are as follows:

1. Clean the wound.
2. Reassess the TBSA.
3. Apply topical antibiotic.
4. Cover the burn (inner layer) with a clean, preferably sterile covering. Bandage the burn wound (outer layer) with a clean bandage to hold it in place and protect from further contamination.
5. Provide pain management.
6. Perform daily bandage changes, following steps 1–5. Sometimes it is difficult to tell the exact depth of burn wounds as they change in appearance every day. Deeper wounds will declare themselves with time making it easier to decide the treatment.

Clean

Clean the burn wound with soap and water while lightly removing any loose skin, dirt and embedded gravel, or clothing. Any soap will suffice, just get the area clean. If in the field, leave blisters intact as they are sterile so the underlying burn will remain clean. If the patient is in a medical facility, blisters larger than 2 cm should be removed with light debridement using scissors to cut off the epidermis.

Reassess

Reassess the burn wound to recalculate the TBSA and estimate burn wound depth. Ask these questions with every bandage change:

- Is there a deterioration of the burn to suggest a deeper burn?
- Is the wound ready for further debridement?
- Is the burn healing?
- Does the type of bandage need to change?
- Is the burn declaring the need for surgical excision and grafting?
- Is there evidence of cellulitis demonstrated by expanding areas of erythema?

Common reasons for changing local burn care include the wound drying out, the patient having a local skin reaction to the topical antibiotic (bacitracin is a typical culprit), or a burn infection being deeper than localized cellulitis.

Antibiotics

Topical antibiotics are the mainstay of burn wound care except for first-degree burns. Topical triple antibiotics include neomycin and bacitracin. Silvadene® (silver sulfadiazine 1%) or Sulfamylon® (mafenide acetate) are premade compounds and will likely be available in limited quantities Silvadene® is on the aircraft carrier (CVN) Authorized Medical Allowance List (AMAL) and should be reserved for deeper burn wound care. Silvadene® is a white cream that is "slathered" onto the wound. It does not desiccate and has good gram positive and negative coverage, but it does not penetrate into the wound. Sulfamylon® penetrates the burn wound and is used for deep burns. It will sting after application, which limits its use in awake patients. Sulfamylon may cause a profound metabolic acidosis; therefore, follow electrolytes and a pH from an arterial blood gas (ABG) if applying large quantities of Sulfamylon®. Silver-impregnated burn coverings such as Aquacel AG®, Acticoat®, or Silverlon® release nanoparticles of silver into the wound which provide antimicrobial coverage. These bandages may be left in place for up to 3 days before changing. The dressing supplies for each platform and mission differ; check to see what is available and "tactically acquire" supplies if necessary.

No systemic antibiotics are indicated in early burn wound care, only for use with later burn wound infections or burn wound sepsis. While low-grade temperature elevations <101 °F are common with burns, temperatures >102 °F should raise the suspicion that the burn wound may be becoming infected.

Bandaging

Burn wounds need to be cleaned, examined, and rebandaged daily. Objective of bandaging is to create a local wound environment that prevents both desiccation and infection. Bandaging uses two distinct layers: inner and outer.

Inner layer: This is a non-adherent layer used to keep the antibiotic directly on the burn. It should be a sterile bandage that can be any non-adherent bandage material. Examples include Xeroform©, Telfa®, or hydrogel material. If none of these are available, regular gauze can be used, but the amount of topical antibiotic placed in the gauze needs to be increased so that the gauze does not become adherent to the burn. The inner layers of the bandage should not go circumferentially around an extremity; they should be individual pieces of inner bandage to allow for soft tissue swelling.

Outer layer: This is a clean bandage that protects the wound from the outside environment. It need not be sterile but needs to be clean. If available, four-inch Kerlix© works well. For example, if bandaging a large area on the chest, take a Kerlix© and unravel it and layer it onto the burn wound over topical antibiotics. Ace wraps or clean sheets cut into six-inch strips also work. Most outer bandages are used circumferentially; take care to wrap snugly but not too tightly to avoid impairing venous return or tissue perfusion.

Some military AMALs will have a "Burn Tec" dressing kit. These bandages are similar to hydrocolloid bandages in civilian use. They are best reserved for partial-thickness burns, superficial or deep, that have a good probability to heal without surgery. The bandage is applied after the wound has been cleaned and mechanically debrided and left in place for 3 days without removal and can be reused for another 3 days if still clean.

Large burns in an austere environment are challenging to provide wound care. These patients will consume large amounts of bandage material, IV fluid, and medications. Therefore, every effort to transport the patient up the echelon of care is essential.

Pain Management

Small burns: Use baseline oral pain control including acetaminophen and NSAIDs. The most pain will come with the cleaning, mechanical debridement, and bandage application, which may merit narcotics. Once the wound is covered and no longer exposed to air the pain will begin to diminish. Keep burned extremities elevated to reduce edema.

Large burns: Full-thickness (third- and fourth-degree burns) are insensate and do not typically require large amounts of pain medications. Patients may need IV narcotics for burn debridement, especially of partial-thickness burns. Maintenance pain control will depend on the depth and TBSA of the burn wound. Morphine, Dilaudid, or Fentanyl can be titrated to effect either as a bolus or as a continuous infusion. Fentanyl has the least amount of cardiodepressant activity and can be titrated if given as a continuous infusion. Intubated patients tend to be patients with large burns or smoke inhalation, typically requiring IV narcotics and may need anxiolytics. The addition of IV lorazepam or midazolam can be used if the patient is anxious, agitated, or has ventilator dyssynchrony. If these agents are utilized, a numeric sedation and analgesic scoring system should be utilized such as the Richmond Agitation and Sedation Scale. Ketamine can also be used for bandage changes.

Preparation for Transport

First and foremost, know the capabilities of the transfer team and the receiving facility to appropriately plan patient care (see Chap. 31). Next, prepare the patient for transfer. Make sure the airway is intact and will remain so for the duration of the transport. If the patient is intubated, make sure the tube is secured (see below), suction equipment is available, and there is an adequate supply of oxygen for the trip. Provide enough IV fluids if needed, but preferably complete any resuscitation prior to a long transport. Bandage all burn wounds, supply pain medication if indicated. Provide blankets to keep the patient warm. If there will be a long transport, make sure there is ample padding to prevent pressure ulcers. Anticipate delays in transport and account for additional supplies as needed (Chap. 31).

Securing Endotracheal Tube (ETT)

Securing the airway is essential for all MEDEVAC patients who are intubated. However, with facial burns or edema of the face due to resuscitation, it becomes more challenging. Tape does not adhere well in either of these situations. A manufactured endotracheal tube (ETT) holder may work up to a point when the facial edema is too great. Simple tracheostomy or cotton ties will work; it is recommended to use dual ties with both ties secured on the ETT and one tie situated above the ears and the remaining under the ears. This attempts to alleviate the problem of a single tie sliding up or down the head and not being in the correct position. Frequent loosening of the ties initially as edema increases is often needed as well as snugging down the ties as the facial edema decreases past the 72-hour mark.

Burn Wound Healing

First Degree: Superficial Burns

These are superficial burns affecting the epidermis. They require cleaning and application of a moisturizing agent twice daily. They require no bandaging and can be exposed to the air. They will heal in 7–10 days on average. Pain control is with acetaminophen or NSAID.

Second Degree: Superficial Partial-Thickness Burns

These burn wounds involve the epidermis and the superficial layer of the dermis. The structural matrix of the skin including blood vessels and nerves are intact to these burns so they are sensate. They require cleaning, debridement of bullae (if

>2 cm), and application of a topical antibiotic ointment, non-adherent covering (e.g., Xeroform© or Telfa®), then a clean bandage to cover the wound. Wound cleaning and bandage changes ideally are done daily. Alternatively, a silver wrap bandage can be applied directly to the burn wound, covered with a clean bandage, and left in place for 3–5 days. Caution should be taken with the initial care of the burn injury to make sure that it is progressing in a favorable direction. Pain control for this burn can be started with acetaminophen and NSAIDs, but may require the addition of a narcotic. These burn wounds will heal over 14–21 days.

Second Degree: Deep Partial-Thickness Burns

These burns affect the epidermis and both superficial and deep dermis. The structural matrix of the skin is injured resulting in altered sensation. They generally require operative excision and placement of a skin graft (autograft). There are some deep partial-thickness wounds that might heal conservatively in situations where the TBSA is small (<10%) or is located on areas of the body that have a thick dermal layer.

Third Degree: Full-Thickness Burns

These wounds involve all three layers of skin. The structural matrix of the skin is destroyed. Blood vessels are thrombosed, and nerve endings are destroyed. These burns require surgical excision and autografting to heal the wound.

Fourth Degree: Burns Involving Structures Deep to the Skin Including Soft Tissue and Bone

These burns involve all layers of the skin and injury into the soft tissue. They are insensate due to the loss of all nerve endings in the burn. These wounds all need surgical debridement, extensive soft tissue wound preparation, and eventual skin grafting.

Burn Pathophysiology

Local Tissue Damage

The cellular pattern of burn injury can be categorized into three major zones of injury: coagulation necrosis, stasis, and hyperemia, similar to cerebrovascular injury (stroke). The central area of the burn wound where the most intense heat source was transferred resulting in the greatest tissue damage or necrosis. Moving peripherally, the next area is the zone of stasis. In this zone, cellular perfusion is compromised and the tissue is tenuous. This is the zone of potentially viable skin and soft tissue that would be put at risk if a perfusion deficit develops. The most distal circumferential area is the zone of hyperemia. Vasodilation occurs in this zone resulting in the hyperemic look to the periphery of the wound. This erythema should not be confused with cellulitis of the wound, which is a low occurrence event and tends to happen days into the burn.

Systemic Capillary Leak

Burn injuries of >20% TBSA are associated with a systemic response. Various inflammatory mediators, cytokines, lymphokines, and tumor necrosis factor are released from the burn tissue leading to a hyperdynamic cardiovascular and hypermetabolic responses. Capillaries develop increased permeability due to an enlargement of the normally tight endothelial junctions. As these junctions widen under the influence of inflammatory mediators, there is a diapedesis of fluid and macromolecules into the interstitium for the first 24–48 h of the burn injury. Once the inflammatory mediator concentration is reduced, the endothelial gap junctions close to their normal aperture and the capillary leak process ceases.

To restate, **this response is not local but a systemic process of edema formation** and tends to become clinically significant with burns >40% TBSA. Therefore, a patient with bilateral lower extremity burns (36% TBSA) and back burns (18% TBSA) totaling 54% TBSA may develop airway compromise as the diffuse edema develops and involves the patient's upper airway far distant to the burn area.

Burn Shock

After the initial burn resuscitation, as the capillary leak progresses, intravascular fluid accumulates in the interstitial space. The circulating plasma volume is decreased, and if not repleted will result in hypotension, poor perfusion to vital organs, and a worsening of the burn wound as the zone of stasis begins to deteriorate due to poor perfusion. A distributive form of shock will ensue and must be addressed. See the resuscitation portion of this chapter for recommendations.

It is imperative that an accurate intake (I) and output (O) flow sheet is maintained. All fluids need to be accounted for in the resuscitation and totaled as the hourly (I). In the early phase of the burn, there is not a lot of fluid loss through the burned skin. The UOP is an accurate marker of clinically significant output and one of the first markers of insufficient resuscitation will be a decrease in the patient's UOP. SBP will decrease with the ongoing third spacing of fluids, reflecting a profound fluid deficit. The clinician's response to this is to increase the resuscitation fluids. It is not a good practice to bolus these patients with fluid. The loss of the bolus fluid is accelerated by the capillary leak problem and the increase in hydrostatic pressure from the fluid bolus will drive more fluid into the interstitium. *The net intravascular fluid gain is less with a bolus approach than by increasing the fluid.*

Burn Wound Infections

Burn Wound Cellulitis

There is localized erythema due to hyperemia and vasodilation around most burns; this does NOT represent infection. Cellulitis involves the epidermis and upper dermal tissues and tends to be seen at >3 days in "dirty" burns and >5 days in clean burns. At 3–5 days the zone of hyperemia has resolved so any new areas of erythema moving outside the original confines of the burn wound likely represent burn wound cellulitis. Treatment of cellulitis includes the administration of antibiotics (first-generation cephalosporin) and assuring the wound is clean.

Burn Wound Infection

This type of infection is seen in deeper burns and represents an infection of the epidermis, dermis, and possibly deeper subcutaneous tissues. It may have erythema or frank purulence emanating from the wound. It tends to occur in deep partial- or full-thickness burns and is indicative of high bacterial wound concentrations. The timeframe is many days post-burn injury, emphasizing the importance of examining, cleaning, and rebandaging burn wounds daily. An unchanged burn bandage can accelerate a wound infection as the bandage provides a dark, moist medium for bacterial growth. If the patient's temperature spikes to >102 °F, examine the burn wound to make sure it is not the culprit. Treatment includes antibiotic therapy and probable surgical debridement.

Burn Wound Sepsis

This is when a burn wound infection results in a systemic infection. The patient's burn microbes have easy access into the capillary system through the burn injury. Bacteremia or burn wound sepsis may develop. It is a virulent and deadly occurrence. The burn wound looks deeply infected, may have purulence or sloughing of the necrotic tissue. **This is a surgical emergency!** The patient needs systemic antibiotics and aggressive surgical wound debridement of the infected tissue.

Types of Burn Injury

Inhalation Injury

Severe inhalation injury occurs in 15% of combat burn injuries. Closed spaces are numerous aboard a surface or subsurface ship. Fire within these areas will place the patient at a greater risk for an inhalation injury due to multiple factors including low ambient oxygen concentration, exposure to the toxic byproducts of combustion and elevated compartment temperature due to the fire. Additional risk factors for inhalation injury include large burns, facial and upper torso burns, loss of consciousness and prolonged extrication. Inhalation injury can be discussed in terms of anatomic or mechanistic injury patterns.

Anatomic: There is supraglottic, subglottic, lower respiratory, and systemic injury. The supraglottic area with its large moist turbinates and hypopharynx can decrease the temperature of the hot inhaled air. Likewise, the nasal hairs trap larger particulate matter before it can enter the lower respiratory tract. The airflow into the hypopharynx is such that additional particulate matter is deposited on the posterior pharyngeal area. If soot is on the posterior hypopharynx, assume a significant inhalation injury is present. Once the lower respiratory tract is entered, the heat is rapidly transferred to distal airways and alveoli.

Mechanistic: There are three types of smoke inhalation injury. In order of occurrence, there is particulate inhalation, toxic inhalation, and thermal inhalation injury.

- Particulate inhalation injury is due to the small particulates of smoke that are inhaled that cause a reactive airway activation. The patient coughs and spits up carbonaceous particulate matter. The treatment is supportive, with bronchodilators and supplemental oxygen to keep the $SpO_2 > 92\%$. With time, most patients clear the episode without progressing further.
- Clinically, there are two common important toxic byproducts of combustion: Carbon monoxide (CO) and cyanide (various compounds).
  - *Carbonmonoxide* is a byproduct of incomplete combustion or auto exhaust, and it is colorless, odorless, and lethal via two deleterious effects. First, hemoglobin has a 200–250 times affinity for CO than for oxygen. Therefore, CO preferentially binds to the iron on the hemoglobin molecule, displacing oxygen and resulting in decreased oxygen delivery to the tissues. Second, CO will competitively bind the cytochrome oxidase enzymes in the Krebs cycle resulting in a reduction in adenosine triphosphate (ATP) production. Symptoms of CO poisoning include headache, dizziness, nausea and vomiting, tachycardia, tachypnea, syncope, seizures, Cheyne-Stokes breathing, coma, bradycardia, hypopnea, and death. Any patient who was in a closed space fire should be assumed to have some degree of CO inhalation injury. Do not be confused by

normal SpO_2 on pulse oximetry. The technology on most oximeters cannot differentiate between oxyhemoglobin and CO-hemoglobin complex, therefore the SpO_2 may be erroneously elevated. The partial pressure of oxygen in the arterial blood (PaO_2) obtained on ABG (if available) is a reliable value. High flow oxygen is the therapy, even it is available in limited quantities in the field. Increasing the concentration gradient in the alveoli will offload CO and improve oxygen delivery. A patient breathing room air will have a CO half-life of 4–6 h. This can be reduced to 60–90 min if the patient is on 100% fraction of inspired oxygen (FiO_2).

– *Cyanide* is released during the combustion of nitrogen and carbon-containing materials such as cotton, paper, wool, silk, and plastics, and it is a colorless gas that releases a bitter almond smell. It interferes with aerobic respiration and ATP production. Symptoms of cyanide poisoning include headaches, vertigo, weakness, dizziness, confusion, pulmonary edema, seizures, apnea, unconsciousness, and cardiac arrest. The best treatment for cyanide poisoning is with the CYANOKIT®, which is hydroxocobalamin (Vitamin B12) that binds to cyanide to form cyanocobalamin, a nontoxic compound. CYANOKIT contains 5 g of hydroxocobalamin and is administered over 15 min. A second dose may be needed in clinically deteriorating patients; in an austere environment, this is not likely to be available. Alternative treatments are amyl nitrate, sodium nitrite, and sodium thiosulfate, if available. High flow oxygen to improve oxygen-carrying capacity of hemoglobin is indicated in all cases. Cyanide toxicity is also discussed in Chap. 29.

- Thermal inhalation injury may be seen in the supraglottic area but is less common in the subglottic and distal airways. If the heat exposure is long, as in the case of a patient enclosed in a closed space fire such as a room or vehicle, then the normal heat exchange mechanism may be overrun resulting in subglottic and lower airway thermal injury. Edema, bronchospasm, inspissation of secretions, sloughing of respiratory epithelium, and mucosal ulcerations all contribute to this injury pattern. Intubation is indicated to provide support to these patients.

Scald Injury

Scald injuries are the most common form of burn injuries in children but are also common in adults. Injuries due to hot water used in cooking, hot beverages, and industrial or occupational activities are leading causes of scalds. Each mechanism of scalding brings liquids of different temperatures in contact with the patient. Hot water for bathing is typically set at 125 °F, and the time for a deep burn to occur at this temperature is 2 min. The same scald burn will occur in 10 seconds (s) at 130 °F and in 2 s at 150 °F. Commercial hot drinks have a serving temperature of around 160–185 °F. Cooking oil from deep fryers is 375 °F and 10 times more viscous than water. Roofing tar is 450 °F and 20 times more viscous than water. The higher viscosity hot liquids will stay in contact with the victim longer and result in deeper burns. Immediate "cooling" of the injured area with a water lavage will limit the extent of the burn.

Steam Injury

Steam injuries often are a result of pressurized steam. In the maritime environment, etiology is commonly steam pressure cookers, propulsion ship engines, and steam heating and hot water systems of shore stations. Pressurized steam is much hotter than steam coming off a boiling pot of water. Steam from boiling water is 212 °F, whereas pressurized steam can be up to 265 °F. One of the occupational risks with steam burns is that the patient is often trapped in a small workspace, making the exposure time to the steam longer. Breathing steam may result in clinically significant inhalation injury due to the high latent heat content capacity of steam. The steam particles overwhelm the patient's nasopharyngeal and upper airway defenses resulting in thermal injury to the entire respiratory tract.

The physical appearance of steam burn injuries can be quite deceiving. Partial thickness steam burns appear erythematous while full thickness steam burns appear white and feel rubbery. These injuries tend to be circumferential due to the behavior of the steam particles in the local environment.

Flame Injury

Flame burns are not all created equal as different substances burn at different temperatures, similar to steam injuries (e.g., cigarette (750–1300 °F), gasoline (1472–2552 °F), and wood (3596 °F)). If the patient's clothes were on fire, they will likely have full-thickness burns. Burn victims with a shirt or blouse on fire are likely to sustain facial burns and inhalation injuries.

Contact/Conduction Injury

Contact burns are as the name implies: burns caused by contact with a heat source. Examples include hot engines, hot deck plates on ships that are sailing in desert climates, steam or hot water lines, and hot pavement in a desert climate. Here the extent of the injury is a product of the temperature of the surface material and the time of the contact. While all trauma protocols for addressing trauma wounds in the field need to be considered, these patients must be moved from the hot surface to prevent a "secondary" burn injury.

Friction Injury

Friction burns are caused by the skin encountering a moving piece of equipment such as a rubber belt or a treadmill or when a patient falls on a rough surface also known as "road rash." The friction generates heat causing a burn injury and the moving parts cause a traumatic tissue injury. It is important to remove the dirt and embedded pieces of material from the injured area, especially those caused by "road rash." It may be necessary to use topical lidocaine on the wound before attempting to clean as the partial-thickness burn wounds will be sensate. If the dirt and other foreign material is not removed, it may become embedded in the wound healing process and remain in the healed skin resulting in a "debris tattoo."

Electrical Injury

Electrical injuries are the result of contact with alternating (AC) or a direct current (DC) source. AC with alternating current direction every 60 cycles facilitates muscle contraction and a similar period of muscle relaxation due to the current directional change. DC is a constant, one-way directional current that results in muscle tetany from constant stimulation. The practical side of this distinction is that with AC current the victim has an opportunity to break away from the current source, whereas with DC the victim tends to stay in contact with the current source due to prolonged flexor muscle contraction. The patient's internal tissue resistance is also a factor for current flow. Muscle and bone are high-resistance tissues and can sustain rapid heat buildup and tissue damage, whereas nerve tissue is one of the lowest resistance tissues, so delicate nerve fibers are often damaged. Generally, if a high current passed from the ipsilateral upper to lower extremity or vice versa, the patient is in a better position than if an electrical current traversed the body from one side to the other, endangering the heart.

Patients who encounter a high voltage electrical source or remain in contact with an electrical source for a longer period may have a more profound injury. The entrance and exit sites tend to have full- or deep partial-thickness burns, which may be diminutive compared to the extent of the internal injury. The soft tissue injury is deep and tends to be localized in the extremity where the entrance wound is found. There are demonstrable motor and sensory abnormalities. An ominous physical sign is to find the extremity (most often hand) in a claw-like position of flexion with no motor function and resistance to passive range of motion. The muscles are "cooked" and in a position of maximal contraction (Fig. 26.3). Patients with these findings will likely require emergency surgery for fasciotomy and soft tissue debridement. They are also at risk for arterial and venous thrombosis in the affected limb. If the radial, ulnar, or brachial arteries have been severely damaged, they may rupture near the 72-hour mark. Any acute bleeding in these wound beds should be assumed to be

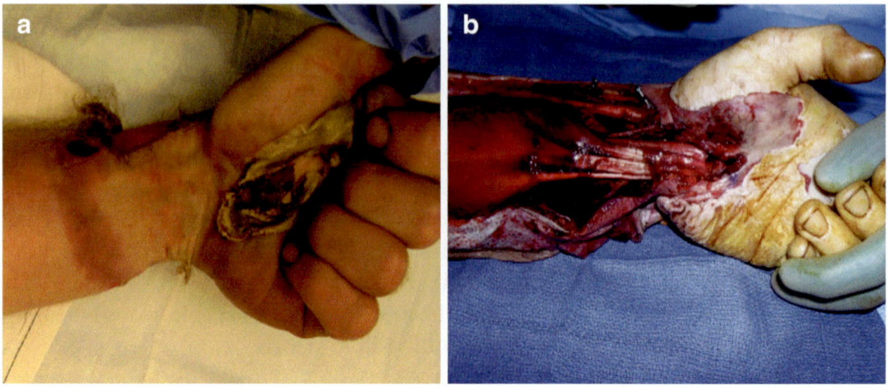

Fig. 26.3 Example of an electrical burn. (**a**) Electrical burn to the right forearm with full-thickness entrance site on palm. Note digit flexion contracture and soft tissue contraction around the wrist. (**b**) Intraoperative photo of the same injury demonstrating a fourth-degree injury. The patient's arm was not salvageable. (Source: Photos courtesy of Bruce Potenza, MD, MPH)

a major arterial bleed and treated aggressively. If an operation is not feasible, put a tourniquet on the extremity and get the patient transported to a higher level of care.

Watch for rhabdomyolysis and follow creatine phosphokinase levels if available. Look for blood in the urine and the development of a dark tan- or red-looking urine. Administer fluids to keep the UOP 100 mL/h.

Two other forms of electrical injury frequently seen with military trauma are arc and flash burns.

Arc: Arc burn is an electrical injury that occurs when the electrical source can send a current through the air and strike a victim. This occurs when there is a short in the electrical system permitting the current to escape its confines. On the victim side they will be close to the electrical source and grounded, most likely working on the piece of equipment. The electrical current will follow the path of least resistance and may arc onto the victim. The arc lasts milliseconds and may cause a "shock-like" feeling and result in a partial-thickness burn.

Flash: Flash electrical burn occurs when there are tiny dust particles in the air, usually when someone is working on a dirty or dusty piece of equipment, usually with a metal tool such as a wrench, and they cause a spark. The spark ignites the dust particles and for a millisecond there is an intense flash emitted as the dust vaporizes. The patient will usually sustain a superficial to deep partial-thickness burn. Some of their clothing may also be burned due to the intense heat, resulting in a patient sustaining flame burns as well. There are no entrance or exit points, only burns from the flash. Care for these burns is no different from any other burn. Think of the flash burn like a single strobe light flash, only this flash is extremely bright and at an extremely high temperature. Remember to do an eye examination; damage to the cornea may occur, and patients typically describe a transient inability to see well. The corneal injury is managed with topical ophthalmic antibiotics and rarely patching of the eye if there is an actual corneal abrasion.

Chemical Injury

The pathophysiology of acid and alkali burn injuries is different from other mechanisms of burn injury. Acid burns denature proteins and result in coagulation necrosis of skin and soft tissue, which *impedes* deeper penetration of the acid. Alkali burns result in liquefaction necrosis, which makes it *easier* for the caustic substance to penetrate deeper into the soft tissue.

The longer any chemical agent is in contact with the skin the deeper the burn, so the initial treatment is copious lavage of the affected area. It is important to remember that the fraction of the chemical agent that has already penetrated the epidermis will continue with tissue destruction until neutralized by the local tissue environment. The injured skin areas are otherwise treated like most other burn injuries.

Three chemical agents are noteworthy for military personnel: hydrogen fluoride (HF), white phosphorus (WP), and cement.

Hydrogen fluoride is a corrosive acid used for cleaning and etching. It is extremely dangerous as it can cause both deep tissue destruction and act as a systemic toxin. This acid is able to penetrate into deep tissues and bone as long as there are active fluoride ions. Bone destruction can be seen long after exposure. Fatal toxicity due to hypocalcemia and hypomagnesemia and hyperkalemia results in cardiac abnormalities including prolonged QT interval and cardiac irritability. Treatment includes copious lavage and the application of a calcium gel or injection of calcium into the injured area to bind with the fluoride ion. A topical calcium gel can be made with 25 mL of 10% calcium gluconate mixed with 75 mL of K-Y Jelly. If the pain persists, consider a calcium injection. Inject a 5–10% calcium gluconate solution into the subcutaneous tissue where the burn occurred using a 25- or 27-gauge needle. In both instances overlap the area of calcium application by at least 1 inch and apply every 4 h.

White phosphorous WP is a common acid agent found in military incendiary shells, fertilizers, and fireworks. When it is exploded via artillery shell at altitude, it lights up the night sky. As it is extremely volatile, it will spontaneously ignite at (86 °F) in the presence of oxygen. Lavage is the first line of care for these patients. Do not try to simply wipe off any residual powder as it may ignite, use only water lavage and wet wipes. Cover the burn with wet bandages and do not let them dry out! Definitive care is to mechanically or surgically debride all the WP particles from the wound bed. The use of copper sulfate is not indicated for this injury. Identification of WP particulates can be accomplished by the use of a Wood's lamp or other ultraviolet source, which will demonstrate a yellow smoldering smoke emanating from the burning skin. This is an indication to get more water over the wound and get the patient into the OR. Where there is smoke there is ongoing tissue destruction. It is a surgical urgency to remove as much of the embedded WP as possible, which may require repeated debridement to accomplish. Particles that are removed in surgery should be placed in a container of water so that they will not ignite on the back table if left open to the air.

Cement is a strong alkali with a pH of 12–14. Construction workers (i.e., Seabees) may get wet cement in their boots or on their pant legs. This should not be allowed to dry on their skin as an alkali burn will develop so they should rinse the cement off their skin. These burns tend to be insidious in the early stage, and patients may not even realize they have been injured. Worse, the patient doesn't rinse off the cement so the contact time can be lengthy. They may present later with skin erythema and pain. At this point, rinse the affected area well and treat the burn as a superficial partial-thickness burn.

Radiation Injury

The containment, decontamination, and overall management of patients with radiation injury are covered extensively in Chap. 29. Radiation burn injuries are initially treated in the same manner as similar depth burn wounds. Radiation injuries are dynamic with cellular damage continuing long due to residual radiation or chromosomal damage. Extreme caution to protect the medical personnel is necessary when working with radiation exposed patients.

Elevated Compartment Pressures and Compartment Syndromes

Elevated tissue pressure in burn injuries develops due to a slightly different mechanism than traumatic injuries. As described in the pathophysiology section, burn injuries >20% TBSA result in a systemic vasodilation, capillary leak syndrome, interstitial third spacing of fluids, and systemic edema. Circumferential or near-circumferential deep partial-thickness and full-thickness burn wounds of the extremity can act to limit the amount of swelling that can occur. As the underlying tissue third spacing and edema formation continues, a point may be reached where the injured skin can no longer stretch to accommodate edema, and the burn wound itself acts as a constricting band on the extremity causing the compartment pressures to increase. Normal compartment pressures are 8–12 cm water (H_2O), and there is little concern for pressures up to 20 cm H_2O. Perfusion pressure at the capillary level may become impaired at levels >20 cm H_2O. Tissue pressures >30 cm H_2O should be considered for escharotomies while between 20–30 cm H_2O can be individualized.

When treating a circumferential extremity burn it is important to keep the extremity elevated. This is much easier in the upper extremities. Once the burn wounds are cleaned and bandaged a sling can be devised to "hang" the extremity from an IV pole. The hand is extended upward as if to wave hello, the elbow bent at 90°, and the upper arm extended at the level of the shoulder.

See Chap. 24 for discussion of the measurement of compartment pressures with both designated and makeshift devices. If one has access to the former, use it and follow the directions.

A second form of compartment syndrome can occur in the abdomen or thorax. The pathophysiology is similar to the same occurrences from trauma or other large-volume resuscitation efforts. During a large burn resuscitation, large amounts of ascitic fluid accompanied by small bowel mesenteric edema and the constrictive nature of the burn may result in abdominal compartment syndrome. Use bladder pressure measurement as a surrogate measurement of intra-abdominal pressure.

The decision to perform an abdominal escharotomy should be made on three factors:

- Total abdominal pressures and trends
- Where the patient is on the resuscitation timeline (end or beginning)-how much more IV fluid will be administered
- Deterioration of physiologic signs (low UOP, decreasing SBP, tachycardia or decreased tidal volumes)

If a point-of-care ultrasound (POCUS) is available and significant ascites is demonstrated, an attempt at paracentesis may be undertaken to relieve some of the pressure. Abdominal pressures >20 cm H_2O should be monitored for a trend upward and at 30 cm H_2O or physiologic signs of deterioration, an abdominal escharotomy should be performed (Fig. 26.4a).

Deep partial- and full-thickness burn wounds to the chest can also affect the chest wall mechanics of intrinsic breathing or ventilator-assisted breathing. The burn wound need not be circumferential, but if it involves most of the anterior and lateral thorax, it is sufficient to restrict normal chest wall movement. Elevated ventilator pressures (peak airway pressures >30 cm H_2O, rising plateau pressures, low exhaled volumes) are markers of physiologic demise. Treatment with escharotomies of the anterior chest wall and extension up onto the neck may be needed to alleviate this condition (Fig. 26.4a).

Escharotomy

Escharotomies are different from fasciotomies. The depth of escharotomy is only through the full thickness of the skin and barely into the subcutaneous fat. Fasciotomies are deeper to release the muscle fascia (see Chaps. 19 and 24). Performing an escharotomy is relatively straightforward requiring only electrocautery and suction, but it should still be done in a formal operating room (OR) setting. To prepare, clean the burn wound with soap and water or betadine. If using the

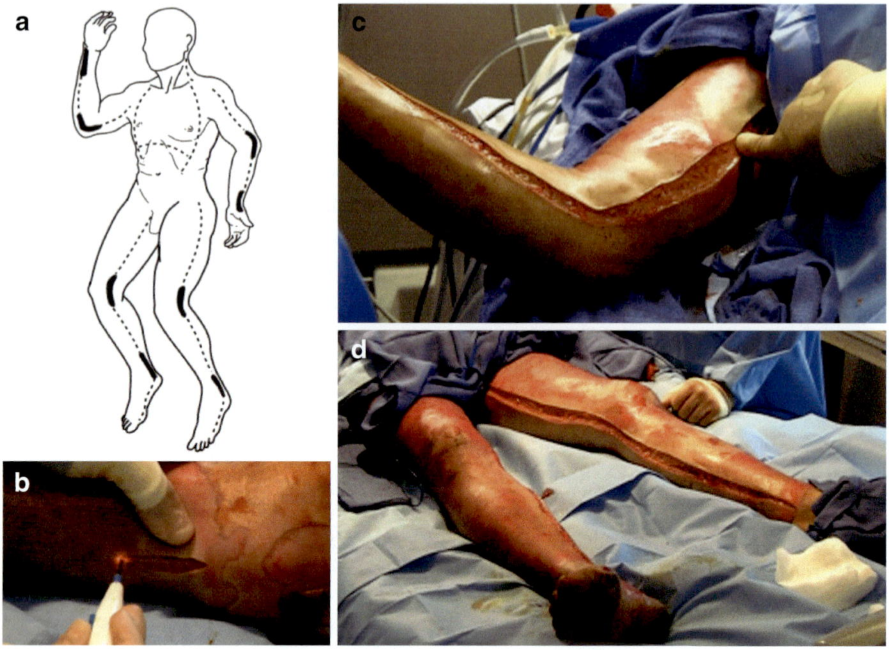

Fig. 26.4 Escharotomy. (**a**) Diagram of Escharotomy incisions. (**b**) Example of left medial lower extremity medial escharotomy. Note how the incision spreads quickly after the escharotomy incision is made. (**c**) Right upper arm medial escharotomy. (**d**) Bilateral lower extremity full-thickness burns with left lower extremity medial escharotomy. (Source: Image and photos courtesy of Bruce Potenza, MD, MPH)

latter, make sure it is dry before using electrocautery as this is an increased fire risk. Draw or visually map out the escharotomy incision line (examples shown in Fig. 26.4). These incisions do not need to be exact as the full-thickness burns will be excised later. If the patient is intubated and sedated, typically some extra IV narcotic is all that is necessary as the wound is insensate. If the patient is awake, use lidocaine with epinephrine. Use electrocautery on coagulation level 40 and slowly incise the full-thickness skin. Obtain hemostasis in real time. Extend the escharotomy 1–2 cm proximal to the burn tissue. Run a finger along the escharotomy incision to feel for any tight bands and incise them with electrocautery as they are dermal bands that may limit release. Bandage the wound with inner and outer layers as described in the bandaging portion of this chapter. Create bandage "windows" over major arteries to facilitate easier serial examinations.

Lateral Orbital Canthotomy Release

Patients with extensive facial edema from burns or resuscitation may develop increased intraocular pressure (IOP) due to edematous, tightly shut eyelids. This is a potentially devastating condition that can lead to blindness due to orbital compartment syndrome. If possible, on the maritime platform, perform serial IOP measurements until the eyelids can easily open and close. Patients with IOP >20 cm H_2O should be considered for a lateral canthotomy release and inferior cantholysis. If IOP measurements are not possible, follow the physical exam. Tightly shut eyelids due to edema translate into increased IOP and should be an indication that a lateral canthotomy and inferior cantholysis may be necessary (Fig. 26.5).

Follow the recommendations in CPG ID 003 (Eye Trauma) available at: https://jts.amedd.army.mil/assets/docs/cpgs/Eye_Trauma_Initial_Care_01_Jun_2021_ID03.pdf

1. Identify the lateral canthus area of the eye. Inject the subdermal area with lidocaine with epinephrine (1:100,000). Extend this infiltration 1–2 cm laterally.
2. Place a small mosquito or snap under the canthus full-thickness skin and lift away from the eye. Clamp the skin for 1–2 min to assist with hemostasis.
3. With scissors, cut the full-thickness skin (lateral canthus) for approximately 1 cm.
4. Grab the lower lateral eyelid with forceps and pull downward where the incision is. Identify a small firm band of tissue along the inferior lateral border of the orbit, which is the inferior lateral canthal ligament that needs to be cut. The ligament is strong and feels like a bowstring.
5. Place scissors across the ligament and cut it completely; the cut is audible as it goes through the ligament.
6. Examine this area again to make sure all of the ligament has been incised. The eye should be mobile laterally. If there is a high IOP the eye should move forward to relieve the pressure.

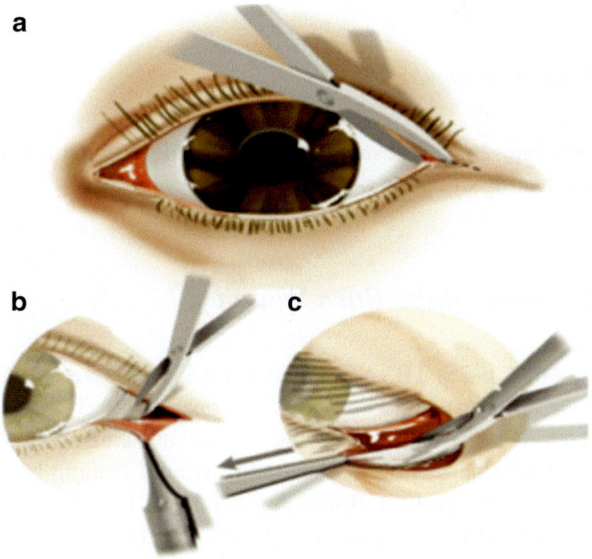

Fig. 26.5 Lateral canthotomy and inferior cantholysis. Note there are two incisions through the (**a**) lateral canthal skin (full-thickness) and (**b**)/(**c**) the inferior canthal ligament. (Source: The Wills Eye Manual. Wolters-Kluwer, used with permission)

7. Repeat on the contralateral side. The areas will not bleed and do not need any hemostatic agents. The combination of the lidocaine and epinephrine with the "crushing" of the tissue will achieve hemostasis.

Post-procedure, administer topical ophthalmic antibiotic lubricant four times daily. Do not place an eye shield over the eyes as this could increase the IOP if contact is made between the shield and the globe.

Technical Procedures Used in Burn Care

Every attempt to transfer a burned injured servicemember up the echelon of care should be the foremost priority. However, there may come a time when the maritime surgical team needs to perform definitive burn wound care such as excision and grafting. The ship may be caring for local nationals (Chap. 35) or there may be no ability to MEDEVAC because of DMO.

Unfortunately, if not at a Role 3 facility, it is unlikely that the materials required to perform these procedures are available for the maritime surgical team. However, in a dynamic multi-domain theater of operations requiring prolonged casualty care, the required equipment may be obtained from a regional Role 3, or for teams on Role 3 hospital ships with the required equipment, the following may be helpful. The members of the maritime surgical team also may not have any recent experience with burn wound procedures. Contact the USAISR Burn Center to have them "talk through" the steps and to be an engaged resource. There are many facets to excision and grafting to make it successful that are beyond the scope of this chapter. This is a brief overview of definitive surgical burn wound care.

Equipment

See Fig. 26.6 for examples of standard equipment used in the excision of burns, harvesting of donor sites, and meshing of grafts.

Excision of the Burn Wound

A small 1–2% TBSA deep burn not located over vital structures (i.e., hands, feet, face, or joint) could be treated nonoperatively if necessary. With good burn wound care, it will heal with some degree of scarring and contracture. Deep partial-thickness burns not demonstrating wound healing by day 7 will likely need to be excised and grafted. Burns that appear to be healing and then start to worsen and develop surrounding erythema may be infected. Excision should be limited to 5%

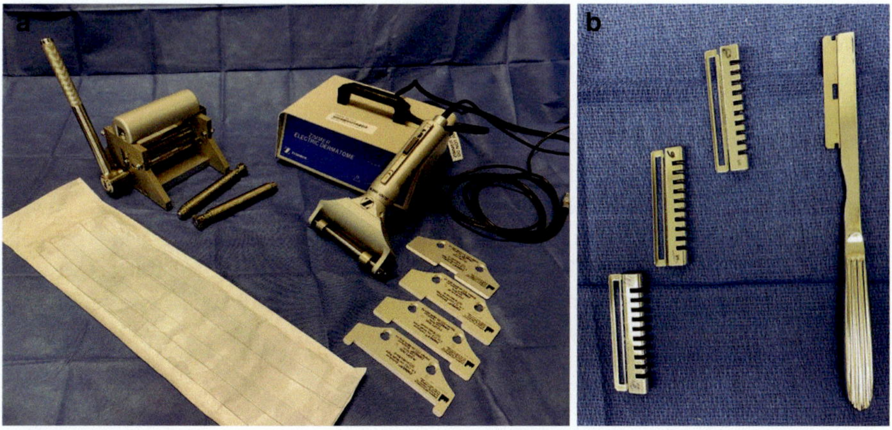

Fig. 26.6 Equipment used for harvesting, meshing, and excising. (**a**) (Left) Skin mesher; roller size determines skin expansion ratio, plastic skin carrier determines skin expansion ratio. (Right) Dermatome for harvesting donor skin. (**b**) Weck or Goulian knives with 0.008–0.012 inch guards. (Source: Photos courtesy of Bruce Potenza, MD, MPH)

TBSA per operation to limit blood loss and operative time. All areas of excision and harvesting should be surgically cleaned and prepped.

To properly excise the burn wound, use a Weck (or Goulian) knife. They are straight razors with a guard that determines the depth of excision. Choose a guard with a depth of 0.008–0.012 in., with deeper burns requiring the larger guard size. Gently but firmly place the blade and guard on the burned skin at a 30–45° angle. Press downward on the burn wound and move the knife in a slicing motion to excise the burn wound. Slowly move the instrument across the entire burn wound. Generally, one can excise a few inches at a time, moving along the burn. Practice ahead of time by trying to excise an orange or apple peel.

The depth of excision should be down to bleeding tissue. If excising a small area (<5% TBSA), no tourniquet is needed so there will be brisk capillary bleeding. Caution; this capillary bleeding can be deceiving and quickly result in significant blood loss. Larger burns (>5% TBSA) should be excised under a tourniquet if possible to minimize blood loss. If no formal orthopedic tourniquet, use a large blood pressure cuff inflated to 100 mm Hg higher than the SBP placed proximal to the sterile extremity field. Try to keep the tourniquet inflated for less than 1 h. When the tourniquet is inflated, the depth of excision is visual as there will not be significant bleeding in the wound bed.

Skin substitutes will likely not be available; therefore, what is excised must be autografted or covered with a temporizing bandage that will promote wound bed growth while waiting for a future skin graft. Smaller burns (2–3% TBSA) can be excised and autografted in one setting. If a skin mesher is available, that number can be extended to 5% TBSA. Otherwise, consider placing a negative pressure dressing (if available) over the excised area to use as a temporizing bandage. Remove in 3 days and re-examine the wound to make certain all the burn wound that is compromised has been excised. Alternately, the excision area of deep partial-thickness burns can be treated with topical antibiotic ointment and Xeroform© gauze. Full-thickness burns can be dressed with wet-to-dry bandaging changed daily to promote granulation tissue growth. These wounds can be managed for up to 2 weeks in this fashion awaiting transfer or to stage autografting. Negative pressure bandage therapy can be used for full thickness wounds for a longer period of time. They are simple and alleviate daily burn wound care. They should be changed every 5 days to provide an opportunity for wound inspection and cleaning.

Harvesting Donor Skin Graft

Skin harvesting is the process of shaving a thin layer of skin for placement on a prepared wound bed. The autograft consists of the entire layer of epidermis and a thin layer of dermis. An electric-powered dermatome is needed for harvesting. Attach the blade in the dermatome and set the depth to 0.010–0.015 in. The final depth of the graft depends on the depth setting and the amount of downward pressure applied to the donor site when harvesting. **It is important to note that no matter how hard one presses it is not possible to get a thicker piece of autograft than the depth setting but if one does not press hard enough it IS possible to get a thinner depth.** There are four size guards to determine the width of autograft, typically a three- or four-inch guard is used.

The best harvest site for small burns is the anterior-lateral aspect of the thigh. There is good thick dermis in this area, and it heals well. The posterior thigh is also good, but more difficult to work on when the patient is in the supine position; however, if the graft site is also posterior then this is a good site. Secondary donor sites include the calves and the posterior torso. If harvesting the posterior torso, try to harvest over the thoracic cage which will assist in providing a firm surface to harvest. The buttocks may be used, but it is a difficult wound site to manage postoperatively.

Prep the donor site as any other surgical field. Use a tumescence solution to limit blood loss and to "firm up" the donor site, which will make using the dermatome easier and limit blood loss. Dilute an epinephrine solution (1 mg per mL as shown in Fig. 26.7) into 1 L of NS. Use a large syringe with a spinal needle or an 18- or 16-gauge needle. Draw up repeated syringes and inject into the subdermal upper-fat layer of the donor site; visualize injecting at the dermal/adipose junction. If in the correct plane, the skin will bulge outward and become firm. Tumesce the entire donor site plus 50% additional area around the periphery.

Place a penetrating towel clip at the proximal and distal ends of the donor area. Have an assistant pull the two towel clamps away from each other so that the donor

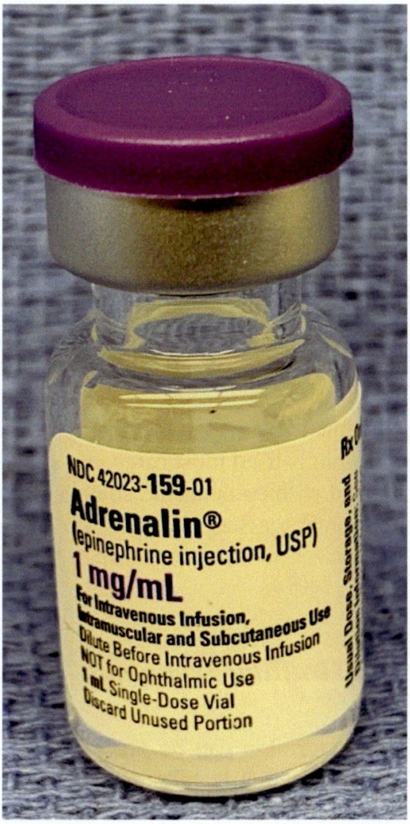

Fig. 26.7 Example of Epinephrine 1 mg/mL concentration. (Source: Photo courtesy of Bruce Potenza, MD, MPH)

skin becomes taut. Place sterile oil or dilute surgical soap on the donor site so the dermatome will slide smoothly over the skin. If this step is skipped, the dermatome will dig into the donor site.

Use the dermatome firmly and smoothly pushing it axially along the donor site to harvest the skin. Watch the skin being harvested to check the depth; if the harvest is only a transparent thin piece of skin, it is too THIN. Strive to have a thin layer of white dermis visible on the autograft when it is harvested. Apply more pressure to the dermatome or increase the setting of the dermatome by another 0.002 in. An assistant can gently pull the autograft out of the dermatome with a forceps during harvest. There should be minimal bleeding at the harvest site if it was tumesced with an epinephrine solution.

Hemostasis

Burn excision and donor site hemostasis is imperative and accomplished in a step-wise fashion. Use a non-adherent gauze as the base layer for hemostasis. Moistened

Telfa© pads are excellent, as they will not stick to the wound when removed. A moistened laparotomy pad will also work but expect some rebleeding with removal. As an adjunct, soak the Telfa© or laparotomy pad in the same epinephrine solution used for tumescence and gently squeeze out the excess. Cover the excised wound base with soaked Telfa© or laparotomy pads then place some dry laparotomy pads on top and wrap snugly with Kerlix©.

Let the tourniquet down and wait 15 min. Then unwrap the Kerlix©, wet down the Telfa© or laparotomy pads with saline, and slowly remove them. The bleeding should have slowed, but this process will likely need to be repeated one or two more times. There may be a need to use spot electrocautery in the excision site to obtain full hemostasis. Before placing a skin graft into the wound bed, achieve meticulous hemostasis, or the graft will "float" and not adhere to the excised wound base resulting in graft loss.

Hemostatic agents for this application may not be available in the field. Topical thrombin is used most often and sprayed or spread directly over the wound and can be used with epinephrine-soaked Telfa© or laparotomy pads. Don't use Surgicel©, Gelfoam©, or Surgifilo©, as the "coagulum debris" all needs to be removed before grating.

Skin Grafting Technique

The donor skin can be placed on the prepared burn wound directly without any meshing, which is called a sheet autograft. If a mesher is available and there is a need to expand the skin to obtain coverage of the burn wound, use a 1:1.5 or 1:2 expansion set. There are two types of meshers, one where the "roller" comes in a predetermined mesh expansion and another where the plastic skin "carrier" has a predetermined expansion size. Look at the end of the roller and it will indicate the expansion for that roller. For example, if the roller number is 2, then it will be expanding the donor skin 1:2. If expansion is needed, it is conventional to use the 1:2 expansion for autografting. Large expansion of 1:3 or 1:4 should not be used in the field as the care of these autografts is very labor intensive.

Moisten the plastic skin carrier for both types of meshers and place the donor skin in it with the dermal side facing the plastic. Use the mesher handle to move the plastic skin carrier through the mesher. Grab the newly meshed skin with a forceps as it comes out from under the roller so that it does not get caught in the roller mechanism.

If no meshing is required, place some linear holes (2–3 mm) in the graft using a #15 blade (1 cm apart) to allow the serum to get out from under the graft. If the skin was meshed, make sure all the hole "interstices" are open. Sometimes the mesher doesn't cut well and the interstices are "stuck" together. Use a #15 blade to open them without cutting the actual skin pattern.

Lay the autograft on the prepared wound bed. When the optimal fit has been obtained, attach the graft to the surrounding healthy skin with a skin stapler or 4-0 nylon sutures spaced 1 cm apart. Place a few additional tacking staples or sutures in the middle of the autograft to hold it in place. Now bandage the autograft.

Bandaging Postoperative Autografts and Donor Sites

Autograft bandaging:

- Option 1: Open a 5 × 9 sheet of Xeroform© and apply a layer of topical antibiotic to the Xeroform© and not directly to the autograft. The layer should be like a thin icing of a cake. Place on the skin topical antibiotic side down, and wrap it in a Kerlix© or equivalent dressing. Leave bandaged for 48 h. Thereafter change daily in the same fashion, applying topical antibiotic to the Xeroform© gauze. If no Xeroform© is available, Adaptec©, Telfa©, or any non-adherent bandage is suitable. Continue for approximately 7 days, longer if meshed to a 2:1 expansion; the endpoint is when the interstices have re-epithelialized.
- Option 2: If a silver-impregnated bandage is available, wrap the autograft with it after it has been moistened to both activate the silver nanoparticles and keep the graft from drying out. Cover with a large cotton bandage or abdominal pads (ABD) and wrap with Kerlix© to keep the silver bandage from moving. Lightly moisten twice a day to keep it moist but not soaking wet.

Donor site bandaging:

- Option 1: Place 5 × 9 sheets of Xeroform© directly onto the donor site, taking care not to overlay one sheet onto the next but also completely covering the donor site. Staple it into place by placing staples every 3–4 in. along the periphery and a few staples in the middle of the Xeroform©. Cover this with a non stick bandage, (Telfa) and then ABD pads and bandage with Kerlix© for 24 h. The outer bandage and Telfa are removed daily for 6–8 h to allow the Xeroform© to dry out and scab over. Rebandaging the donor site at night limits the discomfort to the patient as the site otherwise will stick to the bedsheets. The goal is to have the donor site Xeroform© dry out to facilitate new epithelial cell growth. When the Xeroform© is thoroughly dried around day 14, begin to apply any topical antibiotic, Silvadene®, or petroleum-based skin lotion on the Xeroform©. This process will loosen the Xeroform© from the underlying new skin. Slowly, peel back and remove the Xeroform© and cut off what is easily removed. Try again each day until all of the Xeroform© is removed. Apply topical antibiotic cream to the donor site twice a day until it is all re-epithelialized. Then convert to skin lotion twice a day to keep the donor site moist. Treat any localized erythema as cellulitis with a first-generation cephalosporin or equivalent until the redness has subsided for 3 days. Any pustules that develop under the Xeroform© should be unroofed and topical antibiotics placed over the site.
- Option 2: If a silver-impregnated product is available, cover the donor site and wrap a Kerlix© over it. Moisten twice daily and leave in place for 3–5 days. If

the silver is not kept moist it will adhere to the healing donor site and pull off the newly formed skin. Remove slowly by soaking the silver bandage to loosen it. Make sure the silver wrap is not moving when peeling it off or the newly forming skin may shear away. The wound will stain a dark brown to black from the silver, which is normal. Continue until the wound has re-epithelialized. Lightly clean the wound and remove exudate from the wound bed when the silver bandage gets changed, but do so with great care so as to not wipe off any new epithelial cells.

- Option 3: Small donor site 1–2% TBSA can be covered with large Tegaderm© and wrapped with an ace wrap. Check the wound daily. A seroma will typically form, so make a small cut in the inferior aspect of the Tegaderm© to let it drain and then place some gauze over the Tegaderm© cut and rewrap with the ace. The underlying donor site will be fragile with all types of bandages. Use a topical antibiotic on any sites that are ulcerated, otherwise apply any non-alcohol-based skin moisturizer twice a day for 4 weeks.

Conclusion

Burn care, like trauma care, is a step-wise approach for each clinical situation. Few medical personnel have advanced training or experience treating burns, making this an uncomfortable area for many. If MEDEVAC of wounded servicemembers is available, the maritime surgical team should only need to deal with the initial evaluation and early management of burn patients as they move up the echelons of care, to include assessment of severity, airway management, resuscitation, and basic wound care. However, there may be times when transport is delayed so being able to provide advanced burn care, including decompression of compartment syndromes, simple excision, and skin grafting, will become necessary. Utilize all resources, including this chapter, textbooks, and CPGs. Additionally, internet communication with the USAISR Burn Center will be indispensable; the ability to transmit burn charts, pictures, and laboratory data to obtain guidance in the management of patients will improve the patient's outcome. The maritime surgical team may be deployed, but they are not alone. There are many skilled burn and plastic surgeons who can do amazing things for burned patients in the future, but only the efforts of the maritime surgical team in the first 48 h can give the patient that opportunity!

Declaration of Interest The views expressed in this chapter are those of the authors and do not necessarily reflect the official policy or position of the Department of the Navy, Department of Defense, nor the US Government.

Funding This research did not receive any specific grant from funding agencies in the public, commercial, or not-for-profit sectors.

Conflict of Interest Statement The authors declare no conflict of interest.

Further Reading

Ahuja RB, Gibran N, Greenhalagh, Peck M. ISBI practice guidelines for burn care. Burns. 2016;42:953–1021. https://doi.org/10.1016/j.burns.2016.05.013.

Allorto N, Ateih B, Bolgiani A, Wolf S. ISBI practice guidelines for burn care part 2. Burns. 2018;44:1617–706. https://doi.org/10.1016/j.burns.2018.09.012.

Barillo DJ, Cancio LC, Goodwin GW. Treatment of white phosphorous and other chemical burn injuries at on burn center over a 51-year period. Burns. 2004;30:448–52. https://doi.org/10.1016/j.burns.2004.01.032.

Burn Resuscitation Worksheet. Joint Trauma System. n.d. https://jts.amedd.army.mil/assets/docs/forms/JTS_Burn_Resuscitation_Worksheet.pdf. Accessed 10 Dec 2021.

Cancio LC. Initial assessment and fluid resuscitation of burn patients. Surg Clin North Am. 2014;94(4):741–54. https://doi.org/10.1016/j.suc.2014.05.003.

Cancio LC, Barillo DJ, Kearns RD, Holmes JH. Guidelines for burn care under austere conditions: surgical and nonsurgical wound management. J Burn Care Res. 2017a;38:203–14. https://doi.org/10.1097/bcr.0000000000000368.

Cancio LC, Powell D, Bull K, Keenan S. Burn wound management in prolonged field care (CPG ID:57). 2017b. https://jts.amedd.army.mil/assets/docs/cpgs/Burn_Management_PFC_13_Jan_2017_ID57.pdf. Accessed 10 Dec 2021.

Driscoll KR, Mann-Salinas EA, Boyer NL, Gurney J. Burn care (CPG ID 12). Joint Trauma System clinical practice guideline. 2016. https://jts.amedd.army.mil/assets/docs/cpgs/Burn_Care_11_May_2016_ID12.pdf. Accessed 10 Dec 2021.

Driscoll KR, Nann-Salinas EA, Boyer NL, Pamplin JC, Serio-Melvin ML, Salinas J, Borgman MA, Sheridan RL, et al. Burn casualty care in the deployed setting. Mil Med. 2018;183(suppl_2):448–52. https://doi.org/10.1093/milmed/usy076.

Gensheimer WG, Mazzoli R, Reynolds ME, Shackelford SA. Eye trauma: initial care (CPG ID:03). Pub date 1 June 2021. https://jts.amedd.army.mil/assets/docs/cpgs/Eye_Trauma_Initial_Care_01_Jun_2021_ID03.pdf. Accessed 10 Dec 2021.

Jeschke MG, van Baar ME, Choudry MA, Logsetty S, et al. Burn injury. Nat Rev. 2020;6(11):1–25. https://doi.org/10.1038/s41572-020-0145-5.

Joint Trauma System. Clinical practice guidelines-home page. Clinical practice guidelines (CPGs) - Joint Trauma System (army.mil). n.d. Accessed 10 Dec 2021.

Renz EM, Cancio LC, Barillo DJ, Holcomb JB. Long range transport of war-related burn casualties. J Trauma. 2008;64(2 Suppl):S136–44. https://doi.org/10.1097/ta.0b013e31816086c9.

Chapter 27
Management of the Drowned Patient

Laura M. Adams and Matthew D. Tadlock

You don't drown by falling in the water; you drown by staying there.

Edwin Louis Cole

Author deployment experience	
Laura M. Adams	Trauma/Surgical Critical Care Fellow, University of California San Diego, San Diego, CA, USA, 2020–2022
Matthew D. Tadlock	Flight Surgeon, Carrier Air Wing Three (CVW-3), embarked on the USS *Harry S. Truman* (CVN-75) in support of Operation Iraqi Freedom, Fifth Fleet Area of Responsibility, 2004–2005; supporting Humanitarian Aid Disaster Relief (HADR) operations following Hurricane Katrina, 2005
	Resident Surgeon, USNS *Mercy* (T-AH-19), Pacific Partnership, Micronesia and Papua New Guinea, 2008
	Ship's Surgeon, USS *Carl Vinson* (CVN-70), WESTPAC, INDOPACOM Area of Responsibility, 2011–2012
	Officer in Charge, Forward Resuscitative Surgical System/Shock Trauma Platoon, Charlie Surgical Company, Native Fury, CENTCOM Area of Responsibility, 2016
	Chief of Trauma, NATO Role 3 Multinational Medical Unit, NATO Resolute Support and Operation Freedom's Sentinel, Kandahar Airfield, Afghanistan, 2017–2018
	Staff Surgeon, Expeditionary Resuscitative Surgical System Pacific, 2019–2020; Provided embarked Role 2 Surgical Support, INDOPACOM Area of Responsibility, 2020

L. M. Adams
University of California San Diego, San Diego, CA, USA
e-mail: ladams@health.ucsd.edu

M. D. Tadlock (✉)
Department of Surgery, Naval Medical Center San Diego, San Diego, CA, USA

M. D. Tadlock, A. A. Hernandez (eds.), *Expeditionary Surgery at Sea*,
https://doi.org/10.1007/978-3-031-21893-4_27

BLUF (Bottom Line Up Front)

1. In the deployed maritime environment, drowning events are rare. However, they are associated with a high mortality, particularly "Man Overboard" events. Drowning prevention is the first priority.
2. There is no such thing as "Near Drowning." Correct terminology includes "Non-Fatal Drowning" and "Fatal Drowning."
3. Bradycardia is an ominous sign. It is the prelude to hypoxemic cardiac arrest.
4. Most long-term sequelae from drowning are neurologic in origin. Duration of submersion is a major factor in morbidity and mortality.
5. First responders must first stop the process of drowning while maintaining their own safety. If drowning is the suspected primary cause of unconsciousness, then immediately administer five rescue breaths followed by chest compressions at a 30:2 ratio to rescue breaths.
6. In severely hypoxemic patients, assess and secure the airway FIRST. Have a backup plan for a difficult airway.
7. Hypotensive patients without evidence of traumatic injury are often best managed with isotonic crystalloid resuscitation, supportive care, and treatment of electrolyte derangements as necessary.
8. **Don't Forget: Determine the Underlying Cause of the Drowning.** Depending on the mechanism and operational environment, a drowning patient is a trauma patient and should be treated as such. Remember cervical spine precautions!
9. Surfactant regeneration after drowning takes 48 h; in intubated patients requiring elevated levels of positive end expiratory pressure (PEEP) for appropriate oxygenation, do not wean PEEP or the ventilator until approximately 48 h from the drowning event.
10. Empiric antibiotics for drowning-associated pneumonia are usually not required; however, be aware of atypical causes of pneumonia related to drowning in fresh water, salt water, or contaminated water.
11. In hypothermic patients in cardiopulmonary arrest, cardiopulmonary resuscitation (CPR) should continue until the patient has been rewarmed.

Introduction

Clinical Vignette 27.1

A 35-year-old male was washed overboard by a wave during severe weather while securing equipment on the flight deck of a destroyer (DDG). He was recovered from the ocean within 15 min via Rigid Hull Inflatable Boat (RHIB). Upon evaluation by the Independent Duty Corpsman (IDC), he was awake and alert after an unknown period of loss of consciousness but had pulse oximetry measuring of peripheral saturation of hemoglobin (SpO_2) of approximately 60%. 15% Oxygen therapy was *initiated via non-rebreather mask, a cervical spine collar was placed, and an Advanced Trauma Life Support (ATLS) survey was initiated. No other injuries were identified, and the patient quickly was medically evacuated (MEDEVAC) to a nearby aircraft carrier (CVN) within 30 min of recovery.*

Upon evaluation by the CVN medical department, he was awake and alert despite continued profound hypoxemia so the decision was made to intubate the patient. Prior to intubation a chest X-ray was obtained, which demonstrated significant pulmonary edema. Upon intubation by the ship's certified registered nurse anesthetist (CRNA), a significant amount of salt water drained through the endotracheal tube (ETT). The ETT was then attached to capnography with appropriate color change. No other injuries were found upon repeat ATLS survey. The patient was admitted to the ship's intensive care unit (ICU) for ventilatory management.

Every Sailor who has been deployed on a naval warship has participated in a "Man Overboard" drill after weighing anchor. Although rare, drowning events do occur during routine naval operations, including during small boat operations and severe weather events. A review of Naval Safety Center mishap data from 1970–2020 identified 216 separate drowning events involving 435 Sailors. Of these, 59.7% (260) were fatal drownings. Events labeled as "Man Overboard" were nearly universally fatal. Of 136 "Man Overboard" events involving 137 Sailors, 99.3% were fatal with only one survivor identified in the 50-year review. Table 27.1 lists other causes of identified drowning events: 17 drowning events were classified as suicide (100% fatal); 14 events were weather-related, where rough seas or waves washed Sailors overboard (51.5% fatal); 15 events involved intoxication with alcohol (82% fatal); 9 events occurred during routine small boat operations involving 80 Sailors (14.5% fatal); 6 events occurred pier-side after a fall (100% fatal); 5 events were liberty boat-related (boarding, capsizing, or sinking) involving 131 Sailors (33.6% fatal) [1]. **Given the high mortality of drowning events during routine naval operations, prevention is the first priority when considering drowning in both the civilian and military environment.** All Sailors must adhere to standard shipboard safety protocols to prevent these incidents from occurring! However, the maritime surgical team should always be prepared to care for these critical patients.

Table 27.1 Causes of drowning aboard United States (U.S.) Naval vessels from 1970–2020 [1]

Cause	# Events	# Sailors involved	% Fatal
Man overboard	136	137	99.3% (136)
Suicide	17	17	100%
Weather-related	14	33	51.5% (17)
Alcohol-related	15	17	82% (14)
Small boat operations	9	70	14.3% (10)
Pier side fall	6	6	100%
Liberty boat-related	5	131	33.6% (44)
Other	14	24	66.7% (16)
Total	*216*	*435*	*59.7% (260)*

Drowning

Definition of Drowning

According to the World Health Organization (WHO), drowning is defined as a "process of experiencing respiratory impairment from submersion or immersion in liquid." There are three possible outcomes with drowning:

1. Death
2. Drowning *with* morbidity
3. Drowning *without* morbidity

Terms such as "near drowning," "secondary drowning," "active drowning," "passive drowning," "dry drowning," or "wet drowning" are no longer used. Current accepted terms to describe a drowning event are either "non-fatal drowning" or "fatal drowning." As the term implies, "non-fatal drowning" is when the drowning victim is rescued at any point, thus interrupting the drowning process. "Fatal drowning" refers to the victim's demise at any time [2–5].

Process of Drowning

The process of drowning is described as a continuum. The process begins with either submersion (the victim's airways go below the surface of a liquid) or immersion (liquid is splashed over the victim's airways). In most drowning events, the victim is unable to keep their airway above water resulting in the involuntary aspiration or swallow of water. The first reflex is coughing followed by laryngospasm as the water irritates the oropharynx/larynx. This leads to worsening hypoxemia, resulting in abatement of laryngospasm and further aspiration. The victim experiences a loss of consciousness, bradycardia, and ultimately progresses to pulseless electrical activity (PEA) and hypoxic cardiac death. Some victims are able to voluntarily hold their breath for a period of time but this ultimately leads to hypoxemia, hypercarbia, and acidosis. The hypercarbia from breath-holding results in involuntary inhalation and thus aspiration of water, continuing the vicious cycle of hypoxemia, bradycardia, and death. Of note, as little as 1–2 mL/kg of water need to be aspirated to produce profound hypoxemia. Most victims will aspirate approximately 3–4 mL/kg [2–5].

Shallow Water Drowning

Shallow water drowning can occur with hyperventilation prior to submersion. Hyperventilation decreases partial pressures of carbon dioxide (CO_2) in an attempt to increase breath holds. Hypercapnia drives respiratory actions via central chemoreceptors. By decreasing CO_2 prior to submersion via hyperventilation, the patient becomes hypoxic prior to experiencing an urge to surface and take a breath. This can result in death if not taken out of water prior to loss of consciousness. Prevention and education are the mainstays of management.

Morbidity/Mortality/Complications

Sequelae of drowning include pulmonary edema, metabolic derangements, cardiac dysfunction, and anoxic-ischemic cerebral insult. Most long-term sequelae from drowning are neurological in origin. Duration of submersion is a major factor in morbidity and mortality.

With submersion of 0–5 min, risk of severe neurologic impairment or death is ~10%.
With submersion of 5–10 min, the risk is almost six times greater at 56%.
With submersion of 10–25 min, the risk is 88%.
With submersion >25 min, the risk is 99.9% [4].

Management

First Responder Care

The goal is to stop the process of drowning. First responders should provide flotation devices and attempt to remove the victim from the water. Rescuer safety is a priority in order to prevent more casualties. Rescuers should only go into the water as a last resort. In-water rescue breaths should only be done when immediate extraction is not feasible. In-water chest compressions are not effective and thus should not be performed. Once the victim has been extracted from the water, provide ventilatory support for patients in respiratory distress [4, 5].

Stabilize the cervical spine if there is a concern for injury (e.g., explosion, fall from height, boat accident). Although cervical spine injury in drowning victims is <1%, in the deployed maritime environment drowning victims are likely to also be victims of traumatic injury. Therefore, the initial evaluation should include standard ATLS or Tactical Combat Casualty Care (TCCC) protocols, as depicted in the clinical vignette. However, if drowning is the suspected primary cause of unconsciousness (i.e., there are no outward signs of trauma where the patient is apneic and pulseless) then immediately proceed to administer five rescue breaths followed by chest compressions at a 30:2 ratio to rescue breaths [4]. Be cognizant that these patients are also at a high risk for vomiting; 65% of victims requiring rescue breaths will vomit while 88% of victims receiving chest compressions will also vomit [5]. Once the airway is secure, consider gastric decompression.

Initial Management

Any victim of drowning who required any form of resuscitation should be transported to a hospital for evaluation and monitoring. Similarly, drowning victims on Role 1 platforms should get an emergent MEDEVAC to a higher level of care (shore-based or land-based Role 2 platform or land-based hospital) as soon as practical based on the operational environment. Remember, since hypoxemia is the most common cause of cardiac arrest in the drowning patient, airway must be addressed before circulation [2, 4, 5]. Once the airway is secured, oxygenation will improve resulting in stabilization of the circulatory system.

Whether fresh or salt water, hypotensive drowning victims without evidence of traumatic injury upon initial evaluations should be resuscitated with isotonic crystalloid, typically normal saline [5]. If patients do not respond to appropriate resuscitation, a re-evaluation for traumatic injury should be performed. Drowning victims with persistent hypotension requiring vasopressors without evidence of trauma should be evaluated for sepsis, neurogenic causes, and cardiac etiologies.

In-Hospital Airway Management

If no respiratory distress and/or the patient is asymptomatic, the oxygen can be weaned accordingly. Patients in respiratory distress and a Glasgow Coma Scale (GCS) of 13 or less may be able to be treated with a non-rebreather at 15 L/min to keep $SpO_2 > 95\%$. If available, high flow oxygen by nasal cannula may also help as it theoretically provides some additional positive end expiratory pressure (PEEP). Non-invasive ventilation may also be beneficial (if available), but if the GCS is too depressed or if there is a risk of vomiting, intubation is likely required. If a patient arrives in respiratory distress or with a GCS <8, a definitive airway is required [4].

In a mass casualty incident (MCI), particularly if a traumatic mechanism was related to the drowning event and there is a patient in respiratory distress, initial controlled intubation upon arrival may be prudent to prevent emergent intubation later if the patient's respiratory status rapidly decompensates. As demonstrated by the patient in Clinical Vignette 27.1, patients will usually have pulmonary edema with a significant amount of fluid aspirated and swallowed, therefore rapid sequence intubation (RSI) while maintaining cervical spine precautions is recommended. These patients have a propensity to arrive significantly hypoxemic, even with the use of supplemental oxygen or non-invasive ventilation. Given the possibility for profound hypoxemia and likelihood of a difficult airway, a surgical airway may need to be performed.

Ventilator Management

Drowning victims who require intubation and mechanical ventilation should have an initial arterial blood gas (ABG) obtained (if available) in order to evaluate the adequacy of ventilation, acid-base status, and oxygenation. Standard protective lung ventilation strategies should be used (i.e., low tidal volumes with 6–8 cc/kg of ideal body weight). See Chaps. 20 and 21 for further discussion of ventilator management. As aspiration of liquid can cause washout and destruction of surfactant, 48 h are typically required for surfactant regeneration. Therefore, if intubated patients require increased PEEP (i.e., >5–8 cm water (H_2O)) for hypoxia, continue mechanical ventilation for a minimum of 48 h at the level of PEEP that maintains appropriate partial pressure of oxygen in the arterial blood (PaO_2) prior to attempting a ventilator wean. Premature ventilatory weaning may result in the return of pulmonary edema and hypoxia. Corticosteroids are not recommended for lung protection. If available, consider early bronchoscopy in drowning victims requiring intubation [4, 5].

Considerations in Fresh, Salt, and Contaminated Water

Fresh Water

Patients who aspirate fresh water tend to have worse hypoxemia in comparison to those who have aspirated salt water [6]. With fresh water aspiration, surfactant is washed out resulting in abnormal surface-tension and thus alveolar collapse. Fresh water drowning patients tend to present with lower pH, increased hypoxia (as measured by PaO_2/fraction of inspired oxygen (FiO_2) ratios), worsened hyponatremia, and higher lactate levels compared to salt water drowning victims. Hemolysis can also occur with fresh water aspiration but is generally not clinically relevant. Patients who aspirate large volumes of hypotonic fresh water (>11 mL/kg) can initially present with intravascular hypervolemia. However, if successfully resuscitated, the absorbed aspirated hypotonic fluid can rapidly redistribute, resulting in relative hypovolemia. Initiation of antibiotics is not recommended with aspiration of fresh water [2, 4, 5].

Salt Water

The hypertonicity of aspirated salt water creates an osmotic gradient, resulting in fluid being pulled from the circulation into the alveoli. The result is fluid-filled alveoli and hypovolemia, usually seen in patients who aspirate large volumes of salt water (>11 mL/kg). Initiation of antibiotics is not recommended with aspiration of salt water [2, 4, 5].

Regardless of whether the patient has aspirated fresh or salt water, the victim can develop non-cardiogenic pulmonary edema, decreased lung compliance by 10–40%, and increased ventilation/perfusion mismatch. Interestingly, long-term outcomes are similar between fresh and salt water drowning survivors. Theoretically, a large volume of fresh or salt water aspiration could result in significant electrolyte disturbances; however, drowning survivors typically are unable to aspirate enough fresh or salt water to cause life-threatening electrolyte disturbances [2, 5]. Regardless, electrolytes should be monitored in hospitalized drowning victims, particularly if intubated, and treated accordingly. Once hypoxemia, acidosis, hemodynamic instability, and electrolyte abnormalities have resolved, patients can typically be safely extubated.

Contaminated Water

Patients drowning in contaminated water (e.g., sewage, mud, sand, stagnant water, fuel/petroleum) have an increased risk of lung injury. Aspiration of contaminated water also increases the risk of pneumonia. Some studies recommend early bronchoscopy, specifically in intubated patients, if drowning in contaminated water is suspected. Early bronchoalveolar lavage (BAL) is recommended for removal of large particulate matter and aspirate. However, BAL is not necessarily recommended as a routine preventative treatment for non-fatal drowning patients. See below for discussion of antibiotics.

Atypical Organisms

Most non-fatal drowning victims will not require prophylactic antibiotics. The risk for developing drowning-associated pneumonia is approximately 12% [4]. Given the risk of vomiting, aspiration may be a cause of pneumonia [5]. If it occurs, drowning-associated pneumonia will usually manifest in mechanically ventilated patients after 72–96 h of intubation as pulmonary edema resolves. Patients requiring intubation beyond 48 h after drowning typically have a 34–42% increased risk of developing ventilator-associated pneumonia (VAP) on the third or fourth post-drowning day [4]. Once VAP symptoms develop (e.g., fevers, leukocytosis, new pulmonary infiltrates on chest radiograph), therapeutic bronchoscopy (if available) with bronchoalveolar lavage (BAL) for quantitative cultures should be performed. Broad-spectrum antibiotic coverage is also recommended to cover typical VAP microorganisms.

In general, the use of prophylactic antibiotics and antifungals in drowning victims is not recommended as there is no benefit in reducing the risk of pneumonia or mortality based on available data. Those patients who do indeed develop pneumonia after drowning and were initially placed on prophylactic antibiotics may develop multi-drug resistant infections. Some authors recommend the prophylactic use of antibiotics in non-fatal drowning events occurring in polluted or contaminated water with a high pathogen load.

There are several described organisms that may cause drowning-associated pneumonia. Potentially virulent pathogens known to cause drowning-associated pneumonia include the Aeromonas species. These are water-borne pathogens that belong to the Vibrionaceae family, gram-negative bacilli, and can be seen in contaminated water drowning. Patients with Aeromonas pneumonia have a high rate of positive blood cultures and also a higher mortality rate [7]. Other organisms have been identified to cause pneumonia after drowning in manure or mud-contaminated water such as the fungi *Pseudallescheria boydii* and *Scedosporium apiospermum*. *Burkholderia pseudomallei* has been associated with pneumonia after drowning in rice patties. *Chromobacterium violaceum* can cause pneumonia after drowning in stagnant water and is seen in subtropical and tropical climates, specifically Florida [7–10].

Cold Water

Cold water (0–15 °C) drowning can result in hypothermia. Because of the decrease in metabolic demand from hypothermia, a victim's oxygen and metabolic requirement are also decreased and thus allows for a longer period of submersion with the potential for recovery. Conversely, hypothermia decreases duration of breath holding, decreases the effectiveness of the "diving reflex," and increases the potential for drowning. Severe hypothermia can result in cardiac arrhythmias and cardiac arrest. Rewarming should be initiated immediately. In hypothermic patients in cardiopulmonary arrest, cardiopulmonary resuscitation (CPR) should continue until the patient has been rewarmed. CPR should be terminated after the patient has been rewarmed to 30–33 °C and asystole has persisted for more than 20 min [5]. See Chap. 28 for an in-depth discussion of hypothermia.

Conclusion

Clinical Vignette 27.1 Conclusion

The patient initially had electrolyte derangements, specifically hypernatremia with a sodium of 160. Given the blue water location of the CVN, immediate MEDEVAC to shore was not possible. His pulmonary edema resolved and his electrolyte derangements normalized within 24 h. He was extubated on hospital day #2 and discharged from the ship's ward 1 day after extubation without any sequelae. He returned to full duty on the DDG within 7 days.

Prevention of drowning is the first priority given the high mortality of drowning events in the operational maritime environment. Hypoxemia from drowning can progress to loss of consciousness, bradycardia, and PEA arrest. Therefore, in the unconscious drowning victim airway is the first priority. Drowning can cause significant non-cardiogenic pulmonary edema requiring endotracheal intubation and mechanical ventilation. Ventilated patients requiring elevated levels of PEEP for hypoxemia should not be weaned from the ventilator until stable for 48 h to allow for surfactant regeneration. While the maritime surgical team members may not routinely treat drowned patients on land, this chapter should guide them as they may need to manage these critically ill patients at sea.

Declaration of Interest The views expressed in this chapter are those of the authors and do not necessarily reflect the official policy or position of the Department of the Navy, Department of Defense, nor the US Government.

Funding This research did not receive any specific grant from funding agencies in the public, commercial, or not-for-profit sectors.

Conflict of Interest Statement The authors declare no conflict of interest.

References

1. https://navalsafetycenter.navy.mil.
2. Layon AJ, Modell JH. Drowning: update 2009. Anesthesiology. 2009;110(6):1390–401.
3. Szpilman D, Bierens JJ, Handley AJ, Orlowski JP. Drowning. N Engl J Med. 2012;366(22):2102–10.
4. Szpilman D, Morgan PJ. Management for the drowning patient. Chest. 2021;159(4):1473–83.
5. Parenteau M, Stockinger Z, Hughes S, et al. Drowning management. Mil Med. 2018;183(suppl_2):172–9.
6. Michelet P, Dusart M, Boiron L, et al. Drowning in fresh or salt water: respective influence on respiratory function in a matched cohort study. Eur J Emerg Med. 2019;26(5):340–4.
7. Ender PT, Dolan MJ. Pneumonia associated with near-drowning. Clin Infect Dis. 1997;25(4):896–907.
8. Ender PT, Dolan MJ, Dolan D, Farmer JC, Melcher GP. Near-drowning-associated Aeromonas pneumonia. J Emerg Med. 1996;14(6):737–41.
9. Robert A, Danin PE, Quintard H, et al. Seawater drowning-associated pneumonia: a 10-year descriptive cohort in intensive care unit. Ann Intensive Care. 2017;7(1):45.
10. Tadie JM, Heming N, Serve E, et al. Drowning associated pneumonia: a descriptive cohort. Resuscitation. 2012;83(3):399–401.

Further Reading

Joint Trauma System (JTS), Clinical Practice Guideline (CPG), Drowning Management (CPG ID: 64). https://jts.amedd.army.mil/assets/docs/cpgs/JTS_Clinical_Practice_Guidelines_(CPGs)/Drowning_Management_27_Oct_2017_ID64.pdf.

Chapter 28
Management of Hypothermia and Immersion Injuries

Michael Hight and Kennen Less

Then we plunged into the deep water and all was dark. Cold it was as the tide of death: almost it froze my heart.

The Two Towers, J.R.R. Tolkien

Author deployment experience	
Michael Hight	Dive Medical Officer, 3d Reconnaissance Battalion, 2014–2016; multiple Theater Security Cooperation (TSC) exercises and Korean Marine Exchange, INDOPACOM Area of Responsibility, 2017
	Force Surgeon, 15th Marine Expeditionary Unit, 2019–2021; multiple exercises including WESTPAC, Operation Octave Quartz, and Operation Iron Fist, CENTCOM, INDOPACOM, and AFRICOM Areas of Responsibility, 2019–2021; Special Purpose Marine Air-Ground Task Force Arctic Expeditionary Capabilities, Alaska, 2019; Operation Northern Edge, Alaska, 2021
Kennen Less	Shock Trauma Platoon Emergency Medicine Physician, Combat Logistics Battalion-15, 15th Marine Expeditionary Unit, 2019–2021; multiple exercises including WESTPAC, Operation Octave Quartz, and Operation Iron Fist, CENTCOM, INDOPACOM, and AFRICOM Areas of Responsibility, 2019–2021; Special Purpose Marine Air-Ground Task Force Arctic Expeditionary Capabilities, Alaska, 2019; Operation Northern Edge, Alaska, 2021

M. Hight (✉)
Navy Medicine Readiness and Training Command San Diego, San Diego, CA, USA

K. Less
1st Medical Battalion, Camp Pendleton, CA, USA

M. D. Tadlock, A. A. Hernandez (eds.), *Expeditionary Surgery at Sea*,
https://doi.org/10.1007/978-3-031-21893-4_28

BLUF (Bottom Line Up Front)

1. No matter the clime, hot or cold, prevention of hypothermia is a basic principle of patient care in the deployed environment!
2. A simple system of grading hypothermia can be based on the presence or absence of shivering. Shivering patients have mild hypothermia, non-shivering patients have moderate or more severe hypothermia.
3. Treat hypothermia before frostbite or any other extremity abnormality.

   (a) Mild hypothermia can be treated with passive external rewarming, such as the Hypothermia Prevention and Management Kit (HPMK) or Absorbent Patient Litter System (APLS).
   (b) Moderate hypothermia can be treated with passive plus active external rewarming, such as forced-warm air units or heating pads.
   (c) Severe or profound hypothermia often requires all of the above with invasive internal rewarming techniques with warm water bladder irrigation being the recommendation for deployed teams.

4. Beware of afterdrop: the continued decline of core temperature, despite rewarming. At-risk patients include the injured, energy-depleted, and non-shiver hypothermic patients, or those with interrupted-shiver mechanisms due to medications. These patients require active rewarming measures.
5. When treating freezing extremity injuries such as frostbite, utilize 37–39 °C (98–102 °F) water immersion until the skin has thawed (~15–30 min) and anticipate high pain medication requirements. Do not heat over an open flame.
6. Ensure frostbite patients do not worsen their injury! Avoid nicotine use, rubbing the affected extremity, and thawing a limb that has the potential to refreeze. Prognosis depends on the level of reperfusion cyanosis.
7. For non-freezing cold immersion (NFCI) injuries or warm water immersion foot (WWIF), perform room temperature air drying and anticipate significant pain medication requirements.
8. While frostbite and immersion injuries are similar to a burn injury, wound care is dissimilar and recommendations vary on blister and skin management. Utilize dry dressings and aloe vera for most wounds.
9. Ultimately, the best treatment of frostbite and immersion injuries is prevention.

Introduction

Clinical Vignette 28.1

A healthy 23-year-old active-duty male Marine was performing a nighttime reconnaissance mission of a western Alaska Aleutian Island. While walking along a ridgeline, he accidentally slipped off the edge and fell 30 ft., shattering his ankle upon impact. He was stranded on a small plateau below his comrades and had to wait for a search and rescue (SAR) team. The ambient temperature was −10 °C with a −24 °C wind chill. The patient had multiple layers on but had built up a significant amount of perspiration and began to cool down immediately. It took 60 min for the SAR team to arrive, by which time the patient noted numb fingers and toes in all four extremities. The SAR team loaded the patient into a litter, pulled him up to the level with his team, carried him a few hundred yards, and placed him into a waiting MH-60 for medical evacuation (MEDEVAC).

In the helicopter, the SAR medical technician was able to remove the patient's clothes and place him in a Hypothermia Prevention and Management Kit (HPMK) to start rewarming. A rectal temperature showed a 32 °C core temperature. He was not shivering. The patient was disoriented to place and date but speaking in full sentences. Secondary survey revealed an obviously broken left leg without open injury which was splinted into place; further injuries included frostbite of the nose and fingertips of bilateral hands. Before and after splinting, palpable distal pulses were present in the left leg.

The ocean is a cold and unforgiving place. The maritime surgical team may care for patients that are exposed to the elements from injuries sustained on a ship, after a fall overboard, or during a land-based exercise that are subsequently evacuated to the ship for a higher level of care. Freezing and non-freezing cold injuries (NFCIs) frequently occur in hypothermia patients and require rapid diagnosis and treatment to assure the best possible outcomes. This chapter acts as a guide for the maritime surgical team discussing the pathophysiology, staging, and general treatment strategies for hypothermia, cold immersion injury, frostbite, and NFCI.

Hypothermia

Accidental hypothermia is the unintended decline of at least 2 °C in a patient's core body temperature. Primary accidental hypothermia is associated with environmental exposure. Secondary causes of accidental hypothermia are associated with trauma, sepsis, thermal burns, cold fluid administration, medications, metabolic disorders, central nervous system disease (e.g., stroke, mass, spinal cord lesion), and impaired shiver reflex (malnutrition, physical exhaustion, neuromuscular disorder, extremes of age). Therapeutic hypothermia is the intentional decline of core body temperature in the treatment of certain processes such as post-return of spontaneous circulation (ROSC) care, myocardial infarction, stroke, or other ischemic events.

Over 80% of non-surviving trauma patients had a body temperature of less than 34 °C. Hypothermia can and does occur in both hot and cold climates. Prevention of hypothermia must be emphasized, due to not only the increased morbidity and mortality associated, but also the difficulty, time, and energy required to treat hypothermia and actively re-warm patients.

Pathophysiology

Heat loss occurs via four main methods: conduction, convection, evaporation, and radiation.

- **Conduction** is the loss of heat from direct contact, such as from a warm body to a cold body.
  - This can be mediated via insulation and avoiding contact with cold materials, particularly cold metals.
- **Convection** occurs when cooled fluid comes into contact with a warm body; this can occur with water and air. Water, due to its ability to absorb heat quickly, can result in hypothermia even in temperate conditions if exposure is prolonged.
  - Convective heat loss can be mediated by removal from water, protecting the patient from wind, and covering the patient with warming layers.
- **Evaporation** occurs when a warm, wet body is exposed to air or windy conditions. It is proportional to the time exposed and temperature differences encountered.
  - Evaporation can be mediated by vapor barrier usage.
- **Radiation** occurs when a warm body loses heat via radiating electromagnetic waves.
  - Radiation heat loss can be mediated by keeping room temperatures elevated.

Afterdrop is the continued decline of core temperature after rewarming due to colder blood from the extremities reaching the core after vasodilating due to rewarm. The amount of afterdrop will depend on the stage of hypothermia. Otherwise healthy patients who are uninjured and have the ability to tolerate warmed, sweet drinks will be able to continue shivering and re-warm once removed from the cold stressor. However, injured patients, energy-depleted patients, non-shiver hypothermic patients, or those with interrupted-shiver mechanisms due to medications (e.g., narcotics, sedatives, paralytics) are at significant risk for afterdrop unless active rewarming methods are used.

Staging and Symptoms

The stages of hypothermia are determined by core temperature, worsening as temperature lowers (Table 28.1). **In austere environments, a simple system of grading hypothermia can be based on the presence or absence of shivering.** Shivering is typically present at temperatures greater than 32 °C (i.e., mild stage hypothermia), whereas it is common to see non-shiver hypothermia in temperatures below

Table 28.1 Characteristics of the four stages of hypothermia with recommended rewarming techniques

Stage	Core (°C/°F)	Overview	Rewarming techniques
Mild	35–32/95–89	Conscious *Shivering*	Passive external
Moderate	32–28/89–82	Impaired Not shivering	Passive and active external
Severe	28–22/82–71	Unconscious Vital signs present	Passive and active external Invasive internal if no ECMO or CPB available
Profound	<22/<71	Unconscious No vital signs present	Passive and active external Invasive internal if no ECMO or CPB available

ECMO extracorporeal membrane oxygen, *CPB* cardiopulmonary bypass

32 °C. Non-shiver hypothermia is considered especially dangerous due to the inability to generate heat via muscular contraction and cellular respiration compounded by decreased efficacy of endogenous insulin, resulting in even more rapid declines in core temperature. The patient in the clinical vignette was in moderate stage hypothermia based on temperature, stupor, and absence of shivering.

Mild hypothermia is defined by a core temperature between 35–32 °C. Symptoms include initial increases in blood pressure and heart rate; if continued it will progress to amnesia, poor judgment, bradycardia, and cold diuresis. Moderate hypothermia includes core temperature from 32–28 °C. Symptoms include dilated pupils, stupor, decreased level of consciousness, decreased oxygen consumption, and cardiac dysrhythmias. Paradoxical undressing is associated with peripheral vasodilation that can quicken core temperature decline. Additionally, insulin becomes less effective at temperatures <30 °C. Severe hypothermia consists of core temperatures between 28–22 °C. Symptoms include acid-base disturbances, hyporeflexia, decreased cerebral blood flow, decrease in oxygen consumption, decreased ventricular fibrillation threshold, and decreased cardiac output noted by worsening hypotension and bradycardia. At the extreme lower ranges, corneal reflexes can be absent, and the risk for ventricular fibrillation increases to the point that jostling the patient could incite arrhythmia. Profound hypothermia occurs when the core temperature is less than 22 °C. Little data exists but instances of electroencephalographic silencing, severe bradycardia, and asystole have been noted.

Hypothermia typically generates an initial tachycardia and relative hypertension due to peripheral vasoconstriction, followed by bradycardia, hypotension, and increasing myocardial irritability. Electrocardiography (ECG) changes in hypothermia show prolonged PR and QT intervals with widened QRS complexes. Osborn J-Waves usually occur at less than 32 °C and can be confused with ST elevations, sepsis, benign J-point elevation, and early repolarization among others.

Cold diuresis is the result of increased renal blood flow due to profound peripheral vasoconstriction, resulting in relative core hypervolemia. Cold diuresis can worsen fluid losses in hypothermia and complicate processes such as rhabdomyolysis and increasing blood viscosity. Rhabdomyolysis can present diagnostic uncertainty differentiating frostbite and compartment syndrome in the setting of elevated creatine kinase in the hypothermic patient. Increased blood viscosity, especially below 34 °C, is of special concern in trauma patients as it is a prominent factor in coagulopathy and results in worsened patient outcomes.

Field Passive Rewarming

Prevent further heat loss by drying and covering patients, blocking them from wind, and insulating them from the ground. Wrap them with available materials (e.g., plastic, tarp, space blanket). HPMKs depicted in Figs. 28.1 and 28.2 (used on the patient from Clinical Vignette 28.1) and Absorbent Patient Litter Systems (APLS) depicted in Figs. 28.3 and 28.4 are first line options for rewarming in field environments. If HPMKs or APLS are not available, a field-expedient "hot pocket" can be created by wrapping patients in a wool blanket, space blanket, and body bag. Thankfully, HPMKs and APLS are pervasive in both the conventional and Special Operations Forces (SOF) Authorized Medical Allowance Lists (AMALs) and thus should be readily accessible.

Field Active External Rewarming

Use forced-warm air unit in an HPMK, APLS, or "hot pocket" if available, depicted in Figs. 28.5 and 28.6. Apply additional insulated warm items near areas of high circulation such as neck, groin, and axillae; insulated items reduce chance of

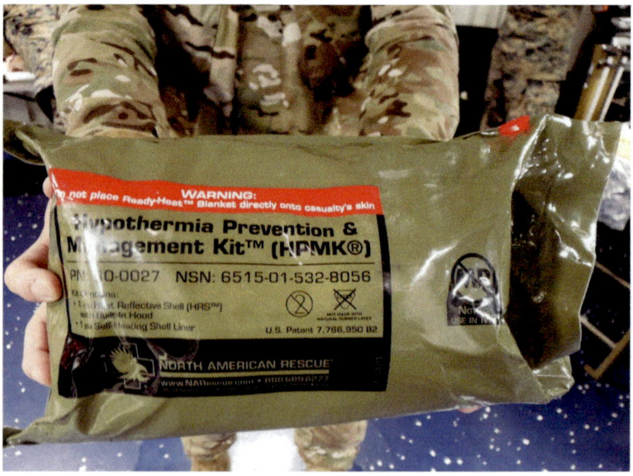

Fig. 28.1 Hypothermia Prevention and Management Kit (HPMK). (Source: Photo courtesy of Michael Hight, DO)

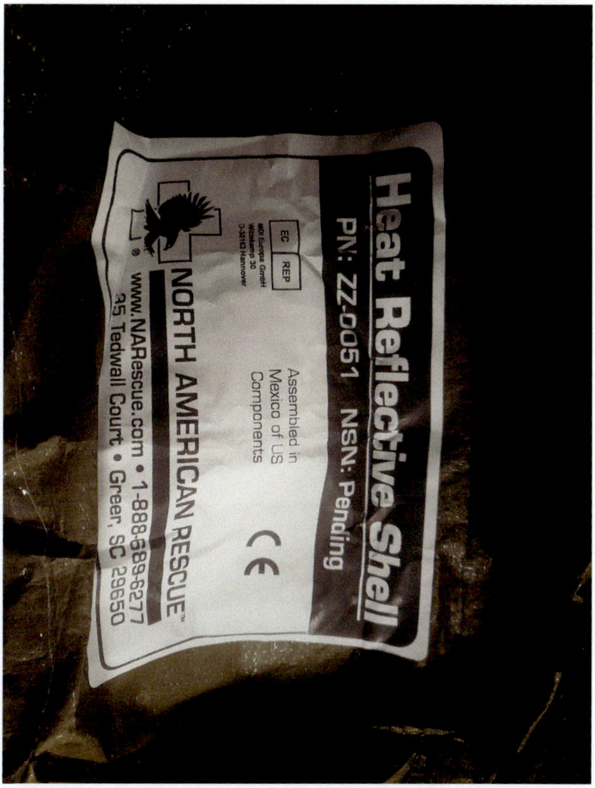

Fig. 28.2 Hypothermia Prevention and Management Kit (HPMK)—heat-reflective shell or "space blanket." (Source: Photo courtesy of Michael Hight, DO)

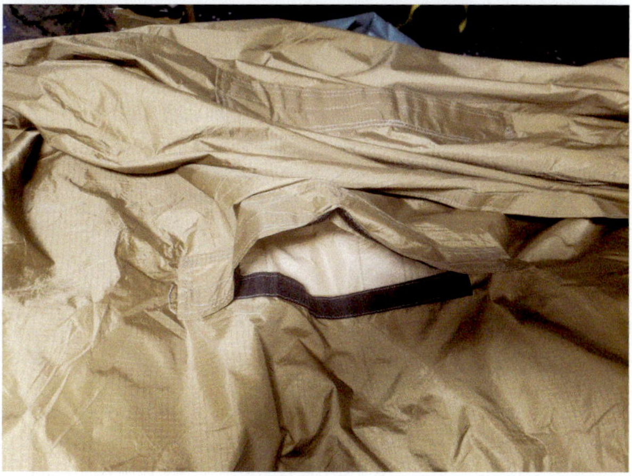

Fig. 28.3 Absorbent Patient Litter System (APLS) pole-free stretcher, with hook-and-loop access for patient. (Source: Photo courtesy of Michael Hight, DO)

thermal burns. Thermal Angel or Belmont Buddy-Lite devices, which warm intravenous (IV) fluids and blood products, should be utilized during treatment and transportation (Figs. 28.7 and 28.8) and are also discussed in Chap. 10.

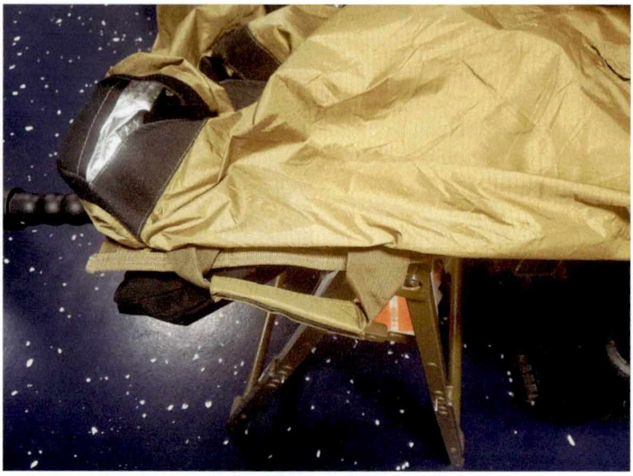

Fig. 28.4 Absorbent Patient Litter System (APLS) pole-free stretcher, with sturdy handles for transport-carry. (Source: Photo courtesy of Michael Hight, DO)

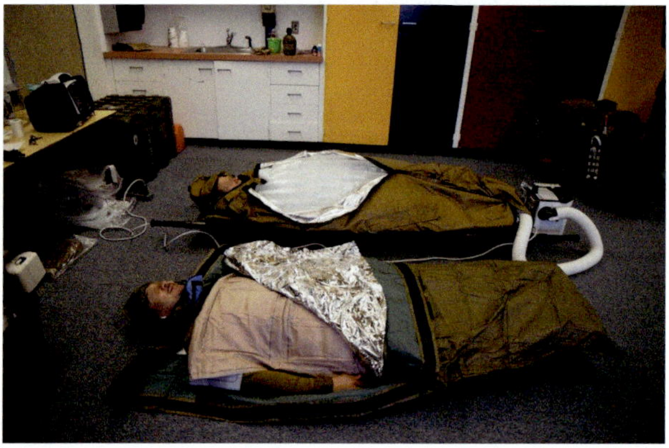

Fig. 28.5 Two patients in makeshift casualty collection point. Patient in foreground using Hypothermia Prevention and Management Kit (HPMK), showing (reflected) outer layer exterior shell, (reflected) middle layer heat-reflective layer of shell, and inner layer self-heating shell liner. Patient in background using Absorbent Patient Litter System (APLS) with forced-warm air unit to provide additional warming opened to show unit within system. (Source: Photo courtesy of Kennen Less, MD)

General Treatment Strategies

As with any field injury or illness, consider scene safety. Handle hypothermic patients carefully, as jostling can induce dysrhythmias due to irritable myocardium. Prevent further heat loss with transport to warm environments, removing wet clothing, covering, and insulating from the ground as discussed above.

Core temperature measurement can be completed in a number of ways: serial core temperatures by rectal probe (ideally at 15 cm depth), indwelling bladder Foley catheter probes, and esophageal probe (in the intubated patient, ideally placed at

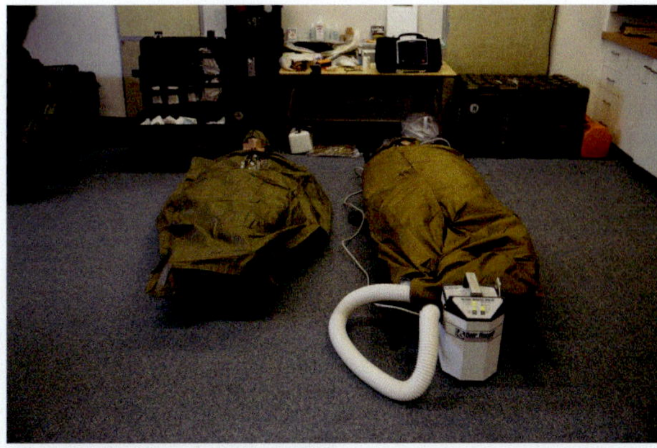

Fig. 28.6 Two patients in makeshift casualty collection point. Patient on left side using Hypothermia Prevention and Management Kit (HPMK). Patient on right side using Absorbent Patient Litter System (APLS) with forced-warm air unit. (Source: Photo courtesy of Kennen Less, MD)

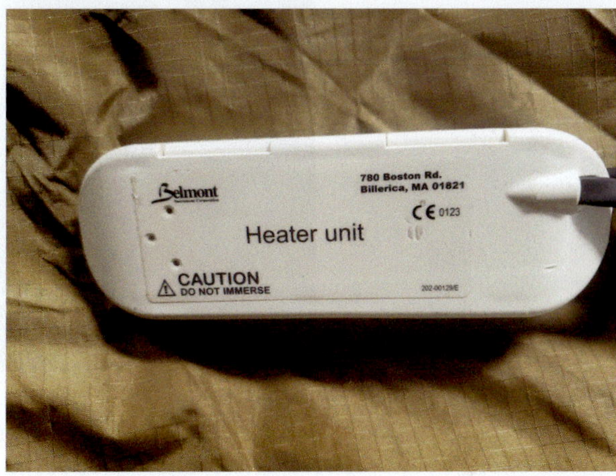

Fig. 28.7 Belmont Buddy-Lite intravenous (IV) fluid heating unit—cartridge site. (Source: Photo courtesy of Michael Hight, DO)

24 cm below the larynx in an adult patient in the lower 1/3 of the esophagus, as this best represents the core temperature based on proximity to the myocardium and pulmonary arteries). TempaDots® and oral/axillary temperatures are unreliable due to vasoconstriction and do not reflect true core temperatures.

For mild hypothermia, encourage the patient to drink warmed, sweet fluids as long as the patient does not have a risk for aspiration. Caffeine and alcohol should be avoided due to associated diuresis. Passive external rewarming techniques should be used, like the HPMK or APLS.

In moderate hypothermia and worse, do not allow oral intake due to aspiration risk. Provide warmed IV fluid administration, preferably warmed dextrose-containing solutions, but know they do not provide significant warming and only reduce the chance of iatrogenic cooling. Avoid lactated Ringer's (LR) due to poor metabolization of lactate by hypothermic livers. Treat with passive plus active external rewarming, such as a forced-warm air unit or heating pads. Continuous cardiac monitoring is indicated due to increased dysrhythmia risk. Vasopressors may be required later in resuscitation after the initial profound peripheral vasoconstriction subsides.

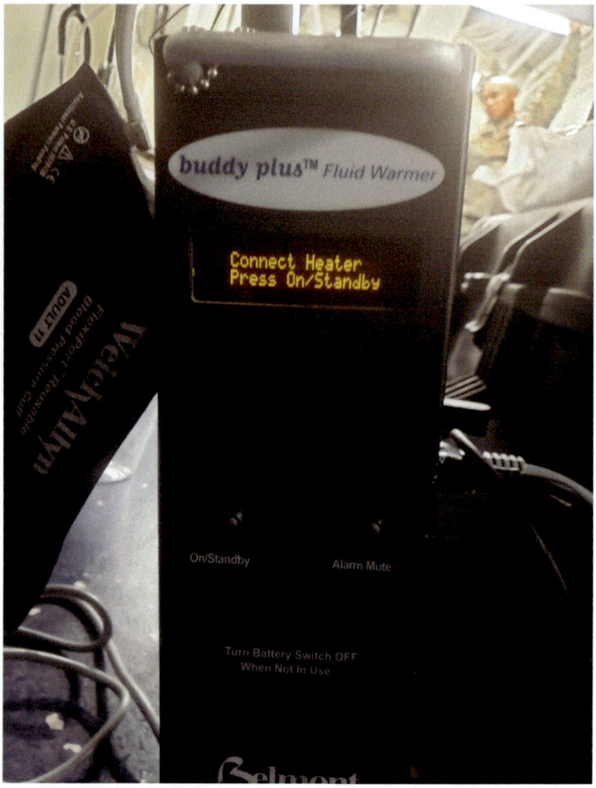

Fig. 28.8 Belmont Buddy-Lite intravenous (IV) fluid heating unit—power unit. (Source: Photo courtesy of Michael Hight, DO)

Severe and profound hypothermia requires all of the above and on land, hospital-based treatments for active internal rewarming, such as cavity lavage, have been replaced by extracorporeal membrane oxygen (ECMO) and warmed cardiopulmonary-bypass (CPB) machines. Obviously, these advanced treatments are not available in the maritime deployed setting. Bladder lavage with warmed normal saline (NS) is associated with decreased morbidity compared to thoracic, peritoneal, gastric, or rectal lavage; thus, it is the recommended technique for the maritime surgical team. Thoracic lavage using single or dual lumen chest tubes is also an option, though is associated with higher morbidity than bladder lavage. Severe and profound hypothermic patients in which rewarming has been unsuccessful should be considered for urgent/priority MEDEVAC to ECMO-capable centers if available.

Routine laboratory testing and imaging is not indicated in pure hypothermia patients but should be considered in undifferentiated patients with abnormal vital signs or altered mental status. The diagnosis of hypothermia is clinical. However, dilemmas may be present when concomitant traumatic, ischemic, infectious, or metabolic derangement processes are present.

Multiple laboratory values are affected by hypothermia. Hematocrit rises ~2% per 1 °C due to decreases in circulating plasma. Electrolytes can be deranged based on peripheral vasoconstriction and IV site hemolysis. Glucose levels can be unpredictable due to initial gluconeogenesis from catecholamine surge followed by increasing insulin resistance at lower core temperatures. Acid-base disturbances are common. Hypothermia can cause an initial tachypnea which drives respiratory alkalosis. Prolonged mild hypothermia may demonstrate a profound metabolic acidosis in response to the initial tachypnea resulting in an acidic pH. Arterial blood gas (ABG) analyzers and coagulopathy tests re-warm samples by convention, which can alter the true value of these laboratory results in the hypothermic patient. Partial pressures of gasses increase in warmer samples compared to the colder in vivo samples.

Cardiopulmonary Resuscitation (CPR) in Hypothermia

Feel for carotid and femoral pulses. Peripheral pulses are often absent due to peripheral vasoconstriction despite central pulses being present. Even in severe hypothermia, if the patient shows signs of life, refrain from Cardiopulmonary Resuscitation (CPR) due to the risk of inducible dysrhythmia. Supporting respirations with bag-valve-mask (BVM) ventilation is appropriate; definitive airways can be secured for standard indications. Resuscitation efforts should be continued for hypothermic patients who are pulseless or have evidence of brain death until at least 32 °C. Patients with obviously non-survivable injuries or potassium >12 mEq/L are candidates for care withdrawal. An exception to the above is a child with rapid accidental hypothermia where prolonged resuscitation efforts may be appropriate.

Cold Water Immersion

The World Health Organization (WHO) estimates over 500,000 annual deaths worldwide due to drowning. According to the Utstein guidelines, drowning refers to "a process resulting in primary respiratory impairment from submersion or immersion in a liquid medium." Submersion is entry into a liquid medium where the body, particularly the head, is below the surface. Immersion is entry in a liquid medium without the head below the surface.

Pathophysiology

The degree of hypoxic insult to the central nervous system determines the ultimate outcome. After entry into a liquid medium, specifically cold water, gasping is due to the cold water shock response. Aspirated liquid contributes to drowning and results in protective laryngospasm reflexes. Water conducts heat 25 times faster than air.

Cold water immersion results in an immediate decline in skin temperatures which is associated with shivering thermogenesis and increased metabolism, tachypnea, tachycardia, and cardiac output. As core temperature drops, decreasing systemic perfusion predominates with bradypnea, bradycardia, and lowered cardiac output.

Non-fatal cases of drowning rarely result in aspiration of more than 3–4 mL/kg. Therefore, the differentiation of fresh versus salt water is less important for patient care scenarios, where larger volumes are needed to see fluid shifts and electrolyte changes comparatively. Any water aspirated, regardless of fresh or salt water, will decrease lung compliance due to washing out surfactant and creating a non-cardiac pulmonary edema and acute respiratory distress syndrome (ARDS). See Chap. 27 for more details on drowning.

General Treatment Strategies

Self-rescue priority is to maintain heat escape lessening posture (HELP) and ensure the head remains out of water. HELP is maintained by holding the knees close to the chest to decrease convection by fluid. If two or more people are immersed, the huddle position is suggested. Children are at greatest risk for hypothermia due to immersion due to increased body surface area relative to volume. In cold water (<10–15 °C), the 1-10-1 rule is a good generality:

- 1 min to calm breathing to prevent aspiration
- 10 min of meaningful movement
- 1 h of consciousness before swim failure and death

Trauma is rarely a result of drowning, but submersion and immersion secondary to trauma is common, especially after diving, falling, and motor vehicle accidents. Standard spinal precautions and MARCH algorithm (Massive Hemorrhage, Airway, Respirations, Circulation, Head Injury/Hypothermia) should be applied if history warrants it, but routine immobilization for all drowning victims is unnecessary. Patients with Glasgow Coma Scale (GCS) scores of ≥13 and pulse oximetry measuring of peripheral saturation of hemoglobin (SpO2) of ≥95% are at low risk for complications. Observation for 4–6 h is indicated. If pulmonary exam reveals adventitious sounds or the patient develops an oxygen requirement, admission and continued observation is warranted.

Patients with GCS ≤13 are at higher risk for complications. Oxygen supplementation and ventilator support are commonly required. High-flow oxygen should be initiated and if adequate oxygenation cannot be maintained, intubation is suggested. Non-invasive positive pressure ventilation (NIPPV) can be considered in patients able to protect their airway from continued aspiration. For those failing high-flow oxygenation and NIPPV, intubation is indicated. See Chap. 27 for a discussion of the treatment of the drowned patient. Standard hypothermia treatments apply (review previously discussed).

Swimming-Induced Pulmonary Edema (SIPE)

Swimming-induced pulmonary edema (SIPE) is common in strenuous surface swimming, especially in cold water. For the military maritime community, it is most commonly seen in Sea, Air, and Land (SEAL) Operators, Marine Special Operations Command (MARSOC) Critical Skills Operators, Marine Combatant Divers, and Self-Contained Underwater Breathing Apparatus (SCUBA) divers. Prior history of SIPE is a significant risk factor. Current data reflects elevated pulmonary artery pressures resulting in vascular stress associated with capillary leakage, increased preload, increased afterload, and higher systemic vascular resistance. Diastolic dysfunction follows, contributing to pulmonary edema, hypoxia, and dyspnea. Treatment includes observation and oxygen supplementation. Rarely, NIPPV will be needed for patients with SIPE.

Frostbite

Frostbite is a clinical condition resulting from prolonged exposure to sub-freezing temperatures. Understandably, its prevalence is highest in the military and outdoor enthusiast populations. It is also more likely to occur in males rather than females, which may be attributed more to their occupations and hobbies than their physiologic vulnerability. Risk factors for occurrence include prior cold injury, being of African descent, fatigue, dehydration, inappropriate clothing, comorbidities such as diabetes or peripheral vascular disease, psychiatric disease, and drug or nicotine use. The severity of injury varies according to ambient temperature, wind chill, length of exposure, altitude, contact with cold items (particularly metals), activity level, and wetting of the skin. Incidence increases dramatically at ambient temperatures below—20 °C, wind speeds of greater than 4.5 m/s (10 mph), and altitudes greater than 5182 m (17,000 ft.). Anatomic areas injured in decreasing order of prevalence are face, hands, then feet, although studies have conflicting incident reports and military studies report higher hand and foot percentages.

Pathophysiology

The pathophysiology of frostbite starts with severe vasoconstriction, followed by formation of ice crystals in extra- and then intra-cellular spaces, coupled with direct cold-induced cell death, and completed by microvascular thrombosis. Injury worsens through treatment as reperfusion incites endothelial damage and brings a cascade of inflammatory mediators (notably arachidonic acid) which increase swelling, cause electrolyte shifts, and lead to further cell death.

There are three zones of frostbite injury:

- **Zone of Coagulation:** most distal, highest morbidity
- **Zone of Stasis:** middle ground, most impacted by quick and thorough treatment
- **Zone of Hyperemia:** most proximal, often heals fully within 2 weeks of injury

Staging and Symptoms

Frostbite classification is broken down by the depth of injury, similar to burn injury (see Chap. 26). Of note, all of these injuries require reperfusion and the healing process to begin before staging can actually be performed. Early staging is difficult due to the time it takes for injuries to develop, and it is recommended to label injuries as either superficial or deep. Up to 65% of patients experience prolonged sequelae, including pain in the form of neuropathy or possible formation of frostbite arthritis, cold intolerance, and hyperhidrosis.

- **First-degree frostbite**, also referred to as "frostnip," is freezing isolated to the epidermis and is associated with pain, numbness, and hyperemia. Desquamation can sometimes occur a few days post-injury. There is no permanent damage.
- **Second-degree frostbite** is freezing of the entire epidermis extending into the dermis. Symptoms are the same as first degree with the added formation of vesicles or large, clear fluid-filled blisters with surrounding erythema. They form 6–24 h after reperfusion occurs.
- **Third-degree frostbite** extends into subcutaneous tissue. Similar to second degree, appearance worsens after reperfusion. However, third-degree frostbite differs in that it forms smaller, blue/black hemorrhagic blisters with frequent ulcer formation. Tissue with third-degree injury is often surrounded by first- and second-degree injury.
- **Fourth-degree frostbite** is a full-thickness injury including tendon, bone, and muscle. Unlike the severe edema of second- and third-degree frostbite, fourth-degree injuries will lack edema and appear severely cyanotic after reperfusion. Days after reperfusion, the skin will appear mummified; these injuries almost always require amputation.

More recently, an updated grading system has been created in an effort to more accurately predict long-term prognosis utilizing the level of reperfusion cyanosis (Table 28.2).

Table 28.2 Frostbite grading system utilizing level of reperfusion cyanosis to predict long-term prognosis

Grade	Level of reperfusion cyanosis	Long-term prognosis
1	None	No amputation
2	Cyanosis of distal phalanx	Minimal distal digit amputation
3	Cyanosis of entire digit	Amputation of digit
4	Cyanosis to carpal/tarsal bones	May result in limb amputation

Diagnosis is made on a clinical basis, and no imaging or laboratory testing is necessary. If there is concern for associated trauma or medical pathology, diagnostics should be steered by those concerns. Photography at the time of arrival is useful to monitor progression of the injured tissues over coming days.

General Treatment Strategies

Treatment priorities should focus on life-threatening abnormalities, particularly hypothermia, before treating frostbite. Do not treat frostbite injuries if there is any chance for refreezing, as this dramatically worsens outcomes. Also attempt to prevent the patient from walking on frostbitten feet or rubbing frozen extremities. Treatment of frostbite is performed by rapid rewarming of the injured tissues in a 37–39 °C (98–102 °F) water bath or warm water-soaked gauze applied to facial tissues.

Rewarming is complete once the extremity is thawed, evidenced by red or purple coloration and softening of the tissue; this typically takes between 15–30 min. Avoid rewarming over a hot air source as this can inflict burn and worsen tissue damage. During the thawing process, **extreme pain should be anticipated, and adequate analgesia is necessary**. Ibuprofen dosed at 12 mg/kg/day in divided doses can be particularly useful, as it treats pain and helps control circulating inflammatory markers after reperfusion. Use of pain-dosed ketamine or opioids is likely necessary, and the decision can be steered by which is most readily available to the deployed provider.

There are no current recommendations for prophylactic antibiotics for any degree of frostbite, and they should be considered only if the patient exhibits signs of infection. The wounds should be dressed with dry bandages similar to burn wound care (see Chap. 26), and use of topical aloe vera with or without a topical antibiotic should be utilized. Tetanus status should be questioned and prophylaxis given to all patients needing a booster. Vasodilators have no evidence to support their use and are not recommended.

If the patient is on the maritime platform for many hours after thawing when the blistering of the higher grades of frostbite start to present, consideration can be given to debriding the injured tissue. While there is no consensus data, the most common recommendation is to debride larger, clear blisters. Some facilities recommend aspirating smaller hemorrhagic blisters, but this is controversial. All third- and fourth-degree frostbite patients should be given urgent/priority MEDEVAC status, whereas most first- and second-degree injuries can be managed on a ship. If prolonged casualty care (PCC) is required (i.e., during distributed maritime operations (DMO)), ensure the patient stays warm, hydrated, and nourished. Dressing changes with aloe/antibacterial cream application should be performed every 6 h.

Land-based hospitals familiar with frostbite treatment may perform computed tomography or magnetic resonance angiography (CTA or MRA) or other advanced imaging to more accurately diagnose microthrombosis associated with frostbite. Those same medical centers will frequently perform intra-arterial tPA (tissue plasminogen activator) in combination with a vasodilator such as papaverine or iloprost (prostaglandin analog). Given the lack of these resources in the typical maritime deployed environment along with restricted blood products in the event of bleeding complications, these options are not recommended.

The best treatment of frostbite is prevention. This starts with adequate protective clothing. Layering should consist of an inner wicking material (e.g., polypropylene fabric) directly over the skin, covered by a middle absorbing fleece layer, and an outermost layer to protect against wind and precipitation. Tight clothing or shoes/boots must be avoided. Facial creams and emollients, although recommended by many companies, are actually contraindicated as there have been findings of worse outcomes with their use. Finally, avoidance of nicotine or any vasoconstrictor is important.

Chilblains

Chilblains, also referred to as "pernio," are localized inflammatory nodules caused by brief exposure to cold moisture at a temperature above freezing. The nodules appear 12–24 h after cold exposure and typically appear as localized plaques or nodules that are pruritic and/or tender to touch. After rewarming, the areas typically turn into blue nodules that can last up to a week. Young women are at highest risk, along with patients with Raynaud's phenomenon or other rheumatologic diseases. These are not permanent and heal after the patient returns to a warm environment with dry clothes. If itching persists, consideration for hydrocortisone cream can be given.

Cold Urticaria

Cold-induced urticaria is a well-recognized reaction secondary to mast cell release of histamine due to the cold. It presents in the typical fashion with scattered skin wheals and associated pruritus. Treatment is best with first-generation antihistamines, but it is best to prevent onset through the use of layering to stay warm. Cold-induced anaphylaxis has been documented, albeit rare, and should be treated as typical anaphylaxis with an EpiPen and antihistamines.

Non-Freezing Cold Injuries (NFCI)

NFCI are injuries relating to prolonged exposure to cold water, specifically 0–15 °C (32–59 °F) water, also referred to as "immersion foot" or the more colloquial term "trench foot." These injuries are rare in the first world, but in the deployed environment the incidence is substantially more commonplace. As their name implies, these are primarily injuries of the distal lower extremity. While both are NFCI, immersion and trench foot differ in that trench foot usually occurs on dry land whereas immersion foot occurs in people sitting in cold water for hours or days at a time (e.g., in a rescue boat after a shipwreck). Injury takes approximately 12 h to occur, although it could be faster given more extreme environmental conditions. Populations at risk are the same as for freezing injuries.

Pathophysiology

The pathophysiology is multifaceted but is most characterized by severe prolonged vasoconstriction eventually causing microvascular thrombosis. Neuronal damage can occur from ischemic injury or directly from cold exposure. Cold-induced vasodilation, also known as the "hunting response," is a phenomenon in some individuals who experience brief episodes of vasodilation of their affected microvasculature in an attempt to improve perfusion distally. It is not ubiquitous across all populations, and studies trend toward better outcomes in those individuals who experience it more frequently.

The injured tissue follows a common disease progression broken down into the following stages. Diagnosis is made clinically and there is no need for blood work or imaging, but again can be performed if there is concern for concomitant trauma or other systemic illness.

- **First-stage NFCI** presents during immersion as erythematous, hyper-perfused tissue, followed by intensely white skin from vasoconstriction. The tissue will be insensate and capillary refill is slow or not present. Gangrene will often be present at this stage.
- **Second-stage NFCI** occurs once the patient is out of the water and dry. The skin will be mottled and pale, often with areas of blue discoloration or mottling. The skin will be cold to the touch, and the tissue will still feel numb to the patient. Pulses may be bounding but capillary refill is extremely slow.
- **Third-stage NFCI** is also known as the "hyperemia" phase and takes place hours or days after rewarming; onset is often abrupt. Patients will experience bright red and edematous tissues, often with various sizes of blister formation. Pulses will be bounding but capillary refill again will be slow due to presumed microvascular damage. Patients often describe new severe pain and a sense of hyperalgesia with any palpation of the area.
- **Fourth-stage NFCI** occurs weeks to years after injury. Skin will have a normal appearance but similar to patients with frostbite injury, NFCI patients may have chronic pain, cold intolerance, and hyperhidrosis. If injury was severe enough, necrosis and auto-amputation can occur.

General Treatment Strategies

Treatment should focus on treating life- or limb-threatening emergencies before focusing on NFCI, including frostbite. Once NFCIs can be addressed, removing wet clothes and drying the patient in room temperature air is paramount. Adequate analgesia is important as rewarming causes severe pain. Elevation of the extremity will help with pain and edema. Avoiding further moisture to the injured areas is also important. Prophylactic antibiotics are not indicated unless there is an obvious nidus for infection, so then the antibiotic choice should cover *Staphylococcus* species, *Streptococcus* species, and *Pseudomonas* species. The significant edema that can occur from NFCI rewarming has been associated with compartment syndrome so the injured extremities should be examined frequently. Prevention focuses on avoiding prolonged moisture exposure and is most successful through frequent changing of socks.

Warm Water Immersion Foot (WWIF)

Warm water immersion foot (WWIF) is extremely similar to NFCI, as it is caused by prolonged exposure (~12 h) to moisture, but the water temperature is above 15 °C (59 °F). Patients with WWIF frequently fully recover, in contrast to its colder relative. Tropical immersion foot (TIF) is the same thing as WWIF but is due to even more prolonged (>72 h) exposure to warm water. The bottom of the feet in both conditions will be wrinkly and white, and patients will describe them as tingling or insensate. TIF is more likely to have severe erythema and edema over the dorsum of the foot. Both conditions are associated with abrasions and ulcerations at shoe/boot pressure points. Infection is more common in WWIF patients, and many patients will present with fevers and inguinal lymphadenopathy. Treatment is the same as for NFCIs. Prevention is performed through frequent changing of socks and attempting to stay dry.

Conclusion

Clinical Vignette 28.1 Conclusion

The patient was transported to a nearby field hospital where he was treated for his trauma, hypothermia, and frostbite. The medical team placed a more appropriate splint on his leg. They continued to utilize the HPMK in addition to a forced-warm air unit, warmed IV fluids, and warm water bladder lavage, resulting in an improvement in his core temperature to 36 °C. Upon rewarming, the patient was more alert and his neurologic status improved. Finally, they placed the patient's frostbitten areas in warm water immersion to thaw.

The patient required orthopedic surgery on his leg the following day. The general surgeon closely monitored the status of his frostbite, as he had a few fingertips with fourth-degree injury. The patient then started his journey via MEDEVAC back to the Continental United States (CONUS) for higher levels of care.

In the vignette, the treatments rendered by the SAR medical technician halted the progression of his hypothermia, and the treatments rendered by the surgical team minimized his morbidity and mortality given his concomitant traumatic injury, hypothermia, and freezing injuries. The expeditionary maritime surgical team may encounter patients suffering from hypothermia, immersion, freezing, or NFCI injuries, either as their sole injury or as part of a complex trauma patient presentation. Education and prevention are crucial for all of these entities. However, if they do occur, treat systemic illness and hypothermia first, followed by frostbite, and finally any concomitant NFCI. Emphasize drying, passive and active rewarming, and prevention of heat loss as soon as possible. The maritime surgical team will likely be involved in the initial intake and stabilization of a patient before they go to a higher level of care, and those crucial interventions can improve outcomes for all entities.

Declaration of Interest The views expressed in this chapter are those of the authors and do not necessarily reflect the official policy or position of the Department of the Navy, Department of Defense, nor the US Government.

Funding This research did not receive any specific grant from funding agencies in the public, commercial, or not-for-profit sectors.

Conflict of Interest Statement The authors declare no conflict of interest.

Further Reading

Bennett B, Holcomb J. Battlefield trauma-induced hypothermia: transitioning the preferred method of casualty rewarming. Wilderness Environ Med. 2017;28:82–9.

Drowning/Near drowning (Chapter 3–5.4). US Navy diving manual, Rev 7, Commander naval sea systems command. 2016.

Global Report on Drowning: World Health Organization. 2020. https://www.who.int/news-room/fact-sheets/detail/drowning.

Joint trauma system, frostbite and immersion foot care. CPG ID59. 2017. https://jts.amedd.army.mil/index.cfm/PI_CPGs/cpgs.

Joint Trauma System. Hypothermia prevention, monitoring and management CPG ID23. 2012. https://jts.amedd.army.mil/index.cfm/PI_CPGs/cpgs.

Joint Trauma System. Drowning management CPG ID64. 2017. https://jts.amedd.army.mil/index.cfm/PI_CPGs/cpgs.

Schmidt AC, Sempsrott JR, Hawkins SC, Arastu AS, et al. Wilderness Medical Society Practice guidelines for the prevention and treatment of drowning. Wilderness Environ Med. 2016;27:236–51. http://www.wemjournal.org/article/S1080-6032(16)00003-X/pdf.

Szpilman D. Drowning. N Engl J Med. 2012;366(22):2102–10. https://doi.org/10.1056/NEJMra1013317.

U.S. Search and Rescue Task Force. Cold water survival. http://ussartf.org.

Chapter 29
Acute Management of Chemical, Biological, Radiological, and Nuclear Exposure at Sea

Jason M. Bowie

Now I am become Death, the destroyer of worlds.

J. Robert Oppenheimer, 1945

Author deployment experience	
Jason M. Bowie	Senior Medical Officer, USS Comstock (LSD-45), WESTPAC in support of the 11th Marine Expeditionary Unit, INDOPACOM Area of Responsibility, 2013–2014.
	Officer in Charge, Role II Light Maneuver Team, forward deployed in support Maritime Security Operations and Navy Special Warfare missions, AFRICOM Area of Responsibility, 2022.

BLUF (Bottom Line Up Front)

1. The most important principle of chemical, biological, radiological, and nuclear (CBRN) exposure in the expeditionary environment is extensive planning, with the ultimate goal being prevention, as exposure can lead to significant morbidity and mortality.
2. Containment and decontamination are key components for managing all CBRN exposures.
3. When CBRN exposure is suspected, first responders should first don personal protective equipment (PPE) and then follow the CRESS algorithm to evaluate patients.
4. After assessment for CBRN exposure, first responders and medical providers should follow the $(MARCHE)^2$ approach to CBRN exposure casualty management.

J. M. Bowie (✉)
Captain James A. Lovell Federal Health Care Center, North Chicago, IL, USA
e-mail: jason.m.bowie.mil@health.mil

M. D. Tadlock, A. A. Hernandez (eds.), *Expeditionary Surgery at Sea*,
https://doi.org/10.1007/978-3-031-21893-4_29

5. Management of CBRN exposure is a complex topic with multiple agents that require varied containment and treatment modalities.
6. Exposures to chemical agents including cyanide, acetylcholinesterase inhibitors, toxic industrial agents (i.e., chlorine), and vesicants (i.e., mustard gas) require rapid identification and treatment based on the specific exposure.
7. The physiologic effects of radiation exposure are rarely identified in the acute setting. Avoiding exposure, wearing appropriate PPE, and limiting overall exposure are key components to mitigating the effects of radiation.
8. Acute exposure to high levels of radiation can cause skin burns and acute radiation syndrome (ARS), characterized by nausea, vomiting, headache, diarrhea, and bone marrow destruction.
9. Chronic exposure to high levels of radiation increases a patient's risk of solid organ or blood cancers as well as cardiovascular disease.

Introduction

The majority of casualties encountered in the expeditionary maritime setting continue to be the result of conventional injuries, but vigilance is required when a chemical, biological, radiological, and nuclear (CBRN) exposure is suspected. The deployed maritime surgical team may be involved in CBRN exposures even in times of peace, and these patients tend to require significantly more resources, time, and training to optimize outcomes. An extensive discussion of this complex topic is outside the scope of this chapter. Instead, it aims to broadly review CBRN exposure and attack, focusing on the roles of the maritime medical and surgical teams during decontamination and management. The Joint Trauma System (JTS) Clinical Practice Guidelines (CPGs) on CBRN injury response and management listed at the end of this chapter provide a more thorough overview.

Operation Tomodachi

In response to the 2011 Tōhoku earthquake and tsunami and subsequent Fukushima Daiichi nuclear disaster, the United States (U.S.) Armed Forces launched an emergency response operation to support disaster relief to Japan and the region. At Fukushima Daiichi, the automatic nuclear reactor earthquake response and flooding from the tsunami led to generator failure and subsequent loss of nuclear reactor cooling, ultimately leading to three reactor meltdowns and three hydrogen explosions. These events led to not only the release of large amounts of atmospheric radiation but also the release of enormous amounts of radioactive isotopes into the nearby Pacific Ocean.

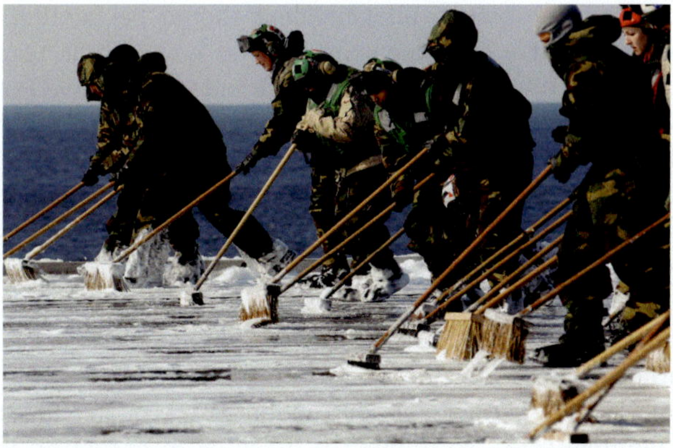

Fig. 29.1 Decontamination efforts during Operation Tomodachi on board Nimitz class aircraft carrier, the USS Ronald Reagan (CVN-76), 2011. (Source: Public domain image, not in copyright. Available at: https://commons.wikimedia.org/wiki/Category:Radiation_decontamination_of_the_USS_Ronald_Reagan)

Operation Tomodachi was a joint operation aimed at providing humanitarian aid and disaster relief (HADR) efforts and search and rescue (SAR) assistance to those affected by the 9.0 magnitude earthquake and resultant tsunami. It involved the deployment of 24 U.S. Navy ships, including the USS Ronald Reagan (CVN-76), 189 aircraft, and a total of over 24,000 American service members. During the course of this effort, monitoring equipment on the USS Ronald Reagan (CVN-76) indicated that the ship was exposed to increased levels of radiation and that several crewmembers had specifically been contaminated during decontamination efforts (Fig. 29.1). Thankfully, no military personnel or members of the local populace died of acute radiation syndrome (ARS). The majority of the acute deaths were attributed to the other disasters surrounding the incident. Long-term effects included an increase in death rates secondary to cancer for the local populace in the years following the disaster. This operation illustrates an example of when U.S. Navy personnel would potentially have a CBRN exposure in the absence of an attack or mishap.

Chemical and Biologic Agent Exposure

Prevention and Planning

The most important principle of CBRN exposure in the expeditionary environment is extensive planning, with the ultimate goal being prevention. Available intelligence should be capable of predicting the likelihood and nature of a chemical or biologic agent attack or exposure. In rare cases, chemical agent exposure can occur accidentally with release of industrial grade chemicals in an uncontrolled setting.

In a high-threat environment, all personnel should be familiar with CBRN-specific personal protective equipment (PPE), and it should be readily available. This PPE is frequently referred to as Mission-Oriented Protective Posture (MOPP) gear. There are multiple MOPP levels, referring to specific levels of readiness. The recommended MOPP level is dictated by the level of concern for a CBRN exposure or attack. Specific MOPP levels do not dictate specific PPE, but rather the availability of and manner by which personnel don their PPE (Fig. 29.2). At sea, personnel typically do not need to carry PPE with them as long as equipment is readily available in spaces at high risk for CBRN exposure such as engine rooms, work spaces, duty stations, mess decks, medical spaces, and flight and well decks. In addition to having appropriate PPE available, it is critical that all personnel know how to safely don and doff masks, overgarments, boots, and gloves. Not all PPE is intuitive and may come in multiple sizes, so training is essential to ensure all individuals are familiar with the available PPE, how it must be worn, and their appropriate size.

In addition to the measures taken to prevent exposure, planning for CBRN casualty evacuation and tracking after exposure must be considered ahead of time. Military medical treatment facilities (MTFs) should help coordinate decontamination and treatment efforts in the field and prepare to receive exposed casualties. MTFs must be aware of their own capacity as well. Chemical and biologic exposure

MISSION-ORIENTED PROTECTIVE POSTURES (MOPP)

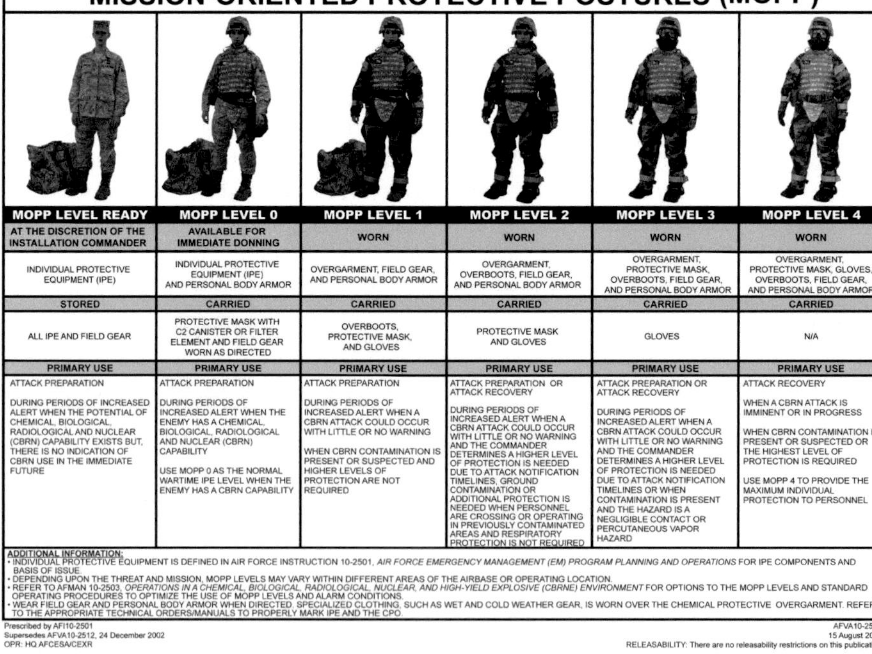

MOPP LEVEL READY	MOPP LEVEL 0	MOPP LEVEL 1	MOPP LEVEL 2	MOPP LEVEL 3	MOPP LEVEL 4
AT THE DISCRETION OF THE INSTALLATION COMMANDER	**AVAILABLE FOR IMMEDIATE DONNING**	**WORN**	**WORN**	**WORN**	**WORN**
INDIVIDUAL PROTECTIVE EQUIPMENT (IPE)	INDIVIDUAL PROTECTIVE EQUIPMENT (IPE) AND PERSONAL BODY ARMOR	OVERGARMENT, FIELD GEAR, AND PERSONAL BODY ARMOR	OVERGARMENT, OVERBOOTS, FIELD GEAR, AND PERSONAL BODY ARMOR	OVERGARMENT, PROTECTIVE MASK, OVERBOOTS, FIELD GEAR, AND PERSONAL BODY ARMOR	OVERGARMENT, PROTECTIVE MASK, GLOVES, OVERBOOTS, FIELD GEAR, AND PERSONAL BODY ARMOR
STORED	**CARRIED**	**CARRIED**	**CARRIED**	**CARRIED**	**CARRIED**
ALL IPE AND FIELD GEAR	PROTECTIVE MASK WITH C2 CANISTER OR FILTER ELEMENT AND FIELD GEAR WORN AS DIRECTED	OVERBOOTS, PROTECTIVE MASK, AND GLOVES	PROTECTIVE MASK AND GLOVES	GLOVES	N/A
PRIMARY USE	**PRIMARY USE**	**PRIMARY USE**	**PRIMARY USE**	**PRIMARY USE**	**PRIMARY USE**
ATTACK PREPARATION DURING PERIODS OF INCREASED ALERT WHEN THE POTENTIAL OF CHEMICAL, BIOLOGICAL, RADIOLOGICAL AND NUCLEAR (CBRN) CAPABILITY EXISTS BUT, THERE IS NO INDICATION OF CBRN USE IN THE IMMEDIATE FUTURE	ATTACK PREPARATION DURING PERIODS OF INCREASED ALERT WHEN THE ENEMY HAS A CHEMICAL, BIOLOGICAL, RADIOLOGICAL AND NUCLEAR (CBRN) CAPABILITY USE MOPP 0 AS THE NORMAL WARTIME IPE LEVEL WHEN THE ENEMY HAS A CBRN CAPABILITY	ATTACK PREPARATION DURING PERIODS OF INCREASED ALERT WHEN A CBRN ATTACK COULD OCCUR WITH LITTLE OR NO WARNING WHEN CBRN CONTAMINATION IS PRESENT OR SUSPECTED AND HIGHER LEVELS OF PROTECTION ARE NOT REQUIRED	ATTACK PREPARATION OR ATTACK RECOVERY DURING PERIODS OF INCREASED ALERT WHEN A CBRN ATTACK COULD OCCUR WITH LITTLE OR NO WARNING AND THE COMMANDER DETERMINES A HIGHER LEVEL OF PROTECTION IS NEEDED DUE TO ATTACK NOTIFICATION TIMELINES, GROUND CONTAMINATION OR ADDITIONAL PROTECTION IS NEEDED WHEN PERSONNEL ARE CROSSING OR OPERATING IN PREVIOUSLY CONTAMINATED AREAS AND RESPIRATORY PROTECTION IS NOT REQUIRED	ATTACK PREPARATION OR ATTACK RECOVERY DURING PERIODS OF INCREASED ALERT WHEN A CBRN ATTACK COULD OCCUR WITH LITTLE OR NO WARNING AND THE COMMANDER DETERMINES A HIGHER LEVEL OF PROTECTION IS NEEDED DUE TO ATTACK NOTIFICATION TIMELINES OR WHEN CONTAMINATION IS PRESENT AND THE HAZARD IS A NEGLIGIBLE CONTACT OR PERCUTANEOUS VAPOR HAZARD	ATTACK RECOVERY WHEN A CBRN ATTACK IS IMMINENT OR IN PROGRESS WHEN CBRN CONTAMINATION IS PRESENT OR SUSPECTED OR THE HIGHEST LEVEL OF PROTECTION IS REQUIRED USE MOPP 4 TO PROVIDE THE MAXIMUM INDIVIDUAL PROTECTION TO PERSONNEL

ADDITIONAL INFORMATION:
- INDIVIDUAL PROTECTIVE EQUIPMENT IS DEFINED IN AIR FORCE INSTRUCTION 10-2501, *AIR FORCE EMERGENCY MANAGEMENT (EM) PROGRAM PLANNING AND OPERATIONS* FOR IPE COMPONENTS AND BASIS OF ISSUE.
- DEPENDING UPON THE THREAT AND MISSION, MOPP LEVELS MAY VARY WITHIN DIFFERENT AREAS OF THE AIRBASE OR OPERATING LOCATION.
- REFER TO AFMAN 10-2503, *OPERATIONS IN A CHEMICAL, BIOLOGICAL, RADIOLOGICAL, NUCLEAR, AND HIGH-YIELD EXPLOSIVE (CBRNE) ENVIRONMENT* FOR OPTIONS TO THE MOPP LEVELS AND STANDARD OPERATING PROCEDURES TO OPTIMIZE THE USE OF MOPP LEVELS AND ALARM CONDITIONS.
- WEAR FIELD GEAR AND PERSONAL BODY ARMOR WHEN DIRECTED. SPECIALIZED CLOTHING, SUCH AS WET AND COLD WEATHER GEAR, IS WORN OVER THE CHEMICAL PROTECTIVE OVERGARMENT. REFER TO THE APPROPRIATE TECHNICAL ORDERS/MANUALS TO PROPERLY MARK IPE AND THE CPO.

Prescribed by AFI10-2501
Supersedes AFVA10-2512, 24 December 2002
OPR: HQ AFCESA/CEXR

AFVA10-2512
15 August 2011
RELEASABILITY: There are no releasability restrictions on this publication

Fig. 29.2 Mission-Oriented Protective Postures (MOPP) from Level Ready to Level 4. (Source: Public domain image, not in copyright. Available at: https://www.446aw.afrc.af.mil/News/Photos/igphoto/2000186472/mediaid/102916/)

casualties are more resource-intensive than typical traumatically injured patients. Medical leaders and planners should be continuously aware of available primary and secondary medical evacuation (MEDEVAC) routes and potential environmental factors. Evacuation platforms can be contaminated during the course of MEDEVAC procedures; therefore, planning for both dirty and clean MEDEVAC platforms is necessary with appropriate vehicle decontamination facilities available during evacuation efforts.

Containment and Decontamination

After a chemical or biologic exposure or attack has occurred, the initial goals of first responders are containment of the threat, isolation of exposed personnel, and decontamination of all individuals and spaces affected by the exposure. As mentioned above, response efforts should proceed in conjunction with a coordinating MTF. Both the ship's line leadership and medical department should have established Standard Operating Procedures (SOPs) for containment and isolation, which should be reviewed and drilled regularly to optimize outcomes. The majority of the medical department involvement in this process is in the decontamination of the individual phase.

To prevent becoming casualties themselves, first responders should don appropriate PPE prior to treating CBRN casualties. Examples of appropriate PPE include M50 masks, Joint Service Lightweight Integrated Suit Technology (JSLIST) chemical and biological protective garments, rubber gloves, and vinyl overboots, as pictured in Figs. 29.1 and 29.2. When CBRN-specific PPE is not available, field-expedient PPE such as nitrile gloves in multiple layers, 6 mm sheeting and bags, and any available respirators or masks should be worn.

To decontaminate individuals, first responders should remove all clothing and equipment from casualties and dispose of these items per SOP. After exposing casualties and removing contaminated garments, appropriate decontamination solutions should be applied. For many agents, time is of the essence. For physical removal and dilution of chemical or biologic agents, copious irrigation with soap and water is recommended. It will not destroy biologic agents though. Decontamination of eye exposure should be with normal saline, water, or eye-specific solutions. Reactive Skin Decontamination Lotion (RSDL) is indicated for decontamination of chemical agents. RSDL comes as a packaged sponge that contains a skin-penetrating reactive agent that deactivates mustard and nerve agents. It should be applied immediately after exposure for best results. The sponge is then used to gently scrub the skin for 2 min; the solution is then removed, reapplied, and left on the intact skin for up to 24 h. RSDL is indicated for intact skin only and should not be used on open wounds or eyes. To destroy most biologic agents, 0.5% hypochlorite solution (created by mixing nine parts water to one part 5% bleach) can be wiped on skin and immediately rinsed with fresh water. This bleach solution should not be used in the chest cavity, abdominal cavity, brain/spinal cord, or eyes.

Management

In the wake of a chemical or biologic exposure or attack, after security has been established and decontamination initiated, casualty management is the next priority. CBRN casualties are often a complex and challenging combination of agent exposure and trauma, requiring significantly more resources, time, and expertise than a conventional trauma patient. In the event of a mass casualty incident (MCI), they require rapid triage by an experienced provider (see Chap. 7). Evaluation for CBRN exposure should follow the CRESS (Consciousness, Respirations, Eyes, Secretions, Skin) acronym (Table 29.1). This acronym is particularly useful for chemical agent exposure, as biological agent exposure typically results in delayed symptom onset and radiation exposure typically only causes acute symptoms at high doses (>6 Gy).

After assessment for CBRN exposure using the CRESS acronym, first responders and medical providers should follow the $(MARCHE)^2$ approach to CBRN casualties. This approach combines the MARCH algorithm for casualty management (Massive hemorrhage, Airway, Respirations, Circulation, and Hypothermia and Head wound) and the addition of CBRN priorities (Mask, Antidotes, Rapid spot decontamination, Countermeasures, Extraction and Evacuation).

Providers and first responders must use clinical judgement when assessing potential CBRN casualties at the point of injury (POI), but priorities remain egress from the threat, donning of PPE, and quickly treating immediate life threats. After egress from a hot zone, responders should begin definitive treatment of life threats including massive hemorrhage and airway and respiratory compromise and apply rapid CBRN antidotes and countermeasures depending on the threat based on the CRESS findings.

Management of exposure to several specific chemical agents is worth discussing individually. Cyanide, nerve agent, pulmonary agent, and vesicant exposures are the most likely agents to be encountered in the deployed maritime environment and are particularly devastating.

Table 29.1 CRESS acronym for specific chemical agent exposures and their findings

Agent	Consciousness	Respirations	Eyes	Secretions	Skin
Nerve	Depressed or unconscious	Increased	Miosis	Increased	Diaphoretic
Cyanide	Depressed or unconscious	Increased	Normal	Normal	Flushed or cyanotic
Chlorine/phosgene	Normal	Increased	Normal	Increased, delayed fluid in lungs	Normal
Vesicants (effects delayed)	Normal	Increased, if vapor	Normal	Increased, delayed fluid in lungs	Normal initially, then blistering

- Cyanide has not been used commonly as a warfare agent, but it has been used as an agent of terrorism on several occasions.
  - Symptoms: Symptoms of cyanide exposure are typically evident within minutes. Patients will experience headache, dizziness, weakness, dyspnea, and diaphoresis. Ultimately, casualties develop tissue hypoxia without cyanosis in conjunction with metabolic acidosis.
  - Management: The key to management of cyanide exposure is rapid recognition as patients will experience a rapid decline to death without treatment. The clinical picture described above combined with arterial blood gasses (ABG) showing metabolic acidosis and elevated lactic acid levels should alert the provider to possible cyanide exposure and lead to rapid intravenous (IV) administration of hydroxycobalamin, commercially available as CYANOKIT®, with concurrent aggressive supportive care with supplemental oxygen even if pulse oximetry measuring of peripheral saturation of hemoglobin (SpO_2) readings is normal. See Chap. 26 for additional discussion.
- Exposure to acetylcholinesterase inhibitors (nerve agents) can be rapidly fatal as well. These agents are chemically similar to pesticide compounds but have been concentrated and modified for increased lethality as agents of warfare.
  - Symptoms: They prevent the breakdown of acetylcholine by binding to acetylcholinesterase leading to a characteristic prodrome of miosis, bradycardia, bronchoconstriction, emesis, lacrimation, salivation, diarrhea, and urination.
  - Management: Inhalational exposure leads to rapid onset of symptoms and can quickly lead to death if not recognized and treated with IV or intramuscular (IM) atropine and pralidoxime (2PAM). If nicotinic effects are present, such as weakness, fasciculations, or seizure, benzodiazepines should be utilized as well.
- Toxic industrial chemicals (pulmonary agents) include phosgene and chlorine and have devastating effects when vaporized. These chemicals are either stored as compressed liquids or refrigerated due to their low temperature of vaporization. Chlorine reacts with moisture in the respiratory system; through hydrolysis it forms hydrochloric acid and hypochlorous acid as well as free radicals that cause cell injury and death. Phosgene participates in acylation to cause protein and lipid denaturation, disruption of cell membrane structures, and disruption of the pulmonary surfactant layer. Additionally, release of these gasses in an enclosed space can cause asphyxiation through the displacement of oxygen.
  - Symptoms: Symptom onset with chlorine exposure is immediate and includes eye pain and lacrimation, headache, dyspnea, cough, tachycardia, tachypnea, and cyanosis. Phosgene symptoms are similar, but tend to have a more insidious onset, starting 2–6 h after exposure.
  - Management: The primary treatments after pulmonary agent exposure are decontamination and supportive. Many patients will develop pulmonary edema within 8 h of exposure so serial chest X-rays and/or intubation may be warranted.

- Mustard gas and other vesicant agents were first developed and used during World War I and are still used in chemical warfare today. These agents can be used in solid, liquid, or gas forms and have been used as recently as the recent conflicts with Islamic State of Iraq and Syria (ISIS).
  - Symptoms: Exposure to these agents is via the skin and causes chemical burns. Second- and third-degree burns as well as corneal erosion typically occur a few hours after exposure. Inhalation or ingestion can result in a similar effect on mucosal surfaces.
  - Management: Decontamination by first responders wearing adequate PPE is the key component of managing vesicant exposure. The agent must be removed within 3 to 5 min to prevent significant absorption. The chemical should then be removed from the skin with a dry cloth and RSDL applied. Eyes should be immediately washed out with copious volumes of water. After decontamination, supportive respiratory and burn care should be initiated. Application of anticholinergic, antibiotic, and steroid ophthalmic ointments is also recommended.

Radiation and Nuclear Agent Exposure

Prevention

Like chemical and biologic agent exposure, the most important component of radiation and nuclear agent exposure management is prevention and planning. Again, all personnel must be trained on the use and wear of available PPE, and it must be readily available. In the shipboard environment, there is a risk of radiation exposure for personnel embarked on nuclear-powered craft. These vessels utilize nuclear reactors to create heat that is transferred from the reactor core to a secondary steam system and used to power the majority of the ship's systems. Reactor plants are shielded in order to minimize radiation exposure to shipboard personnel. Additionally, these ships are designed to maximize the distance between the reactor compartment and duty stations, living quarters, and mess decks. During normal operations, radiation outside the reactor compartment is no greater than natural background radiation. The most likely risk of radiation exposure comes from corrosion and wear products that are carried in coolant from the reactor plant and can become deposited in the piping systems. Personnel can be exposed to these deposited radioactive elements during inspection and maintenance inside the reactor compartment and must take all precautions when performing these tasks.

To measure radiation exposure, thermoluminescent dosimeters (TLDs) are worn by personnel who are at risk for increased radiation exposure, such as individuals involved in reactor compartment inspection or maintenance. Additionally, TLDs are posted at various locations around ships where background radiation should be the only radiation source. These control TLDs are then compared to those worn by shipboard personnel to ensure these personnel are not being exposed to increased radiation doses. It is worth noting that the average annual exposure for shipyard workers and shipboard personnel is significantly less than the annual background radiation that the average American receives. No individuals monitored as part of the Naval Nuclear Propulsion Program have received greater than the annual limit of five Rem, and only four shipboard military personnel have received greater than the quarterly limit of three Rem since monitoring began in 1967. However, embarked personnel may also be asked to respond to radiation incidents, like the Fukushima Daiichi nuclear disaster. Responding to incidents like these, or the more feared nuclear attack, poses a greater risk for radiation exposure than from the ships themselves.

Containment and Decontamination

The primary means of preventing exposure for military personnel is minimizing time near the radioactive source, maximizing the distance from the source, and maintaining shielding to absorb radiation from the source. Additionally, all individuals must limit the risk of internal contamination by preventing ingestion or inhalation of radioactive materials. As with other exposures, response efforts should proceed in conjunction with a coordinating MTF and in line with the previously established local line and medical SOPs for this process, which should be routinely reviewed and drilled.

If asked to respond to a radiation incident and the level of contamination is not known, first responders should don MOPP level 4 PPE such as the JSLIST and appropriate respirators during assessment and decontamination efforts. Additionally, during these efforts, ship's spaces should be periodically surveyed for contamination and the exterior surfaces of the ship decontaminated to remove any loose radiologic debris.

Contaminated personnel should be decontaminated in open air spaces, such as flight decks, by removal and control of any contaminated clothing and washing of the exposed skin and hair using soap and water. Be sure to cover any wounds prior to decontamination process to prevent cross-contamination and ensure gentle decontamination as increased radiation absorption can occur with skin irritation and erythema. Unlike the decontamination for chemical or biologic agents, this process is less urgent in nature. It does not neutralize the particles but does effectively eliminate 95% of the external contamination. When available, a radiation detector can help guide the process.

Management

Following expedited removal from the radiation source and decontamination, much of radiation sickness management is supportive, which is the most likely place the maritime surgical team would be utilized, given their familiarity with

Table 29.2 Dose-effect relationship for whole-body radiation exposure

Dose	Effect
10 cGy	No observable effects
50 cGy	Minor lymphocyte depression
1 Gy	Nausea and vomiting threshold, minor lymphocyte depression No acute deaths
2 Gy	Nausea and vomiting common, moderate lymphocyte depression Few deaths, especially if no combined injuries
3.5–4 Gy	Nausea and vomiting probable, significant lymphocyte depression 50% lethal at 60 days without treatment, more if combined injuries
5–6 Gy	Nausea and vomiting nearly 100%, severe lymphocyte depression 100% lethal at 60 days without treatment, nearly 100% lethal if combined injuries (even with treatment)

cGy centigray, *Gy* gray (1 Gray = 1 Sievert)
Source: Adapted from Flynn DF, Goans RE. Nuclear terrorism: triage and medical management of radiation and combined-injury casualties. Surg Clin N Am. 2006; 86:601–636

critical care medicine and wound care. Supportive care improves survival rates significantly, in particular for patients with a lower and more survivable radiation dose (Fig. 29.2, Table 29.2).

The majority of information about the effect of high-dose radiation exposure comes from the casualties of Hiroshima and Nagasaki, radium dial painters, and residents of islands in the South Pacific that were exposed to high doses of radiation from fallout from early nuclear weapons tests. ARS is divided into hematopoietic, gastrointestinal, and neurovascular syndromes as the dose increases. Each syndrome is then subdivided into four clinical stages: prodromal, latent, manifest illness, and recovery or death. Initial symptoms of exposure to high levels of radiation include headache, nausea, vomiting, and diarrhea, which can start within minutes. Casualties may also experience skin damage similar to superficial second-degree burns in the hours to days after exposure. The primary cause of death from ARS is bone marrow dysfunction and destruction leading to severe infection and spontaneous hemorrhage. Fluid and electrolyte replacement, antimicrobial prophylaxis, meticulous skin/burn care and oral hygiene, isolation and environmental control (to a degree), and antiemetics/antidiarrheals are all interventions that a maritime surgical team can provide, while arrangements are being made to MEDEVAC exposed patients. Upon arrival at a higher level of care treatments will include leuko-reduced and irradiated blood transfusions, true isolation and environmental control, cytokine therapy like granulocyte colony-stimulating factor (G-CSF), or stem-cell transplant. The receiving MTF may also need to manage traumatic injuries that the patients may have concurrently sustained, and these greatly increase the risk of mortality (Fig. 29.2). Closing wounds within 72 h is recommended when possible, as wound healing will be impaired. Additionally, potassium iodide is recommended to decrease the radiation dose absorbed by the thyroid gland.

The predominant latent effect of radiation exposure is development of cancer via damage to cellular deoxyribonucleic acid (DNA). Tissues that are most sensitive to radiation exposure are those that divide rapidly (e.g., bone marrow) or incorporate radioactive ions into their substance (e.g., thyroid gland). All other organs are at risk after significant radiation exposure, but the lung, stomach, colon, bladder, liver, ovary, and breast appear to be at higher risk overall. Individuals exposed to increased radiation doses are also at risk for cataract development, cardiovascular disease, and damage to reproductive cells, which leads to infertility. Due to these significant risks, all personnel with potential for exposure to radiation should undergo radiation physical exams every 2 to 5 years and dosimetry monitoring when entering radiologically controlled areas, as described above.

Conclusion

The first goal of CBRN management remains prevention. Exposure to chemical, biological, radiologic, and nuclear warfare agents can lead to significant morbidity and mortality. All available intelligence should be utilized to mitigate the risk of such exposures. To further mitigate this risk, all first responders and shipboard personnel must be trained on the donning, doffing, and wear of appropriate PPE, and these items must be readily available. While not common, the deployed maritime surgical team may be involved in caring for patients of CBRN exposures, especially if there are concomitant traumatic injuries. Every member of the team must be appropriately trained regarding the necessary response depending on the agent to optimize outcomes on these complex and resource-intensive patients until they can get to a higher level of care.

Declaration of Interest The views expressed in this chapter are those of the authors and do not necessarily reflect the official policy or position of the Department of the Navy, Department of Defense, nor the US Government.

Funding This research did not receive any specific grant from funding agencies in the public, commercial, or not-for-profit sectors.

Conflict of Interest Statement The authors declare no conflict of interest.

Further Reading

Bureau of Medicine and Surgery. NAVMED P-5055, radiation health protection manual. 2018. https://www.med.navy.mil/Portals/62/Documents/BUMED/Directives/All%20Pubs/5055%20(Feb%202011)%20with%20CH-1.pdf?ver=ey1FD5UwePciLs5TCDdN0Q%3d%3d.

Ciottone GR. Toxidrome recognition in chemical-weapons attacks. N Engl J Med. 2018;378:1611–20.

Final Report to the Congressional Defense Committees in Response to the Joint Explanatory Statement Accompanying the Department of Defense Appropriations Act, 2014, Page 90, "radiation exposure". Submitted by the office of the Assistant Secretary of defense for health affairs. 2014.

Flynn DF, Goans RE. Triage and treatment of radiation and combined-injury mass casualties. In: Mickelson AB, editor. Medical consequences of radiological and nuclear weapons. Washington, DC: Borden Institute; 2012. p. 17–30.

Flynn DF, Goans RE. Acute radiation syndrome in humans. In: Mickelson AB, editor. Medical consequences of radiological and nuclear weapons. Washington, DC: Borden Institute; 2012. p. 39–68.

Joint Trauma System. Chemical, biological, radiological and nuclear injury response part I: initial response to CBRN agents clinical practice guideline. 2018. https://jts.amedd.army.mil/assets/docs/cpgs/Chemical_Biological,_Radiological_Nuclear_Injury_Part1_Initial_Response_01_May_2018_ID69.pdf.

Joint Trauma System. Chemical, biological, radiological and nuclear injury response part 2: medical management of chemical agent exposure, Clinical practice guideline. 2022. https://jts.amedd.army.mil/assets/docs/cpgs/Chemical_Biological_Radiological_Nuclear_Injury_Response_Part_2_Medical_Management_25_Mar_2022_ID69.pdf.

Naval Nuclear Propulsion Program. Occupational radiation exposure from U.S. Naval nuclear plants and their support facilities, report NT-19-2. 2019. https://www.energy.gov/sites/prod/files/2019/09/f66/NT-19-2.pdf.

Operation Tomodachi Registry. https://registry.csd.disa.mil/registryWeb/Registry/OperationTomodachi/DisplayAbout?struts.token.name=token&token=G6UTTOJDOF5Y3H4Q0HTSWDNZ9FVOIIKA. Accessed 15 Feb 2022.

Chapter 30
Maritime Prolonged Casualty Care

Jeffrey D. Biberston, Julie A. Darling, and Michael S. Tripp

...the ocean that is open to all, merciful to none, that threatens even when it seems to yield, and that is pitiless always to weakness.

Ernest Shackleton

Author deployment experience	
Jeffrey D. Biberston	Intensive Care Unit Medical Director, forward deployed Naval Hospital Okinawa, Japan, 2020–present
Julie A. Darling	Critical Care Registered Nurse, Fleet Surgical Team-9, 2003–2005; embarked on multiple LHA/LHD platforms, including embarked on the USS Bonhomme Richard (LHD-6) supporting Humanitarian Aid Disaster Relief (HADR) operations following Indian Ocean tsunami, Banda Aceh, Indonesia, 2004; WESTPAC, CENTCOM and INDOPACOM Areas of Responsibility, 2004–2005
	Senior Nurse/Critical Care Registered Nurse, second Medical Battalion, Operation Enduring Freedom, Camp Dwyer, Helmand Provence, Afghanistan, 2009
	Critical Care Subject Matter Expert, USNS Mercy (T-AH-19), Pacific Partnership Subject Matter Expertise Exchange, Nha Trang and Danang, Vietnam, 2017

J. D. Biberston
Navy Medicine Readiness and Training Command Okinawa, Okinawa, Japan

J. A. Darling · M. S. Tripp (✉)
United States Navy Bureau of Medicine and Surgery, Falls Church, VA, USA
e-mail: julie.a.darling.mil@health.mil; michael.s.tripp3.mil@health.mil

M. D. Tadlock, A. A. Hernandez (eds.), *Expeditionary Surgery at Sea*,
https://doi.org/10.1007/978-3-031-21893-4_30

Author deployment experience	
Michael S. Tripp	Intensive Care Unit Medical Director, forward deployed Naval Hospital Guam, 2008–2010
	Intensive Care Unit Department Head, Pulmonologist and Intensivist, NATO Role 3 Multinational Medical Unit, Operation Enduring Freedom, Kandahar Airfield, Afghanistan, 2012
	Undersea Medical Officer and Group Surgeon, Explosive Ordnance Disposal Group ONE, medical operations, INDOPACOM and CENTCOM Areas of Responsibility, 2015–2018
	Head of Undersea Medicine, Radiation Health, and Undersea Independent Duty Corpsmen, United States Navy Bureau of Medicine, Falls Church, VA, USA, 2019–present

BLUF (Bottom Line Up Front)

1. Prolonged Casualty Care (PCC) is any care of casualties where medical evacuation (MEDEVAC) to higher level of care is delayed or unavailable. PCC builds on the principles of Tactical Combat Casualty Care (TCCC) and therefore is a Role 1 contingency capability. However, when resource limitations are imposed by the operational environment, no matter the level of care (e.g., Role 2) the team should switch to a PCC mindset early to conserve available personnel and consumable resources.
2. While any effective medical plan includes PCC as a contingency, PCC is never the primary medical plan.
3. PCC is often delivered by expeditionary teams who may not have requisite training or equipment to provide traditional critical care. Core critical care skills can be practiced anywhere there are critically ill patients. Assessing which skills and outcomes are most essential to the operation is the role of the medical team leaders.
4. The concepts of care standards and minimum/better/best will evolve during a PCC event and should be critically evaluated by both operational and medical leadership.
5. Sepsis is the most common non-hemorrhagic shock likely to be encountered. Protocols should be developed and drilled for its treatment in deployed maritime settings.
6. The use of checklists and algorithms to define the level of care and standards of care available in a given situation is the most effective way to ensure care quality in PCC scenarios.
7. Postoperative patients, particularly those with prolonged operative courses or large abdominal surgeries, may require extensive fluid resuscitation due to fluid losses and shifts. Attention to resuscitation and endpoints such as urine output (UOP) is critical in this population.
8. In the PCC environment (or any environment), multiple endpoints of resuscitation should be used including normalization of capillary refill, urine output, and measurement of lactate if available. In the absence of other monitoring tools and labs, mental status, vital signs, capillary refill, UOP, passive leg raise, and inferior vena cava (IVC) diameter can all be utilized.

9. Be Brilliant in the Basics! Much of the management that prevents patient harm is standard for most critically ill patients and often represented as a daily Intensive Care Unit (ICU) rounds checklist (Table 30.3). All of these actions should be performed in the PCC environment.
10. The Joint Trauma System recently published comprehensive PCC clinical practice guidelines (CPGs) that are available at: https://jts.amedd.army.mil/assets/docs/cpgs/Prolonged_Casualty_Care_Guidelines_21_Dec_2021_ID91.pdf. PCC guidelines build upon Tactical Combat Casualty Care (TCCC) guidelines available at: https://deployedmedicine.com/content/40.

Introduction

Clinical Vignette 30.1

A 22-year-old male Sailor was brought to the medical department of a forward deployed missile frigate staffed by an Independent Duty Corpsman (IDC) and a general medical officer (GMO). He was tachypneic, hypoxemic, and extremely anxious. He had obvious lower extremity swelling which he attributed to "twisting his knee" earlier in the deployment. The ship was actively engaged in maneuvers, and the executive officer (XO) asked for an update on the patient's condition and impact on operations.

How should this patient be managed? Does the patient require medical evacuation (MEDEVAC) from the ship? What resources is this patient likely to need in the short term and long term if no MEDEVAC is available?

Prolonged Casualty Care (PCC) is defined as the need to provide patient care for extended periods of time when MEDEVAC or mission requirements surpass available capabilities and/or capacity to provide that care. In the maritime environment, these situations may be encountered during both peacetime and combat operations. Additionally, medical care in a maritime environment represents a unique challenge where any combination of resource or skill set limitations could impair delivery of conventional medicine. Training and anticipation may allow for some degree of preparation with the understanding that flexibility and creative problem-solving will still be required in periods of extremis and resource limitation, such as during distributed maritime operations (DMO). Advanced procedures, monitoring devices, and therapeutic strategies are often not possible; thus, preparation should be tailored to basic and fundamental strategies that offer the widest degree of clinical applicability with the fewest resources possible. PCC is a mindset for maritime surgical teams that utilizes understanding of basic concepts of critical care, just-in-time training, knowledge of potential injury patterns, and checklist algorithms to optimize patient outcomes and reduce the morbidity and mortality of critically ill patients who require prolonged care at sea.

Recently, the Joint Trauma System (JTS) published comprehensive PCC clinical practice guidelines (CPGs) that cover a wide range of conditions. It is "a consolidated list of casualty-centric knowledge, skills, abilities, and best practices intended to serve as the Department of Defense baseline CPG to direct casualty management over a prolonged period of time in austere, remote, or expeditionary settings, and/or during long-distance movements." An important point emphasized in the PCC CPG is that while PCC should be part of any effective medical plan, it should never be the primary patient care plan. PCC is a contingency capability only when MEDEVAC is not possible due to unexpected changes in the operational environment. The CPG can serve as a guide to PCC for the maritime provider or surgical team and is available at: https://jts.amedd.army.mil/assets/docs/cpgs/Prolonged_Casualty_Care_Guidelines_21_Dec_2021_ID91.pdf

Furthermore, as the PCC guidelines build upon the JTS Tactical Combat Casualty Care (TCCC) guidelines, the maritime provider and surgical team should be familiar with these guidelines as well. They are available at: https://deployedmedicine.com/content/40. As PCC is an extension of TCCC, it is a Role 1 capability typically provided by nonmedical and medical first responders. However, in the DMO environment Role 2 maritime surgical teams may need adapt a PCC mindset when resource limitations are imposed on the operational environment.

Prolonged Casualty Care (PCC) Mindset

Delivery of care will be influenced by the injury and illness patterns, numbers of casualties, and current shipboard operations. If adequate resources, expertise, and MEDEVAC capabilities are available, care can be delivered based on standard operating procedures (SOPs). Resource limitations imposed by significant casualty numbers or acuity, resource, or combat operations will necessitate different priorities. When this happens, a movement toward a PCC mindset should be made early. PCC does not necessarily mean disaster standards of care, but often these scenarios will be superimposed. Priorities including supply and resupply, locations of care delivery, and duration of care expected should be discussed with operational leadership. An up-to-date threat assessment of intended area of operations should be discussed in context on how the current casualty scenario may impact shipboard operations. Despite high levels of uncertainty regarding medical situations, standard categories of preparation will augment capability and potentially reduce morbidity and mortality.

PCC Limitations

Many limitations exist for both acute intensive care unit (ICU) and PCC situations and are additionally discussed in Chap. 20.

Staffing

Healthcare delivery in a maritime environment demands flexibility. Any healthcare team often has a wide spectrum of capability and experience. This variability among members of the healthcare team is often magnified by conventional staffing limitations and imposed resource, resupply, and MEDEVAC limitations. Thus, critical assessment of the team's capabilities and limitations should be undertaken by its leadership prior to deployment. Delivery of care for sustained periods of time in resource-constrained environments will demand individuals utilize skills beyond their traditional roles.

While there is no "recipe" for an ideal healthcare team, there should be adequate representation in experience from providers with experience in management of critically ill patients, perioperative patients, and conventional non-critically ill patients. These providers ideally are separate from the surgical team, to allow for full focus on initial triage and then damage control resuscitation (DCR) and damage control surgery (DCS) for the maritime surgical team (see Chaps. 22 and 23). This model was well utilized and proven during Operation Enduring Freedom (OEF). Obstetrics and pediatrics management represent a less likely required skill set; however, it should still be represented if possible and/or augmented by just-in-time training or virtual consultation (the maritime surgical team's interaction with these specialties is discussed in Chaps. 17 and 34, respectively).

Critical care registered nurses (CCRNs) represent a significant benefit to team dynamics as they are the experts in bedside care of injured and ill patients. CCRNs will be expected to manage complex patients for extended periods of time with minimal physician input during resource-constrained maritime PCC. Thus, ensuring optimal training and experience of CCRNs is crucial to the success of the team both clinically and interpersonally.

Respiratory therapists (RTs) are also a critical asset to any medical team, but are only present on fleet surgical team (FST) platforms currently unless part of an augmentation team. In mass casualty incidents (MCIs) or resource-constrained environments, they should be expected to provide independent ventilator management with minimal oversight from a critical care physician. This skill set includes fundamental understanding of lung-protective strategies, as well as corrections of the various respiratory failure states with various ventilator support techniques. They are also excellent candidates for advanced airway management training.

Skill sets that enhance medical capability and team dynamics should be the focus of formal staff augmentations, such as when teams with critical care physicians, CCRNs, and RTs augmented various maritime platforms for support during the coronavirus disease 2019 (COVID-19) pandemic. Further informal staff augmentation may also be necessary, utilizing capable but nonmedical assets to accomplish tasks with specific just-in-time training that does not require prior medical knowledge (i.e., vital signs, patient positioning). These type of healthcare extenders can increase the capability of the medical team and potentially reserve higher-trained personnel for more advanced medical tasks. A current example is the use of Culinary Specialists on submarines as medical augmentees to the submarine IDC.

Staff should be expected to practice to the limit of their credentials. Predeployment training to targeted personnel is essential to ensure capable staff and available staff are identified. Finally, staffing needs and demands should be continually assessed to ensure proper allocation of skills and appropriate work-rest cycles.

Training

All United States (US) Navy medical personnel need to be trained on medical skills appropriate for their training and mission. In addition to these basic skills, other skills critical for PCC are outlined below.

The critical care team should have procedural competencies in all TCCC skill sets. Hemodynamic monitoring devices (if available) should be functional with accompanied knowledge of setup, troubleshooting, and interpretation. In addition, competency in intravenous (IV) access, resuscitation, and advanced airway management and other procedures is ideal. Ventilator management skills must include setup and technical troubleshooting in addition to clinical management of patients with respiratory failure. Point-of-care ultrasonography (POCUS) should be considered a required imaging modality that offers significant clinical insight as well as procedural augmentation; therefore, this skill set should be taught and competency ensured to all levels of providers caring for critically ill patients.

Peacetime maritime operations usually do not have a significant medical care delivery focus. Critical care cases occurring aboard most vessels represent low frequency but high acuity scenarios usually associated with workplace accidents, which can lead to skill set degradation. Continued real-world clinical experiences in expeditionary relevant care coupled with training and education sessions that represent an opportunity to train with members of the healthcare team on critical skills and scenarios are crucial. Sustainment of critical skills will improve readiness for operations in kinetic environments. Ideally, this training should encompass the continuity of care from point of injury (POI) and initial resuscitative care to patient sustainment and preparation for MEDEVAC. While expeditionary relevant clinical skills performed on real patients can occur at military medical treatment facilities (MTFs) or through partnerships, training should ideally be in the environment where care is expected to be delivered. Scenarios involving PCC should be undertaken to highlight issues of required ongoing training, staff fatigue, and evolving complications.

Equipment

Deployment of medical supplies should be tailored to the skills of the medical team and the expected casualty injury patterns. In the maritime environment, available space, time to replenishment, and shelf life must additionally be considered. Medical teams joining organic shipboard assets must have knowledge of the ship's deployed supply assets to plan for what supply augmentation is necessary to allow for maximal utilization of augmentation skill sets. Supplies and devices which are capable of being prepared and deployed in situations with intermittent environmental controls should be prioritized. Devices and supplies with multiple uses and the ability to be used by multiple levels of staff should be prioritized. Supplies necessary to sustain care with the best evidence are preferred to therapies with narrow indications, even if they are potentially lifesaving in those indications (e.g., biologic therapies and advanced ventilators).

Equipment is only as good as the staff's ability to utilize it. It cannot be emphasized enough: training is perishable and should be an ongoing process. Platform- and scenario-specific training in addition to hands-on experience caring for appropriate patients is essential.

Core Skill Sets

Minimum/Better/Best

The concept of minimum/better/best can be applied to all aspects of critical care planning and delivery in the austere or delayed evacuation environment. Presenting options for decisions regarding personnel and supplies in this manner allows for members of the care team and operational leadership to understand capabilities, limitations, and options for medical operations. This assessment tool is dynamic and changes with resource utilization, duration of casualty event, fatigue of staff, etc. See Table 30.1 for examples of the minimum/better/best model for several aspects of PCC.

Diagnostics/Monitoring

Hemodynamic stabilization can be complex and requires a targeted approach to treatment of the underlying disease state while allowing for restoration of adequate perfusion. Fortunately, basic assessments of perfusion are often easily accomplished by all levels of providers. These include mental status assessment, blood pressure measurement, capillary refill timing, and assessment of peripheral pulses. Peripheral capillary refill assessed at the nailbed is equivalent to serum lactate when used to target fluid resuscitation in septic patients. Central capillary refill is also a measure of hypoperfusion; to assess, put finger pressure on the sternum for 5 s, remove, and time capillary refill. Basic laboratory testing and X-ray capabilities are available on most larger maritime platforms and can be helpful adjunct during initial assessment and resuscitation if available. Invasive measures such as urinary catheter placement should be required skills of all operational medical providers. Advanced or continuous diagnostics and monitoring are not always available but can be of great utility.

Table 30.1 Example of minimum/better/best model for ten aspects of critical care

	Minimum	Better	Best
Monitoring	Obtain, document, and trend vital signs	Pulse oximeter Foley catheter	Portable capnography Portable vital signs monitor with automated features
Diagnostics	Physical examination to identify shock	Noninvasive measures of perfusion such as peripheral or central capillary refill Simple laboratory testing	POCUS to diagnose and manage shock
Fluid resuscitation	Oral intake of water (or via nasogastric tube) Rectal infusion of up to 500 mL/h	Oral intake of electrolyte solution (or via nasogastric tube)	IV or IO fluid resuscitation Isotonic crystalloids (i.e., lactated ringers) Sufficient crystalloid for resuscitation of multiple patients
Blood resuscitation	Plasma and RBCs in a 1:1 ratio Plasma or RBCs alone	Pre-screened type-specific FWB from a WBB Plasma, RBCs, and platelets in a 1:1:1	Cold stored low titer O FWB Pre-screened low titer O FWB from a WBB Sufficient blood supply for resuscitation of multiple patients
Airway	TCCC airway measures Chin lift or jaw thrust Nasopharyngeal airway	LMA Surgical cricothyroidotomy	Endotracheal intubation and trained management of airway complications
Ventilation	BVM ventilation with PEEP valve	BVM with oxygen NIPPV	Mechanical ventilation and trained staff
Sedation and analgesia	TCCC skills, to include use of ketamine	Intermittent narcotics and anxiolytics RSI	IV anesthesia Sedation for ventilated patient
Nursing	Patient warm and dry Basic wound management	Passive ROM Advanced wound management	Preparation for MEDEVAC ERC skills
Procedures	TCCC procedures	Debridement Escharotomy Amputation	Neurosurgical procedures Trauma procedures (e.g., thoracotomy, laparotomy)
Virtual medicine	Asynchronous cellular, satellite, or email	Synchronous cellular or satellite	Real-time mentorship

POCUS point-of-care ultrasound, *IV* intravenous, *IO* intraosseous, *RBC* red blood cells, *WBB* walking blood Bank, *FWB* fresh whole blood, *TCCC* tactical combat casualty care, *LMA* laryngeal mask airway, *BVM* bag-valve-mask, *PEEP* positive end expiratory pressure, *NIPPV* noninvasive positive pressure ventilation, *RSI* rapid sequence intubation, *ROM* range of motion, *MEDEVAC* medical evacuation, *ERC* en route care

Resuscitation

Blood pressure goals should include keeping blood pressures less than the threshold to cause intrinsic vascular injury and high enough to maintain perfusion. Hypotension and shock can be seen with both traumatic and medical illness and can result in multi-organ failure in a short period of time if not managed aggressively. General principles include replacing the thing that is missing, whether that is fluid or blood. Administration of IV fluids is one of the first and most common interventions utilized in the management of hypovolemia. Conditions which may cause ongoing non-hemorrhagic shock in a PCC scenario include severe dehydration from any cause, sepsis, or neurologic injury. Administration of blood products is common in the initial DCR phase of casualty care (see Chap. 23); however, it can also be a part of PCC depending on the patient scenario.

Fluid balance in the ICU can be challenging even in the best-resourced environment. Initial resuscitation often requires some degree of IV fluid or blood product administration, followed by maintenance IV medications with carrier fluids. The risk for hypervolemia is high. The avoidance of excess IV fluid administration greatly benefits patient care and should be reviewed daily. Conversely, intraoperative incessant losses are often under-appreciated by the surgical team after prolonged open thoracic or abdominal operations and may require continued resuscitation with crystalloid or blood products in the postoperative period. **While attempting judicious fluid use in critically ill patients, take care not to under-resuscitate perioperative patients.**

In the absence of more advanced diagnostic and monitoring capabilities, one can perform a passive leg raise (PLR) test to assess the need for fluid resuscitation during ongoing resuscitation as the maneuver provides a temporary natural fluid bolus by returning venous blood to the central circulation. It is ideally assessed with advanced hemodynamic monitoring beyond a blood pressure cuff but may be a valuable physical exam tool in PCC.

1. Avoid inducing pain or sympathetic stimulation that will increase the heart rate.
2. Use the bed to place the patient's head up at 45°. Measure and record blood pressure after approximately 90 s.
3. Use the bed to place the patient supine at 0° in the recumbent position and then raise both legs 45°, and hold for 90 s. Measure and record blood pressure. (If possible, it is ideal to use the bed to elevate the legs. If that is not possible, manually elevate the patient's legs.)
4. Put the legs back down and raise the head of the bed to 45° again. Measure and record blood pressure after approximately 90 s (should return to baseline).

During resuscitation with crystalloid or blood products in the MTF or during PCC, multiple endpoints of resuscitation should be followed in the critically ill or postoperative patient. Postoperative patients, particularly those with prolonged operative courses or large abdominal surgeries, may require extensive fluid resuscitation due to fluid losses and shifts. Attention to resuscitation and endpoints such as urine output (UOP) is critical in this population. In situations where one cannot follow serial lactate values or the patient's acid-base status, common endpoints of resuscitation that can be utilized during PCC include:

- Improved mental status.
- Normalization of blood pressure and heart rate.
- Adequate UOP after appropriate resuscitation (Goal UOP, 0.3–0.5 mL/kg/h).
- Peripheral capillary refill assessed at the nailbed is equivalent to serum lactate when used to target fluid resuscitation in septic patients.
- Negative PLR.
- POCUS respiratory variation of inferior vena cava (IVC) diameter (see Chap. 9): An IVC <1 cm in diameter at its largest during the respiratory cycle and collapsing more than 50% with inspiration suggests hypovolemia. An IVC >2.5 cm in diameter with no respiratory variation suggests hypervolemia. Measurements between those two values are less useful for predicting volume status.

Airway

Airway management strategies will be largely driven by available skill sets. However, there remains an essential inventory of equipment, consumables, and medications to support airway emergencies and maintenance. Bag-valve-mask (BVM) ventilation, supraglottic/laryngeal mask airways (LMAs), direct laryngoscopy, video laryngoscopy, and emergency surgical trans-tracheal approaches to airway management should be represented and trained to (see Chap. 13).

Ventilator

Ventilator management in the PCC environment should be geared toward the type of respiratory failure present, classically broken down into hypoxemic, hypercapnic, or mixed respiratory failure (see Chap. 21). The safest mechanical ventilation strategy is using the mode of ventilation that the healthcare team is most comfortable with and modifying based on expert consultation if available. Ventilators come with various capabilities, with some capable of providing both noninvasive and invasive support. In addition to having knowledge regarding clinical use of the ventilator, knowledge of setup, troubleshooting, and maintenance is critical (see Chap. 21). A variety of airway management and respiratory support techniques within the minimum/better/best construct will likely be required during PCC. Additionally, patients should be triaged on a regular basis to ensure resource allocation, to include personnel, is being optimized for this staff- and resource-intensive skill set.

There are some general principles that will guide the healthcare team toward meeting the goals of mechanical ventilation while maintaining an adequate safety profile. The following lung-protective strategies should be adhered including low tidal volume ventilation (6–8 mL/kg ideal body weight, lower in acute respiratory distress syndrome (ARDS)), avoidance of high plateau pressures (inspiratory pause maneuver less than 30 mmHg), and avoidance of patient-ventilator dyssynchrony. These practice patterns that can be applied to most ventilated patients with slight modifications based on disease process. Hypercapnic respiratory failure can be managed by increasing minute ventilation (Minute ventilation = Tidal Volume × Respiratory Rate) or increasing the difference between the inspiratory pressure (PIP) and the positive end-expiratory pressure (PEEP). In resource-constrained environments, noninvasive ventilation may be a useful adjunct. Patients who traditionally are not thought to be candidates for noninvasive ventilation such as those with altered levels of consciousness may in fact be supported with noninvasive ventilation.

Sedation/Analgesia

Sedation strategies are dependent on both the characteristics of the airway and patient. Endotracheal intubation and airway management require the most extensive sedation skills and equipment. Neuromuscular blockade is helpful at facilitating endotracheal intubation and in some cases facilitating patient-ventilator synchrony. However, it should be used with caution in the operational environment if trained staff and mechanical ventilators are limited as patients are completely dependent upon external support while under the effects of these medications. Patients should be provided analgesia in addition to sedation. Agents such as ketamine and narcotics are readily available and can be provided by non-expert providers with appropriate algorithms.

Common Situations

Infections/Sepsis

Infections represent a significant proportion of admissions in most healthcare settings. Source control and targeted antimicrobial therapy are the standard of care. However, in times of uncertainty, erring on the side of broad-spectrum antibiotics is preferred to delay in care. Prior to underway periods, antimicrobial medications should be reviewed to ensure coverage for a wide variety of organ systems. Antimicrobials for endemic infections such as malaria should also be stocked and staff provided training on their use. Sepsis can result from several highly communicable pathogens such as meningococcus or from bio-terrorism agents like anthrax. Similar patterns of illness in multiple casualties should result in investigation looking for an infectious reservoir or transmissible pathogen, and expert consultation via

Table 30.2 Common sepsis-related organ system complications

System	Complications
Neurologic	Delirium (hyperactive, hypoactive, or mixed)
Cardiovascular	Shock, acute decompensated heart failure, acute coronary syndrome, arrhythmias
Respiratory	Pulmonary edema, acute respiratory distress syndrome, secondary pulmonary infections
Renal	Acute kidney injury, acute tubular necrosis, acute interstitial nephritis

phone, email, or video tele-conferencing should occur if available. Additionally, see Chap. 16 for a discussion of infectious disease at sea.

Sepsis represents a dysregulation of the host immune response to infections. This dysregulation results in a profound inflammatory response manifesting in multiple organ system failure that is the driving factor in mortality associated with sepsis. Table 30.2 lists typical organ system complications associated with the progression of sepsis. Early recognition and initiation of source-specific antibiotics may be challenging but is crucial and lifesaving. In particular, changes in a patient's vital signs from their baseline in the context of an infection should be aggressively evaluated. The general population on a deployed maritime vessel typically has a low resting heart rate so relative tachycardia can be an early sign of concern. Hypotension and shock will require IV fluid resuscitation; however, overuse will further complicate the clinical picture. Targeting endpoints of resuscitation like UOP or capillary refill is critical to avoid over-resuscitation (see Chap. 20). It is often helpful to monitor multiple endpoints of resuscitation (see above) in septic patients.

Fluid resuscitation for non-hemorrhagic shock will frequently be encountered in sepsis, burns, and diarrheal illness. Resuscitation can be accomplished through a variety of methods to include oral, IV, and potentially rectal. Each situation should be evaluated in the minimum/better/best framework. Triaging patients in regard to the need of IV fluids may be necessary. Oral resuscitation is the preferred method in diarrheal illness but is less effective in patients with shock due to reduced perfusion of the gut. Rectal fluid administration is effective, but volume and rapidity of fluid administration are somewhat limited. Solutions for both oral and rectal rehydration can be easily mixed from a variety of readily available supplies such as table salt and baking soda (see Chap. 26 for examples for adult patients and Chap. 34 for examples for pediatric patients). IV fluids should not be mixed or compounded unless personnel are experienced in this and sterility can be assured.

Consideration of early use of vasoactive medications should be considered as part of a measured response to shock and sepsis. Additionally, use of vasoactive medications should be based on experience and understanding of side effect profiles coupled with a targeted treatment of hypoperfusion. Norepinephrine represents the most-used first-line vasopressor in an ICU setting with second-line agents varying depending on the disease process and availability. At a minimum all advanced providers who are deployed on shipboard platforms should be familiar with the vasoactive medicines available to them and their uses.

In settings of fluid- and vasopressor-resistant shock, use of steroids should be considered. However, there should be an attempt to reduce both antibiotics and steroids when possible, as unnecessary use can lead to further complications of the clinical course. An assessment of efficacy should be made no later than the third day of treatment with consideration for cessation, continuation, or modification of therapy.

Cardiovascular/Thromboembolic Disease

Thrombus formation in situ and thromboembolic disease encompass a wide array of disease processes, including ischemic stroke, acute myocardial infarction, and pulmonary embolism (PE). These diseases may be de novo or complications of other injuries. In an austere PCC scenario like the clinical vignette, prompt recognition and initiation of treatment are necessary and often without the full spectrum of diagnostic modalities available. Resources should be available to reference current guidelines and treatment strategies of common cardiovascular conditions, augmenting cardiovascular resuscitation courses and tailored to the medical team's expertise. PE causing hemodynamic collapse as seen in Clinical Vignette 30.1 can also be a catastrophic complication of trauma. Treatment modalities including anticoagulation and potentially thrombolytics should be available. Monitoring for and preventing these complications can be difficult. Simple measures like patient mobilization post-injury may reduce the incidence of this complication.

Burn/Trauma

Trauma and burn injuries are expected during both maritime peacetime and combat operations. The surgical team should be prepared to manage these conditions until stabilized and/or transported to higher echelon of care. Burns and their management are discussed in detail in the JTS CPG and Chap. 26 of this book, to include PCC considerations.

The pathophysiology of burn injuries is complex and represents both an extreme acute inflammatory state with secondary messenger pathways initiating vasodilatory effects, loss of dermal layers resulting in profound desiccation/hypovolemic shock, and hypothermia via insensible losses. Utilization of protocols will reduce the variability of patient care and, in disease states such as burns, should be used unless there exists a specific expertise in managing these patients. In settings of reduced experience with burn management, utilization of approved burn care CPGs and early consultation with recognized Burn Centers should be obtained and are proven to improve outcomes.

Brilliance in the Basics

Long-term management for all critically ill patients is a balance between reversal of adverse pathophysiology, allowance for return to physiologic homeostasis, and avoidance of preventable complications. Much of the management that prevents harm is standard for most critically ill patients and often represented as a daily ICU rounds checklist (see Table 30.3). All of these actions should be performed in the PCC environment.

- Assessment of patient analgesia, typically using nursing-driven standardized tools for the sedated patient, is standard of care for the ICU.
- Daily sedation holidays with coupled ventilator liberation attempts allow for daily neurologic assessment, increase in ventilator-free days, and reduction of the delirium associated with being in an ICU for prolonged periods of time.
- During periods of mechanical ventilation, a ventilator-associated pneumonia (VAP) bundle should be implemented to reduce incidence of VAP. In a PCC environment, this may be as simple as head of bed (HOB) elevation and daily toothbrushing.
- Early mobilization is includes passive range of motion at a minimum or, in very select cases, ambulation while intubated, the latter case only in extremely select cases with a healthcare team with significant experience.
- Nutritional support should be considered early with all patients unless there exists a contraindication. Resource limitations may force creative solutions to nutritional supplementation, and virtual consultation with pharmacists is encouraged.
- Pharmacologic glucose control should be considered with any patient with persistent blood glucose levels persistently above 180 mg/dL.
- Stress ulcer prophylaxis may be indicated for intubated patients in shock, patients with significant burn injuries, and patients with neurologic trauma.

Table 30.3 Example of daily intensive care unit (ICU) rounds checklist

Item	Addressed			Comments
Analgesia optimized	Yes	No	N/A	
Sedation optimized/sedation holiday with neurological assessment	Yes	No	N/A	
Spontaneous breathing trial (SBT)/ventilator-associated pneumonia (VAP) bundle	Yes	No	N/A	
Early mobilization	Yes	No	N/A	
Nutrition	Yes	No	N/A	
Blood glucose control (<180 mg/dL)	Yes	No	N/A	
Stress ulcer prophylaxis	Yes	No	N/A	
Venous thromboembolic (VTE) chemoprophylaxis	Yes	No	N/A	
Invasive tubes/lines/drains (indication)	Yes	No	N/A	
Renal/hepatic function (preserved)	Yes	No	N/A	

- All patients in an ICU setting are considered high risk for VTE and should be started on chemoprophylaxis unless there is a contraindication. In addition, passive mobilization can also help prevent this complication.
- All invasive tubes, lines, and drains should be discussed daily for potential discontinuation as a mechanism of reducing infection rates as well as discomfort to patients. A risk-benefit analysis should be conducted daily for both initiation and discontinuation of all interventions.
- In addition, end-organ damage including kidney and liver injury should be considered daily with discussion of goals of care and need for re-triage. Common disease patterns exist including development of acute kidney and liver injury, either because of underlying disease processes or iatrogenic injury. With identification of end-organ damage, there are often modifications from a medical management perspective that can reduce harm. In addition, discussions regarding resource allocation, triage, and expected patient outcomes must be had.

Preparation for Medical Evacuation (MEDEVAC)

Critically ill patients on platforms with limited resources quickly deplete supplies, making continued medical operations challenging and impacting the ability to care for both current and future casualties. This reality often prompts a request to move toward MEDEVAC as soon as possible. Decisions regarding MEDEVAC are complex to involve both patient and platform considerations. Ultimately, determining where a patient can receive the best care and how they get there will be a shared decision between medical and operational leaders (see Chaps. 1, 6, 14, and 31 for more discussion on this shared decision-making). The maritime surgical team is responsible for the formal assessment of the stability of the patient and their tolerance of transfer. In some situations, patients may be better served by a longer period on a resource-constrained platform than transport to a potentially less secure platform. MEDEVAC is best done by dedicated teams following specific algorithms based on acuity of the patient and capabilities of the en route care (ERC) team (see Chap. 31).

Clinical considerations prior to MEDEVAC include preparation for changes in altitude/oxygen, temperature, and movement. Ideally redundancy of medications and supplies is built into MEDEVAC plans (see Chap. 31). In the event that the transport team is delayed, the physiological impacts on the patient must be considered and planned for. Impacts of loss of supplies and equipment to the evacuating platform will need to be considered and addressed prior to completion of any MEDEVAC operation as MEDEVAC often provides an avenue for resupply if previously arranged.

MEDEVAC should be considered a continuation of PCC rendered while underway. Knowledge of patient transport is a crucial part of PCC preparedness.

Conclusion

Clinical Vignette 30.1 Conclusion

The patient's respiratory failure progressed. His airway was managed with an LMA and oxygen therapy via *a BVM while sedated with ketamine. His shock was treated with IV fluids, and he was treated with systemic anticoagulation for presumed VTE. MEDEVAC was available in 24 h, and the ship's medical staff took shifts with his care assisted by members of the crew.*

PCC scenarios should be expected in the maritime environment due to the large distances and potential for near peer conflict. PCC is one part of the continuum of care in the maritime environment involving POI care, ERC, and definitive care. The concept of DMO demands that medical providers can provide adaptable and scalable patient care models to ensure that combat operations can always continue. By utilizing organic staffing with mission-specific augmentation, the ICU can truly be anywhere. Training personnel to the maximal extent of their credentials and utilizing appropriate virtual mentorship can bridge gaps. PCC is a mindset that should be adopted by all expeditionary medical providers to allow for the best patient outcomes no matter the situation.

Declaration of Interest The views expressed in this chapter are those of the authors and do not necessarily reflect the official policy or position of the Department of the Navy, Department of Defense, nor the US Government.

Funding This research did not receive any specific grant from funding agencies in the public, commercial, or not-for-profit sectors.

Conflict of Interest Statement The authors declare no conflict of interest.

Chapter 31
En Route Care: Shore to Ship, Ship to Ship, and Ship to Shore

Wayne Papalski, Dana Flieger, Ryan Honnoll, and Elliot M. Ross

We can teach anyone in two weeks how to take a kidney out but it takes years to understand why you need to take the kidney. Never sacrifice knowledge of why we do the skill to just focus on doing skills.

Major General Payne

Author deployment experience	
Wayne Papalski	Search and Rescue Medical Technician, Helicopter Anti-Submarine Squadron Five embarked on the USS Dwight D. Eisenhower (CVN-69), Operation Iraqi Freedom, Balad, Iraq, and CENTCOM Area of Responsibility, 2009–2010
	Search and Rescue Medical Technician, Helicopter Sea Combat Squadron Eight Four, Crisis Response Element SOCCENT, Operation Iraqi Freedom, CENTCOM Area of Responsibility, 2010–2011
	Search and Rescue Medical Technician, Helicopter Sea Combat Squadron Eight Four, Operation Iraqi Freedom, CENTCOM Area of Responsibility, 2012–2013
	Search and Rescue Medical Technician, Helicopter Sea Combat Squadron Eight Four, Crisis Response Element SOCCENT, CENTCOM Area of Responsibility, 2012–2013
	Search and Rescue Medical Technician, Helicopter Sea Combat Squadron Eight Four, supporting Humanitarian Aid Disaster Relief (HADR) operations following Hurricane Harvey, College Station, TX, USA, 2017

W. Papalski
Helicopter Sea Combat Squadron-2, Norfolk, VA, USA
e-mail: wayne.n.papalski@navy.mil

D. Flieger
USS Abraham Lincoln (CVN-72), San Diego, CA, USA

R. Honnoll
Helicopter Sea Combat Squadron-22, Norfolk, VA, USA
e-mail: ryan.e.honnoll.mil@us.navy.mil

E. M. Ross (✉)
Expeditionary Medical Facility Jacksonville, Fort Worth, TX, USA
e-mail: elliot.m.ross.mil@us.navy.mil

M. D. Tadlock, A. A. Hernandez (eds.), *Expeditionary Surgery at Sea*,
https://doi.org/10.1007/978-3-031-21893-4_31

Author deployment experience	
	Search and Rescue Medical Technician, Helicopter Sea Combat Squadron Eight Four, supporting Humanitarian Aid Disaster Relief (HADR) operations following Hurricane Dorian, Homestead Air Force Base, FL, USA, 2018
Dana Flieger	Lead En Route Care Critical Care Registered Nurse, Special Marine Air Ground Task Force Crisis Response–Central Command 17.1, Critical Care Nurse augment – 1980th Forward Surgical Team, Operation Inherent Resolve, CENTCOM Area of Responsibility, 2016–2017
	Medical Operations Officer, Special Marine Air Ground Task Force Crisis Response–Central Command 19.1, Operation Inherent Resolve, CENTCOM Area of Responsibility, 2018–2019
	Ship's Nurse, USS Abraham Lincoln (CVN-72), contingency operations, INDOPACOM Area of Responsibility, 2022
Ryan Honnoll	Search and Rescue Medical Technician, 2515th Naval Air Ambulance Detachment, Operation Iraqi Freedom, COB Basra, Iraq, 2009
	Search and Rescue Medical Technician, second Force Reconnaissance 24th Marine Expeditionary Unit (SOC) embarked on the USS Iwo Jima (LHD-7), Operation Iraqi Freedom and Operation Enduring Freedom, fifth Fleet and CENTCOM Area of Responsibility, 2012
	Search and Rescue Medical Technician, Helicopter Sea Combat Squadron-22 DET 3 SAR Detachment embarked on the USS Iwo Jima (LHD-7), Operation Iraqi Freedom and Operation Enduring Freedom, fifth Fleet and CENTCOM Area of Responsibility, 2012
	Search and Rescue Medical Technician, USNS Comfort (T-AH-20), Operation Continuing Promise, fourth Fleet and SOUTHCOM Area of Responsibility, 2015
	Search and Rescue Medical Technician, USNS Comfort (T-AH-20), supporting Humanitarian Aid Disaster Relief (HADR) operations following Hurricane Dorian, Bahamas, 2019
	Search and Rescue Medical Technician, USS Little Rock (LCS-9), JIATF south drug interdiction, SOUTHCOM Area of Responsibility, 2020
	Search and Rescue Medical Technician, USS Detroit (LCS-7), JIATF south drug interdiction, SOUTHCOM Area of Responsibility, 2020
	Search and Rescue Medical Technician, USNS Robert E. Peary (T-AKE-5), Combat Logistics Force, sixth Fleet and EUCOM Area of Responsibility, 2022
Elliot M. Ross	Battalion Surgeon, second Marine Special Operations Battalion, Marine Corps Forces Special Operations Command, Operation Enduring Freedom, Afghanistan and CENTCOM Area of Responsibility, 2010
	Officer in Charge, Expeditionary Resuscitative Surgical System Team 12, 2014; Provided embarked Role 2 Surgical Support, Operation Enduring Freedom, CENTCOM Area of Responsibility, 2014

BLUF (Bottom Line Up Front)

1. Considerations for planning during transport are categorized into groups of concerns: patient access and packaging, equipment organization, and transportation safety.
2. In an effort to optimize transport requirements, the ground/sending team should complete any time- or resource-intensive interventions prior to en route care (ERC) team arrival, including definitive airway management and placement of any appropriate tubes, lines, or drains.

3. The ground/sending team should include any advanced monitoring equipment needed for the transport in the medical evacuation (MEDEVAC) request. Delineation of who is providing blood products should also be determined early.
4. Tasks that must be completed by the ERC team include receiving the patient report from a member of the ground/sending team, performing an assessment of the patient, revalidating the movement of the patient, and verifying correct packaging in preparation for departure.
5. Having a standardized handoff format will benefit both teams and improve the transition of care.
6. Keep it simple! Use practical and manageable interventions to optimize ERC.
7. Package the patient for transport to ensure access to all relevant interventions, organization of resources, and the safety of both the patient and ERC team.
8. Equipment should be fully secured but not resting on the patient. Both patient and equipment need to be secured but also with access for the ERC team members.
9. When planning for any patient transfer, the ERC team should plan for two- to threefold the time that the transport is expected to take when assembling supplies.
10. Transportation safety includes the safety of both the patient and the ERC team's interaction with the patient.
11. All patients shall be provided thermal regulation, as well as visual and auditory protection from the transport environment.

Introduction

En route care (ERC) is the process that provides a continuum of care and coordinates the movement of patients from the point of need to definitive care [1]. Patients are moved only as far rearward as the tactical situation dictates and as clinical needs warrant. Prompt movement of patients to the required level of clinical care is essential to prevent morbidity and mortality, and each service component has aeromedical evacuation (AE), medical evacuation (MEDEVAC), or casualty evacuation (CASEVAC) capability to do so [1, 2]. AE and MEDEVAC both have designated ERC/medical capabilities. CASEVAC is an unregulated movement of casualties without designated ERC/medical capabilities. See Chaps. 1 and 2 for further discussion of transfer between levels of care.

Patient movement consists of three components: medical regulation/mission planning, patient evacuation/mission execution, and ERC. ERC is currently defined in the Department of Defense Dictionary of Military and Associated Terms and JP 4-02 as the continuation of the provision of care during movement (evacuation) between the health service support capabilities in the roles of care, without clinically compromising the patient's condition [1]. ERC involves the provision of transitory medical care, patient holding, and staging capabilities during transport from the point of injury (POI) or onset of disease throughout the continuum of care.

Equally important to the care provided during ERC is the intense preparation required leading up to it. While the complete scope of ERC is far too broad for this book, the purpose of this chapter is to provide a ready resource for the providers who are on the maritime surgical ground/sending team responsible for preparing a patient for ERC and the providers on the maritime surgical team who also may be potentially responsible for caring for a patient through the continuum of care.

En Route Care (ERC) Patient Preparation

Patient preparation for transport is divided into two teams, who are many times different teams communicating with each other but sometimes are the same team with certain members accompanying patients to the next level of care:

- Ground/sending team
- ERC team

Team preparation for patient transport consists of two phases:

- Mission planning phase
- Mission execution phase

The considerations for planning during transport are categorized into groups of concerns:

- Patient access and packaging
- Equipment organization
- Transportation safety, both of the patient and the ERC team

The goal of ERC is to provide the continued level of medical support as the patient is transported throughout the continuum of care. **When planning for any patient transfer, the ERC team should plan for two- to threefold the time that the transport is expected to take.**

En Route Care (ERC) Mission Planning

The mission planning phase begins upon receipt of the 9-Line MEDEVAC request by the ERC team from the ground/sending team. Each aspect of the 9-Line request is important for the transport team. However, particular emphasis is placed on the number of patients, patient precedence, special equipment, and the tactical situation. Accuracy is key as the incoming ERC team must ensure that the patient load will not overwhelm the resources or capability of their team. The ERC team's clear understanding of the situation will lead to their arrival with the correct resources (including medical direction or other specialists, if needed) and ensure the patients are transported to a medical facility with the appropriate capabilities and resources [3, 4]. In the mission planning phase, it is vital for the members of the maritime surgical team, the medical leadership (Senior Medical Officer (SMO) or Officer in Charge (OIC)), and the medical planners (Medical Administrative Officer (MAO) or Medical Regulating Control Officer (MRCO) to work together to communicate with the next facility and/or ERC team. See Chaps. 1 and 6 discussing more about these teams, roles, and discussions.

In an effort to optimize transport requirements, the ground/sending team should also complete any time- or resource-intensive interventions prior to the ERC team's arrival if feasible. This includes definitive airway management, as a difficult airway or ventilator status on the ground will *not* be easier to maintain en route. When tactically possible, optimize patients with secure airway interventions and ventilator support prior to transport. Depending on the length of flight, altitude, and patient condition, consider placing a chest tube prior to transport for a simple pneumothorax, as it may become hemodynamically significant when flying in an unpressurized aircraft. See Chaps. 13, 20, and 21 discussing anesthesia care and airway management, intensive care unit (ICU), and ventilator management at sea, respectively. When available, appropriate, and feasible, the ground/sending team should prepare critically ill patients by inserting Foley catheters, nasogastric/orogastric tubes, and/or advanced vascular access.

The ground/sending team should also include any advanced monitoring equipment needed for the transport in the MEDEVAC request so that no transfer of equipment is needed. If it is not requested, it will not arrive. For trauma and postoperative patients, consider the need for blood products. Optimally, the ground/sending team can provide them, but if they are not available, then the ERC team should request them from their resources as soon as possible as shipboard blood products often require >60 min to prepare [2, 5, 6].

The ERC team should identify the appropriate provider team members based on the 9-line MEDEVAC request, anticipated needs of the patient(s), resources available, and input from the ERC Medical Director (typically an Emergency Medicine Physician). Evidence has shown advanced practice ERC providers can directly impact the outcomes of transported patients, but the United States (U.S.) Navy has identified that there can be gaps in some of the ERC providers' training and competence [2–5, 7, 8]. Use clinical judgment when forming the ERC team as the most experienced providers may perform better than the most trained/educated providers [2, 3].

ERC Mission Execution

During the mission execution phase, time is of the essence. This phase aims to decrease the amount of time spent preparing the patient for movement and rapidly move to the transport phase. Upon the ERC team's arrival to the ground/sending ship, a representative from the ground/sending team should interface with the ERC team to verbally give the pertinent details of the patient and ensure an appropriate patient handoff. Having a standardized handoff format will benefit the teams and improve the transition of care [6]. The ERC team will delineate tasks to ensure an engaged, rapid, thorough handoff is achieved. The ERC team may include the

Table 31.1 En route care (ERC) report tool: MARCHPAWS acronym [9]

	Assessment	Possible interventions to prepare for transport
M	Massive hemorrhage	Elevate, direct pressure, wound packing, hemostatic gauze, pressure dressing, clamp, TXA, tourniquet(s), pelvic sling/junctional tourniquet(s)
A	Airway	Recovery position, sit up and lean forward position, chin lift/jaw thrust, oral/nasal pharyngeal airway, supraglottic airway, endotracheal tube (ETT), cricothyrotomy
R	Respirations	BVM, oxygen, needle decompression, chest seal, finger thoracostomy, tube thoracostomy
C	Circulation	Diagnose and treat shock, IV/IO placement, blood products, calcium
H	Head and hypothermia	Head: Treat increased ICP by securing the airway and keeping SBP >100 mm Hg, $SpO_2 > 93\%$, $ETCO_2$ 30–35 mm Hg Hypothermia: dry patient, insulate, hat, casualty blanket, active warming measures: "Ready Heat" devices, hypothermia prevention management kit (HPMK), advanced patient litter system (APLS)
P	Pain medication	As applicable per protocol
A	Antibiotics	IV/IO/oral for all open combat wounds
W	Wounds	Clean, remove debris, irrigate, dress
S	Splinting	Spinal immobilization per protocol, splints/casts, rigid eye shields

TXA tranexamic acid, *BVM* bag-valve-mask, *IV* intravenous, *IO* intraosseous, *ICP* intracranial pressure, *SBP* systolic blood pressure, SpO_2 pulse oximetry measuring of peripheral saturation of hemoglobin, $ETCO_2$ end-tidal carbon dioxide

tasking of a requesting facility in some aspect of the preparation of the transport patient to expedite movement. Tasks that must be completed by the ERC team include receiving the patient report from a member of the ground/sending team, performing an assessment of the patient, revalidating the movement of the patient, and verifying correct packaging in preparation for departure.

The ERC team guides the report and assessment process. The use of the MARCHPAWS acronym can assist both the ground/sending and the ERC teams in communicating appropriate information in the least amount of time (Table 31.1). At a minimum, for primary survey the ERC team should obtain a full set of vital signs (to include heart rate (HR), systolic blood pressure (SBP), respiratory rate (RR), pulse oximetry measuring of peripheral saturation of hemoglobin (SpO_2), and temperature). Neurologic status can be rapidly assessed using the AVPU mnemonic (alert, voice, pain, unresponsive) and examining the patient's pupils while looking for posturing. Blood glucose testing and electrocardiogram (ECG) should be performed as applicable. For secondary assessment, a head-to-toe exam should be performed. Use of mnemonics like DCAP-BTLS (deformity, contusions, abrasions, punctures/penetrations, burns, tenderness, lacerations, swelling) can focus this exam. Particular attention should be paid to the neurovascular exam of affected extremities.

Often, the priorities of the ground/sending team differ from those of the ERC team. The ERC team should receive the report, ask questions pertinent to the status and transfer of the patient, and then provide an opportunity for the ground/sending team to provide additional information.

Once the report has been completed, the ERC team performs an assessment to confirm findings and assess any interventions. This assessment will develop the "Do

Table 31.2 En route care (ERC) planning tool: patient packaging checklist

Enroute Care Planning Tool Version 2.0 Sep 2018

DO NOW (upon arrival)	**TAKE WITH** (for use in transport)	**Enroute** (during transport and prior to arrival)
M: MASSIVE HEMORRAHGE ☐ Check all bandages, splints, dressings and tourniquets for placement / evidence of ongoing he morrhage. ☐ Assess and mark trauma injuries ☐ Measurement of abd. Girth/distention ☐ Request orders for type and cross-matched blood or O-negative blood fromt the transferring physician. ☐ Request TXA	**M:** ☐ Additional Blood products (Whole blood or 1:1:1) ☐ Tubing ☐ Warmer ☐ Fluid warmer with Battery x 2 ☐ Golden Hour Container	**M:** ☐ Blood products administration ☐ Check all bandages, splints, dressings and tourniquets for placement / evidence of ongoing hemorrhage ☐ Measurement of abd.
A: AIRWAY ☐ Ensure endotracheal tube is secure ☐ Cuff up ☐ Bite block ☐ Document position ☐ Attach ETCO2 monitor ☐ Review chest radiograph, check plaement and function of chest tube/drainage system/ Heimlich valve. ☐ Insert or check NG/OG tube for gastric decompression (unless contraindicatied; cap or place to suction.	**A:** ☐ Extra ETT ☐ Suction soft-tip ☐ 10ml syringe ☐ Bite block ☐ Tape ☐ I-Gel/king LT ☐ BVM	**A:** ☐ Confirm ETT is in appropriate position ☐ Look/feel for symmetric chest wall rise ☐ Verify tube position at teeth ☐ Check ETCO2 ☐ DOPE
R: RESPIRATIONS ☐ Check baseline lung compliance with BVM ☐ Auscultate heart/lung sounds ☐ Calculate/verify tidal volume, rate, I:E, FiO2 and PEEP, theb attach portable ventilator ☐ Request arterial blood gas if > than 30 min since previous ABG	**R:** ☐ O2 for transport ☐ Backup ventilator/BVM ☐ Suction ☐ Needles for decompression	**R:** ☐ Look and feel for chest excursion ☐ Asses for Ventilator Alarms ☐ Check Pulse Ox ☐ Check patients'c color
C: CIRCULATION ☐ Asses distal pulses and neurovascular status prior transport ☐ Ensure IV access x 2 (Minimum). ☐ Remove air from IV bags and pressurize ☐ Review CBC/Chemistry results ☐ LZC Pressure Lines ☐ Label/position Primary Medication Administration Line	**C:** ☐ Vasoactive medications (dopamine, epi, neo, norepi) ☐ Pressure bags ☐ IV fluids and tubing	**C:** ☐ Check temp, pulse BP, and cardiace rhythm ☐ Assess distal, pulse and neurovascuar status during transport. ☐ Assess IV access ☐ LZC Pressure Lines at flight elevation ☐ Check placement of all tubes, lines and & ensure proper functioning
H: HEAD INJURY/HYPOTHERMIA ☐ Conduct baseline neurologic exam: Glasgow Coma Score (GCS) Assess pupil size and response. ☐ Spinal motion restriction or C-collar for transport, unless cleared by transferring physician. ☐ APLS, HPMK, warmed IV fluids, Mechanical warming units, blankets and/or chemical heat packs.	**H:** ☐ 3% NaCl, ☐ Position to account for ICP ☐ Optimze Oxygenation	**H:** ☐ Assess neurologic and sedation status ☐ Assess pupillary response and size ☐ Monitor VS for S/S of ICP ☐ Monitor Temperature Internal Core/External
P: PAIN CONTROL PATIEN SAFETY ☐ Assess pain control, sedation and need for paralysis. re-dose medications if needed before flight. ☐ Ensure the patient is loaded in a manner that allows adequate access to the patient and visibility of monitors and equipment. ☐ Provide eye and ear protection to patient ☐ Review orders and discuss potential en-route problems with the transferring physician. IV medications arrayed for easy access (20ml, 10ml, 5ml, 3ml)	**P:** ☐ Collect all labs, x-rays, pre aid-station/hospital documentation for transport ☐ Reconcile medications; verify allergies and patient's weight ☐ Secure personal effects. ☐ Sedation meds (propofol, ketamine, versed) ☐ Pain meds (fentany, morphine, dilaudid) ☐ Paralytic meds (vecuronium, rocuronium) ☐ Antibiotics	**P:** ☐ Ensure all wires and tubing are accessible and have adequate slack to allow monitors and IVs to be properly positioned and secured ☐ Serial assessments ☐ Prepare patient and give report to receiving facility ☐ **Consider re-dosing sedation/ pain/paralysis meds** ☐ **3 min out package patient in prep for transfer**

PREDEPARTURE CHECK LIST		
Altitude Considerations	Medications (specific for oatient)	Patient Packaging
Required waiting time before transport	Type and number of patients	Additional Medical support/non-medical attendant
Respiratory Support	Monitoring (body systems, medical interventions, etc)	Telephonic consultation
Equipment	Thermal considerations	Transport time and Route of transfer

Source: Government publication, not in copyright. Joint En Route Care Course, En Route Care Planning Tool, Version 2.0 01Sep2018

abd abdomen, *TXA* tranexamic acid, *ETCO*$_2$ end tidal carbon dioxide, *NG/OG* nasogastric/orogastric, *ETT* endotracheal tube, *BVM* bag-valve-mask, *DOPE* displacement, obstruction, pneumothorax, equipment failure, *I:E* inspiratory:expiratory, *FiO*$_2$ fraction of inspired oxygen, *PEEP* peak end expiratory pressure, *ABG* arterial blood gas, *O*$_2$ oxygen, *IV* intravenous, *CBC* complete blood count, *LZC* level, zero, and calibrate, *BP* blood pressure, *APLS* absorbent patient litter system, *HPMK* hypothermia prevention and management kit, *ICP* intracranial pressure, *VS* vital signs, *S/S* signs/symptoms

Now" status of the patient of the ERC planning tool (Table 31.2). The "Do Now" criteria are the current MARCHPAWS findings from the report and assessment that require immediate intervention in order to prepare the patient for transport. As each of the "Do Now" criteria is identified, secondary logistic supplies and assessment needs are developed. During the assessment, ensure that the patient is rolled, all junctional areas are investigated for injuries, and all team members auscultate lung fields, palpate chest for expansion, and assess compliance of bag-valve-mask (BVM) ventilation.

The findings of the ERC patient assessment assist in the validation of the decision to transport the patient. The Joint Trauma System (JTS) Clinical Practice Guideline (CPG) 27 on the Interfacility Transport of patients between theater medical treatment facilities (MTFs) gives clear guidance on the resuscitation goals that should be followed to identify when a patient is safe to transfer. If one or more of these goals is not met, a plan must be developed to optimize the patient in accordance with resources and the tactical situation. This CPG is available at https://jts.amedd.army.mil/assets/docs/cpgs/Interfacility_Transport_of_Patients_between_Theater_Medical_Treatment_Facilities_24_Apr_2018_ID27.pdf

Once the patient is validated for movement, supply need items can be filed under the "Take With" portion of patient transport planning in Table 31.2. The goal of this portion of the planning process is to ask the "What if? "questions for each of the patient's interventions. This item list includes backup support devices, batteries, dressing reinforcement supplies, next step interventions, medications for continued treatment, and pertinent documentation.

The final portion of this process is the development of the "En Route" section of the patient plan (see Table 31.2). This section will develop priority of injury and assessment protocol for the patient while in transport. This is an opportunity for the ERC team to clearly subdivide tasks and ensure that all aspects of the patient's care will be met. It is key to remember that assessment of the critical care transport focuses around five-minute increments (e.g., obtaining vital signs and checking the airway and oxygen pressure checks every 5 min). This creates a pattern repetition or "battle rhythm" for the transport period.

Documentation and reports are developed from the "En Route" portion of the patient transport plan. Depending upon the status and required effort of patient care during transport, documentation on the DD 1380 or DA4700 may prove to be difficult to maintain. At a bare minimum, the ERC team must document vital signs every 5 min (critical patients) or every 15 min (non-critical patients), any administered medication doses/times, and any performed interventions in order to properly transfer the patient and the patient's record.

Keep it simple! **Use practical and manageable interventions to optimize patients en route. Most importantly, the ERC team should agree on a form of reliable communication to use while en route.** This may include internal communication systems or other forms of communication like writing on white boards. ERC is already a complex, fast-paced, high-stakes environment; it is exponentially more complex when communication between ERC team members is hindered.

Transport Planning Concerns

Package a patient for transport to ensure access to all relevant interventions, organization of resources, and the safety of both the patient and ERC team. The personnel, space, and supply constraints on maritime surgical platforms are even MORE

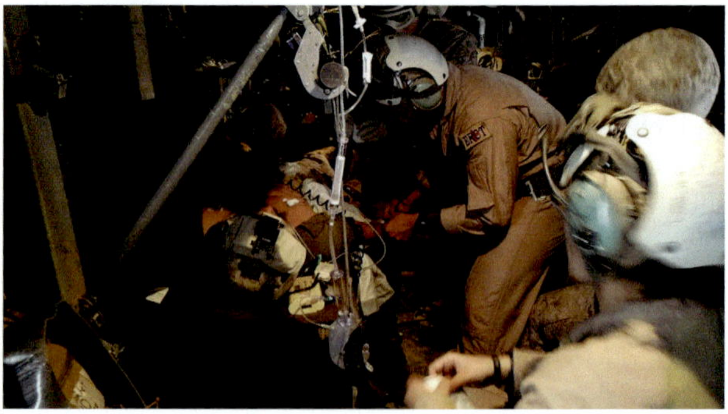

Fig. 31.1 V-22 Patient transport showing space and access limitations. (Source: Photo courtesy of Dana Flieger, CCRN)

constrained during ERC (Fig. 31.1), so every square inch and resource must be as optimized as possible. Time is also an enemy in the provider- and resource-constrained ERC transport environment. The tools performed in the assessment and documented in a checklist like Table 31.2 and/or Table 31.3 can organize preparation and packaging.

Table 31.3 Sample patient transport preparation checklist

PRE-FLIGHT CHECKLIST

(for Critical Care and Post-Surgical Transfers)

Once the decision is mode to transfer a patient and an occepting physicion has been obtained, the following steps will be taken| to prepare the patient for transport:

Initials	Evaluation Steps
	1. Sending location/physician: ____________ Accepting location/physician: ____________ Flight nurse called: name / time: ____________
	2. Anesthesia called: intubation if indicated. **ETT secured/marked**
	3. Patient meets criteria for en route critical care transport: risk documented by sending physician **(POST-OPERATIVE and CC INTRAFACILITY TRANSFER Pre-Transfer Patient Status Requirements)**
	Preparation Steps
	Positioning and Proper Monitoring:
	1. Patient moved to litter (collapsible handles), positioned, padded, strapped, equipment (with necessary attachments) added and secured. 2. For head-injured patients, a pre-sedation neurologic examination will be performed. GCS and neurological exam documented on the en route care form, suggest placing patient sitting at 30°-45°.(For eye injured patients, fox shield in place. For bum patients, **JTS burn sheet initiated.**)
	3. Ventilator switched to PMI vent at least 20-30 min prior to flight and set with transfer settings ordered by physician.
	4. IV / IO access verified, patent, and secured.
	5. Arterial line inserted and secured, if indicated. Transducer accessible
	6. Ventilator tubing checked to be free from obstruction, with $ETCO_2$ and secondary lines attached.
	7. Orogastric or nasogastric tube is inserted (unless contraindicated), placement verified with chest x-ray, and attached to low-intermittent suction.
	8. Chest tubes to water seal/suction (place Heimlich valve for non-atrium chest drainage systems).
	9. Wound vacuum disconnected and stowed.
	10. Foley catheter secured, urine output measured and documented.
	Equipment, Medication, Chart, and Personnel Preparation:
	11. Medications needed for flight prepared and organized.
	12. Flight equipment bag obtained and checked. Backup pulse oximeter readily available.
	13. Complete chart photocopied (induding x-ray cd), patient belongings bagged and tagged. Transfer Document, or other theater / unit approved transfer document, has been initiated.
	14. Earplugs and eye protection for patient and flight nurse.
	15. If facility sends medical attendant, attendant must have relevant personal protective equipment. In a combat environment this includes: Uniform, Kevlar, IBA, Weapon, ID Card, and equipment for transport.
	Ventilator Management:
	16. Blood gas (preferably ABG) obtained, 15 min after initial settings and ventilator changes. All efforts will be made to have a documented blood gas within 30 minutes prior to flight time.
	I7. Adjust ventilator settings and check O_2 tank for length of flight. Resuscitator bag under patient's head with tubing connected to O_2 source, vent tubing free from obstruction.
	Final Verification:
	18. Transferring Physician, Flight Paramedic, ECCN (or Flight Provider) verbally agrees to flight care plan.
	19. Critical Care Transfer Orders reviewed and signed by transferring physician.**(STANDARD ORDER SET for CRITICAL CARE TRANSFERS)**
	20. Enroute CC Transfer Document with completed preflight and enroute care data handed over to and confirmed by receiving provider / facility.

Source: Government publication, not in copyright. U.S. Army Medevac Critical Care Flight Paramedic Standard Medical Operating Guidelines, FY20 Version, Published January 2020
ETT endotracheal tube, *CC* critical care, *JTS* Joint Trauma System, *PMI* pressure muscle index, *IBA* interceptor body armor, *ABG* arterial blood gas, O_2 oxygen, *ECCN* en route critical care nurse

Patient Access and Packaging

Monitors should be placed on the litter structure or attached to a critical care platform transfer device (i.e., Special Medical Emergency Evacuation Device (SMEED)) to ensure that NO EQUIPMENT IS RESTING ON THE PATIENT, that it is fully secured to the litter system, and that all team members have access to the monitors. Securing devices, such as litter straps used for equipment and monitors, should NOT be used for the patient; use separate securing straps and devices for the patient. Patients should be secured with a minimum of two litter restraint straps. See Figs. 31.2, 31.3, and 31.4 for examples of patient packaging for transport.

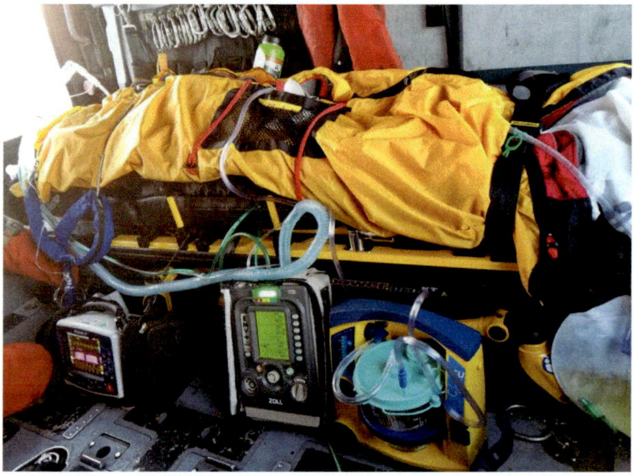

Fig. 31.2 Patient transport with all equipment and cables/lines visible. (Source: Photo courtesy of Wayne Papalski, Search and Rescue Medical Technician)

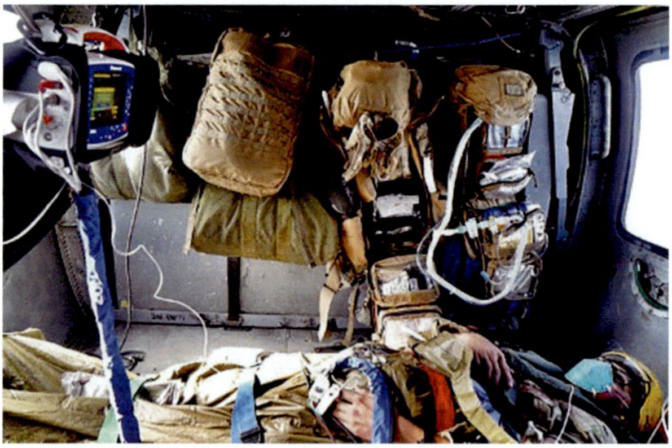

Fig. 31.3 MH-60S En Route Care (ERC) simulation. (Source: Photo courtesy of John Ingraham, Search and Rescue Medical Technician)

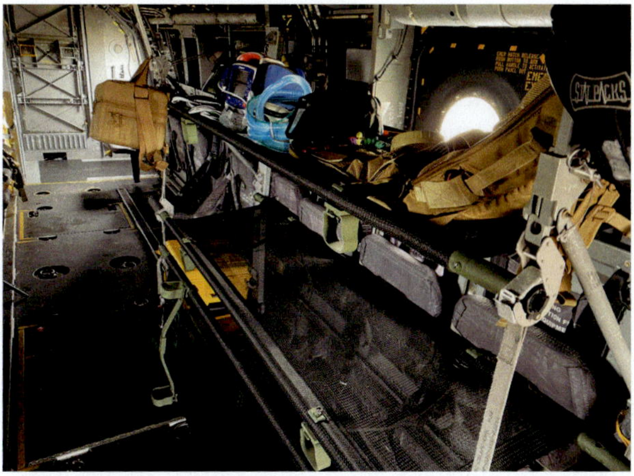

Fig. 31.4 V-22 Transport setup utilizing stanchions. (Source: Photo courtesy of Dana Flieger, CCRN)

Packaging Pearls

- Tubing or wires should be bundled and secured with a litter strap to prevent snagging or disconnection during movement. Intravenous (IV) and intraosseous (IO) tubing should be labeled and secured separately from any suction, ventilation, or drainage tubing.
- Dedicate an IV/IO line for medication administration only. Separate, mark, and place the administration port somewhere accessible to all team members during the transport.
- Predrawn/premixed medications, primed blood and IV tubing, taping of reinforcement bandages near wounds, and prepositioned pelvic binders and tourniquets are all examples of time-saving measures that should be prepared prior to transport.
- Consider placing a loose proximal extremity tourniquet on any extremity that initially had a tourniquet placed and was then transitioned to a pressure dressing to facilitate rapid hemostasis in the event of re-bleed during movement.
- Prepare orogastric/nasogastric tubes with gauze-packed Toomey syringes, and secure with a stopper for emergent and altitude-driven abdominal decompression.
- Thermoregulation is key in combating the lethal triad but difficult to control in the ERC setting. The ground/sending team should make every effort to prepare the patient with thermoregulating devices prior to arrival (see Chap. 28). Initial efforts should focus on monitoring the patient's core temperature, using warmed fluids, and ensuring the patient is adequately protected from the elements.
- For prolonged transports with an airway in place, a c-collar can prevent loss of airway placement in the maritime environment.

Equipment Organization

Inter-facility transport of patients requires high-quality but lightweight monitoring and critical care equipment to ensure safe and successful transport. Certain information such as length of transport, number of patients to be transferred, and severity of patient conditions should be taken into consideration when deciding the type and amount of equipment items to be used. The goal of preparing equipment for patient transport is to ensure all necessary items are accounted for, both consumable and non-consumable [10, 11].

Consumable equipment is that which expires or cannot be reused on another patient. The length of the transport will determine the amounts of fluids, medications, and other consumables that should be brought with the ERC team. At minimum, twice the length of the transport should be planned for when packing these items. Consumables are usually carried by the ERC team members via bag or backpack.

For all non-consumable items, charging batteries fully and performing any function checks should be performed before transport by the ERC team. Although some platforms have the ability to charge the equipment, it is not guaranteed on every platform. These items must be properly inspected and undergo the maintenance requirement recommended by the company of each respective piece of equipment to be safe for use. In general, each patient will require a continuous vital signs monitoring device with both invasive and noninvasive capabilities, external suction machine, and a ventilator (depending on their respiratory status). Models of these pieces of equipment may vary between each service depending on availability. Non-consumable equipment should be secured on the patient litter or transportation device so that all ERC team members can view them during transport. Equipment may be secured down by litter straps, ratchet straps, tape, or other devices (see Figs. 31.2, 31.3, and 31.4 for examples of how equipment is secured).

A sample list of consumables, fluids and medications, and equipment can be found in Table 31.4. Quantities have been left out as it will be different case by case. Although not all items on the list will need to be included for every case, additional supplies needed for potential emergencies during transport should be considered.

Often overlooked, the amount of oxygen required for transport should be calculated prior to initiating movement. The calculation should account for any delays such as waiting on the airfield or ground ambulance movements required from airfield to medical facility. Oxygen expenditure can also be affected by the type of ventilator utilized so understanding the equipment available in advance is critical to planning. Hypoxia can lead to rapid patient deterioration and is generally preventable with proper planning. Resources are available for these calculations; see Table 31.5 for a clinical example.

Table 31.4 Sample en route care (ERC) equipment list

Consumables	*Equipment*
Cricothyrotomy kit	Continuous vital signs monitoring device with defibrillation capacity
Endotracheal tubes (ETT)	Suction machine with backup mechanical device
Supraglottic airway devices (i.e., iGel, King, laryngeal mask airway (LMA))	Ventilator (with airworthiness release (AWR))
Oropharyngeal airway (OPA)	Oxygen tanks
Nasopharyngeal airway (NPA)	*MOVES® system is an alternate to all of the above if available*
Bag-valve-mask (BVM)	IV/intraosseous (IO) fluid warming system
Extra oxygen (O_2) tubing	End tidal carbon dioxide ($ETCO_2$) monitoring device
Soft tip suction (or in-line suction if available)	*Fluids and medications*
Suction tubing	Blood products
Backup handheld suction	Balanced isotonic crystalloids
Tube thoracostomy kit	3% NS
Scalpel	Pain medications
Intravenous (IV) catheter start kits	Sedation medications
10 cc syringes	Advanced cardiovascular life support (ACLS) medications
10 cc normal saline (NS) flushes	
Pressure bag	
IV tubing	
IV fluid warmer tubing and supplies	
Chux pads	
Tourniquets	
Foley kit	
Nasogastric/orogastric tube (NGT/OGT) kit	
Golden Hour container/Vampire Box (if traveling with blood products)	
Approved litter transport system	
Hypothermia management system	
Eye protection	
Ear protection	
Tape	

Table 31.5 Sample oxygen calculation guide [12, 13]

Sample Question: A patient is on a ventilator with an FiO_2 of 60%, TV 450 mL, RR 18. There is a total transport time of 1 h and 45 min (i.e., 105 min). There are 3 D cylinders with 2000 PSI in each available. Is there enough O_2 for transport?	
Conversion factors (constants): D, 0.16; E, 0.28; M, 1.56; H, 3.14	
Step 1: Calculate the Total O_2 available PSI × conversion factor × # cylinders = L Total O_2 available	*Step 1*: 2000 × 0.16 × 3 = 960 L Total O_2 available
Step 2: Calculate the rate of O_2 needed Minute ventilation (i.e., TV × RR) × FiO_2 = L of O_2 needed/min	*Step 2*: 0.450 × 18 × 0.6 = 4.86 L of O_2 needed/min
Step 3: Determine Total O_2 required Rate of O_2 needed × Total transport time = L Total O_2 required (time for pickup to vehicle/aircraft, actual transport time, transport from vehicle/aircraft to next facility)	*Step 3*: 4.86 × 105 = 510.30 L Total O_2 required
Sample question solution: Yes, there is enough oxygen for the transport since there are 960 L available and only 510 L is required	

FiO_2 fraction of inspired oxygen, *TV* tidal volume, *RR* respiratory rate, *PSI* pounds per square inch, *O_2* oxygen

Organization Pearls

- Extra batteries for all electronic devices should be ensured to be sufficient for the duration of transport.
- Additional items should be available for each piece of equipment; therefore, if there is failure or deterioration of the patient, there is a backup plan and the proper materials are available. For example, if the external suction machine fails, a manual suction should be available.
- Ground/sending team should attempt to decrease the fraction of inspired oxygen (FiO_2) requirements in a controlled setting prior to transport to ensure both maintenance of proper oxygen levels and allocation of limited resources en route.

Transportation Safety

Transportation safety encompasses the safety of BOTH the patient and the ERC team. Moving a patient from one echelon of care to another in the military setting requires mitigation of safety risks through the use of personal protective equipment (PPE). PPE is determined in part by the mode of transportation and terrain. PPE must be applied prior to transport. Land, sea, and air are the ways a patient can be transported via ruck, truck, boat, ship, rotary, or fixed wing platforms. Critical thought must be used when considering the appropriate PPE for both the patient and the ERC team, which may include, but is not limited to:

- Hearing protection (single or double)
- Eye protection (may or may not be ballistic grade)
- Cranial protection (helmet or cranial)
- Personal flotation device or life preserver unit (LPU) for overwater flight
- Thermoregulation devices (blankets, "Ready Heat" devices, Hypothermia Prevention and Management Kit (HPMK), Absorbent Patient Litter System (APLS))

Patient safety considerations also must be exercised when moving the patient to, from, and within the transportation platform. Sometimes patient movement is in relatively typical situations (i.e., horizontal loading on a deck to get into an aircraft as depicted in Figs. 31.5 and 31.6). However, it is not uncommon that patient movement occurs at sharp and extreme angles and in precarious situations (Figs. 31.7, 31.8, and 31.9); therefore, both the patient and gear must be properly secured to the litter or sled prior to movement for the safety of both the patient and the ERC team. Consideration must also be given to have adequate numbers of personnel to move a patient from one echelon to another. After the patient is transferred to a platform for transport, the final consideration is to ensure the litter or sled is secured to the conveyance. Though optimal, this final consideration may be omitted for the operational environment.

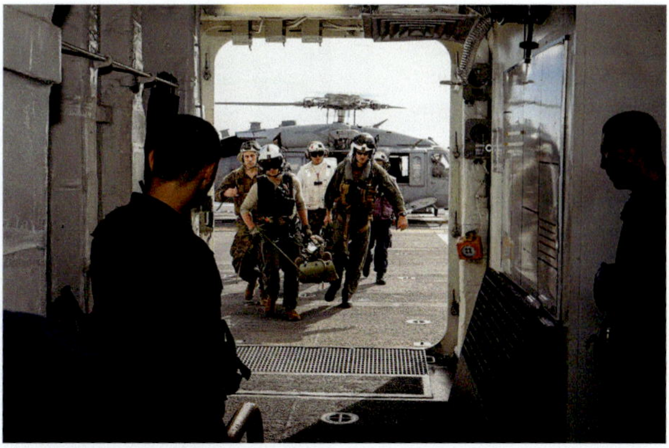

Fig. 31.5 Patient transfer simulation on a Landing Helicopter Dock (LHD) ship. (Source: Photo courtesy of Brock Hite, Search and Rescue Medical Technician)

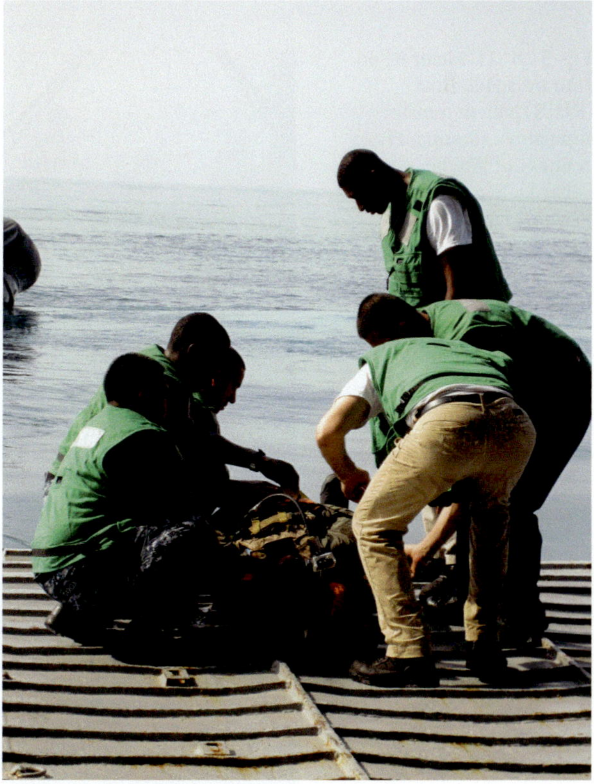

Fig. 31.6 Well deck patient transfer. (Source: Photo courtesy of Wayne Papalski, Search and Rescue Medical Technician)

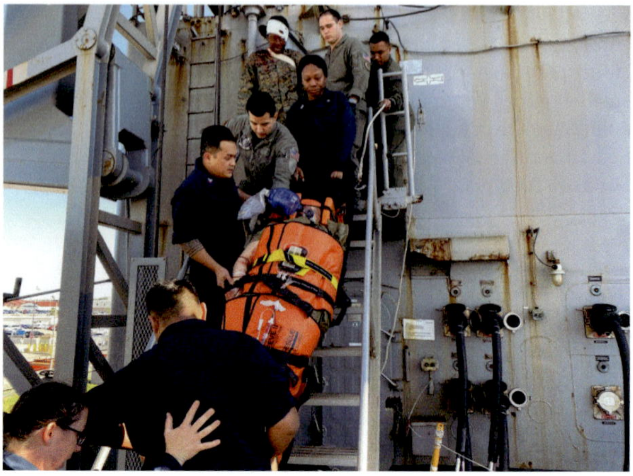

Fig. 31.7 Patient movement down a ladder well of a ship. (Source: Photo courtesy of Wayne Papalski, Search and Rescue Medical Technician)

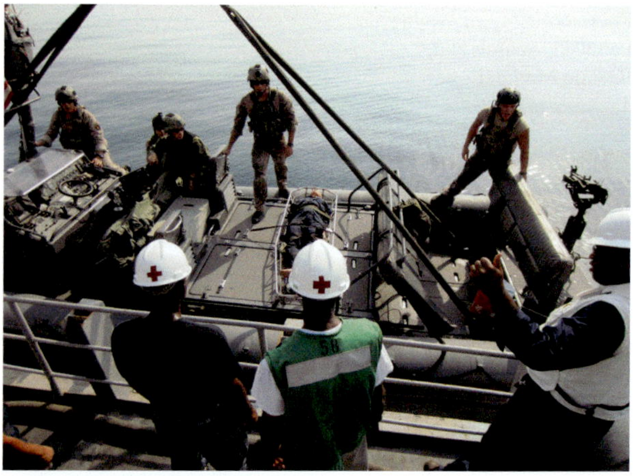

Fig. 31.8 11-Meter Rigid Hull Inflatable Boat (RHIB) patient transfer simulation. (Source: Photo courtesy of Wayne Papalski, Search and Rescue Medical Technician)

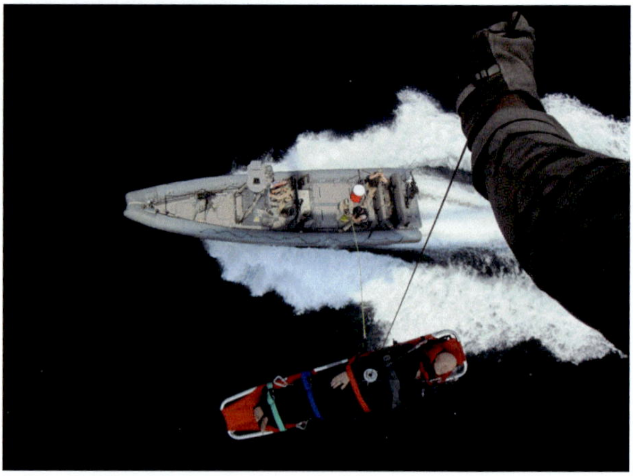

Fig. 31.9 11-Meter Rigid Hull Inflatable Boat (RHIB) patient hoist simulation. (Source: Photo courtesy of Wayne Papalski, Search and Rescue Medical Technician)

The movement of patients from ship to ship/ship to shore can be extremely slow for a multitude of reasons. Many of those have to do with time and distance between vessels when operating independently of each other. A second major consideration is weather. When weather affects the movement of patients via normal means (i.e., helicopter transfer), the movement of patients via smaller craft to ship can be extremely time-consuming. A large portion of that transfer is safety. There are many moving parts to get the patient from one space on a ship to another, to a smaller vessel, transported via open water, then loaded back onto another ship, finally being transferred to a different space on that ship. Each of these locations and during each of these transports, there are countless ways that patient care can deteriorate because of the compromised environment that actively detracts from patient care; refer again to Figs. 31.7, 31.8, and 31.9. It takes 100% of every team member's attention and effort to keep their patients and themselves safe.

Safety Pearls

- Hypothermia management: If ship to ship transfer is happening, there is a reason that air assets are not flying, which could be the weather. Movement via open water is harsh on providers, let alone sick patients. Ensure passive and active warming devices are working and have backups necessary. "Ready Heat" devices do not perform well in salt spray environments so it is essential to ensure they are working properly prior to the start of the transfer.
- Reassess the securing devices after each phase of transport/movement both to ensure that everything is still secure and that all interventions are still in place/ functioning.

Conclusion

ERC involves much more than having a method of transport and a care provider for the journey. This chapter has described a process to avoid errors and provided pearls to improve patient outcomes. With careful planning, communication, and practice, maritime surgical teams can work to achieve the ultimate goal in ERC: delivering patients to the next level of care in better condition than the team received them.

Declaration of Interest The views expressed in this chapter are those of the authors and do not necessarily reflect the official policy or position of the Department of the Navy, Department of Defense, nor the US Government.

Funding This research did not receive any specific grant from funding agencies in the public, commercial, or not-for-profit sectors.

Conflict of Interest Statement The authors declare no conflict of interest.

References

1. Joint Health Services. Joint Publication 4-02. 2017. http://www.jcs.mil/Portals/36/Documents/Doctrine/pubs/jp4_02.pdf. Accessed July 2018.
2. Mabry RL, Apodaca A, Penrod J, Orman JA, Gerhardt RT, Dorlac WC. Impact of critical care–trained flight paramedics on casualty survival during helicopter evacuation in the current war in Afghanistan. J Trauma Acute Care Surg. 2012;73(2):S32–7.
3. Blackman VS, Walrath BD, Reeves LK, Mora AG, Maddry JK, Stockinger ZT. En route care provided by US Navy nurses in Iraq and Afghanistan. Crit Care Nurse. 2018;38(2):e1–6.
4. Walrath B, Mora A, Ganem V, Harper S, Ross E, Kharod C, et al. Navy en route care: a 3-year review of 428 Navy air evacuations. Mil Med. 2017;182(suppl_1):162–6.
5. Andicochea CT, Wilson J, Raetz E, Walrath B. An assessment of flight surgeon confidence to perform en route care. Mil Med. 2019;184(Supplement_1):306–9.
6. Maddry JK, Simon EM, Reeves LK, Mora AG, Clemons MA, Shults NM, et al. Impact of a standardized patient hand-off tool on communication between emergency medical services personnel and emergency department staff. Prehosp Emerg Care. 2020;25:530–8.
7. Laverty C, Tien H, Beckett A, Nathens A, Rivest-Caissy JP, da Luz LT. Primary aeromedical retrieval crew composition: do different teams impact clinical outcomes? A descriptive systematic review. Can J Emerg Med. 2020;22(S2):S89–S103.
8. Snow RW, Papalski W, Siedler J, Drew B, Walrath B. Benefit of critical care flight paramedic-trained search and rescue corpsmen in treatment of severely injured aviators. J Spec Oper Med. 2018;18(1):19–22.
9. TCCC guidelines (November 2020).
10. United States Department of the Air Force. Aeromedical Evacuation Equipment Standards (AFI10–2909). 2013. http://static.e-publishing.af.mil/production/1/af_a3_5/publication/afi10-2909/afi10-2909.pdf. Accessed Apr 2018.
11. Headquarters Department of the Army. Medical evacuation (ATP 4-02.2) Army techniques Publication No. 4-02.2 Aug 12, 2014. http://armypubs.army.mil/doctrine/DR_pubs/dr_a/pdf/atp4_02x2.pdf. Accessed July 2018.
12. Headquarters Department of the Army. Casualty Evacuation (ATP 4-25.13) Army Techniques Publication No. 4-25.13, Feb 9, 2013. https://armypubs.army.mil/epubs/DR_pubs/DR_a/pdf/web/atp4_25x13.pdf. Accessed July 2018.
13. U.S. Department of the Air Force. En route care and aeromedical evacuation medical operations (AFI 41-307). Jan 7, 2017. http://static.e-publishing.af.mil/production/1/af_sg/publication/afi48-307v1/afi48-307v1.pdf. Accessed July 2018.

Part V
Humanitarian and Disaster Relief Missions

Chapter 32
Principles of Elective Navy Humanitarian Missions

Alicia G. Sykes and Romeo C. Ignacio Jr

What have you done for the good of mankind lately?

Dr. Norman McSwain

Author deployment experience	
Alicia G. Sykes	Participated in diplomatic missions, Brazil and Egypt, 2014
	Master of Arts in Global Health, University of California San Diego, San Diego, 2021
Romeo C. Ignacio Jr.	General Medical Officer/Brig Medical Officer, 3D Forces Support Services Group, Camp Hansen, Okinawa, Japan, 1998–1999
	Director of Surgical Services, USNS Mercy (T-AH-19), MERCEX, Preplanning Deployment Team, 2010
	Advance Team Lead Surgeon, Designated Institutional Officer and solo military Pediatric Surgeon, USNS Mercy (T-AH-19), Pacific Partnership, Philippines and Cambodia, 2012
	Covering Ship's Surgeon, USS Kitty Hawk (CV-63), USS Theodore Roosevelt (CVN-71), USS Ronald Reagan (CVN-76), USS Somerset (LPD-25)
	Pediatric Surgeon, surgery outreach missions, Japan, Philippines, Guatemala, and Italy, 2012, 2015–2018
	General Surgeon, USS Somerset (LPD-25), Project UNITAS, Peru, 2018

A. G. Sykes
Navy Medicine Readiness and Training Command San Diego, San Diego, CA, USA
e-mail: alicia.g.sykes.mil@health.mil

R. C. Ignacio Jr (✉)
Division of Pediatric Surgery, Rady Children's Hospital San Diego,
3030 Children's Way, San Diego, CA, USA

Department of Surgery, University of California San Diego School of Medicine,
San Diego, CA, USA
e-mail: r1ignacio@health.ucsd.edu

M. D. Tadlock, A. A. Hernandez (eds.), *Expeditionary Surgery at Sea*,
https://doi.org/10.1007/978-3-031-21893-4_32

BLUF (Bottom Line Up Front)

1. Humanitarian missions will greatly vary depending on the host nation's capabilities, infrastructure, and surgical needs.
2. Quality surgical care is an essential component of humanitarian missions. The surgical capacity to provide care relies on available medical personnel, level of training, surgical equipment, anesthesia support, and ancillary services. Assessment of these resources must be performed prior to deployment.
3. United States (U.S.) military personnel should partner with host nation assets and humanitarian assistance organizations (HAOs) to understand the available resources and build relationships.
4. Significant amounts of planning and communication across and between organizations are essential to optimize the success of any size humanitarian mission, particularly large-scale ones.
5. The humanitarian mission should provide the most care to those in need while minimizing complications, taking postoperative care into consideration.
6. Post-deployment assessments must list best practices, lessons learned, and areas for improvement in preparation for future humanitarian missions.

Introduction

Throughout its history, the United States (U.S.) Navy has engaged in a variety of humanitarian operations. Since its first documented humanitarian action in 1851, the U.S. Navy has continued to carry out humanitarian missions to build upon international partnerships, promote global stability and security, and maintain the operational readiness of military medical personnel [1]. These humanitarian operations include responses to natural disasters and conflicts, rescues at sea, emergency medical assistance, and nation-building activities [2]. More recently, these missions have focused on supporting the establishment and further development of partner nation health systems to promote long-term regional stability and global security [3].

Clinical Vignette 32.1

A U.S. military-sponsored humanitarian mission had a small medical team consisting of one surgeon, two emergency medicine physicians, an anesthesiologist, two nurses, four corpsmen, and limited resources. They were assigned to provide medical support to a local village in a low-income country with limited resources. A three-year-old child with a large empyema who was short of breath and in mild respiratory distress was evaluated.

What considerations must the team consider before treating this child? Should the surgeon or emergency medicine physicians provide care or defer medical treatment elsewhere?

Objectives of U.S. Navy Humanitarian and Civic Assistance (HCA) Missions

The U.S. Navy participates in Foreign Humanitarian Assistance (FHA) operations with the objectives of saving lives, alleviating human suffering, and minimizing the economic costs of conflict, disasters, and displacement [4]. FHA operations are conducted under the direction of the President of the U.S. or the Secretary of Defense and in coordination with local and international stakeholders [4]. Frequently conducted outside of the U.S. and its territories, these missions serve to assist host nation civil authorities or agencies in providing disaster relief, security operations, logistical support (e.g., transportation of supplies or personnel), and medical assistance, among other support activities [4]. These operations may also be conducted concurrently with other Department of Defense (DoD) support missions and activities that support strategic objectives (e.g., providing dislocated civilian support) and enhance theater security (e.g., fostering regional partnerships, providing foreign security assistance, and participating in stability activities) [4].

Encompassed within FHA operations are Humanitarian and Civic Assistance (HCA) and Foreign Disaster Relief (FDR) missions. HCA is provided to build partnerships in order to facilitate cooperation and enhanced interoperability with host and partner nations during times of crisis. These elective operations may utilize U.S. Navy hospital ships, large deck amphibious warfare ships, Maritime Expeditionary Security Forces (MESF), expeditionary medical facilities (EMFs), and forward-deployable preventive medicine units (FDPMUs). On the other hand, FDR operations are conducted in response to natural disasters or international conflict, and any U.S. Navy warship at or near the immediate scene of a foreign disaster can be tasked with participating in these operations as described in Chap. 33 [4].

Health and medical support are essential components of FHA operations. These services include:

- Coordinating actions to prevent or control disease outbreak
- Evacuation or temporary hospitalization of the sick, wounded, or injured followed by a coordinated return to civilian facilities of the host or partner nation
- Distribution of supplies and equipment
- Assistance in reestablishing host nation and donor health sector resources and institutions with primary consideration given to supporting and supplementing any existing medical infrastructure [4]

Surgical care is increasingly being viewed as an essential component of healthcare delivery in military humanitarian missions because high-quality surgical care can facilitate the provision of other vital health services [5]. An estimated 1.4 million deaths could be prevented worldwide with access to essential and emergency surgical care within low- and middle-income countries (LMICs). However, access to surgical care in LMICs remains a challenge as many of these countries lack the necessary medical infrastructure and trained medical personnel [6]. Military humanitarian operations that incorporate surgical care can assist LMICs in building up their local medical infrastructure while helping to alleviate their large surgical burden of disease. These missions can provide a long-lasting impact through the capacity building of the host nation's medical infrastructure and education and training to local medical personnel.

Small- and Medium-Scale HCA Missions

At present, there are no defined size classifications of humanitarian operations. Therefore, the scale of a humanitarian operation depends on the mission's overall objective(s) and the availability of resources and ancillary staff for that mission. Most U.S. missions are in foreign countries, and the needs of the mission often dictate the required personnel and equipment. For example, small-scale missions might include a surgical team with a single surgeon, anesthesia provider, nurse, and corpsman participating in a rescue operation. Medium-scale operations might involve a few more providers in each role. **However, regardless of scale, understanding the host nation's capabilities and appropriately engaging with state and international agencies or organizations are essential to the success of all humanitarian operations.**

Understanding Host Nation Capabilities

During these operations, medical providers are tasked with providing a level of care that meets current U.S. standards of care while at the same time considering the host nation's standards of care and ability to sustain the level of care provided [4]. Therefore, when participating in humanitarian aid and humanitarian operations, military medical providers must consider the expressed needs of the host nation in the context of available resources and local medical infrastructure. Mission planners should anticipate that the healthcare delivery infrastructure in host nations may be austere or nonexistent and should perform early surveying of the host nation in order to identify health and medical needs. This assessment will help coordinate efforts of the local, regional, and international stakeholders [4]. The involvement of host nation leadership and medical care personnel in these missions is pivotal to developing the host nation's medical infrastructure and health system capacity building.

Working with State and International Agencies or Organizations

Various disasters, conflicts, and endemic diseases may affect the ability to provide humanitarian care. The U.S. Department of State (DOS) can provide information on the threat levels and conditions in certain prospective host nations. For this reason, military planners will occasionally work closely with key individuals within the DOS, especially for large-scale humanitarian missions.

Humanitarian assistance organizations (HAOs) may already exist in various foreign countries. There are two types of HAOs: intergovernmental organizations (IGOs) and non-governmental organizations (NGOs). IGOs are entities created by sovereign states through multilateral treaties that act under an agreed treaty that sets up the agencies, organizations, and objectives [7]. Examples of IGOs are the United Nations High Commission on Refugees, the International Committee of the Red Cross, and the World Health Organization (WHO). NGOs, on the other hand, are independent, nonprofit organizations that are predominantly managed by local or international civilian personnel. NGOs provide the majority (>90%) of aid coordinated by the United Nations (UN) [8].

Categories of NGOs are:

- Humanitarian aid
- Advocacy
- Faith-based groups that do not use religion as part of the provided aid
- Missionary groups that seek to spread their religion using humanitarian access to communities

As independent organizations, NGOs usually have no political affiliation. However, because these organizations rely heavily on funding, donor interests or priorities often influence their operations. Therefore, NGO goals may conflict with those of military operations. Strengths of NGOs include their flexibility in being able to perform multiple duties within host nations, their ability to maintain long-term continuity and establish relationships with vulnerable areas, and their capacity to have a specialized response focus, benefit from local resources, and solicit funds to meet needs. Potential weaknesses of NGOs include limited logistical capacity and consequential reliance on military, government, or UN agencies to support large-scale tasks.

Working with host nation assets (medical leadership, host nation ministry, IGOs, or NGOs) may support humanitarian missions and build relationships. However, clear and transparent goals from each participating organization must be established to avoid conflicts in providing care.

Large-Scale HCA Missions

Since 2006, the U.S. Navy hospital ships, the USNS Mercy (T-AH-19) and USNS Comfort (T-AH-20), have regularly deployed in support of large-scale HCA missions. The USNS Mercy (T-AH-19) has deployed periodically to Southeast Asia and Oceania in support of operation "Pacific Partnership," and the USNS Comfort (T-AH-20) has deployed to the Caribbean, Central America, and South America as a part of "Partnership for the Americas," "Operation Continuing Promise," and "Operation Enduring Promise" (Table 32.1). These missions involve coordination

Table 32.1 USNS Mercy (T-AH-19) and USNS Comfort (T-AH-20) large-scale humanitarian and civic assistance (HCA) missions by year

	Large-scale humanitarian and civic assistance mission	
Year	USNS Mercy (T-AH-19)	USNS Comfort (T-AH-20)
2006	Pacific Partnership	
2007		Partnership for the Americas
2008	Pacific Partnership	
2009		Operation Continuing Promise
2010	Pacific Partnership	
2011		Operation Continuing Promise
2012	Pacific Partnership	
2015	Pacific Partnership	Operation Continuing Promise
2018	Pacific Partnership	Operation Enduring Promise

and cooperation between the US military, host and partner nations, and national and international organizations and agencies [4, 5]. Various medical and non-medical personnel from all US military branches, partner nations, and NGOs contribute to the workforce for these missions. These missions typically last between 4 and 5 months and involve 4–12 host nations with an average performance of 51 to 251 operative cases per month.

Medical Capabilities of U.S. Navy Hospital Ships

One unique aspect of the U.S. Navy Fleet is the availability of two dedicated hospital ships, the USNS Mercy (T-AH-19) stationed on the West Coast with homeport in San Diego, CA, and the USNS Comfort (T-AH-20) stationed on the East Coast with homeport in Norfolk, VA [9, 10]. These ships are fully functional, independent, mobile hospitals with their own recurring humanitarian aid mission cycle [5]. Each vessel has 12 operating rooms (ORs), approximately 1000 hospital beds, and 50 casualty-receiving beds [4]. The hospital beds onboard include 20 post-anesthesia care, 80 intensive care, 400 intermediate care, and 500 basic care beds. The capabilities aboard these hospital ships include digital radiological services, a computed tomography (CT) scanner, invasive angiography, a diagnostic and clinical laboratory, a blood bank, a pharmacy, an optometry lab, and two oxygen-producing plants [4]. Both ships also have a helicopter landing deck and side ports to take on patients at sea. Due to their designation as hospital ships and in agreement with the Geneva Convention, they do not possess any offensive weapons, but defensive weapons are available.

The primary mission of U.S. Navy hospital ships is to provide afloat medical capability for acute medical and Level I trauma surgical care for forward deployed operational forces of the military services. The last time that U.S. Navy hospital ships were deployed for this purpose was in 2003 to support Operation Iraqi

Freedom [11]. A secondary mission of these ships is to provide a full-service hospital asset in support of disaster relief, humanitarian aid, and defense support to civil authorities worldwide [5]. For nearly 20 years, U.S. Navy hospital ships have been predominantly utilized to carry out this secondary mission. More recently, these hospital ships have provided limited medical support during the coronavirus disease 2019 (COVID-19) pandemic (see Chap. 33) [12, 13].

The Humanitarian Assistance Survey Team (HAST)

At the request of the United States Agency for International Development (USAID), a Humanitarian Assistance Survey Team (HAST) is organized and deployed to acquire information required for mission planning. The HAST is comprised of medical personnel qualified to conduct health, medical, and environmental vulnerability assessments; engineers along with logisticians, communications experts, transportation management specialists, and force protection experts [4]. This team works with local groups and USAID to assess the ability of the host nation's government to respond to disaster, identify points of contact for coordination and collaboration, determine potential environmental threats, survey local facilities and infrastructure, conduct health and medical assessments, and coordinate specific logistical support to assist with the relief effort [4].

The Advanced Echelon or Advanced Liaison (ADVON) Teams

Advanced Echelon or Advanced Liaison (ADVON) teams also play an essential role in planning U.S. Navy humanitarian missions. ADVON teams consisting of physicians, nurses, and other military personnel deploy several weeks ahead of the humanitarian missions to make preparations. The ADVON team will determine where the missions will take place as well as determine the logistics and organization of the mission. In the weeks before the mission, members of the ADVON team meet with NGOs; host nation directors to include Ministries of Health, Ministers of Education, and Ministers of Internal Affairs; and local healthcare providers, teachers, town officials, and media sources to prioritize healthcare services and determine the best way to organize the medical and surgical mission [14].

Providing Surgical Care

Following the arrival of a U.S. Navy hospital ship deployed on a humanitarian mission, a surgical screening team – consisting of surgery, anesthesiology, cardiology, and radiology providers – evaluates patients onshore and then schedules them for surgery aboard the ship [15]. Host nations may provide a list of surgical candidates to U.S. military medical providers prior to arrival. However, individuals are required to present for preoperative screening in order to be offered surgery. Patients are offered surgery if they met the criteria for same-day surgery or if they will have an anticipated recovery and discharge before ship departure [15]. If the ship is anchored offshore, patients are transported to and from the ship by watercraft or aircraft [15].

Other Aspects of Large-Scale HCA Missions

Large-scale HCA operations are multifaceted missions. While military medical personnel are providing medical and surgical care and participating in shared education and training, other military personnel are engaging in other activities to foster relations and promote the health and security of host nations. These other operations include providing optometry services, providing veterinary care, building local infrastructure (i.e., Seabees), and engaging in public relations activities.

Challenges of HCA Missions

The key to success in military humanitarian deployments is understanding the mission's objectives, understanding the limitations of resources, evaluating the host nation's needs, and participating in cooperative engagement to achieve the goals of the mission. It is crucial to partner with host nations to develop humanitarian aid initiatives, and medical providers must also consider the potential influence of local cultural practices and beliefs. Described challenges of U.S. Navy humanitarian missions include differing objectives and modes of operation, competing missions, inadequate structure and procedures, incompatible communications, overly restrictive security classifications, cultural and religious differences, and bureaucratic and personnel limitations [4]. Host nation priorities can influence mission productivity, and it is essential to participate in cooperative engagement to achieve the goals of the mission. Additional challenges include the relationship between the host nation and the U.S., the staffing and effectiveness of the U.S. embassy, host nation advertising prompting presentation of potential surgical candidates for treatment, in-country U.S. military groups, ministries of health, the availability and cost of supplies and equipment, the effectiveness of communication between mission medical providers onshore and ship-based surgeons, and the distance between the ship at anchor to the various clinics [16].

Deployment Considerations

Capabilities of the Surgical Team

During U.S. Navy HCA missions, U.S. military personnel work together with host nations, partner nations, and NGOs to provide medical, surgical, dental, and veterinary care and resources to host nations [5]. The role of the surgeon and surgical team during these missions is to provide low-risk, high-yield surgical care to individuals living in LMICs while supporting and supplementing existing local medical infrastructure through sharing knowledge and training alongside surgeons from host and partner nations.

The host nation needs will dictate the number of procedures performed on these missions. Additionally, U.S. Navy humanitarian missions are short-term missions (4–5 months), with port visits typically lasting between 4 and 16 days in duration. These time constraints limit the ability of surgeons to perform complex operations or procedures after which patients may require longitudinal follow-up and care. For that reason, the focus of the surgical mission is on the performance of elective operations. Many of the host nations visited by the US Navy hospital ships on these missions lack the healthcare infrastructure and other resources necessary to accommodate long-term postoperative care. If follow-up care is required beyond 2 weeks, efforts are made to establish this care with NGOs or host nation hospitals. However, this varies by country and is dependent on local medical infrastructure.

Screening Criteria for Surgery

Patient selection is a critical task for surgical providers and is especially important while participating in large-scale, foreign HCA missions. Both the capabilities of the hospital ship and a surgical candidate's risk tolerance for elective procedures must be carefully considered [17]. The specialized training of the deployed anesthesia providers and surgical providers will also influence what types of operations can be performed on these missions. Additionally, surgeons must consider the short-term nature of these missions and the ability to coordinate continued care within the medical infrastructure of the host nation when deciding which surgical procedures to offer to those presenting for operative treatment of surgical diseases in host nations. Screening criteria have previously been developed for large-scale HCA missions. Anesthesiologists developed screening criteria on Pacific Partnership 2008 to identify patients who "met criteria for cancellation of cases," and these criteria were later adapted for use during Pacific Partnership 2010 (Table 32.2).

Table 32.2 An example of anesthesia screening criteria for surgery on a large-scale foreign Humanitarian and Civic Assistance (HCA) mission (Source: Reprinted with permission from *Military Medicine*)

System	Criteria for cancellation of cases
Cardiovascular	• HTN: SBP >160 or DBP >90 or PP >80 mm Hg • CAD: myocardial infarction within last 6 months or remote myocardial infarction not revascularized • CHF: evidence of active uncompensated CHF • Arrhythmia: frequent symptomatic palpitations • Tachycardia: resting HR >100 or HR 100–110 (refer to cardiology) • Valvular disease: type III/VI or greater SEM, diastolic murmurs, AS, MR (refer to cardiology)
Respiratory	• Asthma: active wheezing or decreased breath sounds • COPD: symptomatic shortness of breath • OSA: snoring, daytime somnolence, witnessed apneic events • Airway: recognized difficult airways
Endocrine	• DM: fasting blood glucose >300; evidence of end-organ damage • Thyroid: all goiters (refer to cardiothoracic surgery, must have no evidence of thyrotoxicosis) • Obesity: BMI >35
Neurological	• Cerebrovascular: any residual deficit or frequent transient ischemic attacks • Gait disturbances • Seizure: new onset or history of epilepsy
Obstetrics and gynecology	• Pregnant • Breast, ovarian, or cervical cancer • Postpartum <2 months • Counsel if breastfeeding
Oncology	• Any current cancer (unless operative site)
Pediatric	• Age <6 months; advanced cases <2 years • Syndromic appearance • CHD: known lesions/cyanotic history, refer all murmurs to cardiology for evaluation • URI: symptoms within 4 weeks

HTN hypertension, *SBP* systolic blood pressure, *DBP* diastolic blood pressure, *PP* pulse pressure, *CAD* coronary artery disease, *CHF* congestive heart failure, *HR* heart rate, *SEM* systolic ejection murmur, *AS* aortic stenosis, *MR* mitral regurgitation, *COPD* chronic obstructive pulmonary disease, *OSA* obstructive sleep apnea, *DM* diabetes mellitus, *BMI* body mass index, *CHD* congenital heart disease, *URI* upper respiratory infection

Surgical and Medical Civil Action Programs (SURGCAPS and MEDCAPS)

Prospective surgical candidates are evaluated on the arrival of the U.S. hospital ship in shore-based facilities by members of surgical and medical civil action programs (SURGCAP and MEDCAP) [17]. The SURGCAP team consists of 50 to 70 personnel, including surgeons, nurses, surgical technologists, anesthesia providers, internists, cardiologists (with transthoracic echocardiogram capability), translators, lab support, schedulers, hospital administrators, and information technology support [17]. Prospective surgical candidates would then be further evaluated by surgeons and anesthesia providers onboard the U.S. hospital ship. Those deemed as poor surgical candidates by anesthesia but as an acceptable surgical risk by a surgeon would be referred to a Surgical Risk Evaluation Committee.

Subject Matter Expert Exchanges (SMEE)

U.S. Navy humanitarian missions provide a unique setting for the training of medical providers and healthcare personnel within the U.S. military, host nations, and partner nations. During the most recent humanitarian operations—"Pacific Partnership," "Operation Continuing Promise," and "Operation Enduring Promise"—U.S. military healthcare personnel participated in Subject Matter Expert Exchanges (SMEE) with medical providers from host and partner nations. In addition, U.S. Navy surgeons operated alongside surgeons from host and partner nations, which provided an opportunity for surgeons to share knowledge, practices, and skills. This sharing of knowledge supports readiness for U.S. Navy medical personnel and promotes collaboration and partnership between the U.S. and host and partner nations.

Post-deployment

Lessons Learned

Due to the lack of continuity of providers participating in U.S. Navy Humanitarian missions, it is imperative that lessons learned by military teams on these missions be passed on to those who will be participating in these missions in the future. Some past examples include:

- Be flexible. It is not uncommon to experience frequent changes in mission plans at the request of mission leadership, host nation leadership, and mission personnel [18].
- Documentation is extremely important. There is a need for an automated patient tracking system to collect demographic data and clinical information to improve the coordination of longitudinal care and future mission planning.
- Define gaps in care and resources after each mission to decide if future missions should consider additional personnel or equipment to address such deficiencies.
- Local, regional, and country assessments should be evaluated at each mission to determine capabilities and plan for sustainable programs to improve host nation prevention programs, education, and infrastructure.

After Action Reports

Current documentation and dissemination of lessons learned from U.S. Navy humanitarian missions are "highly variable, often lacks transparency, and is not easily accessible" [18]. A variety of resources exist; however, they are not easily accessible nor centralized in one location (e.g., All Partners Access Network, Joint Lessons Learned Information System [JLLIS], Global Health Engagement (GHE) website resource, Global Health eLearning Center, Center for Strategic and International Studies, Military Health System (MHS), and Defense Health Agency (DHA)) [18]. Networking and in-person communications within the GHE community have historically been the best ways to transfer experiential knowledge related to U.S. Navy humanitarian missions [18]. Such exchanges have been made possible through the Asia Pacific Military Health Exchange, GHE Summit, Pacific Partnership Interim and Main Planning Conferences, and MHS Research Symposium [18]. This passing down of knowledge is particularly imperative as military healthcare providers with hospital-based shipboard global health experience will often be selected to plan future missions [18].

Clinical Vignette 32.1 Conclusion

Prior to the humanitarian mission, established guidelines were determined that thoracic operations were beyond the capabilities of the surgical team. However, the team decided to examine the child with the expectation expressed to the host nation physicians that they could not provide emergent thoracic operations. On examination, the child was tachypneic and tachycardic with normal oxygen saturations on room air. Intravenous fluids and antibiotics were administered. A discussion with the host nation physicians and NGOs was performed to arrange for further inpatient care, and the military provided medical transportation to the pediatric ward at a nearby city hospital with full capabilities. An assessment was performed that documented contingent plans in managing pediatric patients in the future at this host nation.

Conclusions

There are many challenges to a successful HCA. Understanding mission goals and host nation expectations is a fundamental requirement before deployment. Medical planners should send teams ahead of time, establish guidelines, and conduct clear, transparent discussions with host nation medical leaders, local governments, partner nations, and NGOs before providing medical care. Surgical team members must not only know their inherent surgical limitations, but they must also consider host nation infrastructure, support from local assets (e.g., IGOs, NGOs, and local healthcare providers), and cultural and religious beliefs that may affect their abilities in providing such care. Post-deployment assessments are mandatory to improve future missions in resource-limited countries.

Declaration of Interest The views expressed in this chapter are those of the authors and do not necessarily reflect the official policy or position of the Department of the Navy, Department of Defense, nor the US Government.

Funding This research did not receive any specific grant from funding agencies in the public, commercial, or not-for-profit sectors.

Conflict of Interest Statement The authors declare no conflict of interest.

References

1. 19th century: humanitarian actions. Naval history and heritage command. https://www.history.navy.mil/content/history/museums/nmusn/explore/photography/humanitarian/19th-century.html. Accessed 5 May 2021.
2. The Navy's Humanitarian Mission. Naval history and heritage command. 2020. https://www.history.navy.mil/browse-by-topic/disasters-and-phenomena/humanitarian-mission.html. Accessed 3 May 2021.
3. Our history. https://www.health.mil/Military-Health-Topics/Health-Readiness/Global-Health-Engagement/Our-History. Accessed 4 May 2021.
4. Joint publication 3-29 foreign humanitarian assistance. 2019. https://www.jcs.mil/Portals/36/Documents/Doctrine/pubs/jp3_29.pdf. Accessed 7 May 2021.
5. Gaidry AD, Lizardo RE, Prieto JM, et al. An analysis of essential pediatric surgical cases encountered during a decade of large-scale military humanitarian aid missions. Mil Med. 2020;185(11-12):e2143–9. https://doi.org/10.1093/milmed/usaa177.
6. Bickler SW, Weiser TG, Kassebaum N, et al. Chapter 2: global burden of surgical conditions. In: Disease control priorities, vol. 1. 3rd ed. Washington: The World Bank; 2015.
7. University of Cincinnati Libraries. Intergovernmental Organizations (IGOs). 2021. https://guides.libraries.uc.edu/igos. Accessed 15 June 2021.
8. Frandsen G. Guide to nongovernmental organizations for the military. Lawry L, ed. 2009. https://fas.org/irp/doddir/dod/ngo-guide.pdf. Accessed 5 May 2021.
9. Military Sealift Command, MSC Public Affairs. Hospital ships T-AH. 2020. https://www.navy.mil/Resources/Fact-Files/Display-FactFiles/Article/2232638/hospital-ships-t-ah/. Accessed 7 May 2021.
10. Surface Warfare Medical Institute. Fleet medicine pocket reference 2016. 2016. https://www.med.navy.mil/sites/nmotc/swmi/Documents/Fleet%20Medcal%20Pocket%20Reference.pdf. Accessed 5 May 2021.
11. Paine GF, Bonnema CL, Stambaugh TA, Capacchione JF, Sipe PS. Anesthesia services aboard USNS COMFORT (T-AH-20) during operation Iraqi Freedom. Mil Med. 2005;170(6):476–82. https://doi.org/10.7205/milmed.170.6.476.
12. Dyer A. Hospital ship mercy returning to San Diego Friday after assisting Los Angeles' COVID-19 response. The San Diego Union-Tribune. https://www.sandiegouniontribune.com/news/military/story/2020-05-14/hospital-ship-mercy-returning-to-san-diego-friday-after-assisting-los-angeles-covid-19-response. Published May 14, 2020. Accessed 7 May 2021.
13. USNS Mercy, USNS Comfort: 2020 COVID-19 Deployment. America's Navy. 2020. https://www.navy.mil/Resources/Blogs/Detail/Article/2268233/usns-mercy-usns-comfort-2020-covid-19-deployment/. Accessed 7 May 2021.
14. Russell M. Pacific partnership 2011 advanced echelon team making final preparations in Vanuatu. Defense visual information distribution service. 2011. https://www.dvidshub.net/news/69351/pacific-partnership-2011-advanced-echelon-team-making-final-preparations-vanuatu. Accessed 7 May 2021.

15. Norris EA, Johnson MS, Mann KE, Pryor HI. Evaluation of surgical caseload aboard the USNS COMFORT (T-AH 20) during enduring promise 2018. Mil Med. 2020;185(3-4):325–7. https://doi.org/10.1093/milmed/usz416.
16. Hartgerink BJ, Chapman LE, Stevenson J, Donahue TF, Pagliara C. Utilization of surgical resources during the USNS COMFORT humanitarian mission to the Americas, June to October 2007. Mil Med. 2010;175(9):638–46. https://doi.org/10.7205/milmed-d-09-00162.
17. Lagrew J, Lujan E, Nelson SC, et al. Pacific partnership 2010: anesthesia support aboard the USNS Mercy humanitarian civic assistance. Mil Med. 2012;177(8):939–46. https://doi.org/10.7205/milmed-d-12-00044.
18. King HC, Bouvier M, Todd N, et al. Shipboard global health engagement missions: essential lessons for military healthcare personnel. Mil Med. 2019;184(11-12):e758–64. https://doi.org/10.1093/milmed/usz113.

Further Reading

Department of Defense Instruction 2205.02: humanitarian and civic assistance (HCA) activities. Effective June 23, 2014. Updated May 22, 2017.
Department of Defense Instruction 2000.30: global health engagement (GHE) activities. Effective July 12, 2017.
Joint Publication 3-29: foreign humanitarian assistance. May 14, 2019.

Chapter 33
Disaster Relief: Lessons Learned

Alfred F. Shwayhat, Daryl B. Fick Jr, Shane Jensen, Matthew D. Tadlock, and Mark S. Johnson

You heard the noise under the ground and its shaking and shaking, and everybody started running. Houses were falling and falling, all the fences were falling, people were falling, people were crying.

Frantz Forestal, survivor of the 2010 Haiti earthquake [1]

Author deployment experience	
Alfred F. Shwayhat	Flight Surgeon, 11th Marine Expeditionary Unit, Air Combat Element, Medium Marine Helicopter Squadron 165 (REIN) embarked on the USS Peleliu (LHA-5), Operation Interfet, East Timor, 1999
	Staff Internist, USNS Comfort (T-AH-20), Partnership for the Americas, Belize, Colombia, Ecuador, El Salvador, Guatemala, Guyana, Haiti, Nicaragua, Panama, Peru, Trinidad and Tobago, and Suriname, 2007
	Senior Medical Officer, Carrier Strike Group One, USS Carl Vinson (CVN-70), Operation Unified Response, Haiti, 2010
	Wing Surgeon, 3rd Marine Aircraft Wing, Marine Corps Air Station, San Diego, California, 2018–2021
	Force Surgeon, Naval Air Forces, Coronado, California, 2021–present

A. F. Shwayhat (✉) · D. B. Fick Jr
Naval Air Forces, Coronado, CA, USA
e-mail: alfred.shwayhat@navy.mil; daryl.b.fick@navy.mil

S. Jensen
Joint Trauma System, San Antonio, TX, USA
e-mail: shane.d.jensen6.mil@health.mil

M. D. Tadlock
Department of Surgery, Naval Medical Center San Diego, San Diego, CA, USA

M. S. Johnson
Navy Medicine Readiness and Training Command Portsmouth, Portsmouth, VA, USA
e-mail: mark.s.johnson9.mil@health.mil

M. D. Tadlock, A. A. Hernandez (eds.), *Expeditionary Surgery at Sea*,
https://doi.org/10.1007/978-3-031-21893-4_33

Author deployment experience	
Daryl B. Fick Jr.	Flight Surgeon, Carrier Air Wing 14 (CVW-14), embarked on the USS Ronald Reagan (CVN-76), 2008-2009; WESTPAC, INDOPACOM Area of Responsibility; supporting Humanitarian Aid Disaster Relief (HADR) operations following Typhoon Fengshen, Philippines, 2008; Operation Enduring Freedom, Afghanistan, 2009
	Lead Internist, Expeditionary Medical Team Mike (EMF-M), COVID-19 Medical Response, Louisiana, USA, 2020
Shane Jensen	Battalion Surgeon, 3rd Battalion 3rd Marines, Operation Iraqi Freedom, Karma and Al Taqaddum, Iraq, 2006–2009
	Resident Surgeon, USNS Mercy (T-AH-19), Pacific Partnership, Vietnam and Cambodia, 2012
	Ship's Surgeon, USS Ronald Reagan (CVN-76), WESTPAC, INDOPACOM Area of Responsibility, 2014–2015
	Staff Trauma/Critical Care Surgeon, USNS Comfort (T-AH-20), supporting Humanitarian Aid Disaster Relief (HADR) operations following Hurricane Maria, Caribbean, 2017
	Chief of Trauma, Tango Rotation Multinational Medical Unit (MMU), NATO Role 3 Kandahar Airfield, Kandahar, Afghanistan, 2018–2019
Matthew D. Tadlock	Flight Surgeon, Carrier Air Wing Three (CVW-3), embarked on the USS Harry S. Truman (CVN-75) in support of Operation Iraqi Freedom, Fifth Fleet Area of Responsibility, 2004–2005; supporting Humanitarian Aid Disaster Relief (HADR) operations following Hurricane Katrina, 2005
	Resident Surgeon, USNS Mercy (T-AH-19), Pacific Partnership, Micronesia and Papua New Guinea, 2008
	Ship's Surgeon, USS Carl Vinson (CVN-70), WESTPAC, INDOPACOM Area of Responsibility, 2011–2012
	Officer in Charge, Forward Resuscitative Surgical System/Shock Trauma Platoon, Charlie Surgical Company, Native Fury, CENTCOM Area of Responsibility, 2016
	Chief of Trauma, NATO Role 3 Multinational Medical Unit, NATO Resolute Support and Operation Freedom's Sentinel, Kandahar Airfield, Afghanistan, 2017–2018
	Staff Surgeon, Expeditionary Resuscitative Surgical System Pacific, 2019–2020; Provided embarked Role 2 Surgical Support, INDOPACOM Area of Responsibility, 2020
Mark S. Johnson	Staff Surgeon, Fleet Surgical Team-4, embarked on the USS Kearsarge (LHD-3), Operation Inherent Resolve, Fifth Fleet Area of Responsibility, 2015–2016
	Staff Surgeon, Role 2 Light Maneuver JMAU Augment, 2016–2017; Provided embarked Role 2 Surgical Support, AFRICOM Area of Responsibility, 2016–2017
	Staff Surgeon, USNS Comfort (T-AH-20), Operation Continuing Promise, Columbia, Ecuador, Peru, Honduras, 2018
	Director of Surgical Services, USNS Comfort (T-AH-20), Operation Enduring Promise, Panama, Columbia, Peru, Costa Rica, Honduras, Grenada, Saint Lucia, Saint Kitts and Nevis, Trinidad and Tobago, Dominican Republic, Jamaica, Haiti, 2019
	Director of Surgical Services, USNS Comfort (T-AH-20), Operation Gotham, New York City, NY, USA, 2020

BLUF (Bottom Line Up Front)

1. Humanitarian Assistance and Disaster Relief (HADR) operations are the second most common of U.S. Navy executed missions, only superseded by wartime missions. The majority of HADR missions are unplanned due to the spontaneity of natural disasters.
2. When responding to an earthquake-specific HADR, prepare for high demand and medical necessity of orthopedic and trauma surgeons, critical care specialists, critical care registered nurses (CCRNs), and corpsmen.
3. On an aircraft carrier, the standard number of pre-assigned medical personnel is not sufficient to handle a simultaneous HADR mission and a ship mass casualty event. Thus, it has to be supplemented like when the USS Carl Vinson (CVN-70) responded to the Haiti 2010 HADR and was supplemented by Fleet Surgical Team-2 (FST-2).
4. Anticipate a twofold increase in disease and non-battle injury (DNBI) clinic visits from military personnel that are deployed to an HADR mission.
5. On a warship it is imperative to identify, screen, enroll, and drill at least 10% of the ship's Sailors into the Walking Blood Bank (WBB) program PRIOR TO DEPLOYMENT. The USS Carl Vinson (CVN-70) activated the WBB an unprecedented five times during the Haiti 2010 HADR.
6. Recognition and understanding of cultural differences and providing clear communication are key foundational principles to successful medical care at a foreign HADR location. Expedite identification of individuals who can provide translational services between relief medical personnel and foreign HADR patients.
7. Ship line/combatant leaders are expected to take the lead of these HADR missions, but training and experience are sparse and sharply contrast with conventional preparation for other conflictual engagements across the globe. Therefore, ship line/combatant and medical leaders must receive standardized training in HADR missions.
8. DO NOT apply the same risk aversion in a disaster relief situation as in a humanitarian assistance mission because they are different. However, they are the same in that every effort needs to be made to maintain the highest standard of care that will be supported by the local system.
9. Aircraft carrier or hospital ship, ACTUAL bed capacity is dependent on patient type, acuity, and manning. Long-term holding capability has severe limitations in both medical and surgical settings.
10. Depending on the region being served, disaster relief missions are less predictable than humanitarian assistance missions. Having surgeons and anesthesiologists who are dual-hatted surgical critical care specialists embarked on hospital ships builds a deeper bench for contingencies.

11. The supporting unit doesn't define what is helpful. Sometimes things that would be considered inappropriate under regular standards of care are what the system needs during a disaster response. Find a way to get to "yes" within the current crisis standards of care.
12. Crisis response manning and standards of care are hard to adapt when goals are not discussed ahead of time.
13. Hospital ships, while broadly capable, require careful consideration of both limitations and strengths when employed outside of their primary combat casualty care mission.
14. Presume there will be critically ill patients; therefore, continuous renal replacement therapy (CRRT) capability is a MUST on hospital ships. The USNS Comfort (T-AH-20) has rectified this and now CRRT capability is standard on all missions.

Introduction

The majority of Humanitarian Assistance and Disaster Relief (HADR) operations involve spontaneous natural disasters that are initially attended to by the closest United States (U.S.) Navy assets. On any given day, there are approximately 100 U.S. ships dispersed throughout the world's oceans [2]. This sets the stage for the U.S. Navy to be geographically poised close to any natural disaster anywhere in the world. Within hours or days, the U.S. Navy can arrive at the coastline of the distressed nation and commence time-critical HADR operations and support. The most likely initial responder to a humanitarian crisis will be a U.S. Navy strike group with its nuclear-powered aircraft carrier and smaller cohort of ships, as was the case of Carrier Strike Group One (CSG-1) embarked on the USS Carl Vinson (CVN-70) during the 2010 Haiti earthquake.

In addition to geographical proximity, another fundamental influence for U.S. Navy HADR missions presented itself in the 2007 Cooperative Strategy for twenty-first-century Seapower. Among the six core capabilities for U.S. Seapower was definitive responses of HADR missions [3]. The circumstances that likely influenced this new strategy stemmed from the humanitarian deployments of the USNS Mercy (T-AH-19) and USNS Comfort (T-AH-20); specifically, Operation Unified Assistance in 2004 was the U.S. military's humanitarian response to the tsunami that struck Northern Indonesia – the deadliest natural disaster to occur worldwide between the years 1980 and 2019.

After 2004 the precedent had been set, and since then the USNS Mercy (T-AH-19) and USNS Comfort (T-AH-20) have participated in regularly scheduled humanitarian missions. For both of these floating hospital ships, the emphasis on HADR missions focused on medical and dental missions planned months to years in advance. However, their scheduled elective humanitarian missions are an overall minority of HADR operations of the U.S. Navy, since the majority of HADR missions are unplanned due to the spontaneity of natural disasters. The short time course to prepare introduces a dynamic number of challenges for the initial military responders to unplanned HADR missions.

The U.S. Navy response to HADR operations is largely dependent upon the capabilities of the ship(s) that arrive at the scene of the humanitarian disaster. The principal strengths of the U.S. Navy response to HADR operations include the capability to provide supplies, clean water, search and rescue, medical and surgical support and treatment, berthing, and personnel support and to do all this with unmatched speed and rapidity. How this unfolds and what burdens are placed on the ship are universally related to the scope and size of the mission.

The dynamic challenges can be understood, and some lessons can be taken through the review of experiences and medical lessons learned of the USS Carl Vinson (CVN-70) medical response to the earthquake in Haiti in 2010 and the USNS Comfort (T-AH-20) responses to Hurricane Maria in Puerto Rico in 2017 and the coronavirus disease 2019 (COVID-19) pandemic in New York City in 2020.

The Earthquake Heard Around the World: Haiti 2010

On the morning of January 12, 2010, the USS Carl Vinson (CVN-70) quietly departed Norfolk, VA, with Commander, Carrier Strike Group One (CSG-1), Commander, Destroyer Squadron One (CDS-1), and Commander, Carrier Air Wing Seventeen (CVW-17) and set out for its deployment around the Horn of South America for a planned homeport change to San Diego, CA. More than two thirds of the medical department's crew were about to undertake their first deployment. Not one had previously served aboard an aircraft carrier and shipboard experience was rare. The ship's medical ward, intensive care unit (ICU), and operating room (OR) had not been used since 2005. The Walking Blood Bank (WBB) was non-existent until immediately prior to the deployment when it was established. On January 12, 2010, at 16:53 local time, a 7.0 magnitude earthquake occurred 16 miles west of Port au Prince, Haiti. Within 48 hours of departing Norfolk, the USS Carl Vinson (CVN-70) received instruction to divert from its deployment and steam at high speed to Port au Prince Harbor. The medical department would soon find itself on the forefront of Operation Unified Response (OUR) and projected to all major television networks and newspapers in 144 countries worldwide [4].

The international response to the 2010 Haiti earthquake included the U.S. military's largest humanitarian effort to date. The catastrophic earthquake accounted for the fourth-highest death toll (316,000 individuals) of all natural disasters to occur throughout the world since 1900 [5]. The robust U.S. naval response to the 2010 Haiti earthquake did not come as a surprise. HADR operations are the second most common of U.S. Navy executed missions, only superseded by wartime missions [6]. This is also not surprising since 44% of the world's population is within 150 kilometers of the coast [7].

Medical Capability Limitations of a US Aircraft Carrier

Humanitarian disasters often fall into one of several categories: geophysical (earthquakes and tsunamis), meteorological (storms and typhoons), hydrological (floods and storm surges), and biological (epidemics and infestations). Disease and injury types that evolve after commencement of the disaster have historically been consistent and predictable, depending on the humanitarian disaster category. For example, after an earthquake occurs, the most common initial injuries are traumatic injuries, often of the lower extremities. This is subsequently followed by infection, predominantly respiratory and digestive diseases.

After the 2010 Haiti earthquake, the most common immediate injuries were not surprisingly injuries of the lower legs, ankle, and foot (36%). This was followed by head injuries (18%) and then abdomen, lower back, lumbar spine, pelvis, and thigh injuries (15% combined) [8]. The traumatic injuries overwhelmingly necessitated medical care within hours to a few days, whereas infectious diseases typically followed an increasing incidence trajectory over days to weeks after the initial earthquake. The cohort of patients that were treated on the USS Carl Vinson (CVN-70) paralleled this blueprint, with an influx of patients with traumatic injuries in the first few days after arrival to the Port au Prince Harbor.

The surge medical capabilities of the USS Carl Vinson (CVN-70) response to 2010 Haiti earthquake initially rested squarely upon the routinely assigned medical personnel. An aircraft carrier's medical department is ideally staffed at a ratio of one corpsman per 150 Sailors and one physician per 1200 Sailors. A typical medical department onboard a deployed US aircraft carrier consists of approximately 50–70 personnel (Table 33.1). This manning accounts for the treatment of routine medical care for 5000+ Sailors on board. It also factors for a mass casualty incident (MCI) on the carrier, such as an aircraft mishap with multiple flight deck injuries. However, the calculus of this equation changed once the USS Carl Vinson (CVN-70) assumed

Table 33.1 Number and type of medical staff on board a US aircraft carrier

# of staff	Medical position description
5	Physicians: 1 senior medical officer (SMO), 1 general surgeon, 1 family medicine physician, and 2 flight surgeons
5	Dentists: 1 oral surgeon and 4 general dentists
1	Physician assistant
1	Independent duty corpsman (IDC)
1	Medical administrative officer (MAO)
1	Radiation health officer (RHO)
1	Psychologist
1	Anesthesia provider
1	Physical therapist
1	Critical care registered nurse (CCRN)
50	Corpsmen (including 1 radiology technician, 2 laboratory technicians, 2 radiation health technicians, 2 surgical technologists (STs), 4 dental technicians)

operations for medical support for Haiti on January 16, 2010. The carrier medical department, without immediate personnel augmentation, was expected to medically flex its capabilities. The mission was to treat any and all Haitian casualties that were brought to its deck in addition to its baseline carrier medical responsibilities. Upon arrival at Port au Prince Harbor, the USS Carl Vinson (CVN-70) was advertised as the only Level II medical/surgical facility available in theater. A higher level of care would not be present until the arrival of the tasked USS Bataan (LHD-5) Amphibious Ready Group and USNS Comfort (T-AH-20), arriving on January 18, 2010, and January 20, 2010, respectively.

The USS Carl Vinson (CVN-70) did have the fortune of receiving an augment team on January 19, 2010, from Fleet Surgical Team-2 (FST-2) that consisted of four individuals: a general surgeon, certified registered nurse anesthetist (CRNA), critical care registered nurse (CCRN), and surgical technologist (ST). Their arrival could not have been more timely, as that same day, an influx of 29 patients were received in a single five-hour period, all with multiple injuries, open fractures, wounds, and illnesses. The patient ages ranged from a two-hour-old infant to a 78-year-old man. Despite the medical augmentation from FST-2, the ship's medical capability still fell short in several ways: an absence of orthopedic and trauma surgeons and critical care specialists, deficient numbers of critical care nursing staff and corpsmen, lack of adequate supplies (i.e., antibiotic therapy), and limited medical space capacity (one OR and three ICU beds).

The benefit of orthopedic and trauma surgeons, critical care specialists, and additional medical support staff (nursing, corpsmen) as part of the initial medical response after an earthquake disaster cannot be overemphasized. The additional staff helps balance the anticipated medical demand signal for traumatic injuries and post-injury critical care, prevents medical personnel fatigue/burnout, and bolsters patient continuity of care. When the USS Carl Vinson (CVN-70) received its initial seven casualties, the surgery team (with only one general surgeon) spent a total of 40 hours operating within a consecutive 48-hour time frame. Two days later, after the additional 29 casualties were received within five hours, only two CCRNs were on hand to provide care for over 30 critical patients. Many of these patients necessitated time-intensive medical care, far exceeding a commonly accepted civilian ICU 1:2 nurse-to-patient ratio. Compounding the challenge was a shortage of medical staff that had prior inpatient experience or significant critical care experience.

In 2010, Navy medicine had not yet implemented the concept of pre-assigned deployment teams, now known as "platforms." The absence of pre-identified medical staff responding to a humanitarian crisis resulted in a time-intensive and laborious process of real-time identification of available individuals to deploy. This process unsurprisingly resulted in deployment delay (often up to several days) of a shore-based medical team to help with HADR missions. At present time, the Navy now assigns medical personnel to specific platforms. As a result, recall of medical personnel to an HADR platform can be performed within 48 h.

In anticipation of a future U.S. Navy HADR medical response to an earthquake, an advanced medical support team can be sent to the responding U.S. aircraft carrier/amphibious assault ship. This medical support team can be sourced from the hospital ship that will ultimately be sent to the HADR location. This shore-based advanced medical team will then transition from the U.S. aircraft carrier/amphibious assault ship to the hospital ship once it arrives on scene. This will bolster patient continuity of care by making transitions of care seamless, as the advanced medical care team will already be familiar with the current cohort of admitted patients.

Although the discussion of the shore-based advanced medical support team included orthopedic and trauma surgeons, critical care specialists, CCRNs, and corpsmen, there are additional critical personnel to be considered. This includes a trained and experienced supervisor to lead the medical effort, a wound care specialist, mental health outreach team, and an infectious disease provider, to name a few. Such proactive bolstering of medical personnel will help reduce the chance that insufficient numbers of medical personnel are the rate-limiting factor to provide initial earthquake HADR medical care.

In hindsight, these aforementioned medical and surgical specialists and additional medical support staff should have been a part of the supplemental medical team that arrived on January 19, 2010. Nonetheless, the Sailors on the USS Carl Vinson (CVN-70) planned appropriately, performed admirably, worked cohesively as a team, and overcame each unpredictable obstacle they encountered. Their unrelenting determination and exhaustive work made the USS Carl Vinson (CVN-70) medical response for Operation Unified Response (OUR) a success. Foresight to adequately bolster medical capability during the initial response with the goal to overshoot and not undershoot medical staff capability is key. **Underestimating the medical demand signal during an HADR mission is a serious and unfixable mistake that can lead to rationed care or no care at all.** Worst of all, this mistake can reduce the medical capability for U.S. Navy vessels to respond to a disaster involving their own personnel.

The USS Carl Vinson (CVN-70) medical department was able to manage the medical care workload between the Haitian casualties and the ship's Sailors. Fortunately, the demand for medical care from Sailors overall remained at its baseline prior to arrival to Port au Prince Harbor as no aviation or other carrier mishap occurred. However, if a ship MCI did occur during treatment of the Haitian casualties, the medical department would have been unlikely to be able to manage both medical crises. As mentioned earlier, a U.S. aircraft carrier medical department is staffed to take care of its Sailor complement and a single MCI (should it arise). The ship's medical department at its standard manning is not appropriately staffed to adequately treat two or more simultaneous MCIs.

Furthermore, an observational health surveillance study completed by the USNS Comfort (T-AH-20) in 2011 (during Operation Continuing Promise) demonstrated that clinic-based disease and non-battle injury (DNBI) rates during an HADR operation were more than two times higher than the rates observed in two non-HADR shipboard studies. The syndrome-specific leading causes of DNBI in order of decreasing prevalence were gastrointestinal, dermatologic, and respiratory conditions [9]. Accounting for up to a twofold increase in DNBI clinic visits from Sailors during an HADR operation provides clear anticipation of increased medical treatment needs for a ship's personnel. This calculus should factor into the number of shore-based medical personnel, supplies, and expertise to be requested by future HADR mission first responders.

What must remain cogent to the ship's Commanding Officer (CO) and Senior Medical Officer (SMO) is the acute awareness that a rapid U.S. Navy response to an HADR mission is filled with medical uncertainty. Daily deckplate reassessment of the ship's medical capacity and capability is a necessity and requires communication up the chain of command. This provides a venue to request more personnel and resources if needed. It also allows a ship's CO increased situational awareness of the HADR mission and opportunity to ensure the medical care needs of the ship's own Sailors can still be met.

Walking Blood Bank (WBB) Activation

Historically, activation of the WBB onboard an aircraft carrier is an infrequent event. Although no official repository of WBB activations is maintained, historical accounts from carrier SMOs prior to 2010 indicate that WBB activation occurs approximately once every 10 years during routine operations. During the 2010 Haiti HADR operation, the USS Carl Vinson (CVN-70) activated the WBB an unprecedented five times. In total, 20 units were drawn and 17 units administered to six critically ill patients [4].

Obligatory to the success of a WBB during deployment is identifying eligible donors prior to deployment. Scheduling WBB drives while pier-side can serve the dual function of screening individuals for the ship's WBB program while also providing local blood banks with a supply of fresh blood donations. At least 10% of the ship's crew should be registered for the WBB program. Given the frequency of rotating personnel, updated records and confirmation of active participants in the program are necessary before going underway. Please see Chap. 23 for more information on shipboard WBB. Once a ship has been given orders to respond to a HADR operation, a WBB simulation event prior to arrival to the HADR location must be performed. This will allow the program to improve upon inefficiencies and identify and act upon training deficiencies prior to a real-time WBB activation. Although there will always be an unknown number of injured casualties for the ship to prepare for, there is no ambiguity that an earthquake HADR will obligate activation of the ship's WBB.

Translation Challenges

Within the USS Carl Vinson (CVN-70) Medical Department After Action Report (AAR), "necessity for effective communication" was one of the top-mentioned lessons learned for all medical staff. It is of no surprise that effective communication was deemed an essential requirement. After all, the U.S. National Patient Safety

Goals have consistently declared "Improving the effectiveness of communication among caregivers" as a top priority [10].

However, communication on a U.S. aircraft carrier's medical department in a foreign port is fundamentally different when compared to a U.S. land-based hospital. The main reason is that English may not be the primary language of the affected nation and routine access to remote translation services, such as phone or video conference, is likely non-existent. In the case of OUR, two languages were spoken in Haiti – Creole and French – with 95% of Haitians speaking Creole as their primary language [11]. The only language translation resources available came directly from the 30 Sailors stationed onboard the ship who were identified and spoke French, Creole, or a combination of both. Their language skills were paramount to providing accurate medical histories, explanation of care, and much needed comfort and compassion to the Haitian casualties. In one case, a woman with a severe and infected pelvic fracture initially refused treatment due to religious beliefs. The family practice physician worked closely with her with the aid of a translator. Effective communication gave the patient a better understanding of the situation, and she ultimately accepted treatment [4].

For any U.S. military force responding to a humanitarian crisis, immediate recognition and identification of translational services is paramount. If no such assisting personnel can be identified on the responding Navy vessel(s), urgency in obtaining this capability is recommended.

Absence of Training Requirements for Leaders

The US Navy/Marine Corps prepares for war and threats of any possible type magnificently. However, while their Maritime Strategy has included HADR missions for two decades, billeting for SMOs of aircraft carrier-based or any other sea-based platform does not include required training for these missions. Furthermore, the overall commanders of these missions are expected to come from the senior ranks of the line officers who are present, but formal preparation for these missions is sparse or non-existent in their training. The nature of HADR missions differs significantly from conventional preparation for conflicts or combat at sea and requires a rapid and seamless shift in paradigm from the medical department being the supporting element to being supported.

Supply Reconnaissance

Supply problems at sea have been around since antiquity. It is essential to have a supply management system already in place before any voyage, with channels and contacts for activation established and supplies frequently monitored for currency. Sole reliance on required protocols and supply lists like the Authorized Medical

Allowance List (AMAL) prior to the ship's projected voyage does not incorporate the most recent medical intelligence at various points along the ship's projected voyage. A HADR mission might not always be predicted, but medical intelligence reports from the region the ship will be voyaging can provide some information on requirements of a disaster relief operation if one were to occur.

For example, the USS Carl Vinson (CVN-70) Medical Department assured the AMAL requirements were met prior to her voyage around the Horn of South America, but obtained additional supplies prior to her voyage based on medical intelligence reports they reviewed. As a result, supplies not listed in the AMAL, such as N95 masks and intravenous (IV) medication for cerebral malaria, were added to the USS Carl Vinson (CVN-70) medical supply inventory and were ultimately utilized in Port au Prince Harbor to treat two patients diagnosed with cerebral malaria [4].

The "Apocalyptic [12]" Aftermath of Hurricane Maria: Puerto Rico 2017

In September 2017 the Category 5 storm Hurricane Maria devastated the Caribbean, and on September 20, 2017, it made landfall in Puerto Rico. The local emergency response and healthcare systems were already hampered by the response and recovery from previous storms and the subsequent flooding and landslides that severely damaged the local infrastructure and power grid. On September 24, 2017, the Governor of Puerto Rico estimated the damage to be over eight billion dollars. The USNS Comfort (T-AH-20) was activated to provide a 250 bed, Role 3 hospital in support of the Federal Emergency Management Administration (FEMA) and Health and Human Services (HHS) response to the disaster [13]. The USNS Comfort (T-AH-20) was ready and manned to deploy 40 hours after receiving notification and set sail on September 29, 2017, with 241 total clinical and supporting personnel. During the Hurricane Maria response, a total of 170 surgical procedures were performed on the USNS Comfort (T-AH-20), and 53 were considered emergent [13].

Humanitarian Assistance Versus Disaster Relief

While HADR missions are often discussed together, humanitarian assistance and disaster relief are two different missions. Humanitarian and Civic Assistance (HCA) missions are elective and pre-planned, designed to build upon international partnerships, promote global stability and security, maintain the operational readiness of military medical personnel, and facilitate interoperability with host and partner nations during crisis response. Generally during elective hospital ship-based HCA missions, the surgical care provided is often limited due to either mission time constraints or the inability to provide appropriate patient follow-up care in the host nation when the hospital ship leaves. Therefore saying "no" to performing certain operations is prudent if postoperatively there is a high likelihood of having a bad complication or poor outcome. Performing complex operations that require complicated long-term follow-up care does not help the host nation and ultimately can cause harm by creating a larger problem if the local system cannot address it (see Chaps. 32 and 36). During elective HCA missions, the operative volume can be high over a short period of time; however, they tend to be low risk, predominantly outpatient surgeries [14].

However, this posture is different during disaster relief missions. Often under these circumstances, the local healthcare systems, which may or may not share the same standards of care as the U.S., are overwhelmed from loss of infrastructure, lack of expertise, or sheer volume of patients exceeding their capacity. This was the case in Puerto Rico after Hurricane Maria in 2017. Greater risk acceptance is paramount when there are no other options. While the mission should do all within available means to uphold the U.S. standard of care, especially when responding within the U.S., crisis standards may need to be implemented as needed but with caution. Two such cases performed during this mission capture this challenge.

Clinical Vignette 33.1

A 30-year-old male presented with tachycardia, fever, borderline hypotension, leukocytosis, and peritonitis. A computed tomography (CT) scan was performed after resuscitation. The patient had splenomegaly with central necrosis and air consistent with an abscess, as well as poorly defined borders at the splenic flexure of the colon and greater curvature of the stomach. It was unclear if the patient had a gastric, colon, or splenic neoplasm, all of which would typically require further workup. He reported multiple trips to local hospitals and had either grown impatient from the wait times or was given antibiotics and discharged without any imaging studies; his experience was likely due to the overwhelmed system and the difficulty performing imaging due to intermittent power outages and the sheer volume of patients. Unfortunately, his delayed presentation due to poor access to care meant he was now presenting with uncontrolled abdominal sepsis. His case was discussed among the surgeons. There was reluctance by some to proceed with surgery, with the concern that if it was a gastric cancer, the resection required may be more than can be handled on the ship or that he would benefit from neoadjuvant treatment under normal standards. However, the decision was made to take him urgently to the OR for source control of his worsening sepsis. At operation there was an enlarged spleen with fistulous connections to both the splenic flexure and the greater curve of the stomach. An en bloc resection was performed with splenectomy, resection of the splenic flexure, and wedge resection of the stomach, with primary anastomosis of the colon. The patient recovered from surgery and by postoperative day #5 was meeting traditional discharge criteria. However, he remained on board an additional week until the pathology results were back; the pathologist on board sent the specimen back to Naval Medical Center Portsmouth due to the limited staining ability available on the ship. The patient had a B-cell lymphoma. This was disclosed to the patient, and he remained on board until one of the physicians, who happened to be a hematologist, was able to secure follow-up for the patient with a local hematologist on the island and communicate the final pathology results for the required follow-up care.

This case highlights the complex pathology that may present during either elective humanitarian mission or disaster relief missions in regions with limited resources. It also highlights an advanced surgical case that might not be appropriate during an elective humanitarian mission where follow-up care may not be able to be set up before the mission ends. However, during a crisis response in a region with an overwhelmed system, not caring for this patient violates the principles of bioethics (see Chap. 36). The first priority is surgical control of sepsis and, after the dust settles, utilizing all available resources to ensure the best long-term care possible.

Clinical Vignette 33.2

A woman in her 60s with a 50-pack-year smoking history presented to a local hospital on the island with a ruptured abdominal aortic aneurysm (rAAA) on computed tomography angiogram (CTA). The local hospital requested assistance from the USNS Comfort (T-AH-20) because they were unable to find a vascular surgeon to support their hospital during the aftermath of Hurricane Maria. A board-certified vascular surgeon had serendipitously brought a few aortic grafts on the ship "just in case." The patient was transferred to the ship and presented tachycardic with mild hypotension. A repeat CTA was performed, showing that the extravasation seen on the local hospital CTA was worsening and that the aneurysm was immediately adjacent to the left renal artery making an endovascular approach impossible, even if it was available. The options were fixed wing transport to Continental US (CONUS) or open repair attempt on the USNS Comfort (T-AH-20). The concern with transport was that she could further rupture and die from hemorrhagic shock en route. It was explained as well that regardless, the intraoperative mortality in this situation was around 50% based on current literature. She chose to receive care on the hospital ship and was taken emergently to the OR with the vascular surgeon assisted by two trauma surgeons and one pediatric surgeon. The patient did well in surgery, there was minimal blood loss, and the case was performed without technical complication. She unfortunately had hypovolemic acute kidney injury due to her initial blood loss exacerbated by the requirement to briefly clamp her left renal artery while the graft was sewn into place; this could not be avoided based on her anatomy. Unfortunately, at the time the ship's ICU did not have the capability to perform continuous renal replacement (CRRT), only intermittent hemodialysis (IHD). From a hemodynamic standpoint, she could not tolerate IHD, and it was stopped multiple times, despite multiple attempts to minimize this effect. Ultimately, she progressed to multiple organ system dysfunction. However, during the 48-hour postoperative period, her family from across the island were able to make it on board the ship. Her husband and family elected to change her to a comfort care status. She ultimately passed on board the ship with her family by her side, who were grateful to have the opportunity to see her again before she passed away.

In a region without appropriate postoperative and follow-up care, this high-risk procedure most assuredly would not be performed during an elective humanitarian mission as the risks and follow-up care would be too much for the local system to absorb. It best exemplifies the difference in risk aversion between humanitarian and disaster relief missions. More importantly it highlights that sometimes the aid provided during a disaster isn't always life-saving but has the potential to offer comfort, dignity, and closure for families that might not be able to receive this level of compassionate care in an overwhelmed system.

This vignette also highlights that hospital ships, while broadly capable, still have limitations that land-based hospitals do not. There was no CRRT capability for this mission. The USNS Comfort (T-AH-20) has rectified this, and now CRRT capability is standard on all missions.

Intensive Care Unit (ICU) Care in a Unique Environment

The care provided to the patient in Clinical Vignette 33.2 was not unique during the USNS Comfort (T-AH-20) response to Hurricane Maria. The crew cared for 36 ICU patients with an average Acute Physiology and Chronic Health Evaluation (APACHE) II score of 30, predicting an overall mortality of 80%. However, the actual ICU mortality for this patient cohort was only 27% [13]. The USNS Comfort (T-AH-20) ICU was staffed by four critical care specialists, including three trauma/critical care surgeons and one anesthesia critical care physician. During the initial mission planning, this ICU staffing was intentional by the Director of Surgical Services (DSS) who believed that a trauma surgeon's expertise might be needed if large volumes of injured patients were going to be treated. A trauma/critical care surgeon can also help cover the general surgery call pool in addition to helping staff the ICU. The anesthesia provider also provided care in both the ICU and OR. Ultimately, few patients with trauma-related issues were cared for on the ship during the mission. However, the ICU, to include the nursing staff and the four critical care specialists with diverse clinical backgrounds, proved to be critical to the mission.

Disaster response teams may have predetermined notions of the kind of care they will provide during disaster relief. **However, since the primary mission is to assist the affected population *now* by supporting an overwhelmed healthcare system based on what it *needs*, "getting to yes" should be the primary response that any unit or platform should take when responding.** During the Hurricane Maria response, the request from the system was to offload their long-term ICU patients in order to make room for more acute patients.

Initially there were six patients, most of whom were admitted with acute exacerbations of their chronic medical conditions, including but not limited to congestive heart failure, chronic obstructive pulmonary disease, and myxedema coma. Most of these patients had evidence of chronic illness and required management of electrolyte abnormalities, input and output monitoring, and other bread-and-butter ICU care. While many of the smaller issues got solved, it became evident that many of the patients received during the mission were not going to get better from their underlying medical conditions. When the families were onboarded, many discussions were had regarding goals of care. In the vast majority of these cases, the families indicated that these conversations were not had previously. This highlights another unique and often overlooked gap in disaster response: in an overwhelmed system, often the most needed aspect of critical care is time-intensive family-centered discussions regarding long-term prognosis and goals of care. This is particularly relevant in a disaster relief setting with communication limitations where it is difficult to locate next of kin.

Additionally, these patients were not receiving a higher level of care on the USNS Comfort (T-AH-20) under traditional definitions, as they were transferred from a local ICU to the hospital ship ICU to create more critical care capacity within the local healthcare system. While some may think it inappropriate to transfer a patient without additional therapeutic options who is likely at the end of their life, this is what the local healthcare system *needed* at the time. If during a crisis response the local system cannot support the discussions and/or the time needed to address these issues, they still need to be done and are integral to the ethical practice of critical care medicine. Providing end-of-life care during this difficult time provides immeasurable value to the system, patients, and their families. Not all help is going to be heroic, but it can always be compassionate and dignified. During a disaster response, get to "yes" and provide the care that is needed.

Beware the Ides of March: The USNS Comfort Augments New York's Medical Care During the COVID-19 Pandemic

On January 9, 2020, the World Health Organization (WHO) announced the first 59 cases of a pneumonia-like illness from what is now called the COVID-19. By March 11, 2020, the WHO formally declared COVID-19 a global pandemic. On March 13, 2020 President Trump declared it a national emergency, unlocking billions of dollars of funding to fight the spread. On March 7, 2020, New York State Governor Cuomo declared a state disaster emergency because COVID-19 was rapidly becoming a crisis in the New York Metropolitan area. In March 2020, the USNS Comfort (T-AH-20) was in a maintenance availability phase. It was rapidly activated to respond to New York City to provide assistance in these early days of the COVID-19 global pandemic.

Activation Without Known Mission Causes Manning Shortages

There are significant challenges in maintaining a ready list of over 1000 personnel who can deploy on less than five days' notice to support hospital ship operations. The nature of the military is that in any large group, approximately 33% will be in transit at any given time, given that the average military member executes a

Permanent Change of Station (PCS) move every three years. This creates a large turnover of personnel, with multiple chains of command responsible for supporting such a large deployment effort. Although Navy medicine is well-equipped to support most key areas, there are some personnel shortages for which it is difficult to obtain sole sourcing from the local military medical treatment facility (MTF), requiring regional and occasionally worldwide support. Some of these critical support areas include hemodialysis technicians and pharmacists (as the Navy has few on active duty, relying instead on civilian MTF staffing for these positions) and critical care specialists (as they were in such high demand during the global pandemic response).

The standard personnel lists for the hospital ships consist of activation levels based on a theoretical bed capacity of 100, 250, 500, or 1000. These lists are based on the anticipated needs for the primary medical mission of Major Combat Operations or MCO (i.e., surgeons, anesthesia providers, nurses, corpsmen), as well as a large number of personnel needed to run the essential non-medical parts of the ship (e.g., galley, laundry, hotel services). These personnel augment the ship's permanent medical crew of 67, called Reduced Operating Status (ROS), who provide caretaker functions when the ship is not activated. For a typical humanitarian mission, the list is then tailored by the hospital ship mission planners, called Full Operating Status (FOS), in order to obtain the skills match needed for the mission at hand.

When the New York mission was assigned, the parameters for the response had not been set, as is typical for a rapidly evolving Disaster Support to Civil Authorities (DSCA) mission. By direction of the CO, the medical personnel list was tailored to reflect what was anticipated for an infectious disease outbreak. Rather than a surgically heavy response, requests were made to support an inpatient medical mission caring for large numbers of critically ill patients, including critical care specialists, CCRNs, internal medicine physicians, and the appropriate support personnel. At the time, all branches of the military were mobilizing rapidly in order to respond to the pandemic, creating multiple personnel shortages in key positions. Due to these shortages, the ship was staffed with a configuration more suited to the MCO mission, with many surgeons and anesthesiologists, both active duty and activated reservists.

The mission parameters were formulated en route to New York over a short transit period, during which the newly formed hospital ship crew also needed to practice for shipboard emergencies and mass casualties, which would shortly become a reality. Instead of multiple combat casualties, the USNS Comfort (T-AH-20) would be providing a mass casualty response in the form of rapid-fire ICU admissions of critically ill patients from the New York hospitals.

During April 2020, the USNS Comfort (T-AH-20) had the highest acuity level of any hospital in the Department of Defense, with a peak of 36 patients on ventilators. With so many critical patients and certain roles with limited numbers, provider and nurse fatigue was becoming a factor. There was also a limited supply of respiratory therapists, three pharmacists, and a single hemodialysis technician on board. During the first week, one of two critical care pulmonologists had to be isolated due to COVID-19 infection, causing an acute shortage in the most necessary physician specialty. Surgeons and anesthesiologists covered down, nurses cross trained on hemodialysis machines, and the midwife ran the casualty receiving operations to get critical patients safely aboard the ship.

Despite the non-MCO nature of the mission, over 110 surgical procedures were performed. The majority were bedside procedures such as tube thoracostomies, flexible endoscopy, and central venous catheter placement. In addition, there were several patients who failed nonoperative management of surgical conditions. There were nine operative wound debridements, seven tracheostomies, three colectomies, three cholecystectomies, two appendectomies, and five miscellaneous procedures, including a complex cranial reconstruction after a decompressive craniectomy for a COVID-19-related thrombotic cerebrovascular accident [15].

Medical Capability Limitations of a Hospital Ship

Although the hospital ships are described as having a capacity of 1000 beds, this is a vast oversimplification. Raw square footage of these vessels is 853,000 over a total of nine decks, which does not account for the ship's infrastructure (e.g., power plant, water production, waste processing). A shore hospital with 1000 bed capacity covers a footprint well over 1.5 million square feet.

The USNS Comfort (T-AH-20) has four ICUs, with a capacity of 20 beds each. The Post Anesthesia Care Unit (PACU) has an overflow capacity for an additional 20 critical care beds. Critical care beds are arranged around a post which contains AC power outlets, oxygen supply, and suction. The ship was initially planned for the much smaller footprint of hospital gurneys or litters rather than the large footprint requirements of a modern ICU bed, making the ship's ICU spaces quite tight. Additionally, the large number of accessory devices such as dialysis machines, infusion pumps, sequential compression devices, ventilators, and the beds themselves demands far more numerous power outlets than the 1980s era designers anticipated. While the ship's power supply is robust, power strips and surge protectors were at a premium in the ICU.

The ship has 12 ORs, one of which is equipped as an interventional radiology suite. There are eight inpatient wards configured as open bays with bunk beds. As configured, of the 1000 available patient beds, 600 are considered appropriate for "minimal care," which assumes a 20:1 patient/nurse ratio and requires that the patient be able to climb into the bed (some are 5 feet above the deck without a ladder). Oxygen delivery on the wards is via one K-type cylinder per four beds, with a single regulator. This required some creative modifications to the regulators whenever more than one patient in four required supplemental oxygen – a common scenario when treating patients affected by a respiratory virus outbreak like COVID-19.

Just-In-Time Supply Limitations

Another area leading to rate limitations was the supply chain. When the hospital ships were designed, medical warehouses with large quantities of supplies existed, and expiration dates were primarily for medications. Current supply systems depend on a demand signal from hospitals to maintain availability of just-in-time consumable goods. For example, if a hospital orders five sets of pressure tubing from a supplier every month, then a small surge in demand can be accommodated; if they suddenly order one thousand, the inventory just isn't there to be had. The hospital ships order very little from their suppliers most of the time until they are actually activated, at which time they order an entire hospital's worth of supplies. In 2020, because the USNS Comfort (T-AH-20) was in a maintenance availability phase, the USNS Mercy (T-AH-19) beat her out of the gate and took most of the available overstock (which was already in high demand from stressed civilian health organizations), complicating the demand problem. Modern critical care also requires many supplies which are outside of the MCO equipment lists, such as chronic wound care supplies, percutaneous tracheostomy sets, hemodialysis tunneled catheters and supplies, ICU supplies for prone positioning, and portable ultrasound machines.

Ongoing Mission Execution Adaptations and Limitations

The first goal during the New York City response was to avoid worsening the problem. Given the high prevalence of COVID-19 in the community, it was assumed that many patients who were thought to be uninfected would in fact be COVID-19 positive. Therefore, rapid testing was used prior to entry into the ship, to enable segregation into COVID-positive and COVID-negative wards. However, the suspicion of asymptomatic infection remained high, so that the terminology evolved to "COVID-ambiguous" rather than "COVID-negative."

Given the shared ventilation systems and close proximity of the crew, the recommendation was initially made for the hospital ship to be used to support overflow care of COVID-negative patients from the New York area. It quickly became apparent that this would not only be impractical due to the high prevalence of COVID-19 in the community, but it would also not meet the needs of the local health system. Therefore, within the first few days of arrival, the USNS Comfort (T-AH-20) began to take care of critical COVID-positive patients as well as "COVID-ambiguous" patients. Social distancing on the hospital ship while in operations was nearly impossible, particularly in the living areas. In order to avoid a large outbreak on board, the CO dispersed the crew, utilizing a local hotel to house medical personnel off the ship. In a disaster response which did not involve a novel infectious disease outbreak, this expensive move would not have been necessary, but in New York, it was critical to maintaining mission effectiveness.

By the end of April 2020, the crew had been operating continuously in the COVID-19 environment for a month, but they were starting to reach some of the limits of the platform. In particular, close proximity of patients in the ICU was becoming untenable; an outbreak of a nosocomial infection was traced to a single cluster of ICU patients, necessitating dispersal into overflow spaces. If there was a need to continue to operate continuously, this outbreak would have at best limited the holding capacity and at worst continued to spread throughout the already maximally utilized ICU. But just as suddenly as it began, it was over. Notification came that the USNS Comfort (T-AH-20) was no longer needed, patient transfers back into the local healthcare system began within 24 h, and they were completed within a few days.

Conclusions

HADR operations are the second most common U.S. Navy executed missions; therefore, it is likely that many surgical team members will be part of one during the course of their career. Disaster relief missions have many parallels to providing combat casualty care in an austere environment and tend to require a robust surgical and critical care capability. The most likely initial responder to a humanitarian crisis will be a U.S. Navy strike group. U.S. Navy hospital ships can be ideal Role 3 platforms to augment disaster relief efforts; however, there can be significant obstacles to provision of modern medical and surgical care outside of their primary capability. This chapter describes details, dynamic challenges, and lessons learned from the U.S. Navy's medical response to three different large-scale events including the catastrophic earthquake in the developing country of Haiti, the "Apocalyptic [12]" Hurricane Maria in Puerto Rico, and the COVID-19 pandemic in the New York Metropolitan healthcare system.

Declaration of Interest The views expressed in this chapter are those of the authors and do not necessarily reflect the official policy or position of the Department of the Navy, Department of Defense, nor the US Government.

Funding This research did not receive any specific grant from funding agencies in the public, commercial, or not-for-profit sectors.

Conflict of Interest Statement The authors declare no conflict of interest.

References

1. Sturcke J. Haiti earthquake: survivors' stories. The Guardian. 2010. https://www.theguardian.com/world/2010/jan/14/haiti-earthquake-survivors.
2. https://news.usni.org/2020/12/14/usni-news-fleet-and-marine-tracker-dec-14-2020.
3. Eden JG. The new maritime strategy – a change for greater relevance? U.S. Army War College. 2008.
4. Shwayhat AF. USS Carl Vinson (CVN-70) Medical Department Southern Seas 2010 Cruise Report. 2010.

5. Cecchine G, et al. The U.S. military response to the 2010 Haiti Earthquake. Rand Corporation. 2013.
6. Greenfield CM, Ingram, CA. An analysis of U.S. Navy humanitarian assistance and disaster relief operations. Calhoun Institutional Archive of the Naval Postgraduate School. 2011.
7. http://www.oceansatlas.org/subtopic/en/c/114/.
8. Kalantar Motamedi MH, Sagafinia M, Ebrahimi A, Shams E, Kalantar MM. Major earthquakes of the past decade (2000-2010): a comparative review of various aspects of management. Trauma Mon. 2012;17(1):219–29. https://doi.org/10.5812/traumamon.4519.
9. Chern A, McCoy A, Brannock T, Martin GJ, Scouten WT, Porter CK, Riddle MS. Incidence and risk factors for disease and non-battle injury aboard the hospital ship USNS COMFORT during a Humanitarian Assistance and Disaster Response Mission, Continuing Promise 2011. Trop Dis Travel Med Vaccines. 2016;2:7. https://doi.org/10.1186/s40794-016-0023-z.
10. National Patient Safety Goals. The Joint Commission. 2021. https://www.jointcommission.org/standards/national-patient-safety-goals/.
11. Chepkemoi J. What languages are Spoken in Haiti? World Atlas. 2019. https://www.worldatlas.com/articles/what-languages-are-spoken-in-haiti.html.
12. Chavez N. Hurricane Maria: Puerto Rico officials describe 'apocalyptic' conditions. CNN World. 2017. https://www.cnn.com/2017/09/24/americas/hurricane-maria-puerto-rico-aftermath/index.html.
13. USNS comfort (T-AH-20) official after action report to hurricane maria response: summary of findings.
14. Jensen S, Tadlock MD, Douglas T, Provencher M, Ignacio RC Jr. Integration of surgical residency training with US military humanitarian missions. J Surg Educ. 2015;72(5):898–903. https://doi.org/10.1016/j.jsurg.2014.12.004.
15. Worlton T, Uber I, Bronaugh S, Liedtke E, Dougherty J, Pinkos K, Weimerskirch B, Johnson M. USNS COMFORT (T-AH 20) surgical services response to the COVID-19 pandemic in New York City. Ann Surg. 2020;272(4):e269–71. https://doi.org/10.1097/SLA.0000000000004320.

Chapter 34
Children in an Operational Environment: Forward Surgical Teams Caring for Pediatric Patients

Robert L. Ricca and Pamela M. Choi

If the operation is difficult, you are not doing it properly.

Alberto Peña

Author deployment experience	
Robert L. Ricca	Ship's Surgeon, USS Harry S. Truman (CVN-75), Operation Enduring Freedom, Mediterranean Sea and Arabian Gulf, 2009–2010
	Role 2 Officer in Charge, Forward Surgical Element Tarin Kowt, Operation Enduring Freedom, Tarin Kowt, Afghanistan, 2013–2014
	Pediatric Surgeon, USNS Spearhead (T-EPF-1), Operation Continuing Promise, Honduras, Guatemala, 2018
Pamela M. Choi	Ship's Surgeon, USS Harry S. Truman (CVN-75), Operation Inherent Resolve, Sixth Fleet Area of Responsibility, 2017–2018

BLUF (Bottom Line Up Front)

1. Coordination with local host nation medical providers is of paramount importance when engaging in medical treatment with pediatric patients. This ensures a successful transition of care and allows for improved management of chronic medical conditions.
2. Intravenous (IV) access can be challenging in the pediatric population, but it is crucial. Plan ahead and have equipment for several options available.

R. L. Ricca (✉)
Prisma Health Upstate, Greenville, SC, USA
e-mail: robert.ricca@prismahealth.org

P. M. Choi
Navy Medicine Readiness and Training Command San Diego, San Diego, CA, USA
e-mail: pamela.m.choi.mil@health.mil

M. D. Tadlock, A. A. Hernandez (eds.), *Expeditionary Surgery at Sea*,
https://doi.org/10.1007/978-3-031-21893-4_34

3. Medication and fluid management in pediatric patients are weight-based. A Broselow tape can be used to provide a rapid estimate of weight based upon a child's length.
4. In children older than 6 months, alternate ibuprofen and acetaminophen postoperatively to maximize pain control and minimize the need for narcotics.
5. Initial fluid resuscitation in pediatric trauma patients is a single 20 mL/kg bolus of isotonic fluid followed by 10–20 mL/kg of packed red blood cells (PRBCs).
6. Balanced fluid resuscitation including PRBCs, fresh frozen plasma (FFP), and platelets is an integral part of pediatric massive transfusion protocol. Whole blood therapy is gaining favor for pediatric trauma patients at some centers.
7. Children should receive isotonic fluid as a maintenance fluid to prevent hyponatremia. Glucose should be monitored and dextrose can be added, especially for young or malnourished children.
8. Beware of hypotension in young children; cardiovascular failure may be imminent! Younger children tend to have a higher resting heart rate; therefore, they are dependent upon systemic vascular resistance.
9. Appropriate management of the pediatric airway is a skill required of all providers caring for children as the most common cause of cardiac arrest in pediatric patients is hypoxia.
10. Primary and secondary surveys in trauma are similar to adults with modifications for anatomic differences and Glasgow Coma Scale (GCS) evaluation.
11. When possible, consider a bowel anastomosis instead of a temporary ostomy as the child may not have the resources for ostomy management or the access to undergo ostomy reversal at a later date.
12. The World Health Organization (WHO) has published a ten-step algorithm for the routine care and treatment of severely malnourished children.
13. A transverse abdominal incision may provide greater exposure in pediatric patients less than 5 years of age.
14. Utilization of an appropriate size chest tube, drain, or urinary catheter is important due to anatomic restrictions. If the appropriate size is not available, different tubes can be used as long as they are the correct size.
15. Do not use mesh when treating pediatric hernias.
16. When treating routine abscess, make a counter incision and bring a vessel loop between these two incisions, and tie it to itself to act as a drain. Avoid large incisions and packing the wound, which can cause unnecessary pain for the child upon removal and be difficult for the families to remove and care for.

Introduction

Forward deployed surgical teams on land and sea that routinely care for adults may find themselves caring for pediatric patients as well, whether it is expected on an elective humanitarian mission or unexpected on a combat support mission. As the adage goes, children are not little adults. Therefore, surgeons and surgical teams need to be ready to care for them well, from gaining vascular access to give weight-based medications and resuscitation to managing the pediatric airway during a trauma to potentially having to have different approaches and incisions. This chapter will serve as a basis for the initial management of pediatric patients in a deployed environment.

Clinical Vignettes

Clinical Vignette 34.1

A 6-year-old male was brought to a Role 2 receiving area after sustaining multiple fragment wounds to the lower extremities due to an improvised explosive device (IED). The child had a partial amputation of the left foot as well as numerous penetrating wounds to both extremities. Tourniquets were applied to both extremities. What should be the initial management to stabilize this patient?

Clinical Vignette 34.2

A 5-year-old female was brought to the receiving area of an elective humanitarian mission for management of a prolapsed ostomy. The child was treated at a host nation hospital for a diagnosis of malrotation with an unknown surgical procedure resulting in an ostomy. The child was markedly malnourished, and a shopping bag was tied around her abdomen to act as an ostomy appliance. The family was asking for assistance in the long-term management of the ostomy.

These vignettes are real-world examples of pediatric patients that have been seen and evaluated by general surgeons and coalition forces in forward operational environments. A well-thought-out initial evaluation plan and resuscitation efforts can provide significant relief to the patient and the family. Coordination with host nation medical providers, including pediatricians and surgeons, is of utmost importance when caring for injured or ill children. This ensures continued management of long-term medical conditions (see Chaps. 32 and 33). Depending upon the mission type (e.g., humanitarian, disaster relief, or combat support), threat level, and security conditions, coordinating surgical management with local resources can offer an opportunity for information exchange with local host nation providers providing significant positive impact especially in humanitarian operations.

Intravenous Access

Vascular access in pediatric patients can be one of the most challenging requests of a pediatric surgeon. Despite the difficulty, vascular access is crucial to the initial resuscitation of a pediatric patient, and a well-thought-out plan is important before embarking upon efforts at vascular access. Ensuring the right equipment is available as well as determining potential second and third options for vascular access will greatly add to success.

For the vast majority of patients seen in a deployed or humanitarian environment, vascular access through the use of a peripheral intravenous (IV) catheter is sufficient for the initial treatment and resuscitation. Common locations for access include the back of the hand, the antecubital space, or the greater saphenous vein. The external jugular vein is easily seen in many pediatric patients and may also be a viable option. In infants, scalp veins may also serve as an option for catheter insertion. Typically, the veins in the leg do not increase in size until the child begins ambulating and therefore can be difficult to find in a small infant.

When placing an IV catheter, it is helpful to have assistance to restrain the patient and the extremity that is being accessed. It is important to pay close attention to the insertion as the "flash" that is seen at the point of entry into the vein may not be as readily apparent as it is in adults. The catheter should thread easily into the vein, and a peripheral flush should be immediately available to test for intraluminal placement. If there is edema present or difficulty flushing the line, then another site should be accessed.

Proper catheter size is vital to the success of catheter placement. Veins in infants will typically accept a 22- or 24-gauge catheter. Young children have veins that will typically allow for a 20- or 22-gauge catheter. Older children and adolescents typically have veins that will accept a 16- or 18-gauge catheter. Once access has been obtained, it is important to adequately secure the catheter with tape or tegaderm. A kerlix or conforming gauze wrapped around the extremity with an arm or leg board will assist with securing the device and ensuring that it does not become dislodged with patient movement.

An intraosseous (IO) line may also be placed if IV access cannot be established or if emergent access is indicated. IOs may be placed in infants as small as 3 kg (15 mm pink needle for 3–40 kg and 25 mm blue needle >40 kg). The best site is the anteromedial aspect of the tibia, 2–3 cm below the tibial tuberosity. An alternate site is the distal tibia, 3 cm proximal to the medial malleolus in the midline. Contraindications to IO placement include fractured/infected limb or prior IO needle insertion in previous 24 h in the same site. Fluids, medications, and blood may all be administered via IO access; however, IO needles are only intended for less than 24-hour use.

Common Medication Doses

Weight-based dosing is the current standard for prescribing all pediatric medications. An accurate weight is essential to appropriate dosing of medication. Children less than 6 months may receive acetaminophen postoperatively; children greater than 6 months may receive acetaminophen and ibuprofen. These medications may be alternated on a scheduled basis every 3 h for the first 48 h following surgery. Prescription oral narcotics are not needed in the vast majority of postoperative patients and should not be prescribed in children under 1 year of age.

The surgeon must recognize that many pediatric patients may only take medication in an elixir form. It is recommended that the surgeon review appropriate dosing guidelines prior to prescribing medication to ensure the appropriate dose. Below are some common medications typically prescribed to the pediatric surgical patient.

- Acetaminophen – 15 mg/kg/dose q6 hours (not to exceed 1000 mg/dose)
- Ibuprofen – 10 mg/kg/dose q6 hours (not to exceed 600 mg/dose)
- Morphine – 0.05 mg/kg IV q2 hours as needed for breakthrough pain
- Roxicodone – 0.1 mg/kg q6 hours as needed for breakthrough pain
- Bupivacaine 0.25% – volume limited to 1 mL/kg
- Bupivacaine 0.5% – volume limited to 0.5 mL/kg
- Ondansetron – 0.1 mg/kg/dose q6 hours (max dose 4 mg)
- Cefazolin – 30 mg/kg IV for perioperative dosing
- Piperacillin/tazobactam – 100 mg piperacillin/12.5 mg tazobactam per kg IV q8 hours (for children greater than 9 months and up to 40 kg)

Fluid and Blood Resuscitation

Fluid resuscitation in pediatric patients is also weight-based. If a weight is not available, use of their length with a Broselow tape or other similar tool can provide an estimate of their weight. Weight-based resuscitation is important for both traumatically injured children and for children who require routine medical or surgical care. The most recent Advanced Trauma Life Support (ATLS) guidelines recommend early intervention with blood products for the fluid management of a traumatically injured child. The initial treatment should be placement of two large-bore IV catheters. Initial fluid resuscitation should consist of an initial weight-based bolus of warmed isotonic crystalloid solution at 20 mL/kg. Following this, initiation of blood products is warranted using a balanced approach [1, 2]. These transfusions are also weight-based and should include the following:

- Packed red blood cells (PRBC) 10–20 mL/kg
- Fresh frozen plasma (FFP) 10–20 mL/kg
- Platelets 10–20 mL/kg

Whole blood has also been increasingly utilized and studied in the pediatric trauma population. Indeed, realistically whole blood may be all that is available in austere environments. Small cohort studies have demonstrated that whole blood may be safely given to children ≥1 year with a maximum dose of 40 mL/kg. Additionally, children who received whole blood had faster resolution of shock with decreased component transfusion [3, 4].

Children receiving IV fluids for maintenance therapy should receive an isotonic crystalloid solution. The authors prefer lactated ringers as it has a lower chloride level and does not usually lead to a metabolic acidosis that can be seen in children who receive large volume resuscitation with normal saline. To calculate the maintenance rate, use the 4:2:1 rule as follows:

1. For the first 10 kg–4 mL/kg
2. For the second 20 kg–add an additional 2 mL/kg
3. For anything above 20 kg–add an additional 1 mL/kg

Furthermore, one can provide gentle resuscitation in children by running maintenance fluids at higher than these calculated rates. For example, in children who present with acute dehydration from appendicitis or other surgical diseases, isotonic crystalloid fluid at 1.25× or 1.5× maintenance can be utilized for resuscitation. Young children should have dextrose added to the crystalloid solution as they may not have the glucose stores to maintain normoglycemia. Routine blood sugar checks are necessary in young children or those with concerns for malnourishment [5].

Pediatric Vitals

Normal vital signs vary by age in the pediatric patient. In general, younger patients tend to have a higher baseline respiratory rate and pulse and a lower baseline systolic blood pressure. Table 34.1 serves as a quick reference [2].

Young children have a higher resting heart rate which limits their ability to increase their heart rate to improve cardiac output. Young children therefore rely heavily upon systemic vascular resistance. Hypotension is therefore an ominous finding and suggests that cardiovascular failure may be imminent.

Table 34.1 Normal ranges for pediatric vital signs

Age	Pulse	Systolic BP (mmHg)	RR	Weight (kg)
0–6 months	110–160	70–90	25–40	4–6
6–12 months	90–140	80–100	25–40	6–10
1–3 years	80–130	90–110	20–30	10–13
3–6 years	70–120	95–115	20–30	13–20
6–12 years	60–110	100–120	15–25	20–40
>12 years	60–100	110–130	12–20	>40

BP blood pressure, *RR* respiratory rate

Anatomical Considerations

There are significant anatomic and physiologic differences that must be considered by the surgical team when caring for children. Most important is the anatomic difference of the pediatric airway. Appropriate management of the pediatric airway is a skill required of all providers caring for children as the most common cause of cardiac arrest in pediatric patients is hypoxia.

Differences in Airway

The anatomic differences in the pediatric patient are most pronounced in younger children. Children have a proportionately larger head compared to their body size with a prominent occiput. This creates a situation where the neck is flexed when the child is placed on a flat surface, increasing the risk of airway obstruction. This also makes alignment of the airway structures more difficult with laryngoscopy. A folded towel or sheet can be placed under the child's shoulder to relieve the obstruction and improve visualization during laryngoscopy. Children also have a relatively larger tongue that adds to the risk of obstruction. Other key anatomic differences include the fact that the airway in children is smaller in diameter and shorter in length when compared to adults. In children, the larynx is also located more anteriorly while the epiglottis is relatively long, floppy, and narrow.

Adequate mask ventilation is a fundamental maneuver. Head tilt, chin lift, and jaw thrust maneuvers can assist with the management during ventilation to overcome the anatomic variations listed above. Additionally, an appropriately sized oral airway can relieve the obstruction from the larger tongue. The size can be approximated by measuring from the anterior gum line to the angle of the mandible. Many children can be managed safely with bag-valve-mask (BVM) ventilation until an individual skilled in pediatric airways can assist. It is of utmost importance to ensure that a child can be safely ventilated using a mask prior to proceeding with a more advanced airway technique [6].

Other Key Anatomic Differences

- The sutures of the skull do not close until about 2 years of age. Evaluation for a bulging (increased intracranial pressure) or sunken (dehydration/malnutrition) anterior fontanelle is an important component of the physical exam in infants.
- Skull fractures with subgaleal hemorrhage in pediatric patients less than 18 months of age can lead to exsanguinating hemorrhage without significant external findings. Serial hemoglobin/hematocrit for 24 h to ensure stability is recommended.

- Children have a proportionately greater body surface area of the skin compared to adults. This can lead to increased heat loss and rapid hypothermia. Therefore, warming of the traumatically injured or critically ill child is important. Burns in children may also be more severe due to this increased body surface area as well as thinner subcutaneous tissue when compared to adults.
- The ribcage is more pliable. Pulmonary contusions may be present even in the absence of rib fractures. The presence of a rib fracture in a young child indicates a significant force was applied.
- The abdominal viscera is less well protected from blunt trauma due to a thin abdominal wall as well as exposed liver and spleen below the costal margin. Bruising or a "seatbelt sign" should raise a concern for intra-abdominal injury in pediatric patients.

Trauma in Pediatric Patients

Primary and Secondary Survey in Pediatric Patients

The primary and secondary survey of pediatric trauma patients is performed in a similar fashion to adults. Recognize the anatomic differences mentioned previously to assist with management and treatment of any abnormal findings. When evaluating the airway, remember that the child has a proportionately larger head and occiput that can lead to obstruction. Place a pad under the back so the patient can align the airway and prevent the flexion of the neck that would lead to airway obstruction. BVM ventilation is the first-line treatment of airway compromise in the pediatric patient. Prior to proceeding with a more advanced airway, ensure that the appropriate size endotracheal tube or laryngeal mask airway is present.

Cricothyroidotomy is usually not performed or required in young children. Typically it can be performed in children older than 12 who have reached adolescence and have a palpable cricothyroid membrane. Due to the high risk of injury to the larynx and surrounding structures, needle cricothyroidotomy is preferred in children younger than 12 years. The trachea is held in place, and the catheter is placed in the middle of the neck at the inferior margin of the cricothyroid member at an angle of 45° while directed caudally. The needle may be removed, and then the catheter may be connected to a bag valve mask.

Assessment of breathing is performed in a similar manner to adults. Again, recognize that the pediatric chest is extremely pliable and a significant force is required for rib fractures to occur; therefore, pulmonary contusions can still be present and clinically significant in the absence of rib fractures. Presently, if needle compression is required, ATLS recommends placement in the second intercostal space midclavicular line. Chest tubes are placed in the same location as adults, usually in the fifth intercostal space anterior to the midaxillary line. It is imperative to tunnel the chest tube due to the thin subcutaneous tissue in children. When evaluating both the airway and breathing of a traumatically injured child, it is important to remember, and to emphasize, **hypoxia is a leading cause of cardiac arrest in pediatric patients**.

Assessment of circulation is dependent upon ensuring appropriate size IV catheter placement, determining the weight of the patient (or using a tool such as a Broselow tape), providing appropriate resuscitation fluids, and determining end goals of resuscitation. Initial resuscitation is performed with an initial 20 mL/kg bolus of isotonic crystalloid solution followed by transfusion of blood products using a balanced weight-based resuscitation protocol. Urine output can be measured to assess resuscitation. Infants should have a urine output of 1–2 mL/kg/h. Toddlers and young children should have a urine output of 1–1.5 mL/kg/h. Teenagers should have a urine output of at least 0.5 mL/kg/h.

Thermoregulation is important in children, and they should be covered quickly to prevent hypothermia and insensible losses.

The secondary survey is also performed in a manner similar to that in adults and should encompass a head-to-toe examination. A chest X-ray as well as pelvis X-ray should be obtained in all trauma patients. Additionally, focused abdominal sonography for trauma (FAST) exams can be performed in children and are an excellent screening tool to determine if there is any sign of intra-abdominal bleeding [1, 2].

Traumatic Brain Injury (TBI) and Pediatric Glasgow Coma Scale (GCS)

Traumatic brain injury (TBI) is one of the most common injuries in the pediatric population, especially with blunt mechanisms to include falls, motor vehicle collisions, or child abuse. Children with TBI should be managed according to the primary and secondary survey previously described. Early recognition and prompt treatment of associated injuries are important due to the profound effect that hypoxia and hypotension have on secondary brain injury; attention to the airway and appropriate fluid resuscitation will improve long-term outcomes in children with TBI. Infrequently, infants can lose a significant volume of blood in the subgaleal space or in the intracranial space due to the open sutures. Assessment of the fontanelle and serial hemoglobins can assist in the evaluation and management of these children. For severely injured children, rapid consultation and evaluation by a neurosurgeon are warranted. Mannitol (1 g/kg) and hypertonic 3% normal saline (bolus 10 mL/kg, continuous infusion 1 mL/kg/h) can be used in the pediatric patient with TBI but should be done with consultation of a neurosurgeon.

When evaluating disability, the Glasgow Coma Scale (GCS) can be used in pediatric patients in a similar manner to adult patients with slight changes. The main variation is in the verbal score, which is dependent upon the age of the patient. Table 34.2 can assist with determining the GCS.

Table 34.2 Glasgow Coma Scale (GCS) for pediatric patients

Eye score	Age <1 year	Age >1 year
4	Spontaneously	Spontaneously
3	To shout	Verbal command
2	To pain	To pain
1	No response	No response

Verbal score	Age 0–2 years	Age 2–4 years	Age >4 years
5	Coos and smiles	Appropriate words	Converses/oriented
4	Cries but consolable	Inappropriate words	Disoriented
3	Inappropriate crying/ screaming	Crying/screaming	Inappropriate words
2	Grunts, restless, or agitated	Grunts, restless, or agitated	Inappropriate sounds
1	No response	No response	No response

Motor score	Age <1 year	Age >1 year
6	Spontaneous movement	Follows commands
5	Localizes pain	Localizes pain
4	Withdraws to pain	Withdraws to pain
3	Abnormal flexion	Abnormal flexion
2	Abnormal extension	Abnormal extension
1	No response	No response

Imaging of patients with TBI has been an ongoing discussion in order to decrease the risks of ionizing radiation by computed tomography (CT) scans. While it is recognized that many deployed surgeons will not have a CT scan available at their disposal, recognition of which children require further imaging or which children can be observed can assist with management and disposition of patients. The Pediatric Emergency Care Applied Research Network (PECARN) has provided guidelines to aid in determining which children will benefit from further imaging [7]. The following patients do not require further imaging of the brain with CT (all criteria must be met):

- GCS 15 with no altered mental status.
- No loss of consciousness (LOC).
- No basilar skull fracture or other fractures in children less than 2 years of age.
- No history of vomiting or severe headache.
- No significant scalp hematoma in children less than 2 years of age.
- Mechanism was not severe.

While these recommendations can guide therapy, when there is doubt especially in a deployed setting, it would be reasonable to obtain further imaging to rule out TBI as many of these patients will not have access to regular follow-up care.

When discussing TBI it is common to evaluate the cervical spine due to the underlying mechanism of trauma. Children should have an appropriately placed cervical collar to immobilize the spine just like adults. The preferred initial radiographic assessment in children is a plain radiograph series of the cervical spine (see Figs. 34.1, 34.2, and 34.3).

CT and magnetic resonance imaging (MRI) may be used after initial plain radiograph series if there are any abnormal radiographic findings. When evaluating the plain radiograph series, recognize that there are radiographic differences seen in children when compared to adults. Pseudo-subluxation is a not uncommon finding. Review of the films with an experienced radiologist is important prior to clearing the cervical spine radiographically. In some children, the cervical spine may be cleared clinically without further imaging [8]. The following criteria must be met:

- GCS 14 or 15
- No neck pain or difficulty with movement
- No torticollis or limited range of motion
- No midline tenderness
- No history of sensory or motor abnormality
- No significant distracting injury

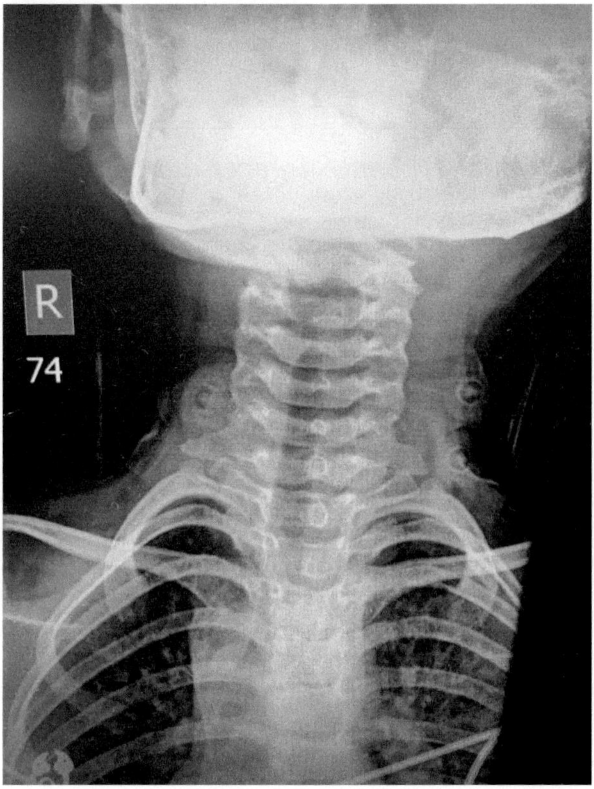

Fig. 34.1 Normal anterior-posterior view of cervical spine of a 7-year-old child (Source: Photo courtesy of Robert L. Ricca, MD)

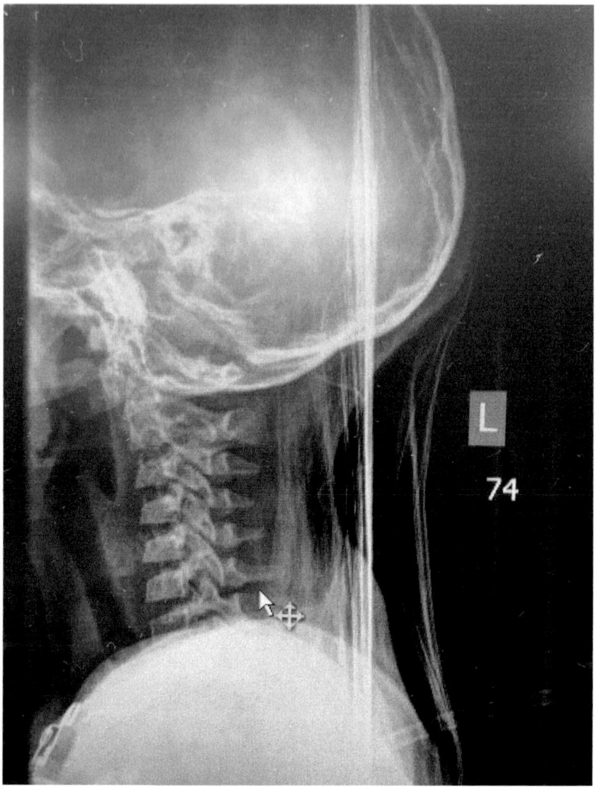

Fig. 34.2 Normal lateral view of cervical spine of a 7-year-old child (Source: Photo courtesy of Robert L. Ricca, MD)

Additional Trauma Surgery Considerations

As noted previously, the initial management of pediatric trauma patients does not differ significantly from that of an adult trauma patient. Similarly, management of penetrating trauma in pediatric patients is similar to that of adult patients. However, when managing a pediatric trauma patient in a host nation, it is important to consider the resources available for the long-term management of these patients and develop relations with host nation resources. It cannot be emphasized enough that the deployed surgeon must understand the resources that are locally available to the patient when planning their operative approach. For example, consider a bowel anastomosis instead of a temporary ostomy when possible as the child may not have the resources for ostomy management (no appliances, inability to maintain hydration) and may not have the ability to undergo ostomy reversal at a later date.

It is worthwhile to note that solid organ injury is managed in a nonoperative fashion in the typical pediatric patient. Splenic salvage has been the mainstay of therapy for pediatric patients and remains so in the United States (U.S.). This requires observation for a period of time to ensure hemodynamic stability. If unstable, splenectomy may be required as the safest option. If possible, post-splenectomy

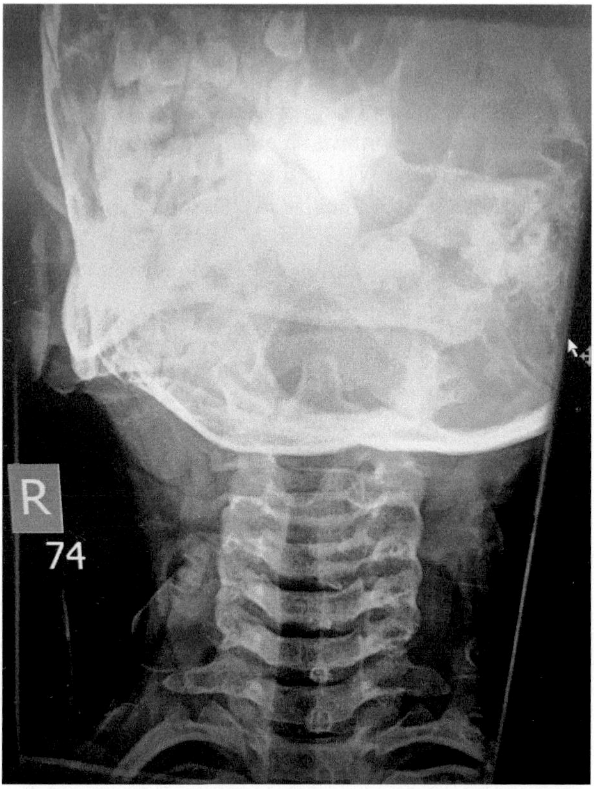

Fig. 34.3 Normal odontoid view of cervical spine of a 7-year-old child (Source: Photo courtesy of Robert L. Ricca, MD)

patients should receive vaccinations for encapsulated organisms as well as receive antibiotic prophylaxis (penicillin) due to the elevated risks of post-splenectomy sepsis in children.

Management of the Malnourished Pediatric Patient

It is not uncommon that a deployed surgical team will encounter host nation individuals who are undernourished. Recognition of their nutritional status and subsequent efforts to optimize nutrition will improve surgical outcomes. On humanitarian missions this can be performed in conjunction with a primary care provider such as a pediatrician. The World Health Organization (WHO) has published a ten-step algorithm for the routine care and treatment of severely malnourished children. The following is a synopsis of these guidelines. The Harriet Lane Handbook of Pediatrics (Cluster and Lao) is also a helpful resource for the management of pediatric patients.

1. Treat and prevent hypoglycemia through either an oral or IV dextrose solution. Routinely check blood sugars with a goal to maintain above 54 mg/dL.

2. Treat and prevent hypothermia. This is especially important for pediatric trauma patients and patients in the operating room (OR) who may become hypothermic due to exposure.
3. Treat and prevent dehydration. Except in cases of shock or trauma, oral rehydration is the preferred method. Rehydration solutions can be prepared and can be found in the WHO guidelines.
4. Treat electrolyte imbalances. Despite a low plasma sodium, malnourished children all have excess body sodium along with low levels of magnesium and potassium. Low sodium rehydration formulas are recommended along with low salt meals.
5. Treat and prevent infection. Malnourished children may not display an immune response to infection. Broad-spectrum antibiotics are routinely indicated on admission.
6. Correct micronutrient deficiencies. Vitamin A supplementation along with multivitamin supplementation will benefit the malnourished child. The WHO guidelines provide a recipe for an electrolyte/mineral solution.
7. Start cautious feeding. If a pediatrician or primary care provider is available, it is warranted to consult them with regard to feeding and fluid management. The WHO recommends the following when beginning enteral feeds in a malnourished child.
   (a) Small, frequent feeds of low osmolarity and low lactose
   (b) Oral or nasogastric feeds (never parenteral preparations)
   (c) 100 kcal/kg/day
   (d) 1–1.5 g protein/kg/day
   (e) 130 mL/kg/day of fluid (100 mL/kg/day if the child has severe edema)
8. Achieve catch up growth.
9. Provide sensory stimulation and emotional support.
10. Prepare for follow-up and recovery.

A thorough review of these guidelines when caring for malnourished children along with routine consultation with primary care providers can optimize outcomes for host nation children requiring surgery who are malnourished [9, 10].

Abdominal Surgical Incisions

Pediatric trauma patients less than 5 years of age tend to have a round or elliptical abdomen. The width of the abdomen tends to be greater than the craniocaudal length of the abdomen. Due to this anatomy, a transverse incision above the umbilicus can be found to provide greater exposure than the classic vertical midline incision. In a trauma environment, it is not inappropriate to perform a vertical midline incision that the adult general surgeon will feel comfortable with. In a non-trauma environment, a transverse incision can be cosmetically appealing using Langer's lines. This will also afford the surgeon with excellent exposure of all four quadrants. When making a right lower quadrant incision for either appendectomy or concern for intussusception, "cheat" higher on the abdomen as it is easier to bring the cecum cranially toward the incision rather than try to bring the cecum down toward an incision that is too low on the abdomen. The following points are essential for a transverse abdominal incision.

1. Begin the exposure approximately 1 cm or one fingerbreadth above the umbilicus.
2. Carry the incision through both rectus muscles for maximal exposure.
3. Tie off and divide the remnant of the umbilical vein.
4. Extend the incision laterally to improve exposure.
5. Close the incision in layers ensuring closure of the posterior and anterior rectus sheath separately.
6. Close the subcutaneous tissue providing a layer between the skin and the abdominal wall fascia. This will help to prevent adherence of the skin to the fascia and poor cosmesis of a sunken scar later in life.

Chest Tubes, Drains, Foleys

Utilization of an appropriate size chest tube, drain, or urinary catheter is important due to anatomic restrictions. Unfortunately, these may not be available within the Authorized Medical Allowance List (AMAL). Urinary catheters, Penrose drains, red rubber catheters, or nasogastric tubes may be used in an emergency setting to meet the needs of the patient. For example, if no chest tube is available, a red rubber catheter or other appropriately sized tube can be used instead. The following provides a general rule of thumb to determine the size of a tube for treatment. Use of the Broselow tape can also serve as a reference.

- Endotracheal tube (ETT) size:
  (Age/4) + 4 for uncuffed tubes (decrease 1/2 size for cuffed tubes)
- Depth of ETT:
  3 times the ETT size (4.0 ETT is usually placed at 12 cm)
- Nasogastric/orogastric tube (NGT/OGT) size:
  2 times the ETT size (4.0 ETT = 8 French NGT/OGT)
- Urinary catheter size:
  2 times the ETT size (4.0 ETT = 8 French Urinary Catheter)
- Chest tube size (trauma):
  4 times the ETT size (4.0 ETT = 16 French Chest Tube)

Any Special Equipment to Bring on the Ship that Is Not in the AMAL Just in Case?

Deployed surgeons routinely commonly face supply issues due to an inability to predict and prepare for all potential injuries or conditions they may face. It is impossible to have a fully stocked OR that one might find in a hospital at home when not deployed. Thankfully, as noted previously, the surgical team can adapt in emergency situations by using other tubes and drains. If there is an expectation that one might face a situation where pediatric patients may need to be cared for, the following items should be considered in addition to the AMAL.

- Broselow bag
- Airway management tools (oral airways, pediatric ventilation masks, pediatric Ambu bag, endotracheal tubes)
- Pediatric IV catheters (22-gauge, 24-gauge)
- WHO guidelines for the treatment of severely malnourished children

Common Surgical Procedures

The following are common pediatric surgery procedures that a general surgeon may need to perform in the deployed environment depending on the mission, medical rules of engagement, and appropriate perioperative support.

Inguinal Hernia

1. Make an incision over the appropriate inguinal canal, typically one fingerbreadth above and lateral to the pubic tubercle.
2. Dissect through Scarpa's fascia to the external oblique aponeurosis.
3. Begin laterally and define the border of the external oblique, eventually identifying the external ring.
4. Open the external ring of the aponeurosis.
5. Split the cremasteric muscles exposing the underlying hernia sac (typically white in appearance).
6. Elevate the spermatic cord and further mobilize the cremasteric muscles creating an inverted V.
7. Isolate the hernia sac on the anteromedial aspect of the cord structures. Ensure identification of the vas deferens and spermatic vessels in a male patient.
8. Divide the hernia sac and dissect it distally to the testicle to prevent hydrocele formation. Dissect it proximally to the internal ring. Twist the hernia sac and close with an absorbable suture – the authors prefer a 3-0 PDS suture with a second 3-0 PDS tie.

9. If the floor is lax, perform a tissue repair – do not use mesh in pediatric patients. With rare exceptions, children under the age of 18 do not require mesh. A Bassini repair involves suturing together the transversalis fascia and inguinal ligament.
10. Close the layers using absorbable sutures.

Umbilical Hernia

1. Make an infra-umbilical incision.
2. Dissect down to the fascia using electrocautery.
3. Dissect circumferentially around the hernia sac using a hemostat or mosquito.
4. Divide the hernia sac from the umbilical stalk, avoiding injury to the stalk.
5. Excise the hernia sac down to the level of the abdominal fascia.
6. Close the hernia defect with interrupted absorbable sutures. Do not use mesh.
7. Reattach the umbilical stalk to the abdominal fascia.
8. Close the incision in layers using absorbable sutures.

Incision and Drainage Abscess

1. Make an incision over the site of maximal fluctuance.
2. Use a hemostat to ensure no loculations are present.
3. Irrigate the wound and send cultures as appropriate.
4. Rather than pack the wound, make a counter incision and bring a vessel loop between these two incisions and tie it to itself to act as a drain. Packing the wound can cause pain for the child upon removal and be difficult for the families to remove and repack. The vessel loop can then be removed in clinic 5–7 days later.

When addressing a perianal abscess seen in a young child (less than 1 year of age), topical lidocaine cream can be applied and a simple stab incision can be used to adequately drain the abscess. In the setting of a recurrent perianal abscess, consider the possibility of a fistula and the need for fistulotomy.

Appendectomy

The vast majority of children can be treated laparoscopically with adult ports/instruments and in the same manner (i.e., 12 mm umbilical port, 5 mm left lower quadrant and 5 mm suprapubic ports). Be mindful that children have thinner abdominal walls so ports do not need to be placed deeply. Remember that there will be smaller working space. If there is any concern about performing this operation laparoscopically, then open appendectomy is an acceptable alternative.

Malrotation/Volvulus

1. Make a transverse right upper quadrant incision. Extend the incision as needed for exposure.
2. Eviscerate the small bowel.
3. Rotate the small bowel counterclockwise ("turning back the hands of time").
4. Assess viability. If needed, create a temporary abdominal dressing (can be as simple as using a cut saline bag to cover the bowel and tucked intra-abdominally while an Ioban can be draped over the abdomen to keep the saline bag in place) for a second look operation.
5. Divide Ladd's bands adhering the colon to the abdominal wall.
6. Widen the mesentery carefully.
7. Perform an appendectomy.
8. Return the small bowel to the right hemi-abdomen with the colon in the left hemi-abdomen. The cecum tends to be in the left upper quadrant providing a wide mesentery.
9. Close the abdomen in layers.

Conclusion

A deployed general surgeon and surgical team may be in the position of having to care for pediatric patients. Children have unique anatomic and physiologic considerations that must be respected by their medical providers, and their evaluation and management must also be tailored accordingly. It is crucial that the deployed surgeon must understand the resources that are locally available to the patient when planning their operative approach and be cognizant of what kind of quality of life these patients may have afterward.

Declaration of Interest The views expressed in this chapter are those of the authors and do not necessarily reflect the official policy or position of the Department of the Navy, Department of Defense, nor the US Government.

Funding This research did not receive any specific grant from funding agencies in the public, commercial, or not-for-profit sectors.

Conflict of Interest Statement The authors declare no conflict of interest.

References

1. Committee on Trauma, American College of Surgeons. Advanced trauma life support student manual. 10th ed. Chicago: American College of Surgeons; 2018.
2. PALS Algorithms 2020. Retrieved from https://www.acls-pals-bls.com/algorithms/pals/.
3. Anand T, Obaid O, Nelson A, Chehab M, Ditillo M, Hammad A, Douglas M, Bible L, Joseph B. Whole blood hemostatic resuscitation in pediatric trauma: a nationwide propensity-matched analysis. J Trauma Acute Care Surg. 2021;91(4):573–8.
4. Leeper CM, Yazer MH, Triulzi DJ, Neal MD, Gaines BA. Whole blood is superior to component transfusion for injured children: a propensity matched analysis. Ann Surg. 2020;272(4):590–4.
5. Feld LG, Neuspiel DR, Foster BA, et al. Subcommittee on fluid and electrolyte therapy. Clinical practice guideline: maintenance intravenous fluids in children. Pediatrics. 2018;142(6):e20183083.
6. Harless J, Ramaiah R, Bhananker SM. Pediatric airway management. Int J Crit Illn Inj Sci. 2014;4(1):65–70. https://doi.org/10.4103/2229-5151.128015.
7. Kuppermann N, Holmes JF, Dayan PS, et al. Pediatric Emergency Care Applied Research Network (PECARN). Identification of children at very low risk of clinically-important brain injuries after head trauma: a prospective cohort study. Lancet. 2009;374(9696):1160–70.
8. Herman MJ, Brown KO, Sponseller PD, et al. Pediatric cervical spine clearance: a consensus statement and algorithm from the Pediatric Cervical Spine Clearance Working Group. J Bone Joint Surg Am. 2019;101(1):e1.
9. Ashworth A, Kahnum S, Jackson A, Schofield C. Guidelines for the inpatient treatment of severely malnourished children. Geneva: World Health Organization; 2003.
10. Balhara KS, Silvestri DM, Tyler Winders W, et al. Global emergency medicine literature review group (GEMLR). Impact of nutrition interventions on pediatric mortality and nutrition outcomes in humanitarian emergencies: a systematic review. Tropical Med Int Health. 2017;22(12):1464–92.

Chapter 35
Avast! Acute Medical Emergencies of Detained Pirates or Local Nationals

Jonathan R. Gower, John S. Parrish, and Amy A. Hernandez

> *A society should be judged not by how it treats its outstanding citizens but by how it treats its criminals.*
>
> *Fyodor Dostoevsky*

Author deployment experience	
Jonathan R. Gower	Battalion Surgeon, 3rd Battalion 1st Marines, embarked with 11th Marine Expeditionary Unit on the USS New Orleans (LPD-18), WESTPAC, INDOPACOM and CENTCOM Areas of Responsibility, 2011–2012
	Resident Surgeon, USNS Mercy (T-AH-19), Pacific Partnership, Indonesia and Malaysia, 2016
	Staff Surgeon, Fleet Surgical Team-3, embarked on the USS Wasp (LHD-1), WESTPAC, INDOPACOM and South America Areas of Responsibility, 2019
John S. Parrish	General Medical Officer/Radiation Health Officer, USS Arkansas (CGN-41), contingency operations, Third Fleet Area of Operations, 1987–1989
	Director of Medical Services, USNS Mercy (T-AH-19), Pacific Partnership, Federated States of Micronesia, Papua New Guinea, Republic of the Philippines, Vietnam, Timor-Leste, 2008
	Director of Medical Operations and Planning, USNS Mercy (T-AH-19), Pacific Partnership, Cambodia, Indonesia, Vietnam, Timor-Leste, 2010
	Pulmonary and Critical Care Subject Matter Expert, USNS Mercy (T-AH-19), Pacific Partnership Subject Matter Expertise Exchange, Qui Nhon, Vietnam, 2011

J. R. Gower (✉) · A. A. Hernandez
Navy Medicine Readiness and Training Command San Diego,
San Diego, USA
e-mail: jonathan.r.gower.mil@health.mil

J. S. Parrish
Department of Pulmonary and Critical Care Medicine, Naval Medical Center San Diego,
San Diego, CA, USA
e-mail: john.s.parrish.civ@health.mil

M. D. Tadlock, A. A. Hernandez (eds.), *Expeditionary Surgery at Sea*,
https://doi.org/10.1007/978-3-031-21893-4_35

Author deployment experience	
	Pulmonary and Critical Care Subject Matter Expert, USNS Mercy (T-AH-19), Pacific Partnership Subject Matter Expertise Exchange, Hanoi, Vietnam, 2013
	Advance Team Medical Planner/Officer, USNS Mercy (T-AH-19), Pacific Partnership, Da Nang, Vietnam and Tacloban, Republic of Philippines, 2014
	Clinical TB/HIV Preceptor, Department of Defense HIV/AIDS Prevention Program (DHAPP), Ghana, 2015–2022
Amy A. Hernandez	Battalion Surgeon, 7th Engineer Support Battalion, Operating Enduring Freedom, Camp Leatherneck, Afghanistan, 2011
	Ship's Surgeon, USS Carl Vinson (CVN-70), WESTPAC, INDOPACOM Area of Responsibility, 2017
	Department Head, Federal Emergency Management Agency (FEMA) and Defense Support of Civilian Authorities (DSCA) COVID-19 Community Vaccination Center mission, St. Louis, MO, USA, 2021

BLUF (Bottom Line Up Front)

1. Approximately 200 piracy incidents occur annually worldwide. Anti-piracy operations continue to be a standing mission of the United States (U.S.) Navy.
2. The Geneva convention, U.S. government, and international community have set standards and rules for the treatment of prisoners, including detained pirates.
3. Detained pirates should be provided the same level of care provided to the service members aboard the vessel.
4. Each vessel should prepare appropriately to plan logistics and establish a standard operating procedure (SOP) in line with the set standards and rules for the treatment and medical care of detainees.
5. All medical personnel who could be required to provide care for detainees should undergo training prior to deployment.
6. At time of initial medical evaluation, detainees should undergo testing, treatment, and isolation if necessary for communicable diseases, specifically tuberculosis (TB) and coronavirus disease 2019 (COVID-19).
7. Mental health is a common issue among incarcerated individuals, and detainees should be screened and monitored for mental health issues both at admission and for the duration of their care.
8. Chronic conditions may be first diagnosed when detainees are brought aboard maritime vessels. Due to the limitation of medical resources aboard each ship, it is not recommended that they start treatment unless it is a direct threat to their lives.

Introduction

Piracy has been present since there have been ships upon the sea, and this is unlikely to end in the coming future. Numerous ships are attacked yearly across the globe. The International Chamber of Commerce (ICC) International Maritime Bureau (IMB) was established in 1981 with the purpose of monitoring and fighting crime on the high seas. Since 1992, the IMB Piracy Report Centre monitors piracy incidents, warns ships in the vicinity of threats, and provides a 24/7 manned operations center [1]. They define piracy as "any illegal acts of violence or detention, or any act of depredation, committed for private ends by the crew or the passengers of a private ship or a private aircraft, and directed on the high seas, against another ship or aircraft." They produce an annual report about the number and location piracy incidents. In 2020, there were 195 piracy incidents worldwide [1]. These numbers have been stable over the last 5 years. The greatest number of incidents occur around the African continent. Despite the ongoing anti-piracy efforts around the world, the number of piracy incidents has remained unchanged.

One of the United States (U.S.) Navy's ongoing global missions is anti-piracy operations. The U.S. has been a part of Combined Task Force 151 since its inception in 2009 with the mission to deter, disrupt, and suppress piracy and armed robbery at sea in the Gulf of Aden, southern Red Sea, and associated waters. With U.S. forces deployed around the world and the continued threat of piracy, treating detained pirates continues to be a possibility for forward deployed medical and surgical teams.

Personnel aboard U.S. and other military ships are required to provide medical care in a unique and challenging environment. Not only are they the sole providers responsible for thousands of service members with limited resources, unknown resupply, and unknown time for medical evacuation, but they may also be tasked with providing medical care for pirates detained during anti-piracy operations at any time. These detainees can be hostile to U.S. military personnel. They are guarded constantly. They can have different cultural backgrounds and speak different languages. Because they often come from low- and middle-income countries (LMIC), they often have had limited access to healthcare throughout their lives and have diseases which medical personnel may have no practical experience treating [2]. This chapter will cover the ethics and level of care required, procedures, training recommendations, and some medical situations that could be encountered in the care of detained pirates.

Clinical Vignette 35.1

"As a very junior Battalion Surgeon stationed aboard the USS New Orleans (LPD-18), I was responsible for the intake and medical evaluation of several Somali pirates detained during anti-piracy operations in the Gulf of Aden. Providing medical care for these detained pirates was a unique challenge. They spoke little English. At times we could not communicate outside of hand gestures because of limited translators. They had to be examined under guard. They were very thin and appeared malnourished. We had no idea what to expect and received no formal training on their intake procedure or ongoing care."

-Jonathan Gower

Clinical Vignette 35.2

"My first utilization tour after completing my surgical residency was as a carrier Ship's Surgeon. As the only male medical officer in the department, I was assigned to perform the initial intake, complete history and physical, and daily medical care of several Somali pirates detained during anti-piracy operations. My role, responsibilities, and documentation requirements were clearly delineated utilizing

contemporary standard operating procedures. Most of what I dealt with were chronic medical conditions such as malnutrition and the chronic sequelae of sexually transmitted infections. At one point a fight broke out between the detainees and I had to repair several lacerations while the patients were under guard. One pirate developed a perirectal abscess requiring surgical drainage. Luckily, he spoke some English, and I was easily able to appropriately go through informed consent process with him. Ultimately, using standard detainee precautions, I performed an incision and drainage of a perirectal abscess in the ship's operating room with anesthesia support without complication. He recovered well and was very thankful for his care."

-Anonymous Ship's Surgeon

Ethics and Level of Care

Healthcare providers have an ethical responsibility to provide adequate medical care for detainees on land or sea. The Geneva convention, U.S. government, and international community have published minimum standards and rules which must be met for their care [3, 4]. These standards and rules do not solely cover their medical care but also the berthing, hygiene, food, and overall care. These documents also delineate areas where medical departments should not take part, such as any level of interrogation or the provision of any information which would aid in interrogation [5].

In general, medical personnel are required to provide the same level of care for detainees as for their own service members. However, this does not mean that every condition or medical problem that these detainees present with will be treated [6]. There will always be limitations to the level of care provided to both service members and prisoners because of the inherent limitations on quantity and types of medicine, diagnostic testing, and therapeutics options. However, the same level of care must be provided of what is available.

Standard Operating Procedures (SOP)

The first time that pirates are captured and brought on board a naval vessel should not be the first time procedures for the care of detainees is discussed. Proper planning should occur and an SOP should be established prior to this type of evolution. As demonstrated in the difference between the clinical vignettes, having preparation and SOP created ahead of time made the difference for medical personnel to feel more confident and supported caring for detainees. All relevant personnel should be involved in the production of this document, including the Commanding Officer (CO), Senior Medical Officer (SMO), Master-at-Arms, etc. All medical personnel should be aware of and trained on these procedures. The following are areas which should be covered under this document [7].

- Berthing: Based on the type of ship, there may be limited capacity in the brig (jail on board a ship); thus, additional holding areas may need to be constructed with similar accommodations, safety, and access to appropriate hygiene and toileting facilities.
- Hygiene: There should be an area appropriate and accessible for hygiene and toileting facilities.
- Food: Food should be provided, taking into consideration any cultural or religious issues if possible.
- Clothing: After detainees arrive and they are searched, they should be placed in clean dry clothing to limit ongoing effects of hypothermia or transmission of communicable diseases.
- Communicable diseases: Detainees should be screened on intake evaluation for any communicable disease if the vessel has the capability to perform this type of testing, particularly highly contagious respiratory diseases such as tuberculosis (TB) or coronavirus disease 2019 (COVID-19). If there is no capability to perform this type of testing on board the vessel, it should be assumed that detained pirates have some form of a communicable disease. Appropriate precautions should be taken to limit spread to the rest of the ship and to other detainees.
- Initial medical intake evaluation: Detainees should undergo a medical evaluation as soon as possible upon arrival on the ship. If possible, translation services should be utilized if appropriate. A complete history and physical should be completed at that time to include an initial assessment of the detainees' medical, dental, and mental health.
- Emergent care: Detainees should have access to medical, dental, and mental healthcare on an emergent or non-emergent basis as needed.
- Daily evaluation: After initial intake, detainees should be evaluated daily for any additional medical, dental, or mental health issues which may arise.
- Medical records: Each detainee should have medical records created which will move with them to their permanent detention facilities. These records should be regarded with the same level of confidentiality as any typical medical record would.

Training

While most medical and surgical trainees and training programs have limited to no experience with the care of pirates, local nationals, or other detainees, the likelihood of encountering them continues to grow while in service with forward deployed units. All medical personnel assigned to maritime vessels should complete regular training on the care and handling of these types of patients. For U.S. Navy medical personnel, resources include Department of Defense (DoD) Instructions 1322.24 Medical Readiness Training and 2310.08 Medical Program Support for Detainee Operations [5, 6]. This is essential to prepare, set expectations, and minimize confusion in order to ensure proper care of these patients.

Specific Medical Situations

In addition to the fact that treatment of these detained pirates is occurring on a vessel with several limitations on resources, they will often have had minimal prior access to healthcare throughout their lives. Many of them have resided in LMIC with limited resources and access to healthcare. These countries have a gross national income of less than $4000 per year according to the World Bank. While conditions and healthcare in these parts of the world are improving over the last several years, there is still an increased incidence of several conditions not commonly seen in the western world. The conditions listed below are pertinent ones which often must be dealt with upon arrival of these detainees, particularly as they relate to their potential surgical care. However, this is not an exhaustive list by any means as the treatment of disease in LMIC could be a textbook unto itself. Refer to Chap. 16 for a more comprehensive list of infectious disease recommendations.

Tuberculosis (TB)

According to the World Health Organization (WHO), one quarter of the world's population has latent tuberculosis infection (LTBI), and there were 10 million cases of active TB and 1.5 million deaths attributed to TB in 2021. Greater than 90% of these cases occur in LMIC. Approximately 4% of these cases are multidrug-resistant TB [8]. Active pulmonary TB is highly transmissible, and its airborne spread would be facilitated by the close quarters found onboard a ship if appropriate precautions are not taken. All detainees should be evaluated for TB at their initial medical intake evaluation. Detainees presenting with productive cough for >3 weeks, hemoptysis, weight loss, breathlessness, and fever or who have physical exam findings suggestive of a pulmonary infection should be suspected of having active TB. Those with suspected TB should undergo a standard evaluation to include chest X-ray and collection of three sputum samples for acid-fast bacilli (AFB) when available. Of note, a Tuberculin Skin Test/Purified Protein Derivative (PPD), although useful in the identification of patients with latent TB, has limited utility in the evaluation of patients with suspected active TB due to low sensitivity and specificity. Detainees whose evaluation demonstrates the presence of active TB would be treated with an extended course of multiple medications, not always available on board a ship. These patients would be considered infectious for a minimum of two weeks after starting effective treatment. Due to limited onboard X-ray and laboratory resources, the initial evaluation for TB may be delayed. Until TB is definitively ruled out, detainees suspected of having TB must be kept isolated from other detainees, and standard precautions should be taken to limit spread to the rest of the ship [8, 9].

Coronavirus Disease 2019 (COVID-19) and Other Communicable Diseases

With the emergence of COVID-19, healthcare providers in the military became much more aware of the risk that new diseases present. Data continues to be gathered on the incidence of COVID-19 worldwide, and access to testing is improving, but due to lack of infrastructure and healthcare resources, the true incidence is unknown in LMIC. The Centers for Disease Control (CDC) and WHO track disease outbreaks throughout the world and should be used as a resource. While COVID-19 testing is currently available on board many U.S. Navy vessels (see Chap. 8), this may not always be true or a new disease may emerge in the future for which a test does not exist. Medical personnel must be aware of novel diseases and mitigate both their spread and consequences to the vulnerable detainee population but also to the ship's personnel, who live in close quarters.

Additionally, detainees may have many other communicable diseases that healthcare providers trained in the western world may not be as familiar with, including but not limited to malaria, cholera, scabies or lice, atypical parasites, etc. [10].

Dehydration and Malnutrition

"Pirate crews are often inadequately provisioned with food and fresh water during their prolonged periods at sea looking for potential targets" [10]. Some may even be hypovolemic and/or in shock on presentation. Resuscitation with isotonic fluid and correction of any severe electrolyte abnormalities should be initiated on intake when appropriate, particularly prior to potential surgical intervention.

Malnutrition continues to be a significant issue in LMIC. The population is not only deficient in calories and proteins but also in micronutrients. Malnutrition is directly responsible for over 300,000 deaths annually, increases susceptibility to and severity of infections, is a major component of illness and death from disease, and is the most important risk factor for the burden of disease in LMIC [11]. This situation is compounded by the fact that pirates from these countries are typically poorly provisioned. Upon intake and throughout their care, their nutritional status and weight need to be assessed, including monitoring for refeeding syndrome. They should be provided with appropriate food and water, and if they have a surgical issue, their nutritional status should be taken into consideration for surgical planning and postoperative care.

A special area regarding nutrition which must be discussed is hunger strikes. They are more common in long-term detention facilities but may still be a situation faced by maritime medical personnel. In situations where there is risk to the detainee's health or life, medical personnel may administer nutrition against the patient's wishes, often through a nasal feeding tube [12].

Dental Health

Dental health is an often-neglected area of global health, particularly in LMIC with minimal access to dental care, affecting 3.5 billion people around the world. Of note, even in the US Adult Correctional System where prisoners have some access to dental care, there is an eightfold increase in the prevalence of dental disease [13]. Oral health can both reflect and affect a patient's overall health in many ways, including nutritional status, postoperative recovery, and risk of developing pneumonia. Therefore, while dental conditions are not often emergent, this should be addressed for detainees if dental care is available.

Mental Health

The incidence of psychiatric conditions in this population is unknown, but detainees subject to confinement should be afforded mental health services as pre-existing mental health issues can become more severe during confinement or new ones can arise. Per instruction and the minimum standard set forth by the international community, detainees should be screened for psychiatric illness during their intake, assessed for it throughout the course of their confinement, and afforded care as appropriate by medical providers available to provide psychiatric services.

Chronic Medical Conditions

Chronic medical conditions present a particular challenge to military personnel in the care of detainees. For example, hypertension and diabetes mellitus are increasing in LMIC. Recent data reports that the prevalence of hypertension in LMIC is approximately 30% and has been increasing [14]. Diabetes rates are similar to that of the western world. There is limited access to pharmaceuticals in these countries, and they are often cost-prohibitive for the impoverished [15]. Therefore, these diseases and others like them often go undiagnosed and untreated. The first time a disease may be diagnosed is when these pirates are detained. They may have limited time on board a vessel, and there is also a limited quantity of medicine on board which could only treat these conditions for short periods of time. Due to the limitations of time, medical supplies, and follow-up care, it is not recommended to treat these chronic conditions unless they are a direct threat to a detainee's life. The diagnosis should be documented in their record so that treatment may be provided when those limitations are mitigated.

Provider and Crew Safety

Due to the potential for exposure to communicable diseases, all healthcare personnel as well as crew members assigned to duties involving close contact with detainees should be instructed in and expected to utilize standard universal precautions during the performance of their detainee-related duties. These precautions should include when appropriate the wearing of gowns, gloves, eye protection, and masks. In addition, detainees with possible TB or viral respiratory infections should wear a mask when near others.

Conclusion

Piracy is an ongoing problem throughout the world. This is unlikely to change, and the U.S. Navy and other militaries are likely to have an ongoing role in global anti-piracy operations. With these operations come detained pirates requiring medical care for a potentially prolonged period of time, which can present several unique challenges. Medical personnel should prepare protocols and undergo training ahead of time to care for detained pirates. The level of care should be equivalent to that of their own service members, paying particular attention to acute and chronic medical, dental, and mental health issues common in people from LMIC without access to care, especially if there are surgical conditions to treat for the maritime surgical team.

Declaration of Interest The views expressed in this chapter are those of the authors and do not necessarily reflect the official policy or position of the Department of the Navy, Department of Defense, nor the US Government.

Funding This research did not receive any specific grant from funding agencies in the public, commercial, or not-for-profit sectors.

Conflict of Interest Statement The authors declare no conflict of interest.

References

1. International ICC, Bureau M. ICC-IMB piracy and armed robbery against ships report 2020. 2020, pp. 1–28.
2. Orach CG. Health equity: challenges in low income countries. Afr Health Sci. 2009;9(Suppl 2):S49–51.
3. Standard Minimum Rules for the Treatment of Prisoners. Nations congress on the prevention of crime and the treatment of offenders. Gene. 1977;2076(1957):1–14.

4. UNODC. United Nations standard minimum rules for the treatment. UNODC. 2015;16487(September):1–36. https://www.unodc.org/documents/justice-and-prison-reform/Nelson_Mandela_Rules-E-ebook.pdf.
5. U.S. Department of Defense. DOD instruction 6025.27 medical ethics in the military health system. 2017.
6. U.S. Department of Defense. DOD instruction 2310.08. Medical Program Support for Detainee Operations. 2019.
7. US Department of Justice Federal Bureau of Prisons. Program statement: patient care. 2014.
8. Tuberculosis, Practical guide for clinicians, nurses, laboratory technicians and medical auxiliaries. Medecins San Frontieres and Partners in Health. 2022 edition. https://medicalguidelines.msf.org/viewport/TUB/latest/tuberculosis-20321086.html
9. WHO Global Tuberculosis Programme & UNHCR. Tuberculosis control in refugee situations: an inter-agency field manual. Geneva: World Health Organization; 1997. https://apps.who.int/iris/handle/10665/63629.
10. Schranz C. The acute medical management of detained Somali pirates and their captives. Mil Med. 2012;177(9):1095–9. https://doi.org/10.7205/milmed-d-12-00130. PMID: 23025141.
11. Müller O, Krawinkel M. Malnutrition and health in developing countries. CMAJ. 2005;173(3):279–86. https://doi.org/10.1503/cmaj.050342.
12. US Department of Justice Federal Bureau of Prisons. Program statement: hunger strikes. 2005.
13. Watt RG, Daly B, Allison P, et al. Ending the neglect of global oral health: time for radical action. Lancet. 2019;394(10194):261–72. https://doi.org/10.1016/S0140-6736(19)31133-X.
14. Saif-Ur-Rahman KM, Hasan M, Hossain S, et al. Non-pharmacological interventions for the prevention of hypertension in low-income and middle-income countries: protocol for a systematic review and meta-analysis. BMJ Open. 2018;8(5):6–11. https://doi.org/10.1136/bmjopen-2017-020724.
15. Chow CK, Ramasundarahettige C, Hu W, et al. Availability and affordability of essential medicines for diabetes across high-income, middle-income, and low-income countries: a prospective epidemiological study. Lancet Diabetes Endocrinol. 2018;6(10):798–808. https://doi.org/10.1016/S2213-8587(18)30233-X.

Chapter 36
Practical Bioethical Principles in the Deployed Maritime Environment

Victoria S. McDonald and Matthew D. Tadlock

God of Battle…Let me never forget that a life or limb is in my keeping and do not let my judgment falter…

A Surgeon's Prayer in Wartime, Col. John J. Moorhead, MD

Author deployment experience	
Victoria S. McDonald	Battalion Surgeon, Combat Logistic Battalion-7, Operation Enduring Freedom, Helmand Province, Afghanistan, 2011
	Resident Surgeon, USNS Mercy (T-AH-19), Pacific Partnership, Fiji and Papua New Guinea, 2015
Matthew D. Tadlock	Flight Surgeon, Carrier Air Wing Three (CVW-3), embarked on the USS Harry S. Truman (CVN-75) in support of Operation Iraqi Freedom, Fifth Fleet Area of Responsibility, 2004–2005; supporting Humanitarian Aid Disaster Relief (HADR) operations following Hurricane Katrina, 2005
	Resident Surgeon, USNS Mercy (T-AH-19), Pacific Partnership, Micronesia and Papua New Guinea, 2008
	Ship's Surgeon, USS Carl Vinson (CVN-70), WESTPAC, INDOPACOM Area of Responsibility, 2011–2012
	Officer in Charge, Forward Resuscitative Surgical System/Shock Trauma Platoon, Charlie Surgical Company, Native Fury, CENTCOM Area of Responsibility, 2016
	Chief of Trauma, NATO Role 3 Multinational Medical Unit, NATO Resolute Support and Operation Freedom's Sentinel, Kandahar Airfield, Afghanistan, 2017–2018
	Staff Surgeon, Expeditionary Resuscitative Surgical System Pacific, 2019–2020; Provided embarked Role 2 Surgical Support, INDOPACOM Area of Responsibility, 2020

V. S. McDonald (✉)
Navy Medicine Readiness and Training Command Camp Pendleton, Camp Pendleton, CA, USA
e-mail: victoria.s.mcdonald2.mil@health.mil

M. D. Tadlock
Department of Surgery, Naval Medical Center San Diego, San Diego, CA, USA
e-mail: matthewtadlockmd@gmail.com

M. D. Tadlock, A. A. Hernandez (eds.), *Expeditionary Surgery at Sea*,
https://doi.org/10.1007/978-3-031-21893-4_36

BLUF (Bottom Line Up Front)

1. Deployed environments can lead to complicated ethical quandaries for surgeons and their teams. Justice, autonomy, nonmaleficence, and beneficence provide the foundation for the ethical practice of medicine and can guide surgical team decision-making during ethical dilemmas. Barriers to adhering to the bioethical principles are commonly system-based factors.
2. During elective humanitarian and disaster relief missions, a top priority in mission planning should be pre-determining eligibility for care (justice).
3. Establishing a pre-designated ethics committee to assist in deliberation and determining appropriate courses of action can prevent the burden of difficult decision-making falling on a single person.
4. For any mission, planning ahead for translation services especially with regard to the informed consent process is imperative (autonomy).
5. The goals of any Humanitarian Assistance and Disaster Relief (HADR) mission should be in line with the goals of the host nation. Developing HADR and Global Health Engagement (GHE) partnerships should be for mutually beneficial goals.
6. Understanding and engaging with the regional medical infrastructure helps surgical teams have good judgment to make decisions for complex patients (nonmaleficence).
7. Topics that incite debate in humanitarian surgery include surgical care for patients with a dismal prognosis, involvement of surgical trainees, and skill sustainment for forward deployed military surgical teams.
8. Follow-up care should be a part of both mission planning and consideration of individual cases (beneficence).
9. Sustainability should be a part of all humanitarian mission planning.
10. Steps that may prevent moral injury of surgical team members when encountering ethical dilemmas include designating an ethics committee, implementing a formal humanitarian ethics curriculum, early surgical team debrief of unexpected or poor outcomes associated with ethical dilemmas, and incorporating ethics discussions into morbidity and mortality process improvement activities.

Introduction

There are four core bioethical principles that guide the ethical practice of medicine and surgery: justice, autonomy, nonmaleficence, and beneficence. Justice is defined as the fair distribution of healthcare resources. Autonomy speaks to the ability to decide for oneself, free from the control of others, with a sufficient level of understanding to provide a meaningful choice. Nonmaleficence echoes the familiar line from the Hippocratic Oath, "Do no harm," via acts of commission or omission.

Beneficence is our *duty* to provide benefit and *intentionally* prevent harm to our patients [1, 2]. "The discipline of surgery places ethical judgment at a premium" [3]. Referring to these four foundational codes can help surgeons make difficult judgment calls, oftentimes in situations with competing priorities where there is no single right answer.

Justice

Clinical Vignette 36.1

A ship is deployed for disaster relief in a developing nation and arrives 48 h after a large-scale natural disaster. Thousands of people need medical care. The ship's capabilities include a three-bed intensive care unit (ICU) and one operating room (OR). Nearby medical facilities are rendered non-functional from the natural disaster. There is no dialysis capability. A patient is brought in after a heroic rescue, having survived being buried in rubble for one week. She had multiple crush injuries and was in florid rhabdomyolysis with associated renal failure [4].

Should this facility accept this patient with a low likelihood of survival, but likely a high resource utilization in a setting of very limited medical resources, at the probable expense of others with a better chance of survival? Or should the facility deny medical treatment in order to save resources for other patients with a better chance of survival, despite search and rescue teams risking their own safety through heroic efforts to save this patient?

Justice, in bioethics, is defined as the fair distribution of healthcare resources. In the immediate sense, this is triage. However, triage in the austere settings of deployment may not be as straightforward as the triage performed in the Level I trauma centers with seemingly limitless resources. "Every mass casualty event raises ethical issues concerning the priorities of treatment…But denying care to some patients for the benefit of others was not a course of action that came readily to physicians accustomed to treating all who seek care" [4].

When planning a surgical mission in an austere environment, there are, by definition, limitations to resources, and this can be a barrier to fulfilling the bioethical principle of justice: limited time at a certain location, limited number of medical personnel, limited OR space, limited amount of surgical consumable items, and limited medications and blood products, to give a few examples. In such instances, it is helpful to pre-determine eligibility for care criteria based on the unique deployment situation and resources. For example, elective humanitarian missions, disaster relief missions, and combat support missions, whether land-based or shipboard, each have different priorities. Triage during elective humanitarian missions should consider short- and long-term outcomes and local cultural norms (see Chap. 32). Triage during disaster relief missions should consider long-term care requirements in the context of host nation resources (see Chap. 33). Combat support missions must follow the medical rules of engagement in their deployed area of responsibility

(AOR). Furthermore, establishing a pre-designated ethics committee can prevent the burden of difficult decision-making falling on a single physician. In situations where multiple medical organizations are working in the same area, every effort should be made to work in concert and appropriately disposition patients depending on each organization's capabilities [3–5]. During disaster relief, the local and regional medical assets frequently shift, and constant re-evaluation of these assets is key. This knowledge can lead to revision of triage, management, and discharge criteria.

Autonomy

Clinical Vignette 36.2

A hospital ship was deployed on an elective humanitarian mission to a non-English-speaking, developing nation. Elective surgeries were planned. Interpreters were used to assist with surgical evaluations and during the consent discussion for recommended surgeries. The interpreters' command of the English language varied greatly during this mission, and accurate translation was sometimes uncertain. At times the host nation surgeons who would be participating in surgeries aboard the hospital ship as a part of the knowledge exchange also acted as interpreters.

Was the patients' autonomy respected without fully bridging the language barrier? Was there a conflict of interest by having host nation surgeons acting as interpreters? Should the mission have aborted if translation capabilities were determined to be insufficient?

Autonomy is the ability to decide for oneself free from the control of others and with a sufficient level of understanding to make a meaningful choice. Military surgeons are frequently deployed to situations where they must provide lifesaving measures to traumatically injured patients. In the situation where a patient presents in extremis and lifesaving interventions need to occur without delay or the injury renders the patient incapable of making decisions for themselves, the surgeon must act in the best interest of the patient and forgo the usual consent discussion [6]. This is an accepted standard of care when practicing in the United States (U.S.) and should be followed when performing surgery anywhere under the American flag.

When considering individual patients in a non-emergent setting, every effort should be made to inform the patient of the risks and benefits of the procedure while remaining sensitive to local cultural norms. Realistic goals of care should be set, and the surgical team's credentials and capabilities should never be misrepresented. Consent discussions should be documented and witnessed [3]. "Should a surgical or other invasive procedure be recommended to the patient…proceeding without a formal consent either written or verbal, and witnessed, may be a medical liability issue, as well as a professional ethics issue if a complication or death results from the procedure" [7].

During any humanitarian mission, identifying interpreters with sufficient fluency in both English and the host nation language can be a challenge and potential barrier to fulfilling the principle of autonomy. Securing proper translation services should be a priority during the planning phase in order to protect patient autonomy. The interpreter should optimally be separate from the surgical team. Relying on a host nation physician to act as interpreter for the informed consent discussion may introduce bias into the conversation as the host nation physician may have secondary gain in performing the surgery with the humanitarian surgeon. On the other hand, the host nation physicians oftentimes have the most fluency in medical English and may provide the most accurate interpretation to the patient. These factors should be weighed when deciding to proceed with elective surgery, and the surgeon should feel confident that the patient understands the risks and benefits of the procedure being performed on them.

Regarding Humanitarian Assistance and Disaster Relief (HADR) missions, the autonomy of the host nation and the host nation's surgeons must be respected. Missions should only go where invited, and the goals of the mission must be in line with the goals of the host nation. Where appropriate, host nation medical personnel should be included to participate in caring for patients [3, 5].

Nonmaleficence

Clinical Vignette 36.3

A 2-month-old Local National girl undergoes medical evacuation to a Role 3 medical facility stood up in support of a combat mission. Mechanism of injury is a blast, which killed both of her parents, and there are no known family members or guardians. Trauma evaluation reveals a skull fracture, comminuted open right femur fracture with significant surrounding soft tissue injury. In the U.S., this patient would have likely been admitted to the pediatric ICU; however, there are no pediatric intensivists nor pediatric nurses on staff at this facility.

Multiple Role 3 staff members raise concerns regarding the facility's ability to care for such a young infant. They are not experienced or credentialled in pediatric care and feel it is unethical to provide substandard care to this patient. Counter arguments from other staff members include that although some staff are not experienced or specifically credentialled in pediatric care, they feel obligated to care for this injured infant because this Role 3 facility is the most capable medical facility in the region. Furthermore, the Role 3 facility has the ability via phone, email, and video telecommunication to reach out to pediatric specialists to assist in the care of this patient.

Nonmaleficence is the bioethical imperative not to intentionally harm patients via acts of commission or omission. In general, surgical care should be restricted to what that the surgical team is competent in based on training, resources, experience, and appropriate standards of care [3]. However, in the instance where a surgeon or surgical team is presented with a patient requiring care beyond their proven competence, the question that must be asked is whether they have a reasonable belief that caring for this patient would be of overall benefit to the patient in comparison with other available options. Is the risk of harm greater to the patient if they are taken care of at this facility or if they are transferred elsewhere [8]? Good judgment and a solid understanding of local and regional resources are crucial. Prioritizing team safety and rest is also essential for the sustainment and health of the team so they can continue to provide quality surgical care.

No surgery is without risk, and complications occur even in the hands of the most skilled surgeons. Furthermore, depending on the deployment mission, surgeons may be geographically isolated, making it difficult to objectively analyze surgical complications and find areas for improvement. It is important to stay engaged with the regional surgical community as technology and operational security allow. Regular participation in a morbidity and mortality conference should be sought with the regional surgical community.

Beneficence

Clinical Vignette 36.4

A 21-month-old boy was brought aboard a hospital ship during an elective humanitarian mission to a developing nation. Nine months prior, this child suffered extensive burns to his face causing severe burn contractures such that he could not entirely close his eyes or mouth. The patient's grandmother, his primary caretaker, consented to contracture release and possible skin grafting with the goal of being able to close his eyes. The surgery was planned for the following day, three days prior to the ship's departure from this location. The surgery was completed without issue, and the child recovered on the ship for the remaining three days that the ship remained at this port. He was then transferred to a local hospital in good condition but still requiring extensive wound management, which may have overburdened local medical capabilities. The long-term outcome for this patient is unknown.

Should this surgery have occurred so close to the time of the hospital ship's departure? Was appropriate follow-up arranged? Should surgical care have been denied because appropriate follow-up may not have been feasible, knowing that this may be the only chance this patient would ever have to undergo this procedure?

Beneficence is the duty to intentionally prevent harm and provide benefit to patients. Beneficence and nonmaleficence occupy opposite sides of the same coin. Surgeons and surgical teams are typically driven by a desire to help patients;

however, in the spirit of intentionally preventing harm, sometimes it is appropriate to abstain from offering surgery to a patient [3]. "Sometimes 'No' is the best answer…never allow providers to do more than they should be doing, given limitations of equipment, time, etc. …Large and complex cases should be reviewed and only performed when the team is convinced that the case can be done safely and that the patient will receive good care when the humanitarian team is no longer on the scene" [5]. Ensuring appropriate follow-up care is one of the biggest barriers to fulfilling the bioethical principle of Beneficence. Leaving behind a labor- and supply-intensive patient burden for the host nation medical system to take care of is one of the cardinal sins of humanitarian surgery. Surgeons should take into consideration local resources when planning surgeries that may require follow up in the local medical system long after the surgical team departs [5].

In order to maximize patient benefit, sustainability should be taken into consideration for every humanitarian mission. Short- or long-term missions should integrate strategies that provide sustained improvement to local healthcare systems. This can be accomplished through education, research, or public health measures [3, 5, 9]. Any research conducted should be ethical and oriented around improvement of long-term outcomes. Patient involvement in research must be voluntary.

Under the topic of beneficence, it is apropos to discuss involvement of trainees and Graduate Medical Education (GME) during humanitarian missions. There is growing interest in global surgery, and many surgical and non-surgical residencies (including Navy GME programs) are offering Global Health Engagement (GHE) rotations. Global humanitarian surgery missions provide surgical residents with opportunities to learn while caring for patients with advanced pathology not typically seen in developed nations. However, as educational as humanitarian surgery may be for the trainees, is involving surgical residents in humanitarian surgery violating the bioethical principle of beneficence by not doing everything to intentionally prevent harm? "With strong mentorship and appropriate supervision, surgical residents can provide the same level of care in the humanitarian setting as in any academic [medical] center in developed nations" [3]. If experiences in GHE are appropriately structured, it allows for the opportunity to teach and review the practical bioethical principles discussed in this chapter, preparing trainees for independent practice in the humanitarian and GHE environment.

Finally, should GHE activities play a role in the military readiness of forward deployable surgical teams? Within military medicine, some look at humanitarian and GHE activities as a way to prevent the attrition of expeditionary relevant skills in forward deployed caregivers, proposing the only way to closely replicate the experience of resource-limited forward deployed surgical environments without actually taking care of combat casualties is through providing medical and surgical care during GHE activities [10, 11]. The bioethical principles of autonomy, nonmaleficence, and beneficence are particularly relevant to the to the discussion of GHE and military medical readiness. First, the primary mission goal cannot be trauma training or clinical experience for military providers. Mission goals must reflect those of the host nation (autonomy). Next, the care provided must be based not only on the appropriate standards of care for the environment and situation, but the surgical care provided must be based on the training and experience that the surgical team *already has*. Sending surgical teams that are not appropriately trained risks harming patients and risks teaching junior and inexperienced forward deployed caregivers incorrectly (nonmaleficence). Finally, GHE surgery missions are enriching experiences with much to gain for the involved surgical teams—trainees, forward deployable units, or otherwise. However, personal gain should never take precedence over what is right for the patient's welfare. It is never ethical to participate in surgical tourism (beneficence) [11]. If Military Medicine's GHE partnerships result in experiences for forward deployed caregivers that help sustain a previously learned combat trauma care skillset while providing a service to partner nations, then like any true partnership, there is mutual benefit.

Ethics Curriculum and Training

It is important to provide a formal ethics curriculum as part of the deployment preparation for surgical teams, trainees, and novices involved in GHE and humanitarian surgery. The goal of this ethics curriculum is reviewing the core bioethical principles in the context of practical application in the deployed environment—humanitarian surgery, disaster relief, or combat support. They are summarized in Table 36.1. These principles are important to review prior to caring for local national patients with different cultural norms, expectations, and follow-on care capabilities available to them. Training in bioethics can help prevent the moral injury that can occur when faced with an ethical dilemma in the deployed setting.

Most deployed surgical teams in any deployed environment have a formal process improvement or morbidity and mortality conference after unanticipated or poor outcomes. Consider incorporating a dedicated discussion about the ethical dilemmas involved in these cases to increase the awareness of the ethical issues inherent in all aspects of humanitarian care and to create a safe space to debrief difficult ethical cases. This last point cannot be overemphasized. When care is withdrawn or there is a poor outcome, often there is misunderstanding by members of the team about why a decision was made or even if the patient was survivable. Debriefing these cases with a focus on ethics in an open forum is critical to maintaining healthy team dynamics and communication skills. It provides a forum for team members to voice concerns, examine ethical dilemmas, correct wrong assumptions, and most importantly decrease the potential moral injury that can occur.

Table 36.1 Practical bioethical principles for the deployed environment

Core bioethical principle	Deployed humanitarian principle
Justice	Triage during elective missions should take into account short- and long-term outcomes and local cultural norms Triage during disaster relief should take into account long-term care requirements in the context of host nation resources. Criteria for eligibility for care should be determined a priori An ethics committee should be identified and pre-designated to assist deliberating ethical dilemmas that may occur Missions from different organizations should be coordinated
Autonomy	Set realistic patient and host nation expectations Do not misrepresent team credentials or capabilities Respect for persons applies to patients and host nation providers Informed consent should be obtained in patient's language and account for cultural norms and religious beliefs. Written documentation of consent should be obtained For humanitarian missions, only go where invited Mission goals must reflect host nation goals
Nonmaleficence	Restrict surgical care/procedures to those that surgeons and surgical teams are competent in, based on training, resources, experience, and appropriate standards of care Use good judgment Consider team safety and rest Ensure strong mentorship and supervision to trainees and inexperienced caregivers Prevent moral injury by providing pre-deployment bioethics review, incorporating ethical dilemmas in morbidity and mortality process improvement activities (consider engaging regional surgical communities), and debriefing controversial ethical dilemmas
Beneficence	Provide the best care possible as permitted by local resources Respect host nation customs without compromising care Ensure appropriate follow-up Personal gain is inherent to missions but should not supersede patient welfare Sustainability should be integral to any mission and can include education, research, and public health measures Research should be ethical and oriented around improvement of long-term outcomes. Involvement should be voluntary

Conclusion

Every deployment is unique in terms of mission objectives, available medical resources, local conditions, individual medical team members, and patients presenting for surgical care. Therefore, there is no single correct answer to any given scenario. At times the four core bioethical principles can seemingly compete with one another. Familiarization with the core bioethical principles can "stimulate moral imagination" and allow surgeons to "enact the highest moral options available in a given situation" [12]. Ultimately, it is the duty of surgeons and surgical teams to take compassionate care of their patients and respect their rights and dignity as fellow humans. "The expectation for observing the fundamental bioethical principles of autonomy, beneficence, nonmaleficence, and justice remains inexplicably joined to expressions of the professional virtues of integrity, truthfulness, compassion and trust" [7].

Declaration of Interest The views expressed in this chapter are those of the authors and do not necessarily reflect the official policy or position of the Department of the Navy, Department of Defense, nor the US Government.

Funding This research did not receive any specific grant from funding agencies in the public, commercial, or not-for-profit sectors.

Conflict of Interest Statement The authors declare no conflict of interest.

References

1. Beauchamp TL, Childress JF. Principles of biomedical ethics. Oxford: Oxford University Press; 2001.
2. Wall A, Angelos P, Brown D, Kodner IJ, Keune JD. Ethics in surgery. Curr Probl Surg. 2013;50(3):99–134.
3. McDonald VS, Ignacio RC, Kuettel MA, Schlitzkus LL, Sullivan ME, Tadlock MD. Practical bioethics for the humanitarian surgeon: the development, implementation and assessment of an ethics curriculum for residents participating in humanitarian missions. J Surg Educ. 2020;77(2):390–403.
4. Merin O, Ash N, Levy G, Schwaber MJ, Kreiss Y. The Israeli field hospital in Haiti–ethical dilemmas in early disaster response. N Engl J Med. 2010;362(11):e38.
5. Welling DR, Ryan JM, Burris DG, Rich NM. Seven sins of humanitarian medicine. World J Surg. 2010;34(3):466–70.
6. Suah A, Angelos P. How should trauma patients' informed consent or refusal be regarded in a trauma bay or other emergency settings? AMA J Ethics. 2018;20(5):425–30.
7. Holt GR. Ethical conduct of humanitarian medical missions: I. Informed consent. Arch Facial Plast Surg. 2012;14(3):215–7.
8. Sheather J, Shah T. Ethical dilemmas in medical humanitarian practice: cases for reflection from Médecins Sans Frontières. J Med Ethics. 2011;37(3):162–5.
9. Younger A, Worlton TJ, Wallace S, Steigleman WA, Ortiz-Pomales Y. Ethical considerations for surgical planners from the lessons learned on USNS COMFORT (T-AH 20) deployment 2019. Mil Med. 2021;186(5-6):117–20.
10. Ratnayake A, Worlton TJ. Intricacies and complexities of maintaining military medical readiness: the Sri Lankan Strategy, in response to "how to maintain the readiness of forward deployed caregivers". J Trauma Acute Care Surg. 2021;91(Suppl 2):S267–8.
11. Tadlock MD. Authors response: "How to maintain the readiness of forward deployed caregivers" or what is the role of global health engagement in military medical readiness? J Trauma Acute Care Surg. 2021;91(Suppl 2):S268–9.
12. Hunt MR. Establishing moral bearings: ethics and expatriate health care professionals in humanitarian work. Disasters. 2011;35(3):606–22.

Appendix A: MacGyver or Tactically Acquire? Maritime "Alternate" Equipment

A paperclip can be a wonderous thing. More times than I can remember, one of these has gotten me out of a tight spot.

There always seems to be a way to fix things. (MacGyver, 1985–1992 Television Series)

MacGyver or Tactically Acquire?

Surgical teams have been deploying on naval warships successfully caring for surgical patients for decades using the equipment, instruments, and consumables in the surgical Authorized Medical Allowance Lists (AMALs) provided to them. To a certain extent, the old saying one may have heard from their parents, "you get what you get and you don't throw a fit," is applicable to the maritime surgical team. However, as discussed in multiple chapters, delays in the supply chain or other unforeseen circumstances historically have caused surgical teams to be innovative and "MacGyver" what they have to care for their patients or go to their local medical treatment facility (MTF) with a large bag in hand to "Tactically Acquire" consumables or expired supplies they may need before deployment as described in Chap. 12. While the practice of tactically acquiring items is not ideal, it is sometimes necessary. More importantly surgical teams should "pay it forward." If the AMAL needs to be changed, work through the formal system to change it (several methods discussed in Chap. 12).

What follows is a summary list of items from their respective chapters that the editors of this book feel maritime surgical teams may need to MacGyver on deployment or tactically acquire before deployment. It is by no means an exhaustive list of what may be needed. The editors also recommend Appendix A from *Front Line Surgery, A Practical Approach* (Martin, Beekley, and Eckert) for a comprehensive list of "field expedient methods in a forward environment" [1].

M. D. Tadlock, A. A. Hernandez (eds.), *Expeditionary Surgery at Sea*,
https://doi.org/10.1007/978-3-031-21893-4

MacGyver

These versatile catheters are typically available on surgical AMALs and have multiple potential uses. Be sure to check for availability, sizes (when applicable), and expiration dates.

- **Vessel Loops**: Besides being used for proximal and distal control of vascular injures, they are useful in other ways.
  - **Temporary Internal Iliac Artery Ligation**: As described in Chap. 22, they can be used for patients in hemorrhagic shock from pelvic fractures; interventional radiology is not an option on naval warships.
  - **Non-cutting Seton** for benign anorectal disease (Chap. 14).
  - **Abscess Management**: As described in Chaps. 14 and 34, can be used in the treatment of abscesses in general for both adult and pediatric patients to minimize painful traumatic dressing changes.
- **Red Rubber Robinson Catheters**:
  - **T-tube:** As described in Chap. 15 and demonstrated in Fig. 15.8, a 14 French Red Rubber Robinson catheter can be fashioned into a T-tube.
  - **Balloon Tamponade Device**: As described in Chap. 22, when holes are cut in a Red Rubber Robinson catheter and it is passed through a Penrose drain, it can be passed into a deep liver tract injury and filled with saline to provide a tamponade effect.
  - **Expeditionary Expedient Rummel Tourniquet for the Pringle Maneuver**: As described in Chap. 22 and demonstrated in Fig. 22.1, a Red Rubber Robinson catheter can be fashioned into a Rummel tourniquet around the portal triad.
  - **Pediatric Chest Tube** (Chap. 34).
- **Foley Catheters**: Make sure to tape over the balloon port so it is not inadvertently deflated.
  - **Cholecystostomy Tube** (Fig. 15.4).
  - **Suprapubic Catheter**: As described in Chap. 17, a Foley catheter can be placed via open suprapubic approach when concern for urethral injury or unable to place urethral catheter.
  - **Bakri Balloon**: As described in Chap. 17, a Foley catheter with a condom can be used as an alternative to a Bakri balloon.
  - **Gastrostomy** or **Jejunostomy Tube** [1].
- **Triple Lumen Central Venous Catheters (CVC)**:
  - **Diagnostic Peritoneal Aspirate**: A CVC can be used when point-of-care ultrasound (POCUS) is not available or equivocal when evaluating abdominal trauma.

- Thoracentesis [1].
- Paracentesis [1].

- **Malecot Catheters**:
  - **Cholecystostomy Tube** (Fig. 15.4).
  - **Gastrostomy Tube** [1].
  - **Abscess Management**: As described in Chap. 14, a Malecot catheter can keep a cavity open after surgical drainage to minimize painful traumatic dressing changes.

These are some work-around solutions for specific surgical consumables that can be lifesaving but may not/are not available on maritime platforms.

- **Appendectomy**: As described in Chap. 14, know multiple ways to perform an appendectomy, including through a right lower quadrant incision. The authors have heard many stories of surgeons meeting their teams on deployment and the surgical staplers being expired or absent.
- **Makeshift Finger Trap Device**: As described in Chap. 19 and demonstrated in Fig. 19.12, a makeshift finger trap device can be fashioned using parachute cord, riggers tape, a nylon strap, and a 10-pound weight.
- **Temporary Abdominal Dressing**: Negative pressure dressings for open abdomens (e.g., the Abthera™ device) are not available on ships. As described in Chap. 22, create one using either a 1010 Steri-Drape™ (3M) or a sterile Mayo table cover, blue towels or laparotomy pads, closed-suction drains, and Ioban™ (3M).
- **Temporary Vascular Shunt**: As described in Chap. 22, intravenous (IV) tubing, nasogastric tubes (NGT), or chest tubes can be cut to length and used as a temporary vascular shunt, depending on vessel size.
- **Temporary Field-Expedient Heimlich Valve**: The finger of a sterile glove with a hole on the end can be attached to a chest tube and used as a Heimlich valve [1].
- **Measuring Extremity Compartment Pressures**: Commercial compartment-measuring devices are typically not available on ships. Chaps. 24 and 26 describe indications for measuring compartment pressures and how to create makeshift ones using electronic pressure transducers (e.g., arterial line). If even those are not available, a makeshift pressure-measuring device can be fashioned using a three-way stopcock connected via IV tubing to an 18-gauge needle, a blood pressure manometer, and saline-filled syringe as demonstrated in Fig. A.1. Use a blood pressure manometer, cut a 6 inch length of rubber tubing, attach it to IV tubing, and plug it into a three-way stopcock. Next, put an 18-gauge needle on the end of another segment of IV tubing and attach it to a different port on the stopcock. Finally, place a saline-filled 10 cc syringe on the final port. Infuse saline halfway up the IV tubing attached to the manometer and its rubber connecting line. Next, locally anesthetize the skin, insert the 18-gauge needle, and flush 5 mL

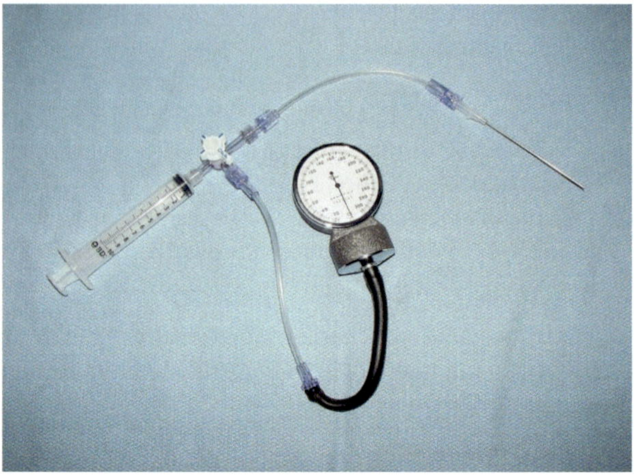

Fig. A.1 Makeshift device for measuring extremity compartment pressures

of saline. Finally, open the stopcock back to the blood pressure manometer line and compress the compartment manually to make sure that the manometer cycles appropriately with increased pressure. Then measure the pressure.

Tactically Acquire

At the time of publication, the following are not available on maritime surgical AMALs. If desired, they should be acquired from another ship or a local MTF.

- **Gastrografin**: Patients with prior abdominal surgery are all over the Fleet! It's not a matter of if, but when a patient with an adhesive small bowel obstruction (SBO) will present to a maritime provider. As discussed in Chap. 14, Gastrografin can be both diagnostic and therapeutic in the management of adhesive SBO.
- **Iohexal (Omnipaque™)**: There are many concentrations available, but the concentration typically used for surgical procedures is Omnipaque™ 240 (Fig. A.2). As described in Chap. 8, it can have many uses for teams that have flat plate X-ray capability.
  - **Intraoperative Cholangiogram**: As described in Chap. 15, use full-strength Omnipaque™ 240 when performing a flat plate cholangiogram.
  - **Retrograde Urethrogram**: As described in Chap. 17, typically Omnipaque™ 240 is diluted 1:1 (50%) with Normal Saline but full strength may be required.
- **Barium**: As described in Chap. 18 and Clinical Vignettes 18.1 and 18.2 and demonstrated in Fig. 18.1, for surgical teams with X-ray capability, barium swallow studies with serial static X-rays can help diagnose a number of upper gastrointestinal disorders and obstruction.

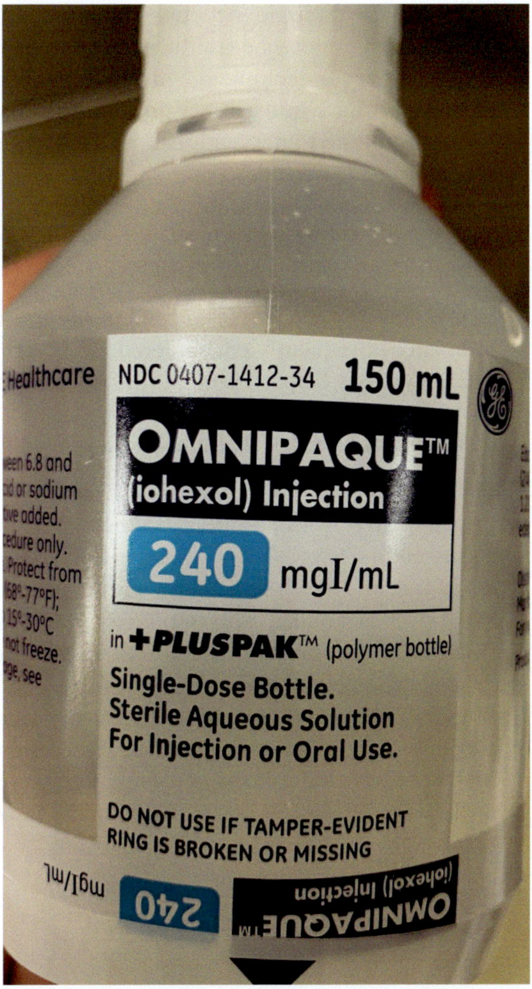

Fig. A.2 Omnipaque™ 240, the concentration typically used for surgical procedures

- **Percutaneous Suprapubic Catheter Kit**: As described in Chap. 17, this could be needed for its intended purpose. As described in Chap. 15, it can also be used as cholecystostomy tube.
- **Endoloop®**: As described in Chaps. 14 and 15, during laparoscopic cases on the ship, PDS® II Endoloops® are invaluable tools to secure the cystic duct stump during cholecystectomy or to secure the appendix at its base before dividing it.
- **Laparoscopic LigaSure™**: Not only do the maritime platforms not have the energy device itself, but they also don't have the electrosurgical unit needed for it to function. Current electrosurgical units are slated to be replaced by LigaSure™ capable ones in 2026 or when they are outside of their lifecycle, and the Maritime Surgery Quality Improvement (MSQI) program is working with Fleet representatives to speed up the transition. The primary argument is that the LigaSure™ device could save time for single surgeon teams during mass casualty incidents

(MCIs) with multiple patients requiring abdominal damage control surgery (DCS), but they can be useful in many types of cases, such as a laparoscopic salpingectomy for ectopic pregnancy described in Chap. 17.

- **Interventional Endoscopy Equipment**: Most shipboard medical departments have very limited interventional endoscopy consumables (if any). As described in Chap. 18, the maritime surgeon could manage a number of conditions requiring interventional endoscopy. At a minimum the authors recommend considering augmenting shipboard endoscopy capabilities with the following:
  - **Grasping Forceps**: Typically only biopsy forceps are available, but larger grasping forceps or raptor forceps are useful for larger food impactions that are not infrequently encountered.
  - **Hemostasis Clips**: Through-the-scope metal clips can be useful to treat gastrointestinal bleeding (GIB).
  - **Injection Needles**: If trained in performing Epinephrine injection, through-the-scope needles can be helpful in the management of some GIB.
- **Resuscitative Endovascular Balloon Occlusion of the Aorta (REBOA)**: As discussed in Chap. 22, if the team is trained in this capability, particularly single surgeon teams likely to manage multiple casualties, this can be a useful hemorrhage control adjunct. Appropriate pre-deployment training is critical.
- **Pediatric Equipment**. Most AMALs do not carry equipment appropriate to care for pediatric patients. However maritime surgical teams are often called on to care for pediatric patients during crisis or contingency operations such as during humanitarian aid disaster relief (HADR) operations. As discussed in Chap. 34, consider acquiring following if there is a pre-existing expectation that maritime surgical teams may be managing pediatric patients:
  - **Broselow bag**
  - **Airway management tools** (oral airways, pediatric ventilation masks, pediatric ambu-bag, endotracheal tubes)
  - **Pediatric IV catheters** (22-gauge, 24-gauge)
- **Head Lamp**: When working in a deep hole, extra light can be very helpful no matter where one is operating. While surgical head lamps cannot be tactically acquired from an MTF, if no head lamps are available in the surgical AMAL, strongly consider purchasing a powerful nonsurgical headlamp. The authors have used the Surefire Maximus™ headlamp, available at: https://www.surefire.com/products/illumination/headlamps/maximus/.

References

1. Appendix A—Improvise, adapt, overcome: field expedient methods in a forward environment. In: Martin MJ, Beekley AC, Eckert MJ, editors. Front line surgery: a practical approach, 2nd ed. Cham: Springer; 2017. p. 869–75.

Appendix B: Sample Packing List for Maritime Deployment

General

- Packing may be different depending on the time of joining the ship—there is a big difference between being in port with unlimited trips to the ship to bring in gear and flying out to meet the team, where there are quantity and weight restrictions.
- Using seabag/flight bag is easiest, but can use whatever bag is allowed. Keep in mind if in uniform, must use military gear.
- For many ship deployments, Amazon or other shipping services are available. Can also have friends and family send packages, which can be pre-staged. Keep in mind that shipping times can be delayed by weeks.
- These are all suggestions; it is impossible to make specific recommendations for every ship, every mission, every time.

Uniforms

Navy Uniform Regulations Website:
https://www.mynavyhr.navy.mil/References/US-Navy-Uniforms/Uniform-Regulations/

- Navy Working Uniform (NWU): Wear in port—recommend at least one set, arrive with rank/corps/warfare devices (if have them) and "U.S. NAVY/LAST NAME" patches already sewn on. **Bring** Enlisted Surface Warfare Specialist (ESWS)/Surface Warfare Medical Department Officer (SWMDO) warfare device patch if plan to obtain qualification on deployment so can sew it on.

M. D. Tadlock, A. A. Hernandez (eds.), *Expeditionary Surgery at Sea*,
https://doi.org/10.1007/978-3-031-21893-4

  - Items required for NWU: NWU cover, tan t-shirts, two velcro patches for the upper sleeves, embroidered slip-on rank/rate insignia (to put onto velcro tab on front of uniform), belt, belt buckle, socks, boots, and boot bands.
  - As needed: NWU Parka ± black fleece (both with embroidered slip-on rank/rate insignia), gloves, etc.

- Flame Resistant Variant (FRV) aka coveralls: Wear underway. Can try on in Navy Exchange (NEX) to get an idea of size if available. They are issued on the ship because they have to be flame-retardant, so are often not available until check in to the ship. **Bring** rank/corps patches on dark blue **or** pins to put on collars. For Expeditionary Resuscitative Surgical System (ERSS) teams augmenting small ships, these uniforms are often provided once onboard, but it is still important to bring rank/corps collar devices (as pins)! Recommend having at least three FRV. Don't need "U.S. NAVY/LAST NAME" or warfare device patches. Get issued Velcro patches with name, rank, which can also include warfare device(s).

  - Items required for FRV: ship ball cap (do not wear on the ship except in certain instances, gets issued), tan t-shirts, belt, belt buckle, socks, boots (no boot bands required).
  - Ship issues a fleece (different than the one for the NWU) to be worn with the FRV.
  - **Bring** at least seven days of undergarments/t-shirts/socks unless plan to do laundry more frequently.

- Belts ± buckles: Be sure to buy the right one! There are different sizes for men and women, different types based on rank, different buckle requirements, and different belt loop sizes on different uniforms.
- Boots: Steel-toed, many options at NEX, check with specific command on policies for brown versus black, bring polish/supplies if plan to do that.
- Navy Physical Training Uniform (PTU): Gear to wear for weigh-in for the Physical Readiness Test (PRT) when applicable.
- Ask command about other required deployment uniforms (service/khaki/white, dress blue, dress white), especially if do not plan to live on the ship.

Clothing

Be sure to plan for weather (e.g., may have left San Diego during warm weather but Korea during winter is cold).

- Civilian clothing worn during port calls or during leisure time on the ship.
- Bring more workout gear than one thinks necessary, check with command on specific regulations (i.e., no tank tops).
- Laundry bag, detergent ± dryer sheets for self-serve laundry (if available).

- Range of comfortable sleeping clothing since berthing/staterooms range from freezing cold to hot and rarely have true temperature control.
- Swimsuit (if plan to swim during any port calls).
- Sunglasses (military-approved if plan to wear in uniform).
- Bag to carry on/off ship in ports if don't want to use military gear.
- As needed: long underwear for prolonged cold weather periods to wear under uniform (issued a fleece coat, but it is bone-chillingly cold in winter in the middle of the ocean).

Technology

Many times, there is ***no Wi-Fi*** *to speak of on the ship!*

Get all cords checked by ship to pass inspections (or hide for inspection).

Figure out how to use cell phone during deployment (e.g., turn off, get SIM cards, get burner phone); on the ship, it may not matter but in port it does.

Be sure all technology apps are PRE-downloaded and functioning on whatever device planned to use for communication, especially FaceTime/Skype!

- Bring all desired technology with charger/cord (**with back-up charger/cord**).
- Bluetooth speakers and/or headphones are awesome for working out/studying/movies, would recommend. However, also **highly** recommend having back-up corded/non-Bluetooth versions, especially headphones, because ships can go into conditions when Bluetooth not allowed.
- Noise-canceling headphones, depending on the location of berthing/stateroom, co-habitants, and ability to sleep with noise.
- Game console with cords/controls, cords to connect computers to TVs to "stream" movies, DVD player to attach to TV if have old-school DVD collection, etc.
- Little flashlight/headlamp in case power goes out on the ship.
- International plug, depending on port calls.

Medical/Surgical

Scrubs are typically provided on larger ships, check with platform.

- Loupes (for surgeons)
- Operating Room (OR) shoes, scrub caps
- Tools of the trade (e.g., stethoscope, shears)
- Medical books (especially surgical subspecialty books like Vascular, Hand, and Urology for surgeons)

- Training supplies (especially for Advanced Trauma Life Support (ATLS)/trauma for surgeons)
- Printer paper (recommend saving a small emergency stash for when the whole ship runs out)
- Signature stamp (for providers)

Paperwork/Administrative

Typically, all papers have already been turned in many times, but will need them again. Promise. Someone will ask for a hard copy and the internet will be down. ***Just bring them****! Best case scenario they get shredded.*

- Hard copies of all pertinent diplomas/certificates/certifications/credentials (e.g., diploma, licensure, Basic Life Support (BLS) certification).
- Hard copies of HIPAA and CYBER AWARENESS annual training (be up to date **before** arrival because internet connection is finicky on deployment).
- Hard copy of orders.
- Hard copy of last Eval/FitRep to make the next cycle smoother.
- Wallet with driver's license and credit cards.
- Common Access Card (CAC).
- Government travel credit card (GTCC).
- Passport! No matter what anyone says, always obtain a civilian passport before deployment. Medical providers at all levels are often asked to travel internationally via commercial airlines to escort patients or for other reasons. Not only can time be saved at airports but interesting travel opportunities can become available if one has a passport.
- Bank information (to get Cash Card, which is how to pay for things on ship) with routing and account numbers.
- Medical/Dental records with Radiation Health/ThermoLuminescent Dosimetry (TLD) information for Radiation Safety as applicable.

Hygiene/Toiletries

Hard to bring enough toiletries for an entire deployment, depending on duration of deployment and amount of use. Can also have them mailed mid-deployment or pick them up in ports.

- Bring all toiletries for hair, teeth, skin, nails, deodorant, hair removal, etc.
  - Ship water is notoriously hard on skin, hair, and lips.
  - Don't forget little things like q-tips, nail clippers, tweezers, chapstick, etc.
  - All the hair stuff to stay in regulations.

- Good Kleenex.
- Robe, shower shoes, ± shower caddy for walk to and from the bathroom.
- GOOD towel (or two), fast-drying preferable.
- Feminine hygiene products as applicable.
- Bring prescriptions for medications (including birth control) or have a plan arranged for them to be sent.
- Sunscreen.
- Fiber! (As every general surgeon knows, this may be the most important thing to pack other than a uniform.)
- If desired: personal supply of over-the-counter medications: **metamucil**, tylenol, motrin, etc.

Berthing/Stateroom

Talk with future co-habitants ahead of time preferably and if possible. Berthing/staterooms differ widely. Many things that make life nicer and easier are technically "not allowed" on the ship, yet many people bring them anyway. If bringing them, be sure to use them safely and hide them for inspections.

- Sheets, pillows, and wool blankets are issued. Many people choose to bring their own of all of those items (may need to hide for inspection). Mattress pad is also recommended by many.
- Blackout curtains/drapes for rack depending on sensitivity to light.
- Ambience lights, decorations, etc. (may need to hide for inspection).
- Magnets, command hooks, etc.
- Combination lock.
- TV monitor (sometimes small one already in staterooms) and/or cords to connect laptop to it.
- Fan and/or space heater (may need to hide for inspection, be sure UNPLUGGED when not in use for safety).
- Clock.
- Rug.
- Clorox wipes (may need to hide for inspection).

Leisure Time

PRE-download shows, movies, podcasts, work-outs, etc. There are typically NO streaming services on the ship and sometimes when out to sea for prolonged periods of time then services go dormant.

- TV shows/movies/podcasts on large external hard drive.
- Packs of cards, small/easy/fun group games (e.g., cards against humanity, bananagrams).

- Photos/child artwork from home to put in workspace and/or berthing.
- Books for personal or professional development (hardcover or e-books).
  - Frequently there is a library with books/movies.
- Binder to put ESWS/SWMDO study materials in.
- Personal pens, journals, notebooks if do not like Navy-issued gear.
- Envelopes, stamps.
  - Frequently Chaplain will have free greeting cards.
- Water bottle(s).
- Coffee/tea cup(s).
- If one likes coffee, many recommend bringing a French press (and coffee) to ensure quality coffee is available during deployment.
- Drink mixes.
- Fun snacks or meal items! Microwaves are usually available in galley or workspaces, can be nice to have something different to eat.
- Condiments of choosing to spice up the food.
- Gum/mints.
- Yoga mat/resistance bands/workout gear of choice if do not want to use the gyms and/or the gyms are not stocked with desired gear.
- Sweat towels for working out.

Appendix C: Glossary of Common Nautical Terms

Author deployment experience	
Radhames E. Lizardo	Battalion Surgeon, 1st Battalion, 12th Marines, Operation Enduring Freedom, Helmand Province, Afghanistan, 2011
	Ship's Surgeon, USS Ronald Reagan (CVN-76), WESTPAC, INDOPACOM Area of Responsibility, 2018

1-MC	1 Main Circuit, public address circuit aboard a ship
3M	Material, Maintenance, & Management system which prolongs the life of the ship
Abandon ship	An imperative to leave the vessel immediately due to overwhelming danger
AFFF	Aqueous Film Forming Foam, used to combat Bravo/Charlie fires
Aft	Toward the stern (rear) of the ship
"Ahoy"	Call for attention
Air Boss	Officer in charge of the Flight Deck
All Hands	The entire Ship's Company
Astern	Behind a ship
"Aye, Aye"	Reply to an order to indicate that it is first heard and understood and second that it will be carried out
Belay	To cancel an order or stop an action, as in "belay the small talk" or "belay my last!"
Berthing	Living/bunking/sleeping spaces on a ship
BDS	Battle Dressing Station, forward medical locations around the ship
Binnacle List	Ship's medical and dental report to include the sick and injured report
Bitter End	Last part or loose end of a rope or cable or anchor

M. D. Tadlock, A. A. Hernandez (eds.), *Expeditionary Surgery at Sea*,
https://doi.org/10.1007/978-3-031-21893-4

Blue Water	Deep water far from land, unable to reach shore with aircraft; only larger, self-sufficient ships can operate on these waters
Boot	Nickname for Sailors fresh out of boot camp or new to first duty station
Bosun	aka "Boatswain," a non-commissioned officer responsible for the ship's rigging and boats
Bow	Forward (front) end of a boat or ship
"Bravo Zulu"	"Congratulations!" or "Good job!"
Bridge	Room from which a ship is commanded
Brig	Jail on a ship
Bulkhead	Vertical partition in a ship aka wall
CBRNE	Chemical, Biological, Radiological, Nuclear and High Explosive
CDO	Command Duty Officer, like the OOD, has delegation from CO
CG	Cruiser Guided Missile ship
CHENG	Chief Engineer of the ship
Chow	Food
CHT	Collection, Holding, and Transfer aka sewage
Cleaning Stations	Field day evolution of a prescribed time in which everyone drops what they're doing and cleans their spaces
Circle William	Preparation for chemical, germ, or nuclear attack
CMC	Command Master Chief (highest-ranking enlisted member of the ship)
CNO	Chief of Naval Operations
CO	Commanding Officer aka "Captain" of the ship
CPO	Chief Petty Officer (E7 enlisted rank), they are rate-specific expert Sailors that are the backbone of the ship and Navy
CoC	Chain of Command
Cofferdam	Narrow vacant space between two bulkheads of a ship
Condition Dog Zebra	Darken Ship, set at sunset
Condition X-Ray	Ship's minimum protective posture, set at pier side or homeport
Condition Yoke	Ship's moderate protective posture, maintained at sea
Condition Zebra	Ship's maximum protective posture, set for GQ/Battle Stations
Colors	Ceremony to lower and raise the U.S. flag
Cover	Head gear, such as uniform hat or ball cap
Crossing the Line	Crossing the Equator, a few variations. There are also several other "fraternities" for similar "milestones" of a Sailor's career. See final reference.
Crow's Nest	Lookout station aloft

CVN	Aircraft Carrier (nuclear-powered)
Davy Jones' Locker	Bottom of the sea
DDG	Destroyer Guided Missile Ship
Deck Hand	Sailor whose job involves aiding in mooring, anchoring, and all evolutions on deck
DC	Damage Control; emergency control of situations that could cause a vessel to sink like fires, floods, etc.
DEERS	Defense Enrollment Eligibility Reporting System
DESRON	Commander of a Destroyer Squadron
DivO	Division Officer
Dog the Hatch	To secure the watertight seals after closing a hatch or door
EMCON	Emissions Condition postures, of which there are several levels
Ensign	Large national flag or O-1 pay grade officer
ESWS	Enlisted Surface Warfare Specialist; qualification that can be attained by medical department enlisted Sailors
"Fair Winds and Following Seas"	Blessing wishing the recipient a safe journey and good fortune
Fantail	Aft-most (rear) deck of a ship aka "poop deck"
Fathom	Nautical unit of length or depth equal to six feet
FFG	Frigate Ship
Field Day	General deep clean of the facility, usually involving all hands
Flight Deck	Flat deck of a vessel used for the launch and recovery of aircraft
Frame	Transverse compartment that gives the hull strength, shape, and specific location; can be located on a map
Forward	Toward the bow (front) of the ship
Focsle	aka "forecastle," forward part of a ship below the main deck, traditional crew's quarters, pronounced "fohk-sul"
FOD Walkdown	Organized and systemic inspection of a flight deck for any Foreign Object Debris (FOD)
FON Ops	Freedom of Navigation operations
Galley	Kitchen
Gangway	Opening in the bulwark of a ship to allow passengers to board or leave the ship
Gator	Ship's Navigator
Geedunk	Refers to ice cream, candy, potato chips, and snack foods from the Ship's Store
General Quarters (GQ)	Full readiness for battle aka "Battle Stations"
Gear Adrift	Items, such as personal gear, not properly stowed

Goat Locker	Mess hall/meeting area reserved for Chief Petty Officers
Gundecking	Filling out a form with imaginary data to satisfy an inspection
Hangar Bay	Main deck of a vessel with a flight deck, where equipment and aircraft are stored
Hatch	Covered opening in a ship's deck through which access is made to a lower or higher deck
Head	Compartment containing toilet facilities
Helm	Steering aka the wheel of the ship
High Seas	aka International Waters, more than 12 nautical miles from a nation state
HYDRA	Hierarchical Yet Dynamically Reprogrammable Architecture aka walkie-talkie aka the "Brick"
Inboard	Toward the centerline of the ship
Jury Rig	Temporary repair to keep a disabled ship sailing until it can make port
Knot	Unit of measurement for vessel movement in the water (1 knot = 1.15 mph)
Kneeknockers	Bottom portion of a watertight door's frame
Ladder	Flight of steps aboard a ship; similarly a stairwell is called a ladder well
Lanyard	Rope that ties something off
Leeward	In the direction that the wind is blowing toward
LHA	Landing Helicopter Assault Ship
LHD	Landing Helicopter Dock Ship
Liberty	Sanctioned absence from ship or station for short time for pleasure rather than business
Liberty Buddies	Sailors who hold each other accountable during port visits
List	Transverse inclination of a vessel (leaning to one side)
Lookout	Sailor assigned to watch surrounding waters for other vessels, hazards, threats, etc.
LPD	Landing Platform Dock Ship
LSD	Landing Ship Dock
LSO	Landing Signal Officer aka "Paddles"
Man Overboard	Sailor who falls, jumps, or is thrown off a vessel into the water
Mess Deck	Place to eat aboard a ship
METOC	Meteorological and Oceanography Officer
Mid-rats	Mid-rations, when mess decks/wardrooms open in the middle of the night
Midshipman	Officer cadet at the Naval Academy

MIO	Maritime Interdiction Operation
MOPP	Mission Oriented Protective Posture, pre-staged CBRNE protective gear
Muster	Roll call
MWR	Morale, Welfare, and Recreation, often the responsibility of the "Fun Boss"
"Nay"	"No," the opposite of "aye"
NEX	Navy Exchange
OOD	Officer of the Deck
Oscar	Man overboard pennant or drill
Padeye	Hook points of a ship's surface used to tie down aircraft with chains
Passageway	aka "p-way," a corridor used for interior horizontal movement aboard ship (similar to hallway ashore)
Pitch	Vertical rise and fall of vessel's bow and stern
Pollywog	One who has never crossed over the Equator
Port	When facing forward, the left side of a ship
PRT	Physical Readiness Test
Quarterdeck	Deck area designated by the CO as the place to host official events
RAS	Replenishment at Sea, resupply a ship during an UNREP (underway replenishment)
RIB	Rigid Inflatable Boat, small boat used for security and search & rescue
River City	Restriction of outgoing communications for security purposes
ROE	Rules of Engagement
Scuttlebutt	Drinking fountain or idle gossip
Shellback	One who has crossed the Equator
Shift Colors	Change arrangement of flags and pennants after getting underway
Ship's Company	All hands permanently attached to a ship or station; aka "the crew"
Shipmate	Fellow Sailor
Shipshape	Neat, clean
Shore Patrol	Temporary assigned personnel when visiting port that ensure Sailors don't get too rowdy on liberty
Sick Bay	Area aboard ship that serves as a hospital or medical clinic
SMO	Senior Medical Officer, in charge of the Medical Department

Smoking lamp	Most navies established regulations restricting smoking to certain areas for safety. Usually, the lamp was located in the forecastle or the area directly surrounding the galley. When particularly hazardous operations or work required that smoking be curtailed (like before drills, refueling, or taking ammunition), the unlighted lamp relayed the message. The smoking lamp has survived only as a figure of speech. When the OOD says "the smoking lamp is out," it means "cease smoking."
SSBN	Sub-Surface Ballistic Missile Submarine
Starboard	When facing forward, the right side of a ship
Staterooms	Living/bunking spaces on a ship for officers
Superstructure	The parts of a ship that project above her main deck
Stern	Rear or back part of a vessel
SWMDO	Surface Warfare Medical Department Officer, qualification that can be attained by medical department officers
SWO	Surface Warfare Officer
TAO	Tactical Action Officer, fights for the ship under supervision of the CO
Territorial Seas	12 nautical miles of waters that extend from a nation's shores that are governed by said nation; all transiting ships must comply with host nation laws
Tonnage	Refers to a ship's displacement in the water or the gross pounds of cargo it is capable of carrying
UA	Unauthorized Absence, not being at appointed place of duty
Vulture's Row	Viewing gallery on an aircraft carrier's tower where a person may watch the flight deck operations
Wake	Trail left by watercraft moving through water
Wardroom	Officers' messing (eating) compartment; collective term used to signify all the officers assigned to a ship
Watch	Usually a 4-hour period into which a day is divided; a particular duty section
Windward	In the direction that the wind is coming from
Working Party	Group of Sailors assigned to a task
XO	Executive Officer; person second in command to CO

References

1. Chrisomalis S. Nautical terms. 2021. http://phrontistery.info/nautical.html. Accessed 11 Oct 2021.
2. Cutler TJ. Appendix K. Glossary of navy terms and acronyms. In: The Bluejacket's manual centennial edition. Annapolis, MD: Naval Institute Press; 2002.

3. Hernandez AA. Surface Warfare Medical Department Officer study guide. 2017.
4. Lizardo RE. Surface Warfare Medical Department Officer study guide. 2018.
5. Page S. Navy lingo decoded: navy terms every sailor should know. 2020. https://www.sandboxx.us/blog/navy-terms-decoded/. Accessed 11 Oct 2021.
6. Valle O. 19 Terms only sailors will understand. 2021. https://www.wearethemighty.com/lists/19-terms-sailors-will-understand/. Accessed 11 Oct 2021.
7. Wikipedia contributors. Glossary of nautical terms. Wikipedia, The Free Encyclopedia. Oct 10, 2021, at 08:21 UTC. Available at: https://en.wikipedia.org/wiki/Glossary_of_nautical_terms. Accessed 11 Oct 2021.
8. Wikipedia contributors. Line-crossing ceremony. Wikipedia, The Free Encyclopedia. Oct 10, 2021, at 10:55 UTC. Available at: https://en.wikipedia.org/wiki/Line-crossing_ceremony. Accessed 11 Oct 2021.

Appendix D: Common Acronyms and References

Common Acronyms

Many common military acronyms are used frequently in several chapters. Some of them are nautical in nature and are also cited in Appendix C, but many are not. While they will always be defined at first use, here is a list for easy reference.

AAR	After Action Report
ACLS	Advanced Cardiac Life Support
AMAL	Authorized Medical Allowance List
AOR	Area of Responsibility
ARG	Amphibious Readiness Group
ATLS	Advanced Trauma Life Support
BAS	Battalion Aid Station
BDS	Battle Dressing Station
CASEVAC	Casualty Evacuation
CATF	Commander, Amphibious Task Force
CCRN	Critical Care Registered Nurse
CNOR	Certified Perioperative Nurse
CoC	Chain of Command
COVID-19	Coronavirus disease 2019
CPG	Clinical Practice Guidelines
CRNA	Certified Registered Nurse Anesthetist
CRTS	Casualty Receiving and Treatment Ships
CSG	Carrier Strike Group
CVN	Aircraft Carrier
DMO	Distributed Maritime Operations
DNBI	Disease and non-battle injury

M. D. Tadlock, A. A. Hernandez (eds.), *Expeditionary Surgery at Sea*,
https://doi.org/10.1007/978-3-031-21893-4

DoD	Department of Defense
EMF	Expeditionary Medical Facility
ERSS	Expeditionary Resuscitative Surgical System
ESG	Expeditionary Strike Group
FFP	Fresh Frozen Plasma
FRSS	Forward Resuscitative Surgical System
FST	Fleet Surgical Team (Forward Surgical Team in Royal Navy or U.S. Army)
FWB	Fresh Whole Blood
GHE	Global Health Engagement
GME	Graduate Medical Education
HADR	Humanitarian Assistance and Disaster Relief
HCA	Humanitarian and Civic Assistance
HMS	Her (or His) Majesty's Ship
IDC	Independent Duty Corpsman
JTS	Joint Trauma System
LHA	Landing Helicopter Assault ship (amphibious assault)
LHD	Landing Helicopter Dock ship (amphibious assault)
LPD	Landing Platform Dock ship (amphibious transport)
MAO	Medical Administrative Officer
MASCAL	Mass Casualty, also known as Mass Casualty Incident (MCI)
MEDEVAC	Medical Evacuation
MEU	Marine Expeditionary Unit
MRCO	Medical Regulating Control Officer
MTF	Medical Treatment Facility (can also be Military Treatment Facility)
NATO	North Atlantic Treaty Organization
OIC	Officer in Charge
OR	Operating Room
PCC	Prolonged Casualty Care
POCUS	Point-of-Care Ultrasound
POI	Point of Injury
PRBC	Packed Red Blood Cells
RFA	Royal Fleet Auxiliary
RN	Registered Nurse
SMO	Senior Medical Officer
SOP	Standard Operating Procedures
SPD	Sterile Processing Department
ST	Surgical Technologist
STP	Shock Trauma Platoon
TAD	Temporary Additional Duty (known as TDY in Army/Air Force)
TCCC	Tactical Combat Casualty Care
U.S.	United States
USMC	United States Marine Corps
USNS	United States Naval Ship
USS	United States Ship
WBB	Walking Blood Bank

Common References and Resources Relevant to Combat Trauma and Expeditionary Surgery

Many references are cited in several chapters. While some are not cited, the editors have compiled a list for easy reference.

Top Knife (Hirshberg and Mattox). The most practical and useful handbook for trauma surgeons and general surgeons taking care of trauma patients.

Joint Trauma System (JTS) Clinical Practice Guidelines (CPGs) homepage at https://jts.amedd.army.mil/index.cfm/PI_CPGs/cpgs. Many specific CPGs are referenced throughout this book and should be downloaded prior to any deployment.

Front Line Surgery, A Practical Approach (Martin, Beekley, and Eckert). The original comprehensive and practical combat trauma handbook. An outstanding resource for any provider taking care of combat trauma patients.

Emergency War Surgery, 5th Edition. An excellent combat trauma and military medicine resource that is routinely updated. Available from the Borden Institute for order or download in PDF format at: https://medcoe.army.mil/borden-tb-ews.

Atlas of Surgical Techniques in Trauma; Second Edition (Demetriades, Inaba, and Velmahos). Provides an excellent step-by-step approach to numerous procedures and exposures relevant to combat trauma and trauma care in general.

ADVISOR system, a 24/7 consultative service (COMM 833-238-7756 or DSN 312-429-9089). Referenced throughout the book, this is an outstanding resource for synchronous and asynchronous consultation from multiple surgical and nonsurgical specialties. At the time of publication, take note that ADVISOR utilizes GTP (Global Teleconsultation Portal), requiring the user to create an account, username, and password at https://path.tamc.amedd.army.mil.

Military Health System (MHS) Virtual Medical Center internal SharePoint site (requires CAC Access): https://info.health.mil/army/VMC/Pages/VMC/OperationalMedicineAdvisor.aspx.

INSTRUCTION 6000.1, the Shipboard Medical Procedures Manual. Differs by region and platform (for example from San Diego: COMNAVAIRPACINST for CVN, COMNAVSURFPACINST/COMNAVSURFLANTINST for the other platforms). Available through chain of command or internet search.

BUMEDINST INSTRUCTION 6700.13, Management and Procurement of Authorized Medical and Dental Allowance Lists. Available through chain of command or Internet search.

War Surgery in Iraq and Afghanistan. Case presentations and numerous photos from combat wounds and management in Iraq and Afghanistan. Available for order through the Borden Institute at: https://medcoe.army.mil/borden-tb-war-surgery-afg-iraq.

Field Management of Chemical and Biological Casualties Handbook. Available from the Borden Institute for order or download in PDF format at: https://medcoe.army.mil/borden-field-mgt-of-cb-casualities.

Pediatric Surgery and Medicine for Hostile Environments (2nd edition). Available from the Borden Institute for order or download in PDF format at: https://medcoe.army.mil/borden-tb-pediatric-surgery.

Out of the Crucible: How the US Military Transformed Combat Casualty Care in Iraq and Afghanistan. Written for a non-medical audience. Covers key lessons and advances during the wars in Iraq and Afghanistan. Available from the Borden Institute for order or download in PDF format at: https://medcoe.army.mil/borden-outofcrucible.

War Wounds: Basic Surgical Management. International Committee of The Red Cross (ICRC) publication on the management of penetrating and blast injuries sustained in third world conflicts. Available for download in PDF format at: https://www.icrc.org/en/publication/0570-war-wounds-basic-surgical-management-principles-and-practice-surgical-management.

Borden Institute Textbooks of Military Medicine. A series of multiple textbooks relevant to military medicine. Available in PDF format at: https://medcoe.army.mil/borden-3-textbooks-of-military-medicine.

Combat Casualty Care: Lessons Learned from OEF and OIF. Another resource that covers all clinical aspects of combat trauma care and can be viewed, downloaded, or ordered free of charge (for military personnel) from the Borden Institute at https://medcoe.army.mil/borden-tb-combat-casualty-care.

Index

M. D. Tadlock, A. A. Hernandez (eds.), *Expeditionary Surgery at Sea*,
https://doi.org/10.1007/978-3-031-21893-4

P

Q

R

S

MIX
Papier aus verantwortungsvollen Quellen
Paper from responsible sources
FSC® C105338

If you have any concerns about our products,
you can contact us on
ProductSafety@springernature.com

In case Publisher is established outside the EU,
the EU authorized representative is:
Springer Nature Customer Service Center GmbH
Europaplatz 3, 69115 Heidelberg, Germany

Printed by Libri Plureos GmbH
in Hamburg, Germany